Delivering Health Care in America

A Systems Approach

FOURTH EDITION

Leiyu Shi, DrPH, MBA, MPA
Professor, Johns Hopkins School of Public Health
Co-Director, Johns Hopkins Primary Care Policy Center for the Underserved
Johns Hopkins University
Baltimore, Maryland

Douglas A. Singh, PhD, MBA
Associate Professor, School of Public and Environmental Affairs
Indiana University South Bend
South Bend, Indiana

JONES AND BARTLETT PUBLISHERS
Sudbury, Massachusetts
BOSTON TORONTO LONDON SINGAPORE

World Headquarters
Jones and Bartlett Publishers
40 Tall Pine Drive
Sudbury, MA 01776
978-443-5000
info@jbpub.com
www.jbpub.com

Jones and Bartlett Publishers Canada
6339 Ormindale Way
Mississauga, Ontario L5V 1J2
Canada

Jones and Bartlett Publishers International
Barb House, Barb Mews
London W6 7PA
United Kingdom

Jones and Bartlett's books and products are available through most bookstores and online booksellers. To contact Jones and Bartlett Publishers directly, call 800-832-0034, fax 978-443-8000, or visit our website www.jbpub.com.

Substantial discounts on bulk quantities of Jones and Bartlett's publications are available to corporations, professional associations, and other qualified organizations. For details and specific discount information, contact the special sales department at Jones and Bartlett via the above contact information or send an email to specialsales@jbpub.com.

ISBN-13: 978-0-7637-4512-7
ISBN-10: 0-7637-4512-X

This publication is designed to provide accurate and authoritative information in regard to the Subject Matter covered. It is sold with the understanding that the publisher is not engaged in rendering legal, accounting, or other professional service. If legal advice or other expert assistance is required, the service of a competent professional person should be sought.

Production Credits
Publisher: Michael Brown
Associate Editor: Katey Birtcher
Production Director: Amy Rose
Production Editor: Tracey Chapman
Marketing Manager: Sophie Fleck
Manufacturing Buyer: Therese Connell
Composition: Publishers' Design and Production Services, Inc.
Cover Design: Kristin E. Ohlin
Cover Image: © Vladimir Ivanov/ShutterStock, Inc.
Printing and Binding: Malloy, Inc.
Cover Printing: Malloy, Inc.

Library of Congress Cataloging-in-Publication Data
Shi, Leiyu.
Delivering health care in America : a systems approach / Leiyu Shi, Douglas A Singh. — 4th ed.
p. ; cm.
Includes bibliographical references and index.
ISBN-13: 978-0-7637-4512-7 (pbk.)
ISBN-10: 0-7637-4512-X (pbk.)
1. Medical care—United States. 2. Medical policy—United States. I. Singh, Douglas A., 1946– II. Title.
[DNLM: 1. Delivery of Health Care—United States. 2. Health Policy—United States. W 84 AA1 S512d 2008]
RA395.A3S485 2008
362.10973—dc22

2007010553

6048
Printed in the United States of America
11 10 09 08 07 10 9 8 7 6 5 4 3 2 1

Contents

Foreword

Describing the US health services system is no easy feat. In one liftable volume, the authors cover the conceptual basis for the system; its historical origins; the structures of ambulatory care, inpatient care, and other important services; the translation of these structures into healthy services themselves; and the manifestations of their impact on costs and quality. They even consider likely future directions. This book thus provides a point of departure for understanding a system that the world views with interest because of its heavy focus on "the market" as the organizing force.

Readers in both the United States and abroad will find it a useful beginning for understanding the basic structures and operations of this very large, and still-growing, sector of the economy. Its extraordinary breadth would be overwhelming in the absence of the organizing schema as presented in the first chapter, which presents a road map for relating the subjects to each other.

Despite the under-recognized failures of the United States in achieving high levels of health as compared with its peers among industrialized nations, and the well recognized fact that is has the highest per capita costs in the world, there is little evidence of a popular movement for targeted change. One reason for this may be the lack of knowledge about the organization and operations of the system. To the extent that this book helps reduce the complexity to the principles, it may go a long way toward providing the basis for a more focused consideration of possible alternatives toward meeting the population's health needs.

Barbara Starfield, MD, MPH University Distinguished Service Professor, Johns Hopkins University

Preface

We continue to see incrementalism at work in the traditional American way to reform the US health care delivery system. Perhaps the most dramatic reform that Medicare has ever undertaken in its 42-year history came about as a result of the Medicare Prescription Drug, Improvement, and Modernization Act of 2003 that added a new Part D to Medicare. Although the program has its critics, it will lower the cost burden for prescription drugs for most elderly Americans. The program also has long-term cost implications for Medicare, particularly when the first wave of baby boomers begins to draw their health care benefits from the Medicare program. Retirement of the baby boomers between 2011 and 2030 is the most worrisome aspect facing future generations. Unprecedented increase in health care expenditures is just one piece of the puzzle. There are other serious questions to be addressed: (1) How will a health care system that is lopsided in its focus on medical specialization deal with a mushrooming sector of the population in which the prevention and management of long-term chronic conditions will be of primary importance? (2) How will the nation deal with the impending shortage of qualified workers in just about every area of health care delivery? (3) What can be done to finance long-term care services that over 20% of the US population will start utilizing around 2020 and beyond? (4) Will the nation be able to afford the ongoing development and use of costly new medical technology that may deliver fewer health benefits in relation to the costs? (5) How will the nation address the increasing costs of health care on the one hand and the need to expand health insurance for the uninsured? These are some of the most critical issues that policymakers, the American public, the providers of health care, and other stakeholders will have to engage in over the next several years. No one has a 'magic bullet' that will adequately address these issues to the satisfaction of all parties concerned. Although some proposals have started to emerge, a detailed discussion of those proposals is beyond the scope of this book. But, the reader should be able to gain a better appreciation of what the main issues are, the factors that fuel those issues, and the factors that may prevent major reforms from taking hold. Other developed nations also face similar dilemmas. However, some of these other nations are ahead of the United States in at least some areas. Most already have universal health insurance and have, for years, employed central planning to limit the availability and use of high-end health care services. Most of these countries also have better developed systems of basic and routine health care services (primary care) that are readily accessible to people. In the United States, primary care is not always readily accessible, sometimes even by those who have good health insurance coverage. Americans take pride in the availability and use of specialized care, but in many instances this care is inappropriately used. A prime example is the misuse of emergency care services in the United States. A lack of basic services and inappropriate use of high-end care is the unfortunate outcome of a free market that does not work very well in health care (Chapter 1 provides an ample discussion of why this is so). We think that sooner rather than later, we will reach a point where the current delivery system, with its focus on specialization, will become unaffordable for most Americans. Some type of rationing will become necessary. However, Americans are not prepared to have the government step in and politicize health care.

Ahead of the 2008 presidential elections, expansion of health care has already become political fodder with most of the presidential hopefuls, and the American media will add their own twists to the issue as we head into the elections. At present, most Americans are relatively well satisfied with their existing employer-sponsored health care arrangements. On the other hand, the people of Massachusetts bought into government-imposed mandates that promise to create a universal insurance system in that state. By creating Medicare Part D, President Bush has perhaps inadvertently triggered the momentum toward further expansion of health insurance. Interestingly, the program was created in an environment marked by tax cuts, but the program's costs will soon start hitting Americans in their pocketbooks. Health insurance for the uninsured is likely to become a hot topic for political rhetoric, but presidential debates aside, we think that at least in the foreseeable future the odds are in favor of the existing private–public system of health care financing and delivery, very similar to the current retirement system which is a combination of private savings, workplace pension (although it has been eroding for some time), and public Social Security.

In its evolution, forces that developed outside the medical and health care arenas have molded health care delivery. We have now reached the corporate era in which health care in the United States, and indeed in many developed and developing nations, is now in the hands of large corporations. Globalization, boosted by advances in global communications, transportation, and trade, has also started to change the way health care is being delivered. In a way, health care itself has started to become globalized and commoditized. The information revolution is another force gripping health care delivery along with its many challenges regarding privacy, security, and confidentiality.

After many years of being regarded as the backwaters of American health care, the public health system has been gaining increasing respect following the 2001 attacks by foreign terrorists and natural disasters from hurricanes Katrina and Rita in 2005. Developing an infrastructure and forging of public–private partnerships to deal with bioterrorism, natural disasters, and potential global threats such as severe acute respiratory syndrome (SARS) and bird flu, are now among the nation's top priorities.

This fourth edition has been updated throughout with the latest pertinent data, trends, and research findings available at the time the manuscript was prepared. As in the previous editions, copious illustrations in the form of examples, facts, figures, tables, and exhibits make the text come alive. Some key additions to the text include: updated information on many developed and developing nations' healthcare systems (Chapter 1); contemporary examples of policy approaches to pressing issues facing the US healthcare delivery system (Chapter 2); the effects of corporatization, information revolution, and globalization on health care delivery (Chapter 3); descriptions of current trends in the US healthcare workforce, including the growing role of hospitalists and the ongoing nursing shortage (Chapter 4); current and future directions in health technology assessment (Chapter 5); Medicare Part D, prospective payment initiatives for inpatient psychiatric facilities and inpatient rehabilitation facilities, and the pay-for-performance initiative (Chapter 6); the role of outpatient and primary care services, with a focus on trends in public payments for home health services (Chapter 7); role of long-term care hospitals and reimbursement for their services (Chapter 8); disease management as a strategy to manage utilization (Chapter 9); an updated and revised discussion of long-term care and its services, and the role of inpatient rehabilitation facilities (Chapter 10); the most recent information on health services for vulnerable populations (Chapter 11); updated information on healthcare costs, access, and quality, including the trend towards pay-for-performance (Chapter 12); discussion of current health policy issues, including state approaches to universal coverage (Chapter 13); and high-deductible health plans, insurance restructuring in Massachusetts, challenges in long-term care, and the era of evidence-based medicine (Chapter 14). In addition, mandates of recent legislation such as the Medicare Prescription Drug, Improvement, and Modernization Act of 2003 and the Deficit Reduction Act of 2005 have been incorporated as warranted by the context.

Aside from the changes, the book retains the original systems framework to discuss the components of US health care delivery. It also retains the original 14 chapters as major themes following the systems model. Our aim in this textbook is to continue to meet the needs of both graduate and undergraduate students. We have attempted to make each chapter complete without making it overwhelming for beginners. Instructors, of course, will choose the sections they decide are most appropriate for their courses.

As in the past, we invite comments from our readers. Communications can be directed to either or both authors:

Leiyu Shi
Department of Health Policy and Management
Bloomburg School of Public Health
Johns Hopkins University
624 North Broadway, Room 409
Baltimore, MD 21205-1996
lshi@jhsph.edu

Douglas A. Singh
School of Public and Environmental Affairs
Indiana University South Bend
Wiekamp Hall, Room 2213
1800 Mishawaka Avenue
P.O. Box 7111
South Bend, IN 46634-7111
dsingh@iusb.edu

We appreciate the work of Patricia Collins in providing invaluable assistance in the review and revision of selected chapters of this book.

List of Exhibits

List of Figures

List of Tables

List of Abbreviations/Acronyms

A

AAs—Asian Americans
AALL—American Association of Labor Legislation
AAMC—Association of American Medical Colleges
AAPIs—Asian American and Pacific Islanders
ACNM—American College of Nurse-Midwives
ACPE—American Council on Pharmaceutical Education
ACS—American College of Surgeons
ADA—Americans with Disabilities Act
ADA—American Dental Association
ADC—adult day care
ADL—activities of daily living
ADN—associate's degree nurse
AFC—adult foster care
AFDC—Aid to Families with Dependent Children
AHA—American Hospital Association
AHRQ—Agency for Healthcare Research and Quality
AIDS—acquired immune deficiency syndrome
ALF—assisted living facility
ALOS—average length of stay
AMA—American Medical Association
ANA—American Nurses Association
APCs—ambulatory payment classifications
APN—advanced practice nurse
AZT—zidovudine

B

BBA—Balanced Budget Act of 1997
BPHC—Bureau of Primary Health Care
BSN—baccalaureate degree nurse

C

C/MHCs—Community and Migrant Health Centers
CAH—Critical Access Hospital
CAM—complementary and alternative medicine
CARE Act—Comprehensive AIDS Resources Emergency Act
CAT—computerized axial tomography
CBO—Congressional Budget Office
CCIP—Chronic Care Improvement Program
CCRC—continuing care retirement community
CDC—Centers for Disease Control and Prevention
CEO—chief executive officer
CEPH—Council on Education for Public Health
CF—conversion factor
CHAMPUS—TriCare program
CHAMPVA—Civilian Health and Medical Program of the Department of Veterans Affairs

CHC—community health center
CIA—Central Intelligence Agency
CMGs—case-mix groups
CMS—Centers for Medicare and Medicaid Services
CAN—certified nursing assistant
CNM—certified nurse midwife
CNSs—clinical nurse specialists
COBRA—Consolidated Omnibus Budget Reconciliation Act of 1985
COGME—Council on Graduate Medical Education
CON—certificate-of-need
COPC—community-oriented primary care
COPD—chronic obstructive pulmonary disease
COTA—certified occupational therapy assistant
COTH—Council of Teaching Hospitals and Health Systems
CPI—consumer price index
CPOE—computerized physician order entry
CPT—current procedural terminology
CQI—continuous quality improvement
CRNA—certified registered nurse anesthetist
CT—computed tomography
CVA—cardiovascular accident

D

DC—Doctor of Chiropractic
DDS—Doctor of Dental Surgery
DHHS—Department of Health and Human Services
DMD—Doctor of Dental Medicine
DME—durable medical equipment
DoD—Department of Defense
DOs—doctors of osteopathy
DPCs—diagnosis-procedure combinations
DPM—Doctor of Podiatric Medicine
DRA—Deficit Reduction Act of 2005
DRGs—diagnostic-related groups
DSM-IV—Diagnostic and Statistical Manual of Mental Disorders
DTP—diptheria-tetanus-pertussis

E

EMB—evidence-based medicine
EBRI—Employee Benefit Research Institute
ECG—electrocardiogram
ECU—extended care unit
ED—emergency department
EEG—electroencephalogram
EHRs—electronic health records
EIAs—enzyme immunoassays
ELISA—enzyme-linked immunosorbent assay
EMT—emergency medical technician
EMTALA—Emergency Medical Treatment and Labor Act
ENP—elderly nutrition program
EPA—Environmental Protection Agency
EPO—exclusive provider organization
EPSDT—Early Periodic Screening, Diagnosis, and Treatment program
ERISA—Employee Retirement Income Security Act
ESP—Economic Stabilization Program

F

FD&C—Federal Food, Drug, and Cosmetic Act
FDA—Food and Drug Administration
FMAP—Federal Medical Assistance Percentage
FQHC—Federally Qualified Health Center
FTE—full-time equivalent
FY—fiscal year

G

GAO—General Accounting Office
GAT—genome amplification testing
GATS—General Agreement on Trade in Services

GDP—gross domestic product
GPs—general practitioners

H

HAART—highly active antiretroviral therapy
HCBW—Home and Community Based Waiver
HCFA—Health Care Financing Administration
HCH—Health Care for the Homeless
HCPP—Health Care Prepayment Plan
HDHP—high-deductible health plan
HEDIS—Health Plan Employer Data and Information Set
HHRG—home health resource group
HI—Hospital Insurance
HIAA—Health Insurance Association of America
Hib—Haemophilus influenzae B
HIPAA—Health Insurance Portability and Accountability Act
HIT—health information technology
HIV—human immunodeficiency virus
HMO—health maintenance organization
HMO Act—Health Maintenance Organization Act
HPSAs—Health Professional Shortage Areas
HPV—human papillomavirus
HRQL—health-related quality of life
HRSA—Health Resources and Services Administration
HSAs—health savings accounts
HSAs—health system agencies
HSIs—Health Status Indicators
HTA—health technology assessment
HUD—Department of Housing and Urban Development

I

IADL—instrumental activities of daily living
ICD-9—International Classification of Diseases, version 9
ICDs—implantable cardioverter defibrillators
ICF—intermediate care facility
ICF/MR—intermediate care facilities for mentally retarded
ICSI IVF—intracytoplasmic sperm injection in vitro fertilization
IDEA—Individuals with Disabilities Education Act
IDS—integrated delivery systems
IDU—injection drug use
IFA—immunofluorescence assay
IHS—Indian Health Service
IMGs—international medical graduates
INS—Immigration and Naturalization Service
IOM—Institute of Medicine
IPA—independent practice association
IRB—Institutional Review Board
IRF—inpatient rehabilitation facility
IS—information systems
IT—information technology
IUDs—intrauterine devices
IV—intravenous

J

JCAHO—Joint Commission on Accreditation of Healthcare Organizations

L

LPN—licensed practical nurse
LTC—long-term care
LTCH—long-term care hospital
LVN—licensed vocational nurse

M

MAC—mycobacterium avium complex
MA-SNP—Medicare Advantage Special Needs Program
MBA—Master of Business Administration

MCOs—managed care organizations
MDS—minimum data set
MDs—doctors of medicine
MedPAC—Medicare Payment Advisory Commission
MEPS—Medical Expenditure Panel Survey
MFS—Medicare Fee Schedule
MHA—Master of Health Administration
MHPs—multiskilled health practitioners
MHPH—1996 Mental Health Policy Act
MHS—multihospital system
MHSA—Master of Health Services Administration
MHSS—Military Health Services System
MLP—midlevel provider
MMA—Medicare Prescription Drug, Improvement, and Modernization Act
MMR—measles-mumps-rubella vaccine
MPA—Master of Public Administration/Affairs
MPFS—Medicare Physician Fee Schedule
MPH—Master of Public Health
MPPRP—Medicare's Physician Payment Reform Program
MR/DD—mentally retarded, developmentally disabled persons
MRHFP—Medicare Rural Hospital Flexibility Program
MRI—magnetic resonance imaging
MSA—medical savings account
MSA—metropolitan statistical area
MSO—management services organization
MTFs—medical treatment facilities
MUAs—Medically Underserved Areas

N

NADSA—National Adult Day Services Association
NAPBC—National Action Plan on Breast Cancer
NASA—National Aeronautic and Space Administration
NAT—nucleic acid testing
NCCAM—National Center for Complementary and Alternative Medicine
NCHS—National Center for Health Statistics
NCQA—National Committee for Quality Assurance
NF—nursing facility
NGC—National Guideline Clearinghouse
NHC—neighborhood health center
NHI—national health insurance
NHS—British National Health Service
NHSC—National Health Service Corp
NIAAA—National Institute of Alcohol Abuse and Alcoholism
NICE—National Institute for Health and Clinical Excellence
NIDA—National Institute on Drug Abuse
NIH—National Institutes of Health
NP—nurse practitioner
NPC—nonphysician clinician
NPP—nonphysician practitioner
NRA—Nurse Reinvestment Act of 2002

O

OAM—Office of Alternative Medicine
OBRA-87—Omnibus Budget Reconciliation Act of 1987
OBRA-89—Omnibus Budget Reconciliation Act of 1989
OBRA-93—Omnibus Budget Reconciliation Act of 1993
OD—Doctor of Optometry
OI—opportunistic infections
OMB—Office of Management and Budget
OPPS—Outpatient Prospective Payment System
OSHA—Occupational Safety and Health Administration
OT—occupational therapist
OWH—Office on Women's Health

P

P4P—pay-for-performance
PA—physician assistant
PACE—Program of All-inclusive Care for the Elderly
PASRR—Preadmission Screening and Resident Review
PCCM—primary care case management
PCGs—primary care groups
PCM—primary care manager
PCP—pneumocystis carinii
PCP—primary care physician
PCT—primary care trust
PEPFAR—President's Emergency Plan for AIDS Relief
PERS—personal emergency response systems
PET—positron emission tomography
PFFS—private fee-for-service
PharmD—Doctor of Pharmacy
PhD—Doctor of Philosophy
PHO—physician-hospital organization
PHS—public health service
PL 107-205—Nurse Reinvestment Act of 2002
PMPM—payment per member per month
PORTS—patient outcomes research teams
POS—point-of-service plan
PPD—per-patient day rate
PPM—physician practice management
PPOs—preferred provider organizations
PPS—prospective payment system
PROs—peer review organizations
PRWORA—Personal Responsibility and Work Opportunity Act
PSO—provider-sponsored organization
PSROs—professional standards review organizations
PsyD—Doctor of Psychology
PTA—physical therapy assistant
PTCA—percutaneous transluminal coronary angioplasty
PTs—physical therapists

Q

QALY—quality-adjusted life year
QDWI—Qualified Disabled and Working Individual Program
QI—qualified individual program
QIOs—Quality Improvement Organizations
QMB—Qualified Medicare Beneficiary program

R

R&D—research and development
RAI—resident assessment instrument
RBRVS—resource-based relative value scales
RFID—radio frequency identification
RICs—rehabilitation impairment categories
RN—registered nurse
RUG-III—Resource Utilization Groups, version 3
RUGs—resource utilization groups
RVUs—relative value units

S

S/HMO—social health maintenance organization
SAMHSA—Substance Abuse and Mental Health Services Administration
SARS—severe acute respiratory syndrome
SAV—small area variations
SCHIP—State Children's Health Insurance Program
SCN—Sentinel Centers Network
SES—socioeconomic status
SHI—socialized health insurance
SIPP—Survey of Income and Program Participation
SLMB—specified low-income Medicare beneficiary
SMI—supplementary medical insurance
SNF—skilled nursing facility
SPECT—single-photon emission computed tomography

SROs—single-room occupancy units
SSI—Supplemental Security Income
STDs—sexually transmitted diseases

T

TAH—total artificial heart
TANF—Temporary Assistance for Needy Families
TCU—transitional care unit
TEFRA—Tax Equity and Fiscal Responsibility Act
TFL—TriCare for Life
TPA—third-party administrator
TQM—total quality management

U

UCR—usual, customary, and reasonable
UR—utilization review

V

VA—Department of Veterans Affairs
VERA—Veterans Equitable Resource Allocation
VHA—Veterans Health Administration
VISN—Veterans Integrated Service Network
VNA—Visiting Nurses Association
VPS—volume performance standard

W

WHO—World Health Organization
WIC—Women, Infants, and Children

Chapter 1

A Distinctive System of Health Care Delivery

Learning Objectives

- To understand the basic nature of the US health care system
- To outline the four key functional components of a health care delivery system
- To discuss the primary characteristics of the US health care system from a free market perspective
- To emphasize why it is important for health care managers to understand the intricacies of the health care delivery system
- To get an overview of the health care systems in other countries
- To introduce the systems model as a framework for studying the health services system in the United States

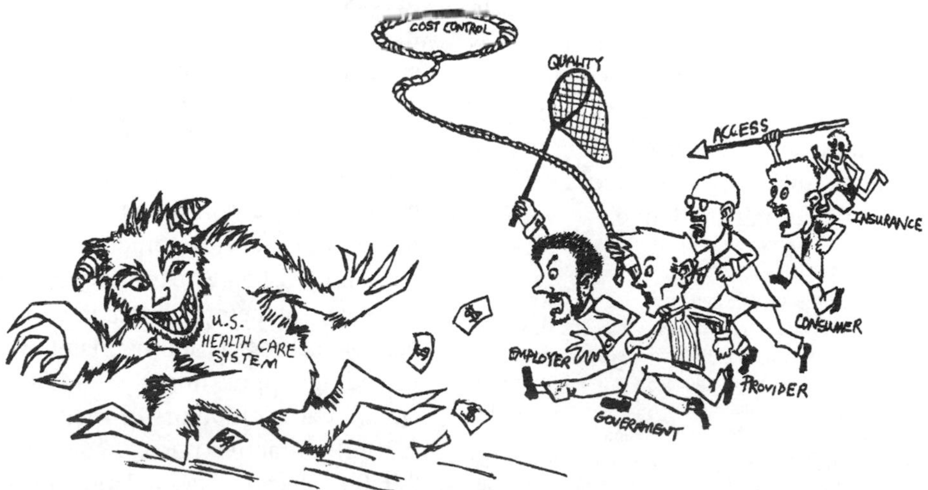

The US health care delivery system is a behemoth that is almost impossible for any single entity to manage and control.

Introduction

The United States has a unique system of health care delivery.* It is unlike any other health care system in the world. Most developed countries have national health insurance programs run by the government and financed through general taxes. Almost all citizens in such countries are entitled to receive health care services. Such is not the case in the United States, where not all Americans are automatically covered by health insurance. The US health care delivery system is not a system in the true sense, even though it is called a system when reference is made to its various features, components, and services. Hence, it may be somewhat misleading to talk about the American health care delivery "system" because a real system does not exist (Wolinsky 1988, 54). The US health care system is unnecessarily fragmented, which is perhaps its central feature (Shortell et al. 1996). The delivery system has continued to undergo periodic changes, mainly in response to concerns with cost, access, and quality. In spite of these efforts, providing at least a basic package of health care at an affordable cost to every man, woman, and child in America remains an unrealized goal. It is highly unlikely that this goal will materialize anytime soon, mainly because expanding access to health care, while containing overall costs and maintaining expected levels of quality, is a daunting challenge.

*The expressions "health care delivery" and "health services delivery" can have two slightly different meanings. In a broad sense, they collectively refer to the major components of the system and the process that enables people to receive health care. In a more restricted sense, they refer to the act of providing health care services to patients, such as in a hospital or physician's clinic. By paying attention to the context, the reader should be able to identify which meaning is intended.

Describing health care delivery in the United States can be a frustrating task. To facilitate an understanding of the structural and conceptual basis for the delivery of health services, this book is organized according to a systems framework presented at the end of this chapter. Also, the mechanisms of health services delivery in the United States are collectively referred to as a system throughout this book.

The main objective of this chapter is to provide a broad understanding of how health care is delivered in the United States. The overview theme provided here introduces the reader to several concepts that are treated more extensively in later chapters.

An Overview of the Scope and Size of the System

Table 1–1 demonstrates the complexity of health care delivery in the United States. Many organizations and individuals are involved in health care. These range from educational and research institutions, medical suppliers, insurers, payers, and claims processors to health care providers. Multitudes of providers are involved in the provision of preventive, primary, subacute, acute, auxiliary, rehabilitative, and continuing care. An increasing number of managed care organizations (MCOs) and integrated networks now provide a continuum of care covering many of the service components.

The US health care delivery system is massive. Total employment in various health delivery settings is approximately 10 million, including approximately 744,000 professionally active doctors of medicine (MDs), 2.2 million active nurses, 168,000 dentists, 226,000 pharmacists, and more than 700,000

Table 1–1 The Complexity of Health Care Delivery

Education/ Research	Suppliers	Insurers	Providers	Payers	Government
Medical schools	Pharmaceutical companies	Managed care plans	***Preventive Care***	Blue Cross/ Blue Shield plans	Public insurance financing
Dental schools	Multipurpose suppliers	Blue Cross/ Blue Shield plans	Health departments	Commercial insurers	Health regulations
Nursing programs	Biotechnology companies	Commercial insurers	***Primary Care***	Employers	Health policy
Physician assistant programs		Self-insured employers	Physician offices	Third-party administrators	Research funding
Nurse practitioner programs		Medicare	Community health centers	State agencies	Public health
Physical therapy, occupational therapy, speech therapy programs		Medicaid	Dentists		
Research organizations		VA	Nonphysician providers		
Private foundations		Tricare	***Subacute Care***		
US Public Health Service (AHRQ, ATSDR, CDC, FDA, HRSA, IHS, NIH, SAMHSA)			Subacute care facilities		
Professional associations			Ambulatory surgery centers		
Trade associations			***Acute Care***		
			Hospitals		
			Auxiliary Services		
			Pharmacists		
			Diagnostic clinics		
			X-ray units		
			Suppliers of medical equipment		
			Rehabilitative Services		
			Home health agencies		
			Rehabilitation centers		
			Skilled nursing facilities		
			Continuing Care		
			Nursing homes		
			End-of-Life Care		
			Hospices		
			Integrated		
			Managed care organizations		
			Integrated networks		

administrators in medical and health care settings. Approximately 325,000 physical, occupational, and speech therapists provide rehabilitation services. The vast array of health care institutions includes 5,760 hospitals, 16,100 nursing homes, and 4,300 inpatient mental health facilities. Nearly 1,000 federally qualified health center grantees, with over 5,700 clinical sites, provide preventive and primary care services to approximately 16 million people living in medically underserved rural and urban areas yearly. Various types of health care professionals are trained in 150 medical and osteopathic schools, 56 dental schools, 91 schools of pharmacy, and more than 1,500 nursing programs located throughout the country. There are 174.5 million Americans with private health insurance coverage, 41.7 million Medicare beneficiaries, and 42.5 million Medicaid recipients. Health insurance can be purchased from over 1,300 health insurance companies and 64 Blue Cross/Blue Shield plans. Multitudes of government agencies are involved with the financing of health care, medical and health services research, and regulatory oversight of the various aspects of the health care delivery system (National Center for Health Statistics 2006; Blue Cross Blue Shield Association 2007; America's Health Insurance Plans 2004; Kaiser Family Foundation Commission on Medicaid and the Uninsured 2005; Kaiser Family Foundation Medicare Policy Project 2005; American Association of Colleges of Pharmacy 2007; American Association of Medical Colleges 2007; American Association of Colleges of Osteopathic Medicine 2007; American Dental Education Association 2007; National Association of Community Health Centers 2006).

A Broad Description of the System

US health care does not consist of a network of interrelated components designed to work together coherently, which one would expect to find in a veritable ***system***. To the contrary, it is a kaleidoscope of financing, insurance, delivery, and payment mechanisms that remain unstandardized and loosely coordinated. Each of these basic functional components—financing, insurance, delivery, and payment—represents an amalgam of public (government) and private sources. Thus, government-run programs finance and insure health care for select groups of people who meet each program's prescribed criteria for eligibility. To a lesser degree, government programs also engage in delivering certain health services directly to the recipients of care, such as veterans, military personnel, and the uninsured who may depend on city and county hospitals or limited services offered by public health clinics. However, the financing, insurance, payment, and delivery functions are largely in private hands.

The market-oriented economy in the United States attracts a variety of private entrepreneurs driven by the pursuit of profits in carrying out the key functions of health care delivery. Employers purchase health insurance for their employees through private sources, and people receive health care services delivered by the private sector. The government finances public insurance through Medicare, Medicaid, and the State Children's Health Insurance Program (SCHIP) for a significant portion of the very low-income, elderly, disabled, and pediatric populations. But, insurance arrangements for many publicly insured people are made through private entities, such as HMOs, and health care services and are rendered by private physicians and hospitals. The blend of public and private involvement in the delivery of health care has resulted in:

- a multiplicity of financial arrangements that enable individuals to pay for health care services
- numerous insurance agencies employing varied mechanisms for insuring against risk
- multiple payers that make their own determinations regarding how much to pay for each type of service
- a large array of settings where medical services are delivered
- numerous consulting firms offering their expertise in planning, cost containment, quality, and restructuring of resources

There is little standardization in a system that is functionally fragmented. The various system components fit together only loosely. Such a system is not subject to overall planning, direction, and coordination from a central agency, such as the government. Due to the missing dimension of system-wide planning, direction, and coordination, there is duplication, overlap, inadequacy, inconsistency, and waste leading to complexity and inefficiency. The system does not lend itself to standard budgetary methods of cost control. Each individual and corporate entity within a predominantly private entrepreneurial system seeks to manipulate financial incentives to its own advantage without regard to its impact on the system as a whole. Hence, cost containment remains an elusive goal. In short, the US health care delivery system is a behemoth that is almost impossible for any single entity to manage and control. It is also an economic megalith. The US economy is the largest in the world and, compared to other nations, consumption of health care services in the United States represents a greater proportion of the country's total economic output. While crediting the system with delivering some of the best medical care in the world, at least according to some standards, it falls short of delivering equitable services to every American.

An acceptable health care delivery system should have two primary objectives: (1) it must enable all citizens to access health care services, and (2) the services must be cost-effective and meet certain established standards of quality. In many ways, the US health care delivery system falls short of these ideals. On the other hand, certain features of US health care are the envy of the world. The United States leads the world in the latest and the best in medical technology, medical training, and research. It offers some of the most sophisticated institutions, products, and processes of health care delivery. These achievements are indeed admirable, but a lot more remains unaccomplished.

Basic Components of a Health Services Delivery System

As illustrated in Figure 1–1, a health care delivery system incorporates four functional components—financing, insurance, delivery, and payment that—that are necessary for the delivery of health services. The four functional components make up the ***quad-function model***. Health care delivery systems differ depending on the arrangement of the four components. The four functions generally overlap, but the degree of overlapping varies between

Figure 1–1 Basic Health Care Delivery Functions.

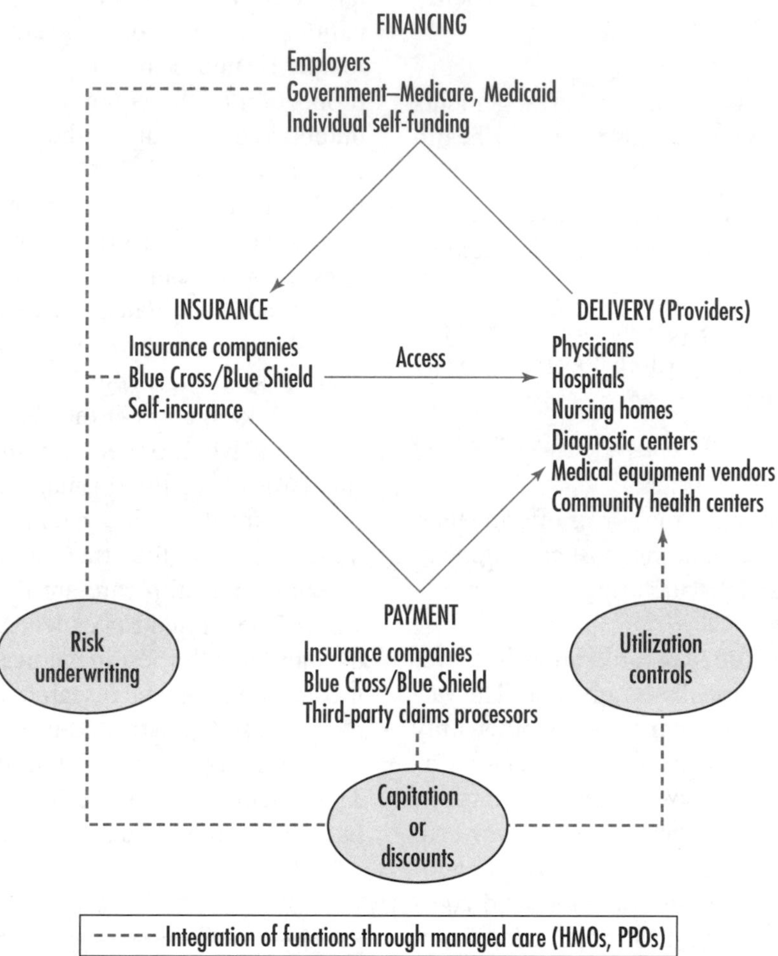

a private and a government-run system and between a traditional health insurance and managed care-based system. In a government-run system, the functions are more closely integrated and may even be indistinguishable. Managed care arrangements also integrate the four functions to varying degrees.

Financing

Health care often requires costly diagnostic tests and procedures and lengthy hospital stays. Financing is necessary to obtain health insurance or to pay for health care services. For most privately insured Americans, health insurance is employer-based; that is, health care is financed by their employers as a fringe benefit. A dependent's spouse or children may also be covered by the working spouse's, or parent's, employer. Most employers, except for the very large ones, purchase health insurance for their employees through an insurance company selected by the employer. In recent years, employers have shifted their purchases from traditional insurance companies to MCOs.

Insurance

Insurance protects the insured against catastrophic risks when needing expensive health care services. The insurance function also determines the package of health services the insured individual is entitled to receive. It specifies how and where health care services will be received. The insurance company or MCO also functions as a claims processor and manages the disbursement of funds to the providers of care.

Delivery

The term delivery refers to the provision of health care services and the receipt of insurance payments directly for those services. Common examples of ***providers*** who deliver care and services include physicians, dentists, optometrists, and therapists in private practices, hospitals, diagnostic and imaging clinics, and suppliers of medical equipment (e.g., wheelchairs, walkers, ostomy supplies, oxygen). With few exceptions, most providers render services to people who have health insurance.

Payment

The payment function deals with reimbursement to providers for services delivered. ***Reimbursement*** is the determination of how much to pay for a certain service. Funds for actual disbursement come from the premiums paid to the insurance company or MCO. In the case of an insurance company, when a covered individual receives health care services, the provider of services either requires payment up front or agrees to bill the insurance company on behalf of the patient. In the former case, the patient files a claim with the insurance company to be reimbursed for a portion of the fees and charges paid to the provider. The most common practice, however, is for the insurance company to pay its portion to the provider directly. When receiving services under a managed care plan, the patient is usually required to pay only a small out-of-pocket amount, such as $15 or $20, to see a physician. The remainder is covered by the managed care plan.

A Disenfranchised Segment

Since the United States has an employer-based financing system, it is not difficult to see why the unemployed generally have no health insurance. However, even some employed individuals may not have health insurance coverage for two main reasons: (1) In most states, employers are not mandated to offer health insurance to their employees; therefore, some employers, due to economic constraints, do not offer it. Some small businesses simply cannot get group insurance at affordable rates and therefore are not able to offer health insurance as a benefit to their employees. (2) In many work settings, participation in health insurance programs is voluntary and does not require employees to join when an employer offers health insurance. Some employees choose not to sign up mainly because they cannot afford the cost of health insurance premiums. Employers rarely pay 100 percent of the insurance premium; most require their employees to pay a portion of the cost, called ***premium cost sharing***. Others require their employees to pay the full cost, in which case health insurance becomes even more unaffordable. Even when the employee has to pay 100 percent of the premium, the benefit is that employees get group rates through their employer that are generally lower than what the rates would be if the employees were to purchase health insurance on their own. Employees who do not have health insurance offered by their employers, or those who are self-employed, have to obtain health insurance on their own. Individual rates are typically higher than group rates and, in some instances, health insurance is unavailable when adverse health conditions are present.

In America, working people earning low wages are the most disenfranchised because most of them are not eligible for public benefits and they cannot afford premium cost sharing. The United States has a significant number of ***uninsured***—those without private or public health insurance coverage. In 2004, the proportion of Americans under age 65 without health insurance was estimated at 41.6 million, or 16–17 percent of the total population (National Center for Health Statistics 2006, 26). The US government finances health benefits for certain special populations, including government employees, the elderly (age 65 and over), people with disabilities, some people with very low incomes, and children from low-income families. The program for the elderly and certain disabled individuals is called ***Medicare***. The program for the indigent, jointly administered by the federal government and state governments, is named ***Medicaid***. The program for children from low-income families, another federal/state partnership, is called the State Children's Health Insurance Program (SCHIP). For such public programs, the government may function as both financier and insurer, or the insurance function may be carved out to an HMO. Private providers, with a few exceptions, render services to these special categories of people. The government pays for the services, generally by establishing contractual arrangements with selected intermediaries for the actual disbursement of payments to the providers. Thus, even in government-financed programs, the four functions of financing, insurance, delivery, and payment may be quite distinct.

Transition from Traditional Insurance to Managed Care

Under traditional insurance, the four basic health delivery functions have been fragmented; that is, the financiers, insurers, providers, and payers have often been different entities, with a few exceptions. For example, self-insured employers, Medicaid in some states, and most participants in Medicare have integrated the functions of financing and insurance. Commercial insurers have integrated the functions of insurance and payment. During the 1990s, however, health care delivery in the United States underwent a fundamental change involving a tighter integration of the basic functions of financing, insurance, payment, and delivery through managed care.

Previously, fragmentation of the functions meant a lack of control over utilization and payments. The quantity of health care consumed refers to ***utilization*** of health services. Traditionally, determination of the utilization of health services and the price charged for each service were left up to the insured individuals and their physicians. Due to rising health care costs, current delivery mechanisms have instituted some controls over both utilization and price.

Managed care is a system of health care delivery that (1) seeks to achieve efficiencies by integrating the basic functions of health care delivery, (2) employs mechanisms to control (manage) utilization of medical services, and (3) determines the price at which the services are purchased and, consequently, how much the providers get paid. The primary financier is still the employer or the government, as the case may be. Instead of purchasing health insurance through a traditional insurance company, the employer contracts with an MCO, such as an HMO or a PPO, to offer a selected health plan to its employees. In this case, the MCO functions like an insurance company and promises to provide health care services contracted under the health plan to the enrollees of the plan. The term ***enrollee*** (member) refers to the individual covered under the plan. The contractual arrangement between the MCO and the enrollee—including the collective array of covered health services that the enrollee is entitled to—is referred to as the ***health plan*** (or "plan," for short). The health plan uses selected providers from whom the enrollees can choose to receive routine services. This primary care provider—often a physician in general practice—is customarily charged with the responsibility to determine the appropriateness of higher level or specialty services. The primary care provider refers the patient to receive specialty services if deemed appropriate.

Managed care integrates the four basic functions of health care delivery. Even though financing is primarily through the employers, health plans set up negotiated fee arrangements through contracts with the providers. The negotiated fee arrangements are based on either capitation or discounts. ***Capitation*** is a payment mechanism in which all health care services are included under one set fee per covered individual. In other words, it is a predetermined fixed payment per member per month (PMPM). As an alternative to capitation, some MCOs negotiate discounts against the providers' customary fees. Generally, HMOs use capitation, whereas PPOs use discounts. Managed care topics are discussed in greater detail in Chapter 9.

Costs are also managed indirectly through control over utilization. The plan underwrites risk; that is, in setting the premiums, the plan relies on the expected cost of health care utilization. There is a risk that expenditures for providing health care services may exceed the premiums collected. The plan thus assumes the role of insurance. The plan pays the providers (through capitation or discounted fees) for services rendered to the enrollees and thus assumes the payment function. Delivery of services may be partially through the plan's own hired physicians, but most services deliver through contracts with external providers, such as physicians, hospitals, and diagnostic clinics.

Primary Characteristics of the US Health Care System

In any country, certain external influences shape the basic character of its health services delivery system. These forces consist of the political climate of a nation, economic development, technological progress, social and cultural values, physical environment, population characteristics, such as demographic and health trends, and global influences (Figure 1–2). The combined interaction of these environmental forces influences the course of health care delivery.

Figure 1–2 External Forces Affecting Health Care Delivery.

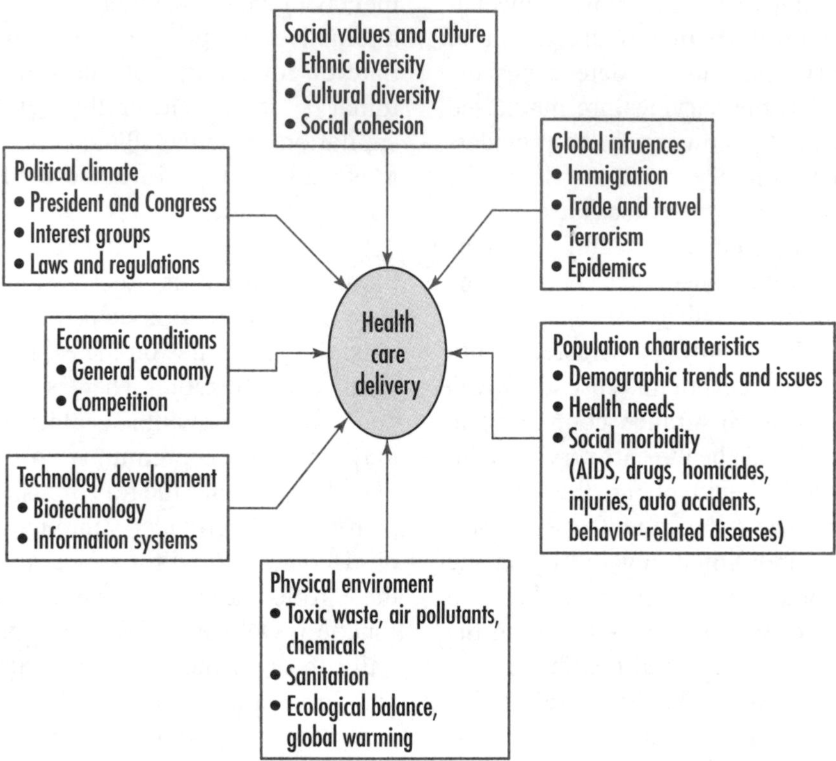

Ten basic characteristics differentiate the US health care delivery system from that of other countries:

1. No central agency governs the system.
2. Access to health care services is selectively based on insurance coverage.
3. Health care is delivered under imperfect market conditions.
4. Third-party insurers act as intermediaries between the financing and delivery functions.
5. Existence of multiple payers makes the system cumbersome.
6. Balance of power among various players prevents any single entity from dominating the system.
7. Legal risks influence practice behavior.
8. Development of new technology creates an automatic demand for its use.
9. New service settings have evolved along a continuum.
10. Quality is no longer accepted as an unachievable goal in the delivery of health care.

No Central Agency

The US health care system is not administratively controlled by a department or an agency of the government. Most other developed nations have national health care programs in which every citizen is entitled to receive a defined set of health care services. Availability of "free" services can break a system financially. To control costs, these systems use ***global budgets*** to determine total health care expenditures on the national scale and to allocate resources within the budgetary limits. Availability of services as well as payments to providers is subject to such budgetary constraints. The government also controls the proliferation of health care services, especially costly medical technology. System-wide controls over the allocation of resources determine to what extent government-sponsored health care services are available to the citizenry. For instance, the availability of specialized services is restricted.

By contrast, the United States has mainly a private system of financing as well as delivery. Private financing, predominantly through employers, accounts for approximately 55 percent of total health care expenditures; the government finances the remaining 45 percent (National Center for Health Statistics 2006, 374). Private delivery of health care means that the majority of hospitals and physician clinics are private businesses, independent of the government. No central agency monitors total expenditures through global budgets and controls the availability and utilization of services. Nevertheless, the federal and state governments in the United States play an important role in health care delivery. They determine public-sector expenditures and reimbursement rates for services provided to Medicaid, SCHIP, and Medicare beneficiaries. The government also formulates ***standards of participation*** through health policy and regulation meaning that providers must comply with the standards established by the government to be certified to provide services to Medicaid, SCHIP, and Medicare beneficiaries. Certification standards are also regarded as minimum standards of quality in most sectors of the health care industry.

Partial Access

Countries with national health care programs provide ***universal access***; that is, health care is available to all citizens. Such is not the case in the United States. ***Access*** means the ability of an individual to obtain health care services when needed. In the United States, access is restricted to: (1) those that have health insurance through their employers, (2) those covered under a government health care program, (3) those who can afford to buy insurance out of their own private funds, and (4) those that are able to pay for services privately. Health insurance is the primary means for ensuring access. Even though the United States offers among the best medical care in the world, such care is generally available primarily to those adequately covered under a health insurance plan or have adequate means to pay for it privately.

As stated earlier, a relatively large segment of the US population is uninsured. For continuous basic and routine care—commonly referred to as ***primary care***—the uninsured are often unable to see a physician unless they can pay the physician's fees or unless they have access to a Federally-Qualified Health Center (FQHC). FQHCs provide primary care and enabling services in medically underserved urban and rural areas, regardless of patients' ability to pay. Uninsured patients, who cannot afford to pay for private physicians and do not have access to free care at a health center, often wait until health problems develop to seek care. At that point, they may be able to receive services in a hospital emergency department, for which the hospital does not receive any direct payments (unless the patient is able to pay). Uninsured Americans, therefore, are able to obtain medical care for acute illness. Hence, one can say that the United States does have a form of universal catastrophic health insurance even for the uninsured (Altman and Reinhardt 1996, xxvi). It is well acknowledged that the absence of insurance inhibits the patient's ability to receive well-directed, coordinated, and continuous health care through access to primary care services and, when needed, referral to specialty services. Experts generally believe that the inadequate access to basic and routine primary care services is one of the main reasons why the United States, in spite of being the most economically advanced country, lags behind other developed nations in measures of population health, such as infant mortality and overall life expectancy.

Imperfect Market

Under national health care programs, patients have varying degrees of choice in selecting their providers; however, true economic market forces are virtually nonexistent. In the United States, even though the delivery of services is largely in private hands, health care is only partially governed by free market forces. The delivery and consumption of health care in the United States do not quite meet the basic tests of a ***free market***, as described below. Hence, the system is best described as a quasi-market or an imperfect market. Following are some key features characterizing free markets.

In a free market, multiple patients (buyers) and providers (sellers) act independently. In other words, in a free market, patients can choose to receive services from any provider. Providers neither collude to fix prices, nor are prices fixed by an external agency. Rather, prices are governed by the free and unencumbered interaction of the forces of supply and demand (Figure 1–3). ***Demand***, in turn, is driven by the prices prevailing in the free market. Under free market conditions, the quantity demanded will increase as the price is lowered for a given product or service. Conversely, the quantity demanded will decrease as the price increases.

At casual observation, it may appear that multiple patients and providers do exist. Most patients, however, are now enrolled either in a private health plan or in government-sponsored Medicare, Medicaid, or SCHIP programs if they meet the eligibility criteria. These plans act as intermediaries for the patients. Also, the consolidation of patients into health plans has the effect of shifting the power from the patients to the administrators of the plans. The result is that, in many respects, the health plans, not the patients, are the real buyers in the health care services market. Private health plans, in many instances, offer their enrollees a limited choice of providers rather than an open choice.

Theoretically, prices are negotiated between the payers and providers. In practice, however, prices are determined by the payers, such as managed care, Medicare, and Medicaid. Because prices are set by agencies external to the market, they are not governed by the unencumbered forces of supply and demand.

For the health care market to be free, unrestrained competition must occur among providers based on price and quality. Generally speaking, free competition exists among health care providers in the United States. The consolidation of buying power in the hands of private health plans, however, is forcing providers to form alliances and integrated delivery systems on the supply side. Integrated delivery systems (discussed in

Figure 1–3 Relationship between Price, Supply, and Demand under Free-Market Conditions.

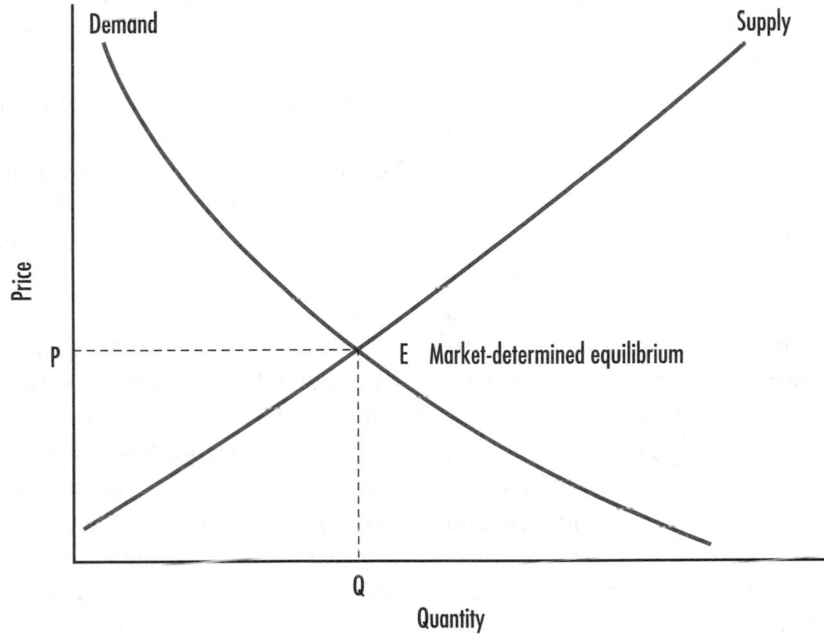

Under free-market conditions, there is an inverse relationship between the quantity of medical services demanded and the price of medical services. That is, quantity demanded goes up when the prices go down and vice versa. On the other hand, there is a direct relationship between price and the quantity supplied by the providers of care. In other words, providers are willing to supply higher quantities at higher prices, and vice versa. In a free market, the quantity of medical care that patients are willing to purchase, the quantity of medical care that providers are willing to supply, and the price reach a state of equilibrium. The equilibrium is achieved without the interference of any nonmarket forces. It is important to keep in mind that these conditions exist only under free-market conditions, which are not characterisitic of the health care market.

Chapter 9) are networks of health services organizations. In certain geographic sectors of the country, a single giant medical system has taken over as the sole provider of major health care services, restricting competition. As the health care system continues to move in this direction, it appears that only in large metropolitan areas will there be more than one large integrated system competing to get the business of the health plans.

A free market requires that patients have information about the availability of various services. In reality, patients do not always have adequate information about services. Technology-driven medical care has become highly sophisticated. New diagnostic methods, intervention techniques, and drugs that are more effective fall in the domain of the professional physician. Also, medical interventions are commonly required in a state of urgency. Hence, patients have neither the skills nor the time and other resources to obtain necessary information when needed. Channeling all health care needs through a primary care provider is likely to reduce this information gap when the primary provider acts as the patient's advocate or agent. On the other hand, the Internet is becoming a prominent source of medical information. Pharmaceutical advertising is also having an impact on consumer expectations.

In a free market, patients have information on price and quality for each provider. The current system has other drawbacks that obstruct information-seeking efforts. Item-based pricing instead of package pricing is one such hurdle. Surgery is a good example to illustrate item-based pricing. Patients can generally obtain the fees the surgeon would charge for a particular operation. But the final bill, after the surgery has been performed, is likely to include charges for supplies, use of the hospital's facilities, and services performed by providers, such as anesthesiologists, nurse anesthetists, and pathologists. These providers, sometimes referred to as ***phantom providers*** functioning in an adjunct capacity, bill for their services separately. Item billing for such additional services, which sometimes cannot be anticipated in advance, makes it extremely difficult to ascertain the total price before services have actually been received. Package pricing and capitated fees can help overcome these drawbacks, but they have made relatively little headway for pricing medical procedures. ***Package pricing*** refers to a bundled fee for a package of related services. In the surgery example, this would mean one all-inclusive price for the surgeon's fees, hospital facilities, supplies, diagnostics, pathology, anesthesia, and postsurgical follow-up. As discussed earlier, with capitation all health care services are included under one set fee per covered individual. Capitation is more all encompassing than package pricing. Whereas package pricing covers services bundled together for one episode, capitation covers all services an enrollee may need during an entire year.

In recent years, quality of health care has received much emphasis. Performance rating of health plans has met some success. However, apart from some sporadic news stories and selectively published health plan, provider, and hospital "report cards," the public still has scant information on the quality of health care providers.

In a free market, patients must directly bear the cost of services received. The purpose of insurance is to protect against the risk of unforeseen catastrophic events. Since the fundamental purpose of insurance is to meet major expenses when unlikely events occur, having insurance for basic and routine health care undermines the principle of insurance. When you buy home insurance to protect your property against the unlikely event of a fire, you generally do not anticipate the occurrence of a loss. The probability that you will suffer a loss by fire is very small. Also, if a fire occurs and causes major damage, insurance will cover the loss, but the policy does not cover routine wear and tear on the house such as chipped paint or a leaking faucet. Health insurance, however, generally covers basic and routine services that are predictable. Health insurance coverage for minor services, such as colds and coughs, earaches, and so forth, amounts to prepayment for such services. Health insurance has the effect of insulating patients from the full cost of health care. There is a ***moral hazard*** that once enrollees have purchased health insurance, they will use health care services to a greater extent than if they were without health insurance. Even certain referrals to higher-level services may be forgone if the patient has to bear the full cost of these services.

In a free market for health care, patients as consumers make decisions about the purchase of health care services. The main factors that severely limit the patient's ability to make health care purchasing decisions have already been discussed. Even with the best intentions, the circumstances surrounding sickness and injury generally prohibit comparative shopping based on price and quality. Further, such information is not easily available. At least two additional factors limit the ability of patients to make decisions. First, decisions about the utilization of health care are often determined by need rather than price-based demand. ***Need*** has generally been defined as the amount of medical care that medical experts believe a person should have to remain or become healthy (Feldstein 1993, 74–75). Needs can also be based on self-evaluation of one's own health status. Second, the delivery of health care can result in demand creation. This follows from self-assessed need, which, coupled with moral hazard, leads to greater utilization. This creates an artificial demand because prices are not taken into consideration. Practitioners who have a financial interest in additional treatments also create artificial demand (Hemenway and Fallon 1985), commonly referred to as ***supplier-induced demand*** or provider-induced demand. Functioning as the patients' agents, physicians exert enormous influence on the demand for health care services (Altman and Wallack 1996). Research studies have pointed to physicians' behavior of creating demand to their own financial benefit (see, for instance, the work of McGuire and Pauly 1991). Demand creation occurs when physicians prescribe medical care beyond what is clinically necessary. It can include practices such as making more frequent follow-up appointments than necessary, prescribing excessive medical tests, and performing unnecessary surgery (Santerre and Neun 1996, 369).

Third-Party Insurers and Payers

Insurance often functions as the intermediary among those who finance, deliver, and receive health care. As discussed earlier, health care is primarily financed by employers in the private sector and by the government in the public sector. Because the government is a large economic machine, it can self-insure against risk. Even though the government assumes the insurance function, payments to providers are generally handled through insurance intermediaries. Some large employers may also be able to self-insure; however, most private employers purchase health insurance from an insurance company or MCO. The employer's role is essentially relegated to selecting health plans and assisting employees with the enrollment process. The insurance company takes over most other administrative functions associated with the plan. The providers as well as the enrollees must comply with the policies set forth by the insurance company in matters associated with the provision of, and payment for, health services. Delivery of health care is often viewed as a transaction between the patient and the provider. But insurance and payment functions introduce a ***third party*** into the transaction (Griffith 1995, 279), the patient being the first party and the provider the second party.

The intermediary role of insurance creates a wall of separation between the financing and delivery functions so that quality of care often remains a secondary concern. In normal economic markets, the consumer is armed with the power to influence demand based on the price and quality of goods and services. Another way to illustrate this concept is to say that, in a free market, consumers vote with their dollar bills for the best candidate among competing products, based on the price and quality of each product. The insurance intermediary generally does not have the incentive to be the patient's advocate on either price or quality. At best, employees can air their dissatisfactions with the plan to their employer, who has the power to discontinue the current plan and choose another company. In reality, however, employers may be reluctant to change plans if the current plan offers lower premiums compared to a new plan. National health care programs have even fewer incentives for promoting quality, although they can contain costs by artificially fixing prices.

Multiple Payers

A national health care system is also sometimes referred to as a ***single-payer system*** because there is generally one primary payer, the government. When delivering services, providers send the bill to an agency of the government that subsequently sends payment to each provider.

By contrast, the United States has a multiplicity of health plans and insurance companies because each employer is free to determine the type of health plan it offers. Each plan spells out the type of services the enrollee can receive. Some plans make an arbitrary determination of how much they will pay for a certain type of service. For Medicare and Medicaid recipients, the government has its own set of regulations and payment schedules.

Multiple payers often represent a billing and collection nightmare for the providers of services. Multiple payers make the system more cumbersome in several ways:

- It is extremely difficult for providers to keep tabs on the numerous health plans. For example, it is difficult to keep up with which services are covered under each plan and how much each plan will pay for those services.
- Providers must hire a battery of claims processors to bill for services and monitor receipt of payments. Billing practices are not always standardized. Each payer establishes its own format.
- Payments can be denied for not following exactly the requirements set by each payer.
- Denied claims necessitate rebilling.
- When only partial payment is received, some health plans may allow the provider to ***balance bill*** the patient for the amount the health plan will not pay. Other plans prohibit balance billing. Even when the balance billing option is available to the provider, it triggers a new cycle of billings and collection efforts.
- Providers must sometimes engage in lengthy collection efforts including writing collection letters, turning delinquent accounts over to collection agencies, and finally writing off as bad debt the amounts that cannot be collected.
- Government programs have complex regulations for determining that payment is made for services actually delivered. Medicare, for example, requires each provider to maintain lengthy documentation on services provided.

When all the costs of billing, collections, bad debts, and maintaining medical records are aggregated for the entire system, the

United States ends up spending far more in ***administrative costs*** than the national health care system of any country in the world.

Power Balancing

The US health services system involves multiple players (not just multiple payers). The key players in the system have been physicians, administrators of health service institutions, insurance companies, large employers, and the government. Big business, labor, insurance companies, physicians, and hospitals make up the powerful and politically active special interest groups represented before lawmakers by high-priced lobbyists. Each player has its own economic interests to protect. Physicians, for instance, want to maximize their incomes and have minimum interference with the way they practice medicine; institutional administrators seek to maximize payment (commonly referred to as reimbursement) from private and public insurers. Insurance companies and MCOs are interested in maintaining their share of the health care insurance market; large employers want to minimize the costs they incur for providing health insurance as a benefit to their employees. The government tries to maintain or enhance existing benefits for select population groups and simultaneously reduce the cost of providing these benefits. The problem is that the self-interests of different players are often at odds. For example, providers seek to maximize government reimbursement for services delivered to Medicare, Medicaid, and SCHIP beneficiaries, but the government wants to contain cost increases. Employers dislike rising health insurance premiums. Health plans, under pressure from the employers, may constrain fees for the providers, who resent any cuts in their incomes.

The fragmented self-interests of the various players produce countervailing forces within the system. One positive effect of these opposing forces is that they prevent any single entity from dominating the system. On the other hand, each player has a large stake in health policy reforms. In an environment that is rife with motivations to protect conflicting self-interests, achieving comprehensive systemwide reforms is next to impossible, and cost containment remains a major challenge. Consequently, the approach to health care reform in the United States is often characterized as incremental or piecemeal.

Legal Risks

America is a litigious society. Motivated by the prospects of enormous jury awards, Americans are quick to drag the alleged offender into the courtroom at the slightest perception of incurred harm. Private health care providers have become increasingly more susceptible to litigation. By contrast, in national health care programs the governments are immune from lawsuits. Hence, in the United States, the risk of malpractice lawsuits is a real consideration in the practice of medicine. To protect themselves against the possibility of litigation, some practitioners engage in what is referred to as ***defensive medicine*** by prescribing additional diagnostic tests, scheduling return checkup visits, and maintaining copious documentation. Many of these additional efforts may be unnecessary; hence, they are costly and inefficient.

High Technology

The United States has been the hotbed of research and innovation in new medical technology. Growth in science and technology often creates demand for new services despite shrinking resources to finance sophisticated care. People generally want "the latest and the best," especially when health insurance would pay for new treatments. Physicians and technicians want to try the latest gadgets. Hospitals compete on the basis of having the most modern equipment and facilities. Once capital investments are made, their costs must be recouped through utilization. Legal risks for providers and health plans alike may also play a role in discouraging denial of new technology. Thus, several factors promote the use of costly new technology once it is developed.

Continuum of Services

Medical care services are generally classified into three broad categories: curative (e.g., drugs, treatments, and surgeries), restorative (e.g., physical, occupational, and speech therapies), and preventive (e.g., prenatal care, mammograms, and immunizations). Health care service settings are no longer confined to the hospital and the physician's office, where many of the aforementioned services were once delivered. Several new settings, such as home health, subacute care units, and outpatient surgery centers, have emerged in response to the changing configuration of economic incentives. Table 1–2 depicts the continuum of health care services.

Table 1–2 The Continuum of Health Care Services

Types of Health Services	Delivery Settings
Preventive care	Public health programs Community programs Personal lifestyles
Primary care	Physician's office or clinic Self-care Alternative medicine
Specialized care	Specialist provider clinics
Chronic care	Primary care settings Specialist provider clinics Home health Long-term care facilities Self-care Alternative medicine
Long-term care	Long-term care facilities Home health
Subacute care	Special subacute units (hospitals, long-term care facilities) Home health Outpatient surgical centers
Acute care	Hospitals
Rehabilitative care	Rehabilitation departments (hospitals, long-term care facilities) Home health Outpatient rehabilitation centers
End-of-life care	Hospice services provided in a variety of settings

Quest for Quality

Even though the definition and measurement of quality in health care are not as clear-cut as they are in other industries, the delivery sector of health care has come under increased pressure to develop quality standards and to demonstrate compliance with those standards. There are higher expectations for improved health outcomes at the individual and the broader community levels. The concept of continuous quality improvement has also received much emphasis in managing health care institutions.

Trends and Directions

Since the final two decades of the 20th century, the US health care delivery system has continued to undergo certain fundamental shifts in emphasis summarized in Figure 1–4. Later chapters discuss these transformations in greater detail and focus on the factors driving them.

Promotion of health at lesser cost has been the driving force behind these trends. An example of a shift in emphasis is the concept of health itself; the focus is changing from illness to wellness. Such a change requires new methods and settings for wellness promotion, although the treatment of illness continues to be the primary goal of the health services delivery system. Many of these changes are interrelated. A change in one area requires a modification in other areas. For example, the system of managed care has been necessary for shifting the emphasis from illness to wellness, from acute care to primary care, and from inpatient to outpatient settings. These fundamental moves will shape the future of the health care system.

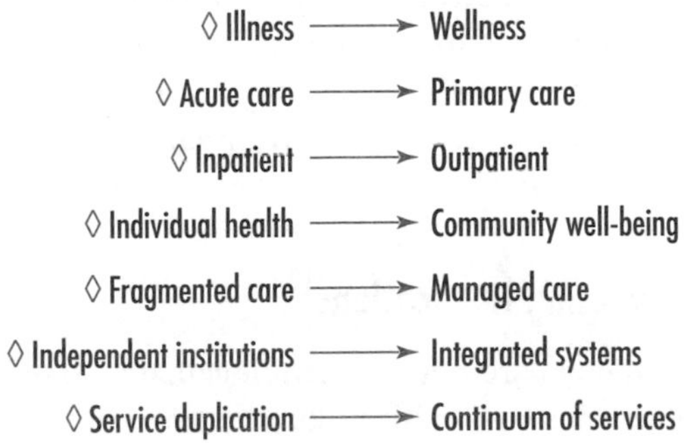
◊ Illness → Wellness
◊ Acute care → Primary care
◊ Inpatient → Outpatient
◊ Individual health → Community well-being
◊ Fragmented care → Managed care
◊ Independent institutions → Integrated systems
◊ Service duplication → Continuum of services

Figure 1–4 Trends and Directions in Health Care Delivery.

Significance for Health Care Practitioners and Policymakers

An understanding of the health care delivery system is essential for managers and policymakers. In fact, an understanding of the intricacies within the health services system would be beneficial to all those who come in contact with the system. In their respective training programs, health professionals, such as physicians, nurses, technicians, therapists, dietitians, pharmacists, and others, may understand their own individual roles, but remain ignorant of the forces outside their profession that could significantly impact current and future practices. An understanding of the health care delivery system can attune health professionals to their relationship with the rest of the health care environment. It can help them better understand changes and their potential impact on their own practice. Adaptation and relearning are strategies that can prepare health professionals to cope with an environment that will see ongoing change long into the future.

Policy decisions to address specific problems must also be made within the broader macro context because policies designed to bring about change in one health care sector can have wider repercussions, both desirable and undesirable, in other areas of the system. Policy decisions and their implementation are often critical to the future direction of the health care delivery system. However, in a multifaceted system, future issues will be best addressed by a joint undertaking that involves a balanced representation of the key players in health services delivery: physicians, insurance companies, managed care organizations, employers, institutional representatives, and the government.

Significance for Health Care Managers

An understanding of the health care system has specific implications for health services managers, who must understand the macro environment in which they make critical decisions in planning and strategic management, regardless of whether they manage a private institution or a public service agency. Such decisions and actions eventually affect the efficiency and quality of services delivered. The interactions between the system's key components and their implications must be well understood because the operations of health care institutions are strongly influenced, either directly or indirectly, by the financing of health services, reimbursement rates, insurance mechanisms, delivery modes, new statutes and legal opinions, and government regulations.

The environment of health care delivery will continue to remain fluid and dynamic. The viability of delivery settings, and thus the success of health care managers, often depends on how the managers react to the system dynamics. Timeliness of action is often a critical factor that can make the difference between failure and success. Following are some more specific reasons why understanding the health care delivery system is indispensable for health care managers.

Positioning the Organization

Health services administrators need to understand their own organizational position within the macro environment of the system. Senior managers, such as chief executive officers, need to evaluate where their organization actually fits in the continuum of services. They must constantly gauge the nature and impact of the fundamental shifts illustrated in Figure 1–4. Managers need to consider which changes in the current configuration of financing, insurance, payment, and delivery might affect their organization's long-term stability. Middle and first-line managers also need to understand their role in the current configuration and how that role might change in the future. How should resources be realigned to effectively respond to those changes? For example, they need to evaluate whether certain functions in their departments will have to be eliminated, modified, or added. Would the changes involve further training? What processes are likely to change and how? What do they need to do to maintain the integrity of their institution's mission, the goodwill of the patients they serve, and the quality of their services? Regardless of the situation, a well thought through and appropriately planned change is likely to cause less turbulence for the providers as well as the recipients of care.

Handling Threats and Opportunities

Changes in any of the functions of financing, insurance, payment, and delivery can present new threats or opportunities in the health care market. Health care managers will be more effective if they proactively deal with any threats to their institution's profitability and viability. Managers need to find ways to transform certain threats into new opportunities.

Evaluating Implications

Managers are better able to evaluate the implications of health policy and new reform proposals when they understand the relevant issues and how such issues link to the delivery of health services in the establishments they manage.

Planning

Senior managers are often responsible for strategic planning regarding which services should be added or discontinued, which resources should be committed to facility expansion, or what should be done with excess capacity. Any long-range planning must take into consideration the current makeup of health services delivery, the evolving trends, and the potential impact of these trends.

Capturing New Markets

Health care administrators are in a better position to capture new health services markets if they understand emerging trends in the financing, insurance, payment, and delivery functions of health care. New opportunities must be explored before any newly evolving segments of the market get overcrowded. An understanding of the dynamics within the system is essential to forging new marketing strategies to stay ahead of the competition and often to finding a service niche.

Complying with Regulations

Delivery of health care services is heavily regulated. Health care managers must comply with government regulations, such as standards of participation, licensing rules, security and privacy laws regarding patient information, and must operate within the constraints of reimbursement rates. The Medicare and Medicaid programs have periodically made drastic changes to their reimbursement methodologies that have triggered the need to make operational changes in the way services are organized and delivered. Private agencies, such as the Joint Commission on Accreditation of Healthcare Organizations (Joint Commission), also play an indirect regulatory role, mainly in the monitoring of quality of services. Health care managers have no choice but to play by the rules set by the various public and private agencies. Hence, it is paramount that health care managers acquaint themselves with the rules and regulations governing their areas of operation.

Following the Organizational Mission

Knowledge of the health care system and its development is essential for effective management of health care organizations. By keeping up to date on community needs, technological progress, consumer demand, and economic prospects, managers can be in a better position to fulfill their organizational missions to enhance access, improve service quality, and achieve efficiency in the delivery of services.

Health Care Systems of Other Countries

Canada and most Western European countries have national health care programs that provide universal access. There are three basic models for structuring national health care systems.

1. In a system under ***national health insurance*** (NHI), such as in Canada, the government finances health care through general taxes, but the actual care is delivered by private providers. In the context of the quad-function

model, NHI requires a tighter consolidation of the financing, insurance, and payment functions coordinated by the government. Delivery is characterized by detached private arrangements.

2. In a ***national health system*** (NHS), such as the one in Great Britain, in addition to financing a tax-supported NHI program, the government also manages the infrastructure for the delivery of medical care. Under such a system, the government operates most of the medical institutions. Most health care providers, such as physicians, either are government employees or are tightly organized in a publicly managed infrastructure. In the context of the quad-function model, NHS requires a tighter consolidation of all four functions.

3. In a ***socialized health insurance*** (SHI) system, such as in Germany, government-mandated contributions, by employers and employees, finance health care. Private providers deliver health care. Private not-for-profit insurance companies, called sickness funds, are responsible for collecting the contributions and paying physicians and hospitals (Santerre and Neun 1996, 134). In a socialized health insurance system, insurance and payment functions are closely integrated, and the financing function is better coordinated with the insurance and payment functions than it is in the United States. Delivery is characterized by independent private arrangements. The government exercises overall control.

In the remainder of this book, the terms "national health care program" and "national health insurance" are used generically and interchangeably to refer to any type of government-supported universal access health care program. Table 1–3 presents selected features of the national health care programs in Canada, Germany, and Great Britain compared to the United States. Following is a brief discussion of health care delivery in some selected countries from various parts of the world to illustrate the application of the three models discussed above and to provide a sample of the variety of healthcare systems in the world.

Australia

In the past, Australia switched from a universal national health care program to a privately financed system. Since 1984, it has returned to a national program called Medicare financed by income taxes and an income-based Medicare levy. The system is built on the philosophy of everyone contributing to the cost of health care according to his or her capacity to pay. In addition to Medicare, approximately 43 percent of Australians carry private health insurance (Australian Government 2004).This private health insurance covers gaps in public coverage, such as dental services, and covers care received in private hospitals (Willcox 2001). Acquiring private health insurance is voluntary, but is strongly encouraged by the Australian government through tax subsidies for purchasers and tax penalties for nonpurchasers (Healy 2002). Public hospital spending is funded by the government, but private hospitals offer better choice. Costs incurred by patients receiving private medical services, whether in or out of the hospi-

Table 1–3 Health Care Systems of Selected Industrialized Countries

	United States	Canada	Great Britain	Germany
Type	Pluralisitic	National health insurance	National health system	Socialized health insurance
Ownership	Private	Public/Private	Public	Private
Financing	Voluntary, multipayer system (premiums or general taxes)	Single-payer (general taxes)	Single-payer (general taxes)	Employer-employee (mandated payroll contributions and general taxes)
Reimbursement (hospital)	Varies (DRG, negotiated fee-for-service, per diem, capitation)	Global budgets	Global budgets	Per diem payments
Reimbursement (physicians)	RBRVS, fee for service	Negotiated fee for service	Salaries and capitation payments	Negotiated fee for service
Consumer co-payment	Small to significant	Negligible	Negligible	Negligible

Note: RBRVS, resource-based relative value scale.

Source: Data from R.E. Santerre and S.P. Neun, *Health Economics: Theories, Insights, and Industry Studies,* p. 146, © 1996, Irwin.

tal, are reimbursed in whole or in part by Medicare (Healthcare Costs 2002). Private patients are free to choose and/or change their doctors. The well-organized medical profession in Australia is composed mainly of private practitioners who provide care predominantly on a fee-for-service basis (Hall 1999; Podger 1999).

Canada

Canada implemented its national health insurance system—referred to as Medicare—under the Medical Care Act of 1966. Currently, Medicare is composed of 13 provincial and territorial health insurance plans sharing basic standards of coverage as defined by the Canada Health Act (Health Canada 2006). The bulk of financing for Medicare comes from general provincial tax revenues; the federal government provides a constant amount that is independent of actual expenditures. The public pays for nearly 70 percent of total health care expenditures in Canada. The remaining 30 percent, paying for supplementary services such as drugs, dental care, and vision care, is financed privately (Canadian Institute for Health Information 2005). Provincial and territorial departments of health have the responsibility to administer medical insurance plans, determine reimbursement for providers, and deliver certain public health services. Provinces are required by law to provide reasonable access to all medically necessary services and to provide portability of benefits from province to province. The program provides comprehensive coverage, but excludes dental care. Coverage for home health care and prescription drugs varies across the provinces. To cover these exclusions, many Canadians have supplemental coverage through private insurance provided by employers. Patients are free to select their providers (Akaho et al. 1998). Several provinces have established contracts with providers in the United States for certain specialized services. However, contrary to popular perceptions, few Canadians have to obtain health care services in the United States due to waiting times or unavailability of technology in their own country (Katz et al. 2002).

Nearly all the Canadian provinces (Ontario being one exception) have resorted to regionalization by creating administrative districts within each province. The objective of regionalization is to decentralize authority and responsibility to more efficiently address local needs and to promote citizen participation in health care decision-making (Church and Barker 1998). The majority of Canadian hospitals are operated as private nonprofit entities run by community boards of trustees, voluntary organizations, or municipalities, and most physicians are in private practice (Health Canada 2006). Most provinces use global budgets and allocate set reimbursement amounts for each hospital. Physicians are paid fee-for-service rates negotiated between each provincial government and medical association (MacPhee 1996; Naylor 1999).

Over the years, federal financial support to the provinces was drastically reduced. Under the increasing burden of higher costs, certain provinces, such as Alberta and Ontario, have started small-scale experimentation with privatization. However, in 2003, the Health Council of Canada, comprised of representatives of federal, provincial, and territorial governments, as well as health care experts, was established to assess Canada's health care system performance and establish goals for improvement. The Council's 2003 First Ministers' Accord on Health Care Renewal created a five-year, $16 billion Health Reform Fund targeted to improving primary health care, home care, and catastrophic drug coverage (Health Council of Canada 2005).

China

Since the economic reforms initiated in the late 1970s, health care in the People's Republic of China has undergone significant changes, most prominently reflected in health insurance and health care delivery. In urban China, health insurance has evolved from a predominantly public insurance (either government or public enterprise) system to a multi-payer system. Government employees are covered under government insurance as a part of their benefits. Employees for public enterprises are largely covered through public enterprise insurance, but the actual benefits and payments vary according to the financial well-being of the enterprises. Employees of foreign businesses or joint ventures typically are well insured through private insurance arrangements. Almost all of these plans contain costs through a variety of means such as experience-based premiums, deductibles, co-payments, and health benefit dollars (i.e., pre-allocated benefit dollars for health care that can be converted into income if not fully used). The unemployed, self-employed, and employees working for small enterprises (public or private) are largely uninsured. They can purchase individual or family plans in the private market or pay for services out of pocket.

In rural China, except for a few well-to-do communities, fee-for-service has replaced the cooperative medical system. Health insurance is not mandatory. In 2002, the Chinese government introduced a new basic insurance plan for poor, rural citizens. Under this plan, the government provides the equivalent of $2.50 a year to cover basic insurance, which the plan holder matches with $1.25. These plans do not cover primary care services or drugs; rather, they cover only inpatient services, with a very high deductible (Blumenthal and Hsiao 2005).

Health care delivery has also undergone significant changes. The former three-tier referral system (primary, second, tertiary) has been largely abolished. Patients can now go to any hospital of their choice as long as they are insured or can pay out of pocket. As a result, large (tertiary) hospitals are typically overutilized whereas smaller (primary and secondary) hospitals are underutilized. Use of large hospitals contributes to medical cost escalation and medical specialization. In rural China, the cooperative medical system run by "barefoot" doctors (peasant paramedics) has been abolished. "Barefoot" doctors either have changed their profession or have received further training to become licensed physicians to practice in rural hospitals or private clinics.

Major changes in health insurance and delivery have made access to medical care more difficult for the poor and uninsured. As a result, wide and growing disparities in health care access, quality, and outcomes are becoming apparent between rural and urban areas and between the rich and the poor. It remains uncertain whether China will continue its current course of medical specialization and privatization, or restore its previously integrated health care delivery system aimed at achieving universal access. The recent SARS epidemic serves as a wake-up call to the government, which now recognizes the importance of a well-developed public health infrastructure. To this end, the government has created an electronic disease reporting system based at the district level. In addition, each district in China now has a hospital dedicated to infectious disease. However, flaws in the system, particularly in monitoring infectious disease in the remote localities that comprise some districts, remain (Blumenthal and Hsiao 2005).

Germany

The German health care system is characterized by socialized health insurance (SHI) financed by pooling employer and employee premium contributions. Nonprofit sickness funds manage the social insurance pool. About 88 percent of the population has been enrolled in a sickness fund; another 11 percent of Germans either have private health insurance or are government workers with special coverage provisions. Less than 0.2 percent of Germans are uninsured (Busse 2002). Sickness funds act as purchasing entities by negotiating contracts with hospitals. To control costs, the system employs global budgets for the hospital sector and places annual limits on spending for physician services. During the 1990s, Germany adopted new legislation to promote competition among sickness funds (Brown and Amelung 1999).

Great Britain

Britain follows the national health system (NHS) model. Coincidentally, the British health delivery system is also named NHS (National Health Service), which marked 50 years of existence in 1998. The NHS is founded on the principles of primary care and has a strong focus on community health services. The system owns its hospitals and employs its hospital-based specialists and other staff on a salaried basis. The primary care physicians, referred to as general practitioners (GPs), are mostly private practitioners.

Since 1991, the NHS has undergone some major transformations initiated by former Prime Minister Thatcher and continued by Tony Blair's Labor government. The quasi-market reforms initially resulted in the creation of primary care groups (PCGs), which brought local GPs, community nurses, and other health care and social services professionals under semiautonomous local health care delivery units. Local health authorities had fiscal and management responsibilities for most PCGs (Bindman et al. 2001).

In recent years, PCGs have evolved into primary care trusts (PCTs) in England, local health groups in Wales, health boards in Scotland, and primary care partnerships in Northern Ireland. PCTs have geographically assigned responsibility for community health services, and each person living in a given geographic area is assigned to a PCT. A typical PCT is responsible for approximately 50,000–250,000 patients (Dixon and Robinson 2002). PCTs function independently of the local health authorities and are governed by a consumer-dominated board. A fully developed PCT has its own budget allocations used for both primary care and hospital-based services. In this respect, PCTs function like MCOs in the United States.

It is also of interest to note that 11.5 percent of the British population holds private health care insurance (Dixon and Robinson 2002), and approximately 2.2 billion pounds are spent annually in the acute sector of private health care (Doyle and McNeilly 1999).

Israel

Until 1995, Israel had a system of universal access based on the German model of SHI financed through an employer tax and income-based contributions from individuals. The insurance function was managed by four sickness funds. In 1995, the country legislated an NHI program replacing the citizens' sickness fund contributions with a specific health tax, which is an earmarked payroll tax. In addition, general tax revenue supplements the health tax revenue. The contribution of general tax revenue toward the NHI depends on the yearly, government-determined level of NHI funding. The employer tax for health care was abolished in 1997; as a result, the share of general tax revenue as a percentage of total health care financing rose from 26 percent in 1995 to 46 percent in 2000 (Rosen 2003).

The insurance function and the delivery of care are still in the hands of the sickness funds. Citizens can enroll in any of the four sickness funds, which are nonprofit, independent legal entities operating within a regulatory framework defined by the government. The funds compete based on client satisfaction and provide a minimum, predefined basic package of health care services. The sickness funds also sell private health insurance to supplement the basic package.

Unlike Germany, approximately 85 percent of the general hospital beds in Israel are owned by the government and the General Sick Fund, the largest of the four sickness funds. Hospitals are reimbursed under the global budget model (Chinitz and Israeli 1997). There was a major effort in the early

1990s to shift hospitals from government ownership to independent, nonprofit trusts, but this endeavor failed due to the opposition of health care unions. Despite this, government hospitals have been granted far more autonomy in the intervening years (Rosen 2003).

Japan

Since 1961, Japan has been providing universal coverage to its citizens through two main types of health insurance schemes. The first one is an employer-based system modeled after Germany's SHI program. The second is a national health insurance program. Generally, large employers (with more than 300 employees) have their own health programs. Nearly 2,000 private, nonprofit health insurance societies manage insurance for large firms. Smaller companies either band together to provide private health insurance or belong to a government-managed plan. Day laborers, seamen, agricultural workers, the self-employed, and retirees are covered under the national health care program. Individual employees pay roughly 8 percent of their salaries as premiums and receive coverage for about 90 percent of the cost of medical services, with some limitations. Dependents get a little less than 90 percent coverage. Employers and the national government subsidize the cost of private premiums. Coverage is comprehensive, including dental care and prescription drugs. Patients are free to select their providers (Akaho et al. 1998; Babazono et al. 1998). Providers are paid on a fee-for-service basis with little control over reimbursement (McClellan and Kessler 1999).

Several health policy issues have emerged in Japan in the past few years. First, since 2002, some business leaders and economists have urged the Japanese government to lift its ban on mixed public and private payments for medical services, arguing private payments should be allowed for services not covered by medical insurance (i.e., services involving new technologies or drugs). The Japan Medical Association and Ministry of Health, Labor, and Welfare have argued against these recommendations, stating such a policy would favor the wealthy, create disparities in access to care, and could be a risk to patient safety. While the ban on mixed payments has not been lifted, Prime Minister Koizumi expanded the existing "exceptional approvals system" for new medical technologies in 2004, which will allow private payments for selected technologies not covered by medical insurance at hospitals meeting certain conditions (Nomura and Nakayama 2005).

Another recent policy development in Japan is hospitals' increased use of a new system of reimbursement for inpatient care services, called diagnosis-procedure combinations (DPCs). The DPC system, spearheaded by the Ministry of Health, Labor, and Welfare, started in 2003 with 82 hospitals. Using DPC, hospitals receive daily fees for each condition and treatment, regardless of actual provision of tests and interventions, proportionate to patients' length of stay. It is theorized that the DPC system will incentivize hospitals to provide more efficient, higher quality care to patients (Nomura and Nakayama 2005).

Singapore

Prior to 1984, Singapore had a British-style NHS program where medical services were provided mainly by the public sector and financed through general taxes. Since then, the nation has designed a system based on market competition and self-reliance. Singapore has achieved universal access through government policy requiring mandatory private contributions but little government financing. The program, known as Medisave, mandates every working person, including the self-employed, to deposit a portion of earnings into an individual Medisave account. Employers are required to match employee contributions. These savings can only be withdrawn (1) to pay for hospital services and some selected expensive physician services, and (2) to purchase a government-sponsored insurance plan (called Medishield) for catastrophic (expensive and major) illness. For basic and routine services, people are expected to pay out of pocket. Those who cannot afford to pay receive government assistance (Hsiao 1995). In 2002, the government introduced ElderShield, which defrays out-of-pocket medical expenses for the elderly and severely disabled people requiring long-term care (Singapore Ministry of Health 2004). The fee-for-service system of payment to providers is prevalent throughout Singapore (McClellan and Kessler 1999).

Developing Countries

Developing countries containing 84 percent of the world's population, claim only 11 percent of the world's health spending. Yet, these countries account for 93 percent of the worldwide burden of disease. The six developing regions of the world are East Asia and the Pacific, Europe (mainly Eastern Europe) and Central Asia, Latin America and the Caribbean, the Middle East and North Africa, South Asia, and Sub-Saharan Africa. Of these, the latter two have the least resources and the greatest health burden. On a per capita basis, industrialized countries have six times as many hospital beds and three times as many physicians as developing countries. People with private financial means can find reasonably good health care in many parts of the developing world. The majority of the populations, however, have to depend on limited government services that are often of questionable quality as evaluated by Western standards. As a general observation, government financing for health services increases in countries with higher per capita incomes (Schieber and Maeda 1999).

The Systems Framework

A system consists of a set of interrelated and interdependent components designed to achieve some common goals, and the components are logically coordinated. Even though the various functional components of the health services delivery structure in the United States are at best only loosely coordinated, the main components can be identified by using a systems model. The systems framework used here helps one understand that the structure of health care services in the United States is based on some foundations, provides a logical arrangement of the various components, and demonstrates a progression from inputs to outputs. The main elements of this arrangement are system inputs (resources), system structure, system processes, and system outputs (outcomes). In addition, system outlook (future directions) is a necessary element of a dynamic system. This system's framework has been used as the conceptual base for organizing later chapters in this book (see Figure 1–5).

Figure 1–5 The Systems Model and Related Chapters.

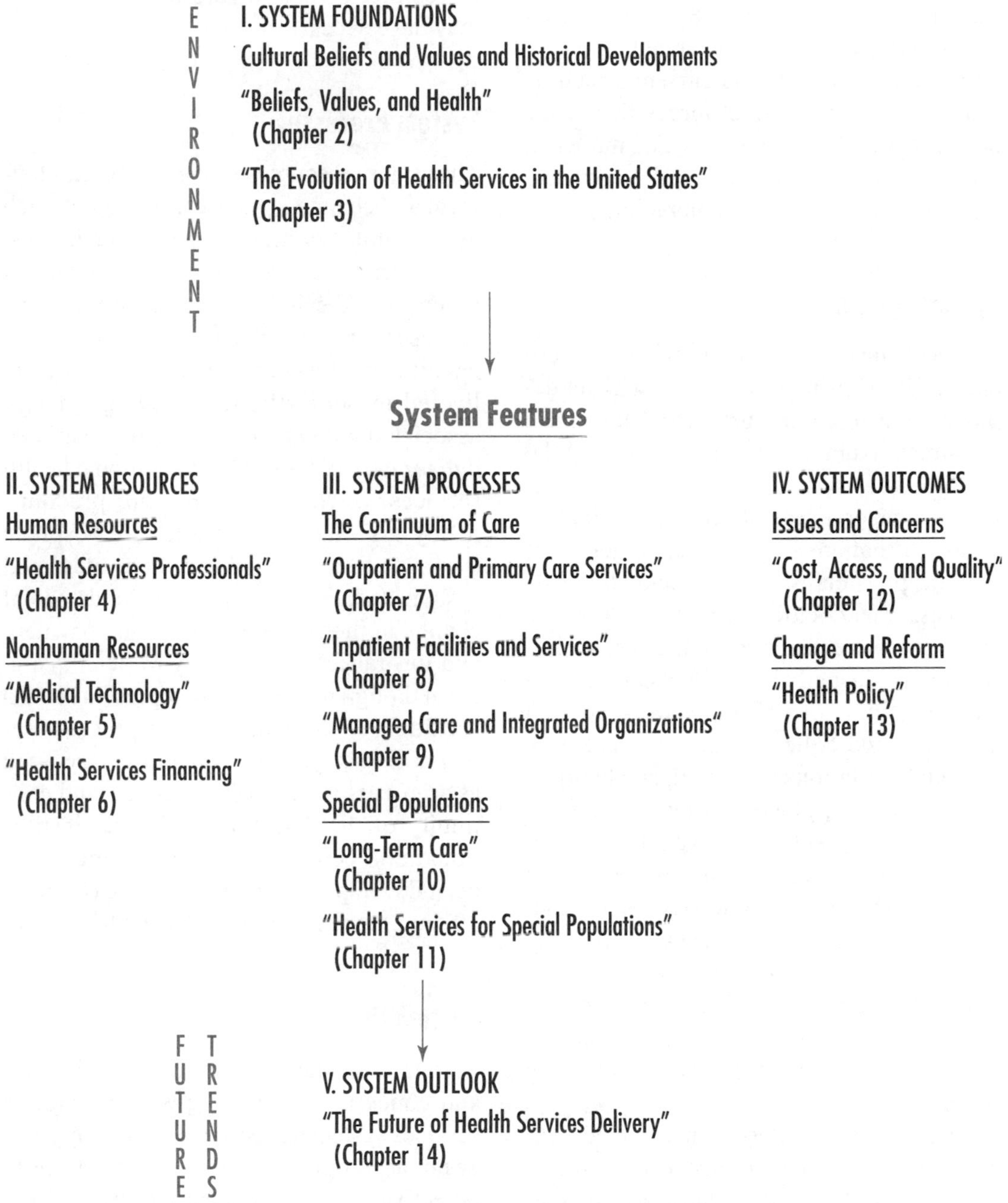

ENVIRONMENT

I. SYSTEM FOUNDATIONS

Cultural Beliefs and Values and Historical Developments

"Beliefs, Values, and Health" (Chapter 2)

"The Evolution of Health Services in the United States" (Chapter 3)

System Features

II. SYSTEM RESOURCES

Human Resources

"Health Services Professionals" (Chapter 4)

Nonhuman Resources

"Medical Technology" (Chapter 5)

"Health Services Financing" (Chapter 6)

III. SYSTEM PROCESSES

The Continuum of Care

"Outpatient and Primary Care Services" (Chapter 7)

"Inpatient Facilities and Services" (Chapter 8)

"Managed Care and Integrated Organizations" (Chapter 9)

Special Populations

"Long-Term Care" (Chapter 10)

"Health Services for Special Populations" (Chapter 11)

IV. SYSTEM OUTCOMES

Issues and Concerns

"Cost, Access, and Quality" (Chapter 12)

Change and Reform

"Health Policy" (Chapter 13)

FUTURE TRENDS

V. SYSTEM OUTLOOK

"The Future of Health Services Delivery" (Chapter 14)

System Foundations

The current health care system is not an accident. Historical, cultural, social, and economic factors explain its current structure. These factors also affect forces that shape new trends and developments, and those that impede change. Chapters 2 and 3 provide a discussion of the system foundations.

System Resources

No mechanism for health services delivery can fulfill its primary objective without deploying the necessary human and nonhuman resources. Human resources consist of the various types and categories of workers directly engaged in the delivery of health services to patients. Such personnel—that include physicians, nurses, dentists, pharmacists, other doctoral trained professionals, and numerous categories of allied health professionals—usually have direct contact with patients. Numerous ancillary workers, such as billing and collection agents, marketing and public relations personnel, and building maintenance employees, often play an important but indirect supportive role in the delivery of health care. Health care managers are needed to manage various types of health care services. This book discusses primarily the personnel engaged in the direct delivery of health care services (Chapter 4). The nonhuman resources include medical technology (Chapter 5) and health services financing (Chapter 6).

Resources are closely intertwined with access to health care. For instance, in certain rural areas of the United States, access is restricted due to a shortage of certain categories of health professionals. Development and diffusion of technology also determine the caliber of health care to which people may have access.

System Processes

The system resources influence the development and change in physical structures, such as hospitals, clinics, and nursing homes. These structures are associated with distinct processes of health services delivery, and the processes are associated with distinct health conditions. Most health care services are delivered in noninstitutional settings mainly associated with processes referred to as ***outpatient care*** (Chapter 7). Institutional health services, or ***inpatient care***, are predominantly associated with acute care hospitals (Chapter 8). Managed care and integrated systems (Chapter 9) represent a fundamental change in the financing (including payment and insurance) and delivery of health care. Even though managed care represents an integration of the resource and process elements of the systems model, it is discussed as a process for the sake of clarity and continuity of the discussions. Special institutional and community-based settings have been developed for long-term care (Chapter 10) and mental health (Chapter 11).

System Outcomes

System outcomes refer to the critical issues and concerns surrounding what the health services system has been able to accomplish, or not accomplish, in relation to its primary objective. As indicated earlier, the primary objective of any health care delivery system is to provide, to an entire nation, cost-effective health services that meet certain established standards of quality. The previous three elements of the systems model play a critical role in fulfilling this objective. Access, cost, and quality are the main outcome criteria for evaluating the success of a health care delivery system (Chapter 12). Issues and concerns regarding these criteria trigger broad initiatives for reforming the system through health policy (Chapter 13).

System Outlook

A dynamic health care system must be forward-looking. In essence, it must project into the future the accomplishment of desired system outcomes in view of anticipated social, cultural, and economic changes. Chapter 14 discusses these future perspectives.

Summary

The United States has a unique system of health care delivery. The basic features that characterize this system, or patchwork of subsystems, include: the absence of a central agency to govern the system, unequal access to health care services due to lack of health insurance for all Americans, health care delivery under imperfect market conditions, existence of multiple payers, third-party insurers functioning as intermediaries between the financing and delivery aspects of health care, balancing of power among various players, legal risks influencing practice behavior, new and expensive medical technology, a continuum of service settings, and a focus on quality improvement. No country in the world has a perfect system. Most nations with a national health care program also have a private sector that varies in size. The developing countries of the world face serious challenges due to scarce resources and strong underlying needs for services.

Health care administrators must understand how the health care delivery system works and evolves. Such an understanding improves their awareness of the position their organization occupies within the macro environment of the system. It also facilitates strategic planning and compliance with health regulations, enabling them to deal proactively with both opportunities and threats, and enabling them to effectively manage health care organizations. The systems framework provides an organized approach to an understanding of the various components of the US health care delivery system.

Under free-market conditions, there is an inverse relationship between the quantity of medical services demanded and the price of medical services. That is, quantity demanded goes up when the prices go down and vice versa. On the other hand, there is a direct relationship between price and the quantity supplied by the providers of care. In other words, providers are willing to supply higher quantities at higher prices, and vice versa. In a free market, the quantity of medical care that patients are willing to purchase, the quantity of medical care that providers are willing to supply, and the price reach a state of equilibrium. The equilibrium is achieved without the interference of any non-market forces. It is important to keep in mind that these conditions exist only under free-market conditions, which are not characteristic of the health care market.

Test Your Understanding

Terminology

access
administrative costs
balance bill
capitation
defensive medicine
demand
enrollee
free market
global budget
health plan
inpatient care
managed care
Medicaid
Medicare
moral hazard
national health insurance
national health system
need
outpatient care
package pricing
phantom providers
premium cost sharing
primary care
provider
quad-function model
reimbursement
single-payer system
socialized health insurance
standards of participation
supplier-induced demand
system
third party
uninsured
universal access
utilization

Review Questions

1. Why does cost containment remain an elusive goal in US health services delivery?
2. What are the two main objectives of a health care delivery system?
3. Name the four basic functional components of the US health care delivery system. What role does each play in the delivery of health care?
4. What is the primary reason for employers to purchase insurance plans to provide health benefits to their employees?
5. Why is it that despite public and private health insurance programs, some US citizens are without any coverage?
6. What is managed care?
7. Why is the US health care market referred to as "imperfect"?
8. Discuss the intermediary role of insurance in the delivery of health care.
9. Who are the major players in the US health services system? What are the positive and negative effects of the often-conflicting self-interests of these players?
10. What main roles does the government play in the US health services system?
11. Why is it important for health care managers and policymakers to understand the intricacies of the health care delivery system?
12. What kind of a cooperative approach do the authors recommend for charting the future course of the health care delivery system?
13. What is the difference between national health insurance (NHI) and a national health system (NHS)?
14. What is socialized health insurance (SHI)?

REFERENCES

Akaho, E. et al. 1998. A proposed optimal health care system based on a comparative study conducted between Canada and Japan. *Canadian Journal of Public Health* 89, no. 5: 301–307.

Altman, S.H., and U.E. Reinhardt. 1996. Introduction: Where does health care reform go from here? An uncharted odyssey. In *Strategic choices for a changing health care system*, eds. S.H. Altman and U.E. Reinhardt, xxi–xxxii. Chicago: Health Administration Press.

Altman, S.H., and S.S. Wallack. 1996. Health care spending: Can the United States control it? In *Strategic choices for a changing health care system*, eds. S.H. Altman and U.E. Reinhardt, 1–32. Chicago: Health Administration Press.

American Association of Colleges of Osteopathic Medicine. 2007. *http://aacom.org/colleges*.

American Association of Colleges of Pharmacy. 2007. *http://aacp.org/issi/membership/schools.asp*.

American Association of Medical Colleges. 2007. *http://aamc.org/medicalschools.htm*.

American Dental Education Association. 2007. *http://adea.org/DMS/instlinks/default.htm*.

America's Health Insurance Plans. 2004. *2002 AHIP survey of health insurance plans: Chart book of findings*. Washington, DC: America's Health Insurance Plans.

Australian Government, Department of Health and Ageing. May 2004. Australia: Selected health care delivery and financing statistics. Available at: *http://www.health.gov/au*. Accessed September 2006.

Babazono, A. et al. 1998. The effect of a redistribution system for health care for the elderly on the financial performance of health insurance societies in Japan. *International Journal of Technology Assessment in Health Care* 14, no. 3: 458–466.

Bindman, A.B. et al. 2001. Primary care groups in the United Kingdom: Quality and accountability. *Health Affairs* 20, no. 3: 132–145.

Blue Cross Blue Shield Association. 2007. *http://www.bcbs.com/coverage/find/plan*.

Blumenthal D., and W. Hsiao. 2005. Privitization and its discontents—The evolving Chinese health care system. *New England Journal of Medicine* 353, no.11:1165–70.

Brown, L.D., and V.E. Amelung. 1999. "Manacled competition". Market reforms in German health care. *Health Affairs* 18, no. 3: 76–91.

Busse, R. 2002. Germany. In Dixon, A., and E. Mossialos, eds. *Health care systems in eight countries: Trends and challenges*. London: The European Observatory on Health Care Systems, London School of Economics & Political Science, 47–60.

Canadian Institute for Health Information. 2005. *National health expenditure trends, 1975–2005*. Ottawa: The Institute, pp. iii, 7.

Chinitz, D., and A. Israeli. 1997. Health reform and rationing in Israel. *Health Affairs* 16, no. 5: 205–210.

Church, J., and P. Barker. 1998. Regionalization of health services in Canada: A critical perspective. *International Journal of Health Services* 28, no. 3: 467–486.

Dixon, A., and R. Robinson. 2002. The United Kingdom. In Dixon, A., and E. Mossialos, eds. *Health care systems in eight countries: Trends and challenges*. London: The European Observatory on Health Care Systems, London School of Economics & Political Science, 103–14.

Doyle, Y.G., and R.H. McNeilly. 1999. The diffusion of new medical technologies in the private sector of the U.K. health care system. *International Journal of Technology Assessment in Health Care* 15, no. 4: 619–628.

Feldstein, P.J. 1993. *Health care economics*. 4th ed. New York: Delmar Publishing.

Griffith, J.R. 1995. *The well-managed health care organization*. Ann Arbor, MI: AUPHA Press/Health Administration Press.

Hall, J. 1999. Incremental change in the Australian health care system. *Health Affairs* 18, no. 3: 95–110.

Health Canada. 2006. Available at: *http://www.hc-sc.gc.ca/hcs-sss/medi-assur/index_e.htmlwhich*. Accessed September 2006.

Health Council of Canada. 2005. Annual Report 2005. Available at: *http://www.healthcouncilcanada.ca/en/index.php?option=com_content&task=view&id=51&Itemid=50*. Accessed September 2006.

Healthcare Costs. *http://www.networkmigration.co.za/australia/health.html*. Accessed December 2002.

Healy, J. 2002. Australia. In Dixon, A., and E. Mossialos, eds. *Health care systems in eight countries: Trends and challenges*. London: The European Observatory on Health Care Systems, London School of Economics & Political Science, 3–16.

Hemenway, D., and D. Fallon. 1985. Testing for physician-induced demand with hypothetical cases. *Medical Care* 23, no. 4: 344–349.

Hsiao, W.C. 1995. Medical savings accounts: Lessons from Singapore. *Health Affairs* 14, no. 2: 260–266.

Kaiser Family Foundation Commission on Medicaid and the Uninsured. 2005. *Medicaid enrollment in 50 states: June 2005 data update. http://kff.org/medicaid/7606.cfm*.

Kaiser Family Foundation Medicare Policy Project. 2005. *Medicare Chart Book, 2005. http://kff.org/medicare/7284.cfm*.

Katz, S.J. et al. 2002. Phantoms in the snow: Canadians' use of health care services in the United States. *Health Affairs* 21, no. 3: 19–31.

MacPhee, S. 1996. Reform the watchword as OECD countries struggle to contain health care costs. *Canadian Medical Association Journal* 154, no. 5: 699–701.

McClellan, M., and D. Kessler. 1999. A global analysis of technological change in health care: The case of heart attacks. *Health Affairs* 18, no. 3: 250–257.

McGuire, T.G., and M.V. Pauly. 1991. Physician response to fee changes with multiple payers. *Journal of Health Economics* 10, no. 4: 385–410.

National Association of Community Health Centers (NACHC). 2006. *A sketch of community health centers: Chart book, 2006*. Washington, DC: NACHC.

National Center for Health Statistics. 2006. *Health, United States, 2006: With chartbook on trends in the health of Americans*. Hyattsville, Maryland: Department of Health and Human Services.

Naylor, C.D. 1999. Health care in Canada: Incrementalism under fiscal duress. *Health Affairs* 18, no. 3: 9–26.

Nomura, H., and T. Nakayama. 2005. The Japanese healthcare system. *BMJ* 331:648–9.

Podger, A. 1999. Reforming the Australian health care system: A government perspective. *Health Affairs* 18, no. 3: 111–113.

Rosen, B. 2003. In Tomson, S. and E. Mossialos (eds.) *Health care systems in transition: Israel*. Copenhagen: European Observatory on Health Care Systems.

Santerre, R.E., and S.P. Neun. 1996. *Health economics: Theories, insights, and industry studies*. Chicago: Irwin.

Schieber, G., and A. Maeda. 1999. Health care financing and delivery in developing countries. *Health Affairs* 18, no. 3: 193–205.

Shortell, S.M. et al. 1996. *Remaking health care in America: Building organized delivery systems*. San Francisco: Jossey-Bass Publishers.

Singapore Ministry of Health. 2004. *Medisave, Medishield and other subsidy schemes: Overview*. Available at: *www.moh.gov.sg/corp/financing/overview.do*. Accessed September 2006.

Willcox, S. 2001. Promoting private health insurance in Australia. *Health Affairs* 20, no. 3: 152–161.

Wolinsky, F.D. 1988. *The sociology of health: Principles, practitioners, and issues*. 2nd ed. Belmont, CA: Wadsworth Publishing Company.

PART I

System Foundations

Chapter 2

Beliefs, Values, and Health

Learning Objectives

- To understand the concepts of health and sickness
- To examine the determinants of health
- To explore the American beliefs and values governing the delivery of health care
- To appreciate the implications of the above concepts for medical care delivery and for the promotion of health and prevention of disease
- To develop a position on the equitable distribution of health services
- To understand some basic measures of health status and health services utilization

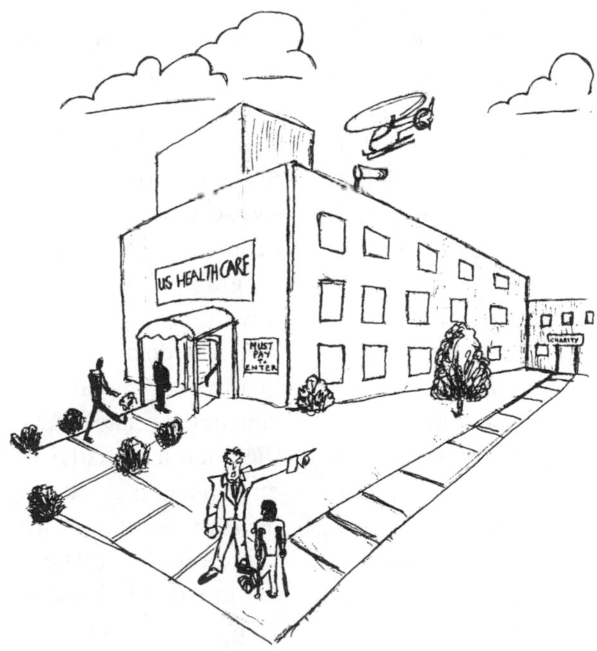

"This is the market justice system. Social justice is over there."

Introduction

From an economic perspective, curative medicine seems to produce decreasing returns in health improvement with increased health care expenditures (Saward and Sorensen 1980), and there is increased recognition of the benefits to society from the promotion of health and prevention of disease, disability, and premature death. Although the financing of health care has mainly focused on curative medicine, some strides are being made toward an emphasis on health promotion and disease prevention. Progress in this direction has been slow because of the social values and beliefs that emphasize disease rather than health. The common definitions of health, as well as measures for evaluating health status, reflect similar inclinations. This chapter proposes a holistic approach to health, although such an ideal would be very difficult to fully achieve. For example, it is not easy for a system to enact a change in self-imposed risk behaviors among the population. Regardless, the health care delivery system must allocate resources and take other measures to set a change in course. The 10-year *Healthy People* initiatives, undertaken by the US Department of Health and Human Services since 1980, illustrate steps taken in this direction, even though these initiatives generally have been strong in rhetoric but weak in strategy.

Beliefs and values ingrained in the American culture have also been influential in laying the foundations of a system that has remained predominantly private, as opposed to a tax-financed national health care program. Discussion on this theme begins in this chapter and continues in Chapter 3 where failures of past proposals to create a nationalized health care system are discussed in the context of cultural beliefs and values. Social norms also help explain how society views illness and the expectations it has of those who are sick.

This chapter further explores the issue of equity in the distribution of health services using the contrasting theories of market justice and social justice. The conflict between market and social justice is reflected throughout US health care delivery. For the most part, strong market justice values prevail, particularly during economic recessions. However, some components of health care delivery in the United States do reflect strong social justice values. This chapter concludes with an overview of measures commonly used to understand the health status of a population.

Significance for Managers and Policymakers

Materials covered in this chapter have several implications for health services managers and policymakers. (1) The health status of a population has a tremendous bearing on the utilization of health services, assuming that the services are readily available. Planning of health services must be governed by demographic and health trends and initiatives toward reducing disease and disability. (2) The concepts of health, its determinants, and health risk appraisal should be used to design appropriate educational, preventive, and therapeutic initiatives. (3) There is a growing emphasis on evaluating the effectiveness of health care organizations based on the contributions they make to community and population health. The concepts discussed in this chapter can guide administrators in implementing programs of most value to their communities. (4) The exercise of justice and equity in making health care available to all Americans remains a lingering concern. This monumental problem will require a joint undertaking from providers, administrators, policymakers, and other key stakeholders. (5) Quantified measures of health status and utilization can be used by managers and policymakers to evaluate the adequacy and effectiveness of existing programs, plan new strategies, measure progress, and discontinue ineffective services.

Basic Concepts

Health

In the United States, the concepts of health and health care have largely been governed by the ***medical model***, or more specifically, the biomedical model. The medical model presupposes the existence of ***illness*** or ***disease***. It, therefore, emphasizes clinical diagnosis and medical interventions to treat disease or symptoms of disease. The medical model defines health as the absence of illness or disease. The implication is that optimum health exists when a person is free of symptoms and does not require medical treatment. However, it is not a definition of health in the true sense, but a definition of what ill health is not (Wolinsky 1988, 76). Accordingly, prevention of disease and health promotion is relegated to a secondary status. Therefore, when the term "health care delivery" is used, in reality, it refers to medical care delivery.

Medical sociologists have gone a step further in defining health as the state of optimum capacity of an individual to perform his or her expected social roles and tasks, such as work, school, and doing household chores (Parsons 1972). A person who is unable (as opposed to unwilling) to perform his or her social roles in society is considered sick. However, this concept also tends to view health negatively because many people continue to engage in their social obligations despite suffering from pain, cough, colds, and other types of temporary disabilities, including mental distress. In other words, a person's engagement in social roles does not necessarily signify that the individual is in optimal health.

An emphasis on both physical and mental dimensions of health is found in the definition of health proposed by the Society for Academic Emergency Medicine, according to which health is "a state of physical and mental well-being that facilitates the achievement of individual and societal goals" (Ethics Committee, Society for Academic Emergency Medicine 1992). This view of health recognizes the importance of achieving harmony between the physiological and emotional dimensions.

Currently, the World Health Organization's (WHO) definition of health is most often cited as the ideal for health care delivery systems. WHO defines health as "a complete state of physical, mental, and social well-being, and not merely the absence of disease or infirmity" (WHO 1948). WHO's definition specifically identifies social well-being as a third dimension of health. In doing so, it emphasizes the importance of positive social relationships. Having a social support network is positively associated with life stresses, self-esteem, and social relations. The social aspects of health also extend beyond the individual level to include responsibility for the health of entire communities and populations. WHO's definition recognizes that optimal health is more than a mere absence of disease or infirmity. Since it includes the physical, mental, and social dimensions, WHO's model can be referred to as the biopsychosocial model of health. WHO has also defined a health care system as all the activities whose primary purpose is to promote, restore, or maintain health (McKee 2001). As this chapter points out, health care should include much more than medical care. Thus, ***health care*** would include a variety of services believed to improve a person's health and well-being.

In recent years, a growing interest has emerged in ***holistic health***, which emphasizes the well-being of every aspect of what makes a person whole and complete. Thus, ***holistic medicine*** seeks to treat the individual as a whole person (Ward 1995). Holistic health incorporates the spiritual dimension as a fourth element—in addition to the physical, mental, and social aspects—as necessary for optimal health (Figure 2–1). A growing volume of medical literature points to the healing effects of a person's religion and spirituality on morbidity and mortality (Levin 1994). Numerous studies point to an inverse association between religious involvement and all-cause mortality (McCullough et al. 2000). Religious and spiritual beliefs and practices have shown a positive impact on a person's physical, mental, and social well-being. They may affect the incidences, experiences, and outcomes of several common medical problems (Maugans 1996). For instance, people with high levels of general religious involvement are likely to suffer less from depressive symptoms and disorders (McCullough and Larson 1999). Spiritual well-being has been recognized as an important internal resource for helping people cope with illness. For instance, a study conducted at the University of Michigan found that 93 percent of the women undergoing cancer treatment indicated that their religious lives helped them sustain their hopes (Roberts et al. 1997). Studies have found that a large percentage of patients want their physicians to consider their spiritual needs, and almost half expressed a desire that the physicians should pray with them if they could (see Post et al. 2000). However, many physicians feel that spiritual matters fall outside their expertise, or that they would be intruding into patients' private lives. Also, caution about ethical issues and religious coercion are valid concerns. Referral to a chaplain or pastoral leader is often a more appropriate alternative (Post et al. 2000).

Figure 2–1 The Four Dimensions of Holistic Health.

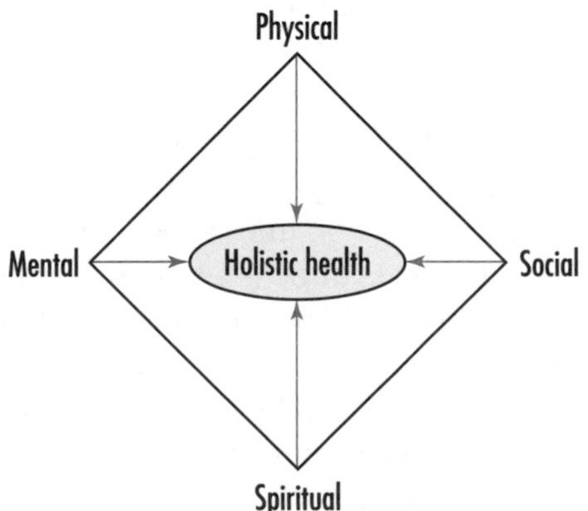

The spiritual dimension is frequently tied to one's religious beliefs, values, morals, and practices. More broadly, it is described as meaning, purpose, and fulfillment in life; hope and will to live; faith; and a person's relationship with God (Marwick 1995; Ross 1995; Swanson 1995). A clinically tested scale to measure spiritual well-being includes categories such as belief in a power greater than oneself, purpose in life, faith, trust in providence, prayer, meditation, group worship, ability to forgive, and gratitude for life (Hatch et al. 1998).

Some of the nation's leading medical schools now offer courses that explore spiritual issues in health care and how to address such issues in patient care delivery (American Physical Therapy Association 1997). Spiritual assessment instruments have been developed to assist physicians and other clinicians in spiritual history taking (Maugans 1996; Puchalski and Romer 2000). The Committee on Religion and Psychiatry of the American Psychological Association has issued a position statement to emphasize the importance of maintaining respect for a patient's religious/spiritual beliefs. For the first time, "religious or spiritual problem" has been included as a diagnostic category in DSM-IV.* The holistic approach to health also alludes to the need for incorporating alternative therapies (discussed in Chapter 7) into the predominant medical model.

Tamm (1993) observed that different groups in society—including physicians, nurses, and patients—look at health and disease from partly different vantage points, those that are holistic and those that emphasize illness and disease. Such tensions can have significant implications for the delivery of health services, especially in a pluralistic society such as the United States. Although the medical model plays a key role in the delivery of health care, integration of the concepts of holistic health can optimize well-being and promote early recovery from sickness.

Illness and Disease

Once the existence of illness and/or disease is recognized, it triggers care seeking and care utilization behaviors. Health services professionals diagnose illness and prescribe treatment mainly to ease symptoms. In most cases, once relief is obtained, the individual is declared well, regardless of whether or not the underlying cause of disease is cured.

The terms "illness" and "disease" are not synonymous, although they are often used interchangeably as they will be throughout this book. Illness is recognized by means of a person's own perceptions and evaluation of how he or she feels. For example, an individual may feel pain, discomfort, weakness, depression, or anxiety, but a disease may or may not be present. From a sociocultural standpoint, people consider themselves ill when they feel they are not quite able to perform the tasks or roles that society expects from them (Wolinsky 1988, 82). For example, due to a severe headache, a person may feel unable to go to work or attend school. The person may take pain medication and rest. If symptoms persist, the person may seek professional medical help. During an initial visit, a primary care physician may find nothing wrong physically. The person may still suffer from pain and discomfort and may forego engagement in social roles, but the person is not declared diseased. He or she may subsequently be referred to a neurologist—a specialist in diseases of the nervous system—who may discover some nervous disorder and prescribe treatment. At this point, the person is declared diseased. Thus, the determination that disease is present is based on professional evaluation, rather than the patient's. It reflects the highest state of professional knowledge, particularly that of the physician, and it requires therapeutic intervention (May 1993). In this example, both illness and disease were found to be present, but that is not always the case. Certain diseases, such as hypertension (high blood pressure), are asymptomatic and not always

*Diagnostic and Statistical Manual of Mental Disorders is the most widely recognized system of classifying mental disorders.

manifested through illness. A hypertensive person has a disease but may not know it. Thus, it is possible to be diseased without feeling ill. Likewise, one may feel ill and yet not have a disease.

Diseases are often caused by more than a single factor. For example, the mere presence of tubercle bacillus does not mean that the infected person will develop tuberculosis. Other factors, such as poverty, overcrowding, and malnutrition, may be essential for the disease to develop (Friedman 1980, 3). One useful explanation of disease occurrence (for communicable diseases in particular) is provided by the tripartite model sometimes referred to as the Epidemiology* Triangle (Figure 2–2). Of the three elements in the model, the ***host*** is the organism—generally, a human—that becomes sick. However, for the host to become sick, at least one factor, an ***agent***, must be present, although presence of an agent does not ensure that disease will occur. In the above example, tubercle bacillus is the agent for tuberculosis. Other examples are chemical agents, radiation, tobacco smoke, dietary indiscretions, and nutritional deficiencies. Factors associated with the host include genetic makeup, level of immunity, fitness, and personal habits and behaviors. Such factors are associated with the contracting of an agent or making the agent active. The third factor, ***environment***, is external to the host. The environment is a moderating factor that can either enhance or reduce susceptibility to disease. It includes the physical, social, cultural, and economic aspects of the environment. Sanitation, air pollution, cultural beliefs, social equity, social norms, and economic status are examples. Because the three factors commonly interact to produce disease, the model has important implications for disease prevention. ***Risk factors***—attributes that increase the likelihood of developing a particular disease or negative health condition at some time in the future—can be traced to the agent, the host, and/or the environment. A risk factor can be associated with any of the factors listed earlier, such as tobacco smoke or poor diet (associated with the agent), genetic makeup or levels of fitness (associated with the host), and poor sanitation or low socioeconomic status (associated with the environment). Preventive interventions to eliminate risk factors constitute an important strategy to reduce occurrence of disease and to promote better health.

*The study of the nature, cause, control, and determinants of the frequency and distribution of disease, disability, and death in human populations (Timmreck 1994, 2).

Behavioral Risk Factors

Certain individual behaviors and personal lifestyle choices represent important risk factors for illness and disease. For example, smoking has been identified as the leading cause of preventable disease and death in the United States because it significantly increases the risk of heart disease, stroke, lung

Figure 2–2 The Epidemiology Triangle.

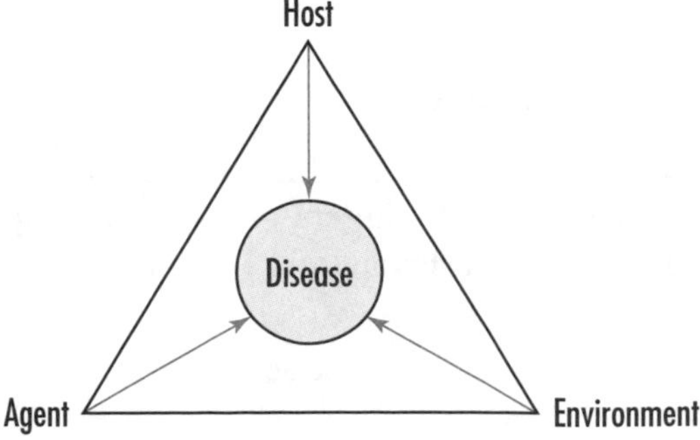

cancer, and chronic lung disease (Centers for Disease Control and Prevention 1999). Substance abuse, inadequate physical exercise, a high-fat diet, irresponsible use of motor vehicles, and unsafe sex are additional examples of behavioral risk factors. (Table 2–1 presents the percentage of the US population with selected behavioral risks.)

Acute, Subacute, and Chronic Conditions

Disease can be classified as acute, subacute, or chronic. An ***acute condition*** is relatively severe, episodic (of short duration), and often treatable (Timmreck 1994, 26). It is subject to recovery. Treatments are generally provided in a hospital. Examples of acute conditions are a sudden interruption of kidney function or a myocardial infarction (heart attack). A ***subacute condition*** is between acute and chronic but has some acute features (Thomas 1985). It can be a postacute condition requiring treatment after discharge from a hospital. Examples include ventilator and head trauma care. A ***chronic condition*** is less severe but of long and continuous duration (Timmreck 1994, 26). The patient may not fully recover. The disease may be kept under control through appropriate medical treatment, but if left untreated, the condition may lead to severe and life-threatening health problems. Examples are asthma, diabetes, and hypertension. Contributors to chronic disease include ethnical, cultural, and behavioral factors, and the social and physical environment, discussed later in this chapter.

Table 2–1 Percentage of Population with Behavioral Risks

Behavioral Risks	Percentage of Population	Year
Alcohol (12 years and over)	50.3	2004
Marijuana (12 years and over)	6.1	2004
Cocaine use (12th graders)	2.3	2005
Cocaine use (10th graders)	1.5	2005
Cocaine use (8th graders)	1.0	2005
Cigarette smoking (18 years and over)	20.8	2004
Hypertension (20–74 years)	25.3	2001–04
Overweight (20–74 years)	66.0	2001–04
Serum cholesterol (20–74 years)	16.0	2001–04

Note: Data are based on household interviews of a sample of the civilian noninstitutionalized population 12 years of age and over in the coterminous United States.

Source: Data from National Center for Health Statistics. *Health, United States, 2006.* Hyattsville, MD: Department of Health and Human Services, 2006. pp. 266, 271, 273, 279, 287.

Health Promotion and Disease Prevention

As discussed earlier, the medical model of health and health care emphasizes clinical interventions once disease has been diagnosed. The ***wellness model***, on the other hand, emphasizes efforts and programs geared toward prevention of disease and maintenance of an optimum state of well-being. It is well recognized that medical care alone cannot promote health. To promote optimum health, a health care delivery system must provide medical treatment but also use disease prevention and health promotion strategies. The two should complement each other.

The concept of health promotion and disease prevention is built on three factors: (1) An understanding of risk factors associated with host, agent, and/or environment. Risk factors and their health consequences are evaluated through a process called ***health risk appraisal***. Only when the risk factors and their health consequences are known can interventions be developed to help individuals adopt healthier lifestyles. (2) Interventions for counteracting the key risk factors include two main interventions: (a) behavior modification geared toward the goal of adopting healthier lifestyles and (b) therapeutic interventions. Both are discussed in the next paragraph. (3) Adequate public health and social services, as discussed later in this chapter, includes all health-related services designed to minimize risk factors and their negative effects in order to prevent disease, control disease outbreaks, and contain the spread of infectious agents. The goal is to maximize the health of a population.

Various avenues can be used for motivating individuals to alter behaviors that may contribute to disease, disability, or death. Behavior can be modified through educational programs and incentives directed at specific high-risk populations. In the case of cigarette smoking, for example, health promotion aims at building people's knowledge, attitudes, and skills to avoid or quit smoking. It also involves reducing advertisements and other environmental inducements that promote nicotine addiction. Financial incentives, such as a higher cigarette tax, are used to discourage purchase of cigarettes.

Therapeutic interventions generally fall into three areas of preventive effort: primary prevention, secondary prevention, and tertiary prevention.

Primary prevention refers to activities undertaken to reduce the probability that a disease will develop at some point in the future (Kane 1988). Its objective is to restrain the development of a disease or negative health condition before it occurs. Therapeutic intervention would include physicians' efforts to assist their patients in smoking cessation (Breslow 1989). Smoking cessation can prevent lung cancer; an increase in physical activity can prevent heart disease; teen driver education can prevent disability and death from auto accidents; and safety practices can reduce serious injuries in the workplace. Prenatal care is associated with lower infant mortality rates. Immunization has had a greater impact on prevention against childhood diseases and mortality reduction than any other public health intervention, besides clean water (Plotkin and Plotkin 1999). Hand washing, refrigeration of foods, garbage collection, and protection of the water supply are other examples of primary prevention (Timmreck 1994, 15). There have been numerous incidents where emphasis on food safety and proper cooking could have prevented outbreaks of potentially deadly episodes, such as those caused by E coli.

Secondary prevention refers to early detection and treatment of disease. Health screenings and periodic health examinations are examples. The main objective of secondary prevention is to block the progression of disease or an injury from developing into an impairment or disability (Timmreck 1994, 17). Screening tests, such as hypertension screening, Pap smears, and mammograms, have been instrumental in prescribing early treatment.

Tertiary prevention refers to rehabilitative therapies and the monitoring of health care processes to prevent complications or to prevent further illness, injury, or disability. For example, regular turning of bed-bound patients prevents pressure sores; infection control practices in hospitals and nursing homes are designed to prevent ***iatrogenic illnesses***, that is, illnesses or injuries caused by the process of health care. Tertiary prevention may also involve patient education and behavior change to prevent recurrence of disease (Timmreck 1994, 17). Examples include nutrition counseling or smoking cessation to keep disease in check.

As shown in Table 2–2, prevention, early detection, and treatment efforts helped reduce cancer mortality quite significantly between 1991 and 1995. This decrease was the first sustained decline since recordkeeping was instituted in the 1930s. The decline in breast cancer has been credited to early detection and treatment advances. The drop in cervical cancer has been attributed to the widespread use of Pap screening. Later data, however, show that the declines in cancer death rates are moderating, most likely due to other factors, such as aging.

Table 2–2 Annual Percent Decline in Cancer Mortality 1991–2003

Type of Cancer	1991–95	1994–2003
All cancers	3.0	1.1
Breast cancer	6.3	2.5
Cervical cancer	9.7	3.6
Ovarian cancer	4.8	0.5
Prostate cancer	6.3	3.5

Source: Data from National Center for Health Statistics of the Centers for Disease Control and Prevention, National Cancer Institute, SEER Cancer Statistics Review, 1975–2003 (Table I–7).

Developmental Health

Development refers to growth in skill and capacity to function normally (Hancock and Mandle 1994). Early childhood development influences a person's health in later years. The foundations laid in the early years often determine the individual's future adjustments to life (Berger 1988) and shape individual behaviors. Children who fail to acquire certain skills in childhood often have real difficulties as adults (Wynder and Orlandi 1984). The importance of early childhood development has important implications for health services delivery in two main areas: (1) Expectant mothers need adequate prenatal care. The health promotional needs of the expectant mother and the fetus are so closely intertwined that they must be considered a unit (Hancock and Mandle 1994). (2) Adequate childcare is needed, especially during the first few years of growth. Immunization, nutrition, family and social interaction, and health care are key developmental elements until a child reaches adulthood. Preventable developmental disabilities impose an undue burden on the health care delivery system.

Public Health

Almost all Americans consider public health important. However, public health remains poorly understood by its prime beneficiaries, the public, as well as by many of its dedicated practitioners. For some people, public health evokes images of a massive social enterprise or welfare system. To others, the term describes the professionals and workforce responsible for dealing with important health problems that confront the population. Still another image of public health is that of a body of knowledge and techniques that can be applied to health-related problems (Turnock 1997, 2–7). None of these ideas adequately reflects what ***public health*** is.

Two definitions have been found to be particularly helpful in characterizing public health. The first, by the Institute of Medicine (IOM), proposes that the mission of public health is to fulfill "society's interest in assuring conditions in which people can be healthy" (IOM 1988, 7). Public health deals with broad societal concerns about ensuring conditions that promote optimum health for society as a whole.

The practices of medicine and public health have followed divergent paths, mainly due to a lack of an infrastructure to support collaboration between the two sectors (Lasker et al. 1998). As a point of distinction, it can be said that medicine focuses on the individual patient—diagnosing symptoms, treating and preventing disease, relieving pain and suffering, and maintaining or restoring normal function. Public health, on the other hand, focuses on populations (Lasker 1997, 3). The emphases in modern medicine are on the biological causes of disease and developing treatments and therapies. Public health focuses on identifying the environmental, social, and behavioral risk factors that cause disease and on developing and implementing population-based interventions to minimize the risk factors (Peters et al. 2001). While medicine focuses on the treatment of disease and recovery of health, public health deals with various efforts to prevent disease and promote health.

To promote and protect society's interest in health and well-being, public health must influence the social, economic, political, and medical care factors that affect health and illness. Public health activities can range from providing education on nutrition to passing laws that enhance automobile safety. Public health includes dissemination to the public and to health professionals of timely and appropriate information about important health issues. Another distinguishing characteristic of public health is the broader range of professionals involved, compared to the delivery of medical services. The medical sector encompasses physicians, nurses, dentists, therapists, social workers, psychologists, nutritionists, health educators, pharmacists, laboratory technicians, health services administrators, and so forth. In addition to these professionals, public health also involves professionals such as sanitarians, epidemiologists, statisticians, industrial hygienists, environmental health specialists, food and drug inspectors, toxicologists, and economists (Lasker 1997, 3).

The second definition, given more than eight decades ago, characterizes public health as the science and art of preventing disease, prolonging life, and promoting health and efficiency through organized community effort (Winslow 1920). Accordingly, public health is a broad social enterprise that seeks to apply the current knowledge pertaining to health and disease in ways that will have the maximum impact on the health status of a population (Turnock 1997, 10).

Health Protection

Environmental health has been an integral component of public health ever since John Snow, in the 1850s, successfully traced the risk of cholera outbreaks in London to the

Broad Street water pump (Rosen 1993). Since then, ***environmental health*** has specifically dealt with preventing the spread of disease through water, air, and food (Schneider 2000). Environmental health science, along with other public health measures, was instrumental in reducing the risk of infectious diseases during the last century. For example, in 1900, pneumonia, tuberculosis, and diarrhea along with enteritis were the top three killers in the United States (Centers for Disease Control and Prevention 1999); that is no longer the case today (see Table 2–3). With the rapid industrialization during the 20th century, environmental health faced new challenges due to serious health hazards from chemicals, industrial waste, infectious waste, radiation, asbestos, and other toxic substances. Due to actual and potential industrial accidents, a third major role of public health emerged—that of health protection (in addition to prevention and health promotion). However, due to the complexity of dealing with numerous toxins, many environmental responsibilities were specifically assigned to newly created agencies, such as the Environmental Protection Agency (EPA) and the Occupational Safety and Health Administration (OSHA). Rapid cleanup, evacuation of the affected population, and transfer of victims to medical care facilities have been the main types of response when accidents occur. Firefighters, police, paramedics, and other civil defense agencies cooperate in such efforts and coordinate functions with local medical centers and public health agencies.

Since the horrific events of what is now commonly referred to as 9/11 (September 11, 2001), America has opened a new chapter in health protection. As the nation was still recovering from the shock of the attacks on New York's World Trade Center, attempts to disseminate anthrax through the US Postal

Table 2–3 Leading Causes of Death, 2003

Cause of Death	Deaths	Percentage
All causes	2,448,288	100.0
Diseases of the heart	685,089	28.0
Malignant neoplasms	556,902	22.7
Cerebrovascular diseases	157,689	6.4
Chronic lower respitory diseases	126,382	5.2
Unintentional injuries	109,277	4.5
Diabetes mellitus	74,219	3.0
Influenza and pneumonia	65,163	2.7
Alzheimer's disease	63,457	2.6
Nephritis, nephrotic syndrome, and nephrosis	42,453	1.7
Septicemia	34,069	1.4

Source: Data from National Center for Health Statistics. *Health, United States, 2006.* Hyattsville, MD: Department of Health and Human Services, 2006, p. 187.

Service were discovered. In June 2002, President Bush signed into law the Public Health Security and Bioterrorism Response Act of 2002. The term ***bioterrorism*** encompasses the use of chemical, biological, and nuclear agents to cause harm to relatively large civilian populations. Dealing with such a threat requires large-scale preparations, which include appropriate tools and training for workers in medical care, public health, emergency care, and civil defense agencies at the federal, state, and local levels. It requires national initiatives to develop countermeasures, such as new vaccines, a robust public health infrastructure, and coordination between numerous agencies. It requires an infrastructure to handle large numbers of casualties and isolation facilities for contagious patients. Hospitals, public health agencies, and civil defense need to be linked together through information systems. Containment of infectious agents, such as smallpox, would require quick detection, treatment, isolation, and organized efforts to protect the unaffected population. To address these issues, President Bush has proposed substantial increases in funding for bioterrorism.

Even broader provisions are contained in the Homeland Security Act of 2002, signed into law in November 2002. The legislation calls for a major restructuring of the nation's resources with the primary mission of helping prevent, protect against, and respond to any acts of terrorism in America. The legislation is also designed to enhance the nation's ability to prevent and detect bioterrorist attacks. For example, it calls for improved inspections of food products entering the United States. It provides for better tools to contain attacks on the food and water supplies, protect the nation's vital infrastructures, such as nuclear facilities, and track biological materials anywhere in the United States. Chapter 14 discusses future trends and the changing role of public health to address such potential threats.

To prevent the introduction, transmission, and spread of severe acute respiratory syndrome (SARS), a contagious disease that is accompanied by fever and symptoms of pneumonia or other respiratory illness, President Bush signed an Executive Order on April 4, 2003, to designate SARS as a communicable disease for the apprehension, detention, or conditional release of individuals with SARS. The order also covers other suspected communicable diseases that include cholera, diphtheria, infectious tuberculosis, plague, smallpox, yellow fever, and viral hemorrhagic fevers such as Ebola.

The global threat of avian influenza has also solicited a public health and government response. The Centers for Disease Control and Prevention launched a website dedicated to educating the public about avian influenza, how it is spread, and past and current outbreaks. The website contains specific information for health professionals, travelers, the poultry industry, state departments of health, and people with possible exposures to avian influenza (Centers for Disease Control and Prevention 2007). In January 2006, President Bush pledged $334 million to support the global campaign against avian influenza through improved surveillance and response systems, assistance to countries threatened by the virus, and public awareness campaigns (White House 2006).

Quality of Life

The term ***quality of life*** is used in a denotative sense to capture the essence of overall satisfaction with life during and following a person's encounter with the health care delivery system. Thus, the term is employed in two different ways. First, it is an indicator of how satisfied a person was with the experiences while receiving health care. Specific life domains, such as comfort factors, respect, privacy, security, degree of independence, decision-making autonomy, and attention to personal preferences are significant to most people. These factors are now regarded as rights that patients can demand during any type of health care encounter. Second, quality of life can refer to a person's overall satisfaction with life and with self-perceptions of health, particularly after some medical intervention. The implication is that desirable processes during medical treatment and successful outcomes would subsequently have a positive effect on an individual's ability to function, carry out social roles and obligations, and have a sense of fulfillment and self-worth.

Determinants of Health

The determinants of health—factors that influence individual and population health status—are well established. Starfield (1973) suggested that health status is determined by a confluence of factors that can be classified into four major categories: (1) a person's individual behaviors, (2) genetic makeup, (3) medical practice, and (4) the environment. The Centers for Disease Control and Prevention (CDC) (1979) estimated that 50 percent of premature death in the US population was directly related to individual lifestyle and behaviors, 20 percent was attributed to an individual's inherited genetic profile, and only 10 percent could be ascribed to inadequate access to medical care. The remaining 20 percent of premature mortality could be attributed to social and environmental factors (Figure 2–3).

In 1974, Blum (1981) proposed an "Environment of Health" model later called the "Force Field and Well-Being Paradigms of Health" (Figure 2–4). Blum proposed four major inputs that contributed to health and well-being. These main influences (called "force fields") are the environment, lifestyle, heredity, and medical care, all of which must be considered simultaneously when addressing the health status of an individual or a population. The four wedges in Figure 2–4 represent the four major force fields. The size of each wedge signifies its relative

Figure 2–3 Relative Contribution of the Four Health Determinants to Premature Death.

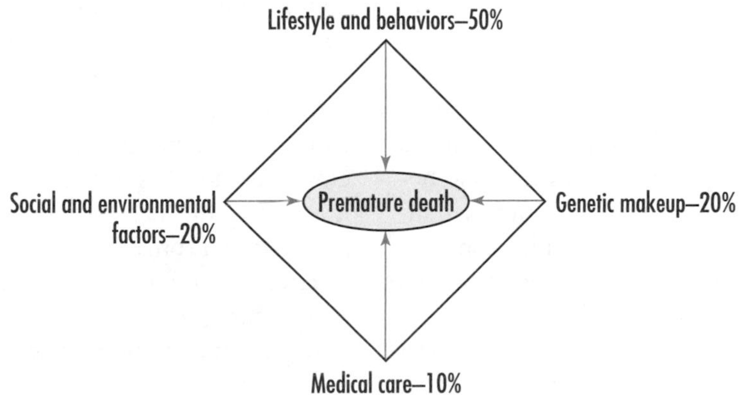

Figure 2–4 The Force Field and Well-Being Paradigms of Health.

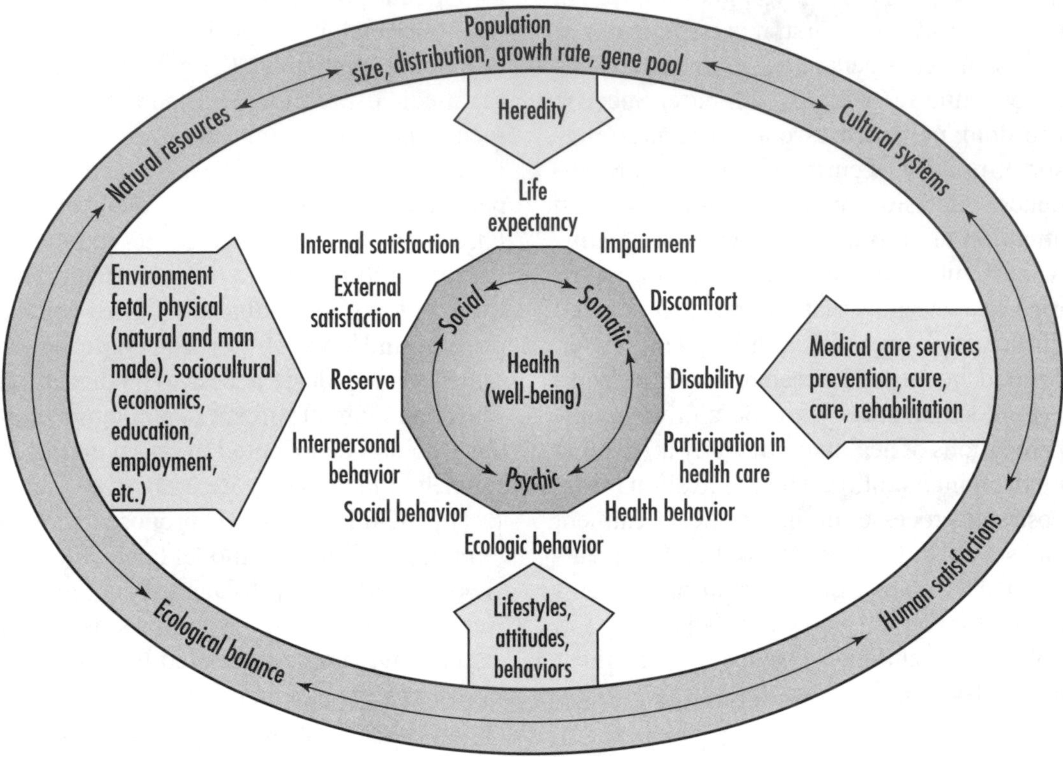

Source: Reprinted with permission from H.L. Blum, *Planning for Health,* © 1981, Human Sciences Press.

importance. Thus, the most important force field according to this model is the environment, followed by lifestyles and heredity. Medical care has the least impact on health and well-being. Although both CDC and Blum models point to the same four factors, they are slightly different. The CDC model emphasizes causes leading to premature death and points to individual lifestyle behaviors as the main contributor. Blum's model emphasizes overall well-being, including health, and points to environmental factors as the main contributors.

The determinants of health have made a major contribution to the understanding that a singular focus on medical care delivery is unlikely to improve the health status of any given population. Instead, a more balanced approach to public policy addresses broad social and economic concerns in society. The following discussion and examples show that, regardless of the type of health care system a nation may have, social policies must address a multiple of factors for improving the health and well-being of a population. From a health care delivery perspective, the goal of providing adequate primary care to everyone may be more important than providing access to the latest technology.

Environment

Environmental factors encompass the physical, socioeconomic, sociopolitical, and sociocultural dimensions. Among physical environmental factors are air pollution, food and water contaminants, radiation, toxic chemicals, wastes, disease vectors, safety hazards, and habitat alterations. The relationship of socioeconomic status (SES) to health and well-being may be explained by the general likelihood that people who have better education also have higher incomes. They live in better homes and locations where they are less exposed to environmental risks, have better access to health care, and are more likely to avoid risk behaviors, such as smoking and drug abuse. The relationship between education and health status has been well established. Less educated Americans die younger compared to their better educated counterparts. Diseases mainly responsible for this disparity in mortality are ischemic heart disease, lung cancer, stroke, pneumonia, congestive heart failure, and lung disease, which are, incidentally, all smoking-related diseases (Tanne 2002). Unemployment may affect social health because of reduced social functioning, mental health because of increased levels of stress, and physical health due to various stress-related illnesses.

A significant body of literature in recent years has demonstrated the association of income inequality with a variety of health indicators, such as life expectancy, age-adjusted mortality rates, and leading causes of death (Kaplan et al. 1996; Kawachi et al. 1997; Kennedy et al. 1996; Mackenbach et al. 1997). The greater the economic gap between the rich and the poor in a given geographic area, the worse the health status of the population in that area will be. It has been suggested that wide income gaps produce less social cohesion and greater psychosocial stress and, consequently, poorer health (Wilkinson 1997). For example, social cohesion, characterized by a hospitable social environment in which people trust each other and participate in communal activities, is linked to lower overall mortality and better self-rated health (Kawachi et al. 1997; Kawachi et al. 1999). Researchers have postulated that the political and policy context that creates income inequality is a precursor to health inequalities (Dye 1991). Political traditions more committed to redistributive policies, such as those followed by social democratic governments, are generally more successful in improving the health of populations, such as reducing infant mortality (Navarro and Shi 2001). However, even countries, such as Britain, Australia, Denmark, and Sweden, with national health insurance programs experience persistent and widening disparities in health according to socioeconomic status (Pincus et al. 1998). Pincus and colleagues proposed that poor health in sociologically disadvantaged populations results more from unfavorable social conditions and ineffective self-management than from limitations in access to medical care.

The availability of primary care may serve as one alternative pathway through which income inequality influences population-level health outcomes. Shi and colleagues (1999, 2001) examined the joint relationships among income inequality, availability of primary care, and certain health indicators. The results indicate that the availability of primary care physicians, in addition to income inequality, significantly correlates with reduced mortality, increased life expectancy, and improved birth outcome. In another study using the 1996 Robert Wood Johnson Community Tracking Study household survey, they also examined whether income inequality and primary care, measured at the state level, predict individual morbidity, as measured by self-rated health status while adjusting for potentially confounding individual variables (Shi et al. 2002). The results of the study indicate that the distributions of income and primary care in states were significantly associated with individuals' self-rated health. There was a gradient effect of income inequality on self-rated health, and individuals living in states with a higher primary care physician-to-population ratio were more likely to report good health than those living in states with a lower ratio. These studies made the authors conclude that from a policy perspective, improvement in individuals' health is likely to require a multipronged approach that addresses individual socioeconomic determinants of health, social, and economic policies that affect income distribution and strengthens primary care aspects of health services.

The environment can also have a significant influence on developmental health. It has been shown, for example, that children who are isolated and do not socialize much with their peers tend to be overrepresented in groups of delinquents and adults with mental health problems (Wynder and Orlandi 1984). Current research points out that the experiences that children receive and the way adults interact with them in the early years have a major impact on children's mental and emotional development. Neuroscientists have found that good nurturing and stimulation in the first three years of life—a prime time for brain development—activate neural pathways in the brain that might otherwise atrophy, and may even permanently increase the number of brain cells. Hence, the importance of quality of childcare provided in the first three years of life is monumental (Shellenbarger 1997).

Lifestyle

Lifestyle or behavioral risk factors were discussed earlier. This section provides some illustrations of how lifestyle factors are related to health. Studies have shown that diet and foods, for example, play a major role in most of the significant health problems of today. Heart disease, diabetes, stroke, and cancer are but some of the diseases with direct links to dietary choices. Throughout the world, incidence and mortality rates for many forms of cancer are rising. Yet research has clearly indicated that a significant portion of cancer is preventable. The role of diet and nutrition in cancer prevention has been one of the most exciting and promising research areas over the past few years. Researchers now estimate that 40 percent to 60 percent of all cancers, and as many as 35 percent of cancer deaths, are linked to diet (American Institute for Cancer Research 1996). Current research also shows that a diet rich in fruits, vegetables, and low-fat dairy foods, and with reduced saturated and total fat can substantially lower blood pressure. Thus, a nutritional approach can be effective in both preventing and treating hypertension (Appel et al. 1997). The role of exercise and physical activity as a potentially useful, effective, and acceptable method for reducing the risk of colon cancer is also significant (Macfarlane and Lowenfels 1994). Research findings have also confirmed the association between recreational and/or occupational physical activity and a reduced risk of colon cancer (White et al. 1996).

Heredity

Heredity is a key determinant of health because genetic factors predispose individuals to certain diseases. For example, cancer occurs when the body's healthy genes lose their ability to suppress malignant growth or when other genetic processes stop working properly, although this does not mean that cancer is entirely a disease of the genes (Davis and Webster 2002).

A person can do little about the genetic makeup one has inherited. However, lifestyles and behaviors that a person may currently engage in can have significant influences on future progeny. Advances in gene therapy hold the promise of treating a variety of inherited or acquired diseases.

Medical Care

Even though the other three factors are more important in the determination of health, well-being, and susceptibility to premature death, medical care is nevertheless a key determinant of health. Both individual and population health are closely related to having access to adequate preventive and curative health care services. Despite the fact that medical care, compared to the other three force fields, has the least impact on health and well-being, the American public's attitudes toward improving health are based on more medical research, development of new medical technology, and spending more on high-tech medical care. Yet, significant declines in mortality rates were achieved well before the modernization of Western medicine and the escalation in medical care expenditures.

Overarching Factors and Implications for Health Care Delivery

The force fields illustrated in Blum's model (Figure 2–4) are affected by broad national and international factors, such as a nation's population characteristics, natural resources, ecological balance, human satisfactions, and cultural systems. Among these factors can be included the type of health care delivery system. Historically, public health and environmental interventions, such as improved nutrition, sanitation, and immunization, have contributed to significant declines in mortality. Currently, tobacco use, diet and activity patterns, microbial and toxic agents, alcohol and drug abuse, firearms, sexual behavior, and motor vehicle accidents continue to impose a substantial public health burden. Yet the preponderance of health care expenditures is devoted to the treatment of medical conditions (e.g., heart disease, cancer, and stroke) rather than to the prevention and control of factors that produce those medical conditions in the first place. This misdirection can be traced to the conflicts that often result from the beliefs and values ingrained in the American culture.

Cultural Beliefs and Values

Cultural beliefs and values are among the overarching factors that influence the key determinants of health, according to Blum's model. A value system orients the members of a society toward defining what is desirable for that society. It has been observed that even a society as complex and highly differentiated as the United States can be said to have a relatively well-integrated system of institutionalized common values at the societal level (Parsons 1972). Although such a view may still prevail, the American society now has several different subcultures that have grown in size due to a steady influx of immigrants from different parts of the world. There are sociocultural variations in how people view their health and, more important, how such differences influence people's attitudes and behaviors concerning health, illness, and death (Wolinsky 1988, 39).

As pointed out in Chapter 1 (see Figure 1–2), societal values and cultural beliefs are among the external forces that influence how health care is delivered. Decisions about who will receive what type of services can often be culture based. For example, cross-cultural perspectives show wide variations among countries in the way people prioritize who should receive scarce medical resources. In traditional Indian and Chinese cultures, boys are valued more than girls are. Girls are more likely to suffer from poor nutrition and lack of health care. Other culture-based differences exist among some African tribes in how they distribute scarce medical resources among those who may be in equal need of those services (Brown 1992). Modernization, education, and adoption of Western values are changing some of the cultural orientations toward the use of health care in these countries. On the other hand, certain beliefs and values remain firmly ingrained despite modern influences. In a multicultural society such as the United States, beliefs and values in certain groups that are foreign to the Western culture need to be treated with sensitivity by the providers of health care.

The current system of health services delivery traces its roots to the traditional beliefs and values espoused by the American people. The value and belief system governs the training and general orientation of health care providers, type of health delivery settings, financing and allocation of resources, and access to health care. Health care systems in other countries also reflect deeply rooted beliefs and values that, largely, make people oppose any major reforms. For example, Canadians are very much opposed to some recent proposals recommending an increased role of private sector companies in the delivery of health services. Canadians also prefer increased spending on health and social programs than receiving a tax cut from the government. Americans, on the other hand, are skeptical of any heavy-handed government involvement in the health care system.

Some of the main beliefs and values predominant in the American culture are outlined below:

1. A strong belief in the advancement of science and the application of the scientific method to medicine were instrumental in creating the medical model that primarily governs health care delivery in the United States. In turn, the medical model has fueled the tremendous growth in medical science and technological innovation. As a result, the United States has been leading the world in new medical breakthroughs. These developments have had numerous implications for health services delivery:
   a. They increase the demand for the latest treatments and raise patients' expectations of finding a cure.
   b. Medical professionals have been preoccupied almost exclusively with clinical interventions, whereas the holistic aspects of health and

use of alternative therapies have been deemphasized.

c. Health care professionals have been trained to focus on physical symptoms.

d. Few attempts have been made to integrate diagnosis and treatment with health education and disease prevention.

e. The concern with nonhealth has funneled most research efforts away from the pursuit of health into development of sophisticated medical technology. Commitment of resources to the preservation and enhancement of health and well-being has lagged far behind.

f. Medical specialists using the latest technology have been held in higher esteem and have earned higher incomes than general practitioners and health educators.

g. The desirability of health care delivery institutions, such as hospitals, is often evaluated by their acquisition of advanced technology.

h. While biomedicine has taken central stage, diagnosis and treatment of mental health have been relegated to a lesser status. Difficulties linking certain behaviors to mental disorders have been at least partially responsible for the secondary status of mental health services in the health care delivery system.

i. The biomedical model has also isolated the social and spiritual elements of health.

2. America has been a champion of capitalism. Due to a strong belief in capitalism, health care has largely been viewed as an economic good (or service), not as a public resource.

3. A culture of capitalism promotes entrepreneurial spirit and self-determination. Hence, individual capabilities to obtain health services have largely determined the production and consumption of health care—which services will be produced, where, and in what quantity, and who will have access to those services. Some key implications are:

   a. Financing of health care through individual health insurance coverage has made access to health care a social privilege.

   b. A clear distinction exists between the types of services for poor and affluent communities and between those in rural and urban locations.

   c. The culture of individualism emphasizes individual health rather than population health. Medical practice, therefore, has been directed at keeping the individual healthy rather than keeping the entire community healthy.

4. A concern for the most underprivileged classes in society—the poor, the elderly, the disabled, and children—led to the creation of the public programs Medicare, Medicaid, and SCHIP.

5. Principles of free enterprise and a general distrust of big government have kept the delivery of health care largely in private hands. Hence, a separation also exists between public health functions and private practice of medicine.

A Social Model of Health

The social model of health views health and well-being in terms of a person's capacity to function socially and to perform the expected societal roles was discussed earlier. A person unable to perform the social roles is declared sick and is expected to adopt the sick role (Wolinsky 1988, 82). Parsons (1972) also viewed illness as a socially institutionalized role type that has four specific features: (1) The sick individual is not held responsible for his or her sickness. (2) Being sick is recognized as the legitimate basis for society to exempt the individual from his or her social role obligations. (3) The individual is exempted from social roles on the condition that he or she recognizes that being sick is undesirable and that the individual has the obligation to try to get well. (4) The sick individual must seek competent help and cooperate with medical agencies trying to help the individual get well.

The model has two important implications for health care delivery. First, the primary focus is on the individual. Societal roles are mainly passive and consensual: agreeing to release the individual from his or her social obligations and, because illness is only partially and conditionally legitimated (Parsons 1972), maintaining some sort of surveillance over the individual to ensure that he or she is carrying through with the sick role obligations. More important, society is not required to furnish medical services. The sick individual must seek appropriate medical care and comply with the prescribed regimen. Family members or significant others may assist the individual.

Second, the social model assumes that the sick role obligations are carried out within the context of the medical model of health services delivery. Parsons implied that even though people have an obligation to prevent threatened illness (Parsons 1972), society does not hold the individual responsible for his or her diseased condition. Even though personal lifestyles and behaviors can substantially increase the risk of high-cost illness, society does not impose any sanctions on the individual for diseases acquired as a direct result of personal indiscretions. The reason, perhaps, is that society also does not assume any responsibility for providing medical care. It is interesting to note that in recent debates and court cases seeking damages for treatment costs for certain groups of smokers who developed lung disease, society has put the entire blame on the tobacco industry while absolving the individual smokers of any personal responsibility.

Equitable Distribution of Health Care

Scarcity of economic resources is a central economic concept. From this perspective, health care can be viewed as an economic good. Two fundamental questions arise with regard to how scarce health care resources ought to be used. (1) How much health care should be produced? (2) How should health care be distributed? The first question concerns the appropriate combination in which health services ought to be produced in relation to all other goods and services in the overall economy. If more health care is produced, people will have to forgo some other goods, like food, clothing, and transportation. The second question affects individuals at a more personal level. It deals with who can receive which type of medical services and who will be restricted from accessing services.

The production, distribution, and subsequent consumption of health care must be perceived as equitable. No society has found a perfectly equitable method to distribute limited economic resources. In fact, any method of resource distribution leaves some inequalities. Societies, therefore, try to allocate resources according to some guiding principles acceptable to each society. Such principles are generally ingrained in a society's value and belief system. It is generally recognized that not everyone can receive everything medical science has to offer. The fundamental question that deals with distributive justice or equity is who should receive the medical goods and services that society produces (Santerre and Neun 1996, 7). By extension, this basic question about equity includes not only who should receive medical care but also which type of services and in what quantity.

A just and fair allocation of health care poses conceptual and practical difficulties; hence, a theory of justice needs to resolve the problem of health care allocation (Jonsen 1986). The principle of justice derives from ethical theories, especially those advanced by John Rawls, who defined justice as fairness (Darr 1991). Even though various ethical principles can be used to guide decisions pertaining to just and fair allocation of health care in individual circumstances, the broad concern about equitable access to health services is addressed by the theories referred to as ***market justice*** and ***social justice***. These two contrasting theories govern the production and distribution of health care services.

Market Justice

The principle of market justice ascribes the fair distribution of health care to the market forces in a free economy. Medical care and its benefits are distributed based on people's willingness and ability to pay (Santerre and Neun 1996, 7). In other words, people are entitled to purchase a share of the available goods and services that they value. They are to purchase these valued goods and services by means of wealth acquired through their own legitimate efforts. This is how most goods and services are distributed in a free market. The free market implies that giving people something they have not earned would be morally and economically wrong.

Chapter 1 discussed several characteristics that describe a pure market. Those market characteristics are a precondition because market justice requires that health care be delivered in a free market. In addition, the principle of market justice is based on the following key assumptions:

- Health care is like any other economic good or service. If health care was considered different from other economic products, it could not be governed by free market forces of supply and demand.
- Individuals are responsible for their own achievements. When individuals pursue their own best interests, the interests of society as a whole are best served (Ferguson and Maurice 1970).
- People make rational choices in their decisions to purchase health care products and services. People demand health care because it can rectify a health problem and restore health, can reduce pain and discomfort and make people feel better, and can reduce anxiety about their health and well-being. Therefore, people are willing to purchase health care services. Grossman (1972) proposed that health is also an investment commodity. People consider the purchase of health services

as an investment. For example, the investment has a monetary payoff when it reduces the number of sick days, making extra time available for productive activities, such as earning a living. Or it can have a utility payoff—that is, a payoff in terms of satisfaction—when it makes life more enjoyable and fulfilling.

- People, in consultation with their physicians, know what is best for themselves. This assumption implies that people place a certain degree of trust in their physicians and that the physician-patient relationship is ongoing.
- The marketplace works best with minimum interference from the government. In other words, the market rather than the government can allocate health care resources in the most efficient and equitable manner.

The classical ethical theory known as ***deontology*** may be applied to market justice. Deontology asserts that it is an individual's duty (from the Greek word "deon") to do what is right. The results are not important. Deontology emphasizes individual responsibilities as in a physician-patient relationship. A physician is duty-bound to do whatever is necessary to restore a patient's health. The patient is responsible for compensating the physician for his or her services. The destitute and poor may be served by charity, but deontology largely tends to ignore the importance of societal good. It does not address what responsibilities people have toward the society.

Market justice may also be associated with the libertarian view that equity is achieved when resources are distributed according to merits. That is, health care should be distributed according to minimum standards and financed according to willingness to pay. According to this view, equality in health status need not be a central priority (Starfield 1998).

Under market justice, the production of health care is determined by how much the consumers are willing and able to purchase at the prevailing market prices. It follows that in a pure market system, individuals without sufficient income face a financial barrier to obtaining health care (Santerre and Neun 1996, 7). Thus, prices and ability to pay ration the quantity and type of health care services people would consume. The uninsured and those who lack sufficient income to pay privately generally face barriers to obtaining health care. Such limitations to obtaining health care are referred to as "rationing by ability to pay" (Feldstein 1994, 45), ***demand-side rationing***, or price rationing.

The key characteristics and their implications under the system of market justice are summarized in Table 2–4. Market justice emphasizes individual rather than collective responsibility for health. It proposes private rather than government solutions to social problems of health.

Social Justice

The idea of social justice is at odds with the principles of capitalism and market justice. The term "social justice" was invented in the 19th century by the critics of capitalism to describe the good society (Kristol 1978). According to the principle of social justice, the equitable distribution of health care is a societal responsibility. This can best be achieved by letting a central agency, generally the government, take over the production and distribution functions. Social justice regards health care as a social good—as opposed to an economic good—that should be

Table 2–4 Comparison of Market Justice and Social Justice

Market Justice	Social Justice
Characteristics	
• Views health care as an economic good	• Views health care as a social resource
• Assumes free-market conditions for health services delivery	• Requires active government involvement in health services delivery
• Assumes that markets are more efficient in allocating health resources equitably	• Assumes that the government is more efficient in allocating health resources equitably
• Production and distribution of health care determined by market-based demand	• Medical resource allocation determined by central planning
• Medical care distribution based on people's ability to pay	• Ability to pay inconsequential for receiving medical care
• Access to medical care viewed as an economic reward of personal effort and achievement	• Equal access to medical services viewed as a basic right
Implications	
• Individual responsibility for health	• Collective responsibility for health
• Benefits based on individual purchasing power	• Everyone is entitled to a basic package of benefits
• Limited obligation to the collective good	• Strong obligation to the collective good
• Emphasis on individual well-being	• Community well-being supersedes that of the individual
• Private solutions to social problems	• Public solutions to social problems
• Rationing based on ability to pay	• Planned rationing of health care

collectively financed and available to all citizens regardless of the individual recipient's ability to pay for that care. Canadians and Europeans, for example, long ago reached a broad social consensus that health care was a social good (Reinhardt 1994). Public health also has a social justice orientation (Turnock 1997). Under the social justice system, inability to obtain medical services because of a lack of financial resources is considered unjust. A just distribution of benefits must be based on need, not simply on one's ability to purchase in the marketplace (demand). Need for health care is determined either by the patient or by a health professional. The principle of social justice is also based on certain assumptions:

- Health care is different from most other goods and services. Health-seeking behavior is governed primarily by need rather than by how much it would cost.
- Responsibility for health is shared. Individuals are not held totally responsible for their condition because factors outside their control may have brought on

the condition. Society feels responsible for a lack of control of certain environmental factors, such as economic inequalities, unemployment, unsanitary conditions, or air pollution.

- Society has an obligation to the collective good. The well-being of the community is superior to that of the individual. An unhealthy individual is a burden on society. A person carrying a deadly infection, for example, is a threat to society. Society, therefore, is obligated to cure the problem by providing health care to the individual because by doing so the whole society would benefit.
- The government, rather than the market, can better decide, through rational planning, how much health care to produce and how to distribute it among all citizens.

Social justice is consistent with the theory of ***utilitarianism***, a teleological principle (from the Greek, "telos," meaning end). Utilitarianism emphasizes happiness and welfare for the masses; it ignores the individual. Society's goal is to achieve the greatest good for the greatest number of people. In this case, the greatest good for the greatest number of people is thought to be achieved when the well-being of the whole community supersedes the well-being of individuals. By implication, the government is thought to distribute health care resources more equitably than the market.

Social justice finds its ethical roots in the egalitarian view that equity is achieved when resources are distributed according to needs. That is, more resources are made available to populations that need more services because of their greater social or health disadvantage (Starfield 1998).

Under social justice, how much health care to produce is determined by the government; however, no country can afford to provide unlimited amounts of health care to all its citizens (Feldstein 1994, 44). The government then also finds ways to limit the availability of certain health care services by deciding, for instance, how technology will be dispersed and who will be allowed access to certain types of high-tech services, even though basic services may be available to all. This concept refers to ***planned rationing***, ***supply-side rationing***, or nonprice rationing. The government makes deliberate attempts, often referred to as "health planning," to limit the supply of health care services, particularly those beyond the basic level of care. The main characteristics and implications of social justice are summarized in Table 2–4.

Justice in the US Health Delivery System

As discussed in Chapter 1, the market for health care delivery in the United States cannot be regarded as a pure market. It is characterized as a quasi or imperfect market. Hence, elements of both market justice and social justice exist, but the principles of market justice prevail. In some areas, the principles of market justice and social justice complement each other. In other areas, the two conflict.

Health Insurance

In a society with strong market justice values, individuals paying for their own care would predominantly finance the medical care system. A multitude of private health insurance plans would prevail. In a society with strong social justice principles, the government through general tax revenues would finance the medical care system (Long 1994, 30).

In the United States, the principles of market justice and social justice complement each other with private, employer-based health insurance for mainly middle-income Americans (market justice), publicly financed Medicaid, Medicare, and SCHIP coverage for certain disadvantaged groups, and workers' compensation for those injured at work (social justice). The two principles collide, however, regarding the large number of uninsured who cannot afford to purchase private health insurance and do not meet the eligibility criteria for Medicaid, Medicare, SCHIP, or other public programs. Americans have not been able to resolve the question of who should provide health insurance to the uninsured.

Organization of Health Care Delivery

In a market justice-dominant society, the number and type of physicians produced by the educational system are determined by the desires of would-be physicians and their assessment of the chances of future success. Physicians themselves decide where they will be located to practice, without necessarily taking into account the needs of the population (Long 1994, 31–32). Physicians are compensated mostly on a fee-for-service basis, the fees being established by the physicians themselves. Similarly, hospital location and operations are influenced by financial viability without regard to duplication or shortages of services and technology. In a society with strong social justice values, the number, type, and location of physicians and hospitals, reimbursement to providers, and distribution of medical technology are determined by the government, supposedly based on the health needs of the populations.

In the United States, private and government health insurance programs enable the covered populations to have access to health care services delivered by private practitioners and private institutions (market justice). Tax-supported county and city hospitals, public health clinics, and community health centers can be accessed by the uninsured in areas where such services are available (social justice). Publicly run institutions generally operate in large inner cities and certain rural areas. Conflict between the two principles of justice arises in small cities and towns and large rural sections where such services are not available. Medicare and Medicaid make their own determinations on how much to pay for the services. These characteristics do not fully harmonize with the pure market justice principles.

Equality in the US Health Care Delivery System

Equity advocates argue that health insurance should be universally extended to all Americans (Santerre and Neun 1996, 7). Major health care reform proposals to establish universal access were advanced shortly after Bill Clinton became president in 1992. The first lady, Hillary Rodham Clinton, took the lead in championing the cause. In a speech delivered to the American Medical Association on June 13, 1993, Mrs. Clinton said, "We must guarantee all Americans access to a comprehensive package of [health] benefits, no matter where they work, where they live, or whether they have ever been sick before" (Clinton 1995, 6). In response to such proposals, a market advocate labeled the Clinton health plan as radical because under such a policy proposal "every person would have the same comprehensive coverage designed by the government, regardless of their health status, health habits, and preferences for insurance coverage. The only individual choice would be to select more or less expensive versions of this same coverage, like the opportunity to choose first class or coach but not the destination of a flight" (Niskanen 1995, 15). As discussed earlier, such American ideals reflect strong individualistic values underlying market justice.

The health policy agenda of George W. Bush, the president succeeding Bill Clinton, has adhered to these individualistic values. The major elements of Bush's health platform include: (1) the promotion of Health Savings Accounts (HSAs), which allow people to create tax-free accounts to pay for out-of-pocket medical expenses; (2) efforts to increase "transparency" (i.e., readily available information) in health care pricing and quality, to allow people to make better decisions about their health care choices; and (3) the endorsement of Health Information Technology (HIT) to "facilitate the rapid exchange of health information" (White House 2007). The President has also called for expansion of the Community Health Center program providing preventive and primary health care services to an estimated 16 million people in underserved communities who otherwise would lack access to care. This initiative seems more oriented toward social justice than Bush's other initiatives. However, community health centers derive a significant proportion of their operating revenues from Medicaid reimbursements. During Bush's tenure as president, Medicaid cuts at the federal and state levels, coupled with rising health care costs and increasing numbers of uninsured people, have threatened health centers' efforts to provide care to vulnerable populations (National Association of Community Health Centers 2005).

Americans have a tradition of reliance on individual responsibility and a commitment to the ideal of a limited national government, which are more in accord with the principles of market justice than social justice. In contrast, Western Europe, Canada, and most developed countries have adopted a public policy of universal access. Even though they reflect social justice values, such policies were not motivated primarily by concerns about justice and equality but by social objectives: to have a more productive labor force, to have a healthy citizenry for national defense, and to bring stability against social unrest (President's Commission 1983, 14).

Equality of individuals has always been a prominent American value, but "the traditional emphasis has been on equal civil and political liberties rather than on economic equality" (President's Commission 1983, 14). Social justice represents an effort to stretch the idea of justice to cover economic equality as well (Kristol 1978). If health care is regarded as a basic right, then an important measure of a just system of health care allocation would be equal access to medical services. In the United States, this ideal of equality obscures when it comes to equal access to comprehensive medical care (Brown 1992).

Distributional Efficiency

Equity requires distributional efficiency, which deals with the amount of resources to allocate and how to distribute them. Since resources are scarce, equity requires that their distribution be efficient, otherwise some people may be denied the benefit of the wasted resources. At a more practical level, resources equate to total expenditures for delivering health care. Market justice assumes that the market would handle the distribution of resources most efficiently, that is, market forces would govern allocation of health dollars. Market justice advocates would also argue that the government is inefficient and resorts to rationing to cover up its inefficiencies. However, in evaluating efficiency, a greater emphasis is being placed on health outcomes. From this perspective, the United States has failed to achieve distributional efficiency, compared to other industrialized nations. The United States tops all other countries in per capita expenditures on health care (see Table 12–2), but the American population as a whole lags far behind in key indicators of health, such as life expectancy and infant mortality. This largely attributes to significant disparities in health within US subpopulation groups (e.g., racial/ethnic groups, socioeconomic groups, etc.; see Chapter 11).

Limitations of Market Justice

The principles of market justice work well in the allocation of economic goods when their unequal distribution does not affect the larger society. For example, based on individual success, people live in different sizes and styles of homes, drive different types of automobiles, and spend their money on a variety of things, but the allocation of certain resources has wider repercussions for society. In these areas, market justice has severe limitations:

1. Market justice principles generally fail to rectify critical human concerns. Pervasive social problems, such as crime, illiteracy, and homelessness, can significantly weaken the fabric of a society. Indeed, the United States has recognized such issues and instituted programs based on social justice to combat the problems through added police protection, publicly supported education, subsidized housing, and, more recently, national initiatives against terrorism. Health care is an important social issue because it not only affects human productivity and achievement, but it also provides basic human dignity.
2. Market justice does not always protect a society. Individual health issues can have negative consequences for society because ill health is not always confined to the individual. The acquired immune deficiency syndrome (AIDS) epidemic is an example in which society can be put at serious risk. Initial spread of the SARS epidemic in Beijing was largely due to patients with SARS symptoms being turned away by hospitals since they were not able to pay in advance for the cost of the treatment. Similar to clean air and water, health care is a social concern that, in the long run, protects against the burden of preventable disease and disability, a burden that is ultimately placed on the shoulders of society.
3. Market justice does not work well in health care delivery. The decade of the 1990s was characterized by unprecedented economic growth and creation of wealth in the United States. This period of prosperity, however, did not reduce the number of Americans without health insurance. In a nation where the benefits of health care are employment based,

this condition is truly a paradox given a low rate of unemployment compared to many other industrialized nations. The experience clearly shows that equitable delivery of health care requires social justice-based solutions.

Integration of Individual and Community Health

In recent years, it has been recognized that the typical emphasis on the treatment of acute illness in hospitals, biomedical research into disease, and high technology has not improved the population's health. The notable concern to contain rising health care costs and a paradigm shift toward delivery of health services through managed care have also prompted a reevaluation of the traditional medical model. It has been proposed that the medical model should be replaced with a disease-prevention, health-promotion, or primary care model (Shortell et al. 1995). More precisely, this is a call for integration of the two models rather than a total abandonment of the medical model in favor of the other. Society continues to need the benefits of modern science and technology for the treatment of disease. Disease prevention, health promotion, and primary care can prevent certain health problems from occurring, delay the onset of disease, and prevent disability and premature death. An integrated approach will not make disease, disability, and death go away; but it will improve the overall health of the population, enhance people's quality of life, and conserve health care resources.

An integrated approach must go beyond a simple merger of the medical and wellness models. The real challenge for the health care delivery system is to incorporate these models within the holistic context of health. The Ottawa Charter for Health Promotion, for instance, mentions caring, holism, and ecology as essential issues in developing strategies for health promotion (de Leeuw 1989). "Holism" and "ecology" refer to the complex relationships that exist among the individual, the health care delivery system, and the physical, social, cultural, and economic environmental factors. "Environment," in this context, could be viewed as an extension of the social dimension of health discussed earlier in this chapter. In addition, as the increasing body of research points out, the spiritual dimension must be incorporated into the integrated model.

Another equally important challenge for the health care delivery system is to focus on both individual and population health outcomes. The nature of health is complex, and the interrelationships among the physical, mental, social, and spiritual dimensions are not well understood. How to translate this multidimensional framework of health into specific actions that are efficiently configured to achieve better individual and community health is the greatest challenge any health care system could possibly face.

For an integrated approach to become reality, resource limitations would make it necessary to deploy the best US ingenuity toward health-spending reduction, elimination of wasteful care, promotion of individual responsibility and accountability for one's health, and improved access to services. In a broad sense, these services include medical care, preventive services, health promotion, and social policy to improve education, lifestyles, employment, and housing (Figure 2–5). The Ottawa Charter has proposed achieving health objectives through social public policy and community

Figure 2–5 Integrated Model for Holistic Health.

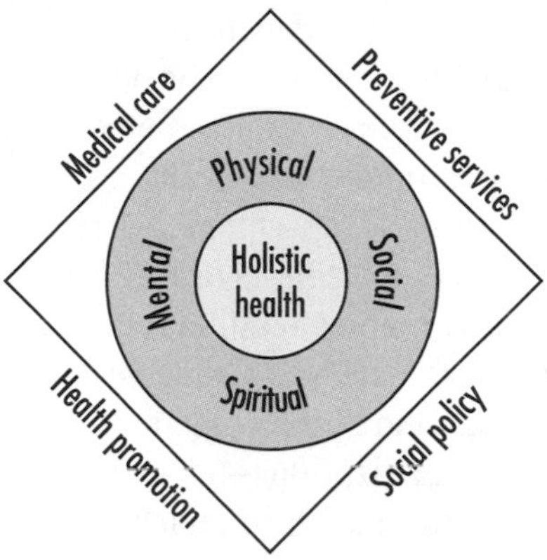

action. An integrated approach also necessitates creation of a new model for training health care professionals by forming partnerships with the community (Henry 1993). The following paragraphs describe examples of community partnership reflected in community health assessment and Healthy People initiatives.

Community Health Assessment

Community health assessment is a method used to conduct broad assessments of populations at a local or state level. For integrating individual and community health, the assessment is best conducted by collaboration among public health agencies, hospitals, and other health care providers. Community hospitals in particular are increasingly held accountable for the health status of the communities in which they are located. To fulfill this mission, hospitals must first conduct a health assessment of their communities. Such an assessment provides a broad perspective of a population's health, and it also points to specific needs that health care providers can address. It can help pinpoint interventions that should be given priority to improve the population's health status, or to address critical issues pertaining to certain groups within the population. Measures of health status discussed later in this chapter are essential to conduct a community health assessment. It also requires an evaluation of health determinants and utilization of medical care services.

Healthy People Initiatives

Since 1980, the United States has undertaken 10-year plans outlining certain key national health objectives to be accomplished during each of the 10-year periods. These initiatives have been founded on the integration of medical care with preventive services, health promotion, and education; integration of personal and community health care; and increased access to integrated services. Accordingly, the objectives are developed by a consortium of national and state organizations, under the leadership of the US Surgeon General. The first of these programs, with objectives for 1990, provided national goals for reducing premature deaths and for preserving the independence of older adults. Next, *Healthy People 2000: National Health Promotion and Disease Prevention Objectives*, released in 1990, identified health improvement goals and objectives to be reached by the year 2000. As part of this process, standardized Health Status Indicators (HSIs) were developed to facilitate the comparison of health status measures at national, state, and local levels over time. According to the final review published by the National Center for Health Statistics (2001), the major accomplishments of Healthy People 2000 included: surpassing the targets for reducing deaths from coronary heart disease and cancer; meeting the targets for incidence rates for AIDS and syphilis, mammography exams, violent deaths, and tobacco-related deaths; nearly meeting the targets for infant mortality and number of children with elevated levels of lead in blood; and making progress in reducing health disparities among special populations.

Healthy People 2010: Healthy People in Healthy Communities, launched in January 2000, continues in the earlier traditions as an instrument to improve the health of the American people in the first decade of the 21st century. The context developed in national objectives for *Healthy People 2010* differs from the framework of *Healthy People 2000*. Advanced preventive therapies, vaccines and pharmaceuticals, and improved surveillance and data systems are now available. Demographic changes in the United States reflect an older and more racially diverse population. Global forces, such as food supplies, emerging infectious diseases, and environmental interdependence, present new public health challenges. The objectives also define new relationships between public health departments and health care delivery organizations (Department of Health and Human Services 1998). *Healthy People 2010* specifically emphasizes the role of community partners—such as businesses, local governments, and civic, professional, and religious organizations—as effective agents for improving health in their local communities. In addition, the objectives for 2010 specifically focus on the determinants of health discussed earlier.

Figure 2–6 presents the graphic framework for *Healthy People 2010*. The two over-

Figure 2–6 Healthy People 2010: Healthy People in Healthy Communities.

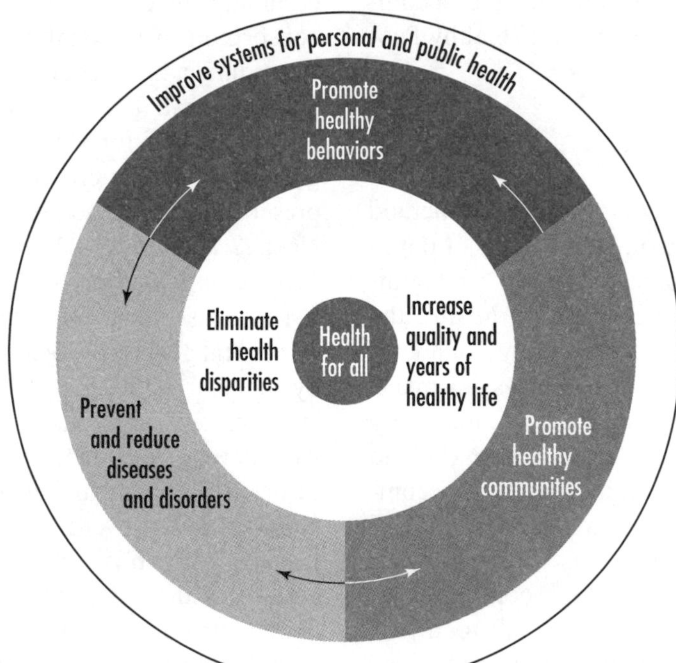

Source: Reprinted from *Healthy People 2010 Objectives: Draft for Public Comment,* Department of Health and Human Services.

arching goals designed for achievement by *Healthy People 2010* are (Department of Health and Human Services 2000):

- ***Increase Quality and Years of Healthy Life.*** The first goal is to help individuals of all ages increase life expectancy and improve their quality of life. In particular, differences in life expectancy among populations suggest a substantial need and opportunity for improvement. At least 18 countries with populations of one million or more have life expectancies greater than the United States for both men and women. Similar to life expectancy, various population groups show dramatic differences in quality of life. A disproportionate number of Americans in low-income households, women, and those living in rural areas report their health status as fair or poor. These findings lead to the second goal.
- ***Eliminate Health Disparities.*** The second goal of *Healthy People 2010* is to eliminate health disparities among different segments of the population. These include differences that occur by gender, race or ethnicity, education or income, disability, living in rural localities, or sexual orientation. The greatest opportunities for reducing health disparities are in empowering individuals to make informed health care decisions and in promoting communitywide safety, education, and access to health care.

To realize these two broad goals, 28 focus areas were identified as measureable targets by the year 2010 (see Exhibit 2–1).

Exhibit 2–1 *Healthy People 2010* Focus Areas

1. Access to Quality Health Services
2. Arthritis, Osteoporosis, and Chronic Back Conditions
3. Cancer
4. Chronic Kidney Disease
5. Diabetes
6. Disability and Secondary Conditions
7. Educational and Community-Based Programs
8. Environmental Health
9. Family Planning
10. Food Safety
11. Health Communication
12. Heart Disease and Stroke
13. HIV
14. Immunization and Infectious Diseases
15. Injury and Violence Prevention
16. Maternal, Infant, and Child Health
17. Medical Product Safety
18. Mental Health and Mental Disorders
19. Nutrition and Overweight
20. Occupational Safety and Health
21. Oral Health
22. Physical Activity and Fitness
23. Public Health Infrastructure
24. Respiratory Diseases
25. Sexually Transmitted Diseases
26. Substance Abuse
27. Tobacco Use
28. Vision and Hearing

Source: Department of Health and Human Services. *Healthy People 2010* (Conference Edition, in Two Volumes). Washington, DC: January 2000.

Using data gathered through January 2005, the Department of Health and Human Services released a Midcourse Review of progress toward achieving the *Healthy People 2010* goals. With regard to the initiative's first overarching goal (Increase Quality and Years of Healthy Life), the Midcourse Review reported life expectancy continues to increase, but significant gender and racial/ethnic differences remain. In addition, the United States continues to have lower life expectancy than many other developed nations. Two quality of life measures (i.e., expected years in good or better health and expected years free of activity limitations) improved slightly while a third quality of life measure (i.e., expected years free of selected chronic diseases) declined slightly (Department of Health and Human Services 2006).

With regard to the second overarching goal of *Healthy People 2010* (Eliminate Health Disparities), the Midcourse Review reported very little progress has been made. While there were reductions in several health areas with disparities, there were increases in disparities in other health areas. The Midcourse Review noted that the lack of data on education, income, and other socioeconomic factors for many *Healthy People 2010* objectives has limited our capabilities to plan programs that are effective in reducing and eliminating disparities (Department of Health and Human Services 2006).

Measures of Health Status

Certain quantitative measurements commonly apply to health, health status, and the utilization of health care. It is one thing to conceptually define health but quite a different thing to measure health status or the health state of a population. The conceptual approaches for defining health and its distribution help form a vision for the future, but objective measures are needed to evaluate the success of various programs and to direct future planning activities. Practical approaches for measuring health are, however, quite limited, and mental health is more difficult to quantify and measure than physical health. Measures of physical and mental health presented in this section are basic measures in common use. An objective evaluation of social and spiritual health is even more obscure. Approaches presented for quantifying the latter are mere illustrations.

The concept of population as it applies to population health has been borrowed from the disciplines of statistics and epidemiology. The term "population" is not restricted to describing the total population. Although commonly used in that way, the term may also apply to a defined subpopulation, for example, age groups, marital categories, income levels, occupation categories, racial or ethnic groups, a group of people having a common disease, people in a certain risk category, or people in a certain community or geographic region of a country. The main advantage of studying subpopulations is that it traces the existence of health problems to a defined group in the total population. It avoids concealing serious problems in a minority group within the favorable statistics of the majority. By pinpointing health problems in certain well-defined groups, appropriate interventions and new policy initiatives can be deployed in the most effective manner.

Evaluation of Health Status

Measures in health status are determined largely by how health is defined (Siegmann 1979). Mainly because of the emphasis on the biomedical dimensions, measurement of health status is disease oriented. Health status is often interpreted through ***morbidity*** (disease and disability) and ***mortality*** (death) rates because positive health indicators are lacking. Health status and longevity are two positive indicators in common use.

Table 2–5 Life Expectancy at Birth—1999 and Future Projections

Year	Total	Male	Female
1999	76.7	73.9	79.4
White	77.3	74.6	79.9
Black	71.4	67.8	74.7
2003	77.5	74.8	80.1
White	78.0	75.3	80.5
Black	72.7	69.0	76.1
2010	77.9	74.1	80.6

Sources: Data from National Center for Health Statistics, *Health, United States, 1996–97; Injury Chartbook.* Hyattsville, MD: Public Health Service, 1997, p. 108; *Health, United States, 2002,* p. 116; and *Health, United States, 2006,* p. 176.

Health Status

Self-perceived health status commonly uses an indicator of health and well-being. For example, respondents are asked to rate their health as excellent, very good, good, fair, or poor. Self-perceived health status is highly correlated with many objective measures of health status. It is also a good predictor of patient-initiated physician visits, including general medical and mental health visits.

Longevity

Life expectancy, or a prediction of how long a person will live, is widely used as a basic measure of health status. The two common measures are life expectancy at birth (Table 2–5), or how long a newborn can expect to live, and life expectancy at age 65, or expected remaining years of life for someone at age 65. These measures are actuarially determined and published by government agencies, such as the National Center for Health Statistics.

Morbidity

The measurement of morbidity or disease, such as cancer or heart disease, is expressed as a ratio or proportion of those who have the problem and the population at risk. The ***population at risk*** includes all the people in the same community or population group who can acquire a disease or a condition (Smith 1979). Incidence and prevalence are two widely used indicators for the number of ***cases***, that is, people who acquire a negative health condition, such as victims of disease or disability. ***Incidence*** counts the number of new cases occurring in the population at risk within a certain period, such as a month or a year (Smith 1979) (see Formula 2–1). Incidence describes the extent to which, in a given population, people who do not have a disease develop the disease during the specified period (Timmreck 1994, 5). Incidence is particularly useful in estimating the magnitude of conditions of relatively short duration. Successful health promotion and disease prevention programs are those that result in decreased incidence because they prevent new cases (Ibrahim 1985, 20). High levels of incidence may suggest an impending ***epidemic***, that is, a large number of people who get a specific disease from a common source. The second measure of morbidity, ***prevalence*** determines the total number of cases at a specific point in time in a defined population (see Formula 2–2). Prevalence is useful in quantifying the magnitude of illnesses of a relatively long duration. Successful treatment programs are those that result in decreased prevalence by shortening the duration of illness (Ibrahim 1985, 20–21). Both incidence and prevalence rates can apply to disease, disability, or death.

The calculation of rates often requires dividing a small number by a large number representing a defined population. The result is a fraction. To make the fractions meaningful and interpretable, they are multiplied by 100 (to get a percentage), 1,000 (to get a rate per 1,000), 10,000 (to get a rate per 10,000), or a higher multiple of 10.

Formula 2–1

Incidence = Number of new cases during a specified period/Population at risk

Formula 2–2

Prevalence = Total number of cases at a specific point in time/Specified population

Disability

Disease and injury can lead to temporary or permanent, as well as partial or total, disability. Although the idea of morbidity includes disabilities as well as disease, there are some specific measures of disability (or dysfunction). Some of the common measures are days of bed confinement, number of days missed from work or school, and number of days of restricted activity. All measures are in reference to a specific time period, such as one year.

One of the most widely used measures of physical dysfunction among the elderly is the ***activities of daily living (ADL)*** scale. The ADL scale is appropriate for evaluating disability in both community-dwelling and institutionalized adults. The classic ADL scale, developed by Katz and colleagues, included six basic activities to determine whether an individual needs assistance. The six basic activities were eating, bathing, dressing, using the toilet, maintaining continence, and transferring from bed to chair (Katz and Akpom 1979). To evaluate disability in community-dwelling adults, a modified Katz scale is commonly used. It consists of seven items (Ostir et al. 1999). Five of these items—feeding, bathing, dressing, using the toilet, and transferring—have been retained from the original Katz scale. The additional two items are grooming and walking a distance of eight feet. Thus, it includes items measuring self-care and mobility. The ADLs identify personal care functions with which a disabled person may need assistance. Depending on the extent of disability, met personal care needs through adaptive devices, care rendered by another individual, such as a family member, or care in a nursing facility.

Another commonly used measure of physical function is the ***instrumental activities of daily living (IADL)***. This scale measures activities that are necessary for living independently in the community, such as using the telephone, driving a car or traveling alone in a bus or taxi, shopping, preparing meals, doing light housework, taking medicine, handling money, doing heavy housework, walking up and down stairs, and walking a half-mile without help. These 10 items categorize activities the person is (a) able or (b) unable to do. IADLs typically require higher cognitive functioning than ADLs and, as such, are not purely physical tests of functional disability. IADLs are not generally used in institutional settings because institutionalized persons are not required to perform many IADL tasks (Ostir et al. 1999). The IADL scale measures the level of functioning in activities that are important for self-sufficiency but are less basic than ADLs.

Mortality

Death rates are computed in different forms as indicators of population health. ***Crude rates*** refer to the total population; they are not specific to any age groups or disease categories (Formula 2–3).

Formula 2–3

Crude death rate = Total deaths (usually in one year)/Total population

Specific rates are useful because death rates vary greatly by race, sex, age, and type of disease or condition. Specific rates allow health care managers to target their programs at the appropriate population subgroups (Dever 1984, 75). Examples of specific rates are age-specific mortality rate (Formula 2–4) and cause-specific mortality rate (Formula 2–5). The age-specific mortality rate provides a measure of the risk (or probability) of dying when a person is in a certain age group. The cause-specific mortality rate provides a measure of the risk (or probability) of dying from a specific cause. Table 2–3 provides the 10 leading causes of death in the United States.

Formula 2–4

Age-specific mortality rate = Number of deaths within a certain age group/Total number of persons in that age group

Formula 2–5

Cause-specific mortality rate = Number of deaths from a specific disease/Total population

Infant mortality rate (actually a ratio, Formula 2–6) is another important indicator. It reflects the health status of the mother and the child through pregnancy and the birth process. It also reflects the level of prenatal and postnatal nutritional care (Timmreck 1994, 106).

Formula 2–6

Infant mortality rate = Number of deaths from birth to one year of age (in one year)/Number of live births during the same year

Demographic Change

In addition to measures of disease and mortality, changes in the composition of a population over time are also important in planning of health services. For example, the migration of the elderly to the southern states requires planning of adequate retirement and long-term care services in those states. Population change involves three components: births, deaths, and migration (Dever 1984). Longevity is also an important factor that determines demographic change. For example, lower death rates, lower birth rates, and greater longevity together indicate an aging population. Measures of death were discussed previously. This section presents measures of births and migration.

Births

Natality and fertility are two measures associated with births. ***Natality***, or birth rate, is useful in assessing the influence of births on demographic change and measured by the crude birth rate (Formula 2–7).

Formula 2–7

Crude birth rate = Number of live births (usually in one year)/Total population

Fertility refers to the capacity of a population to reproduce (see Formula 2–8 for fertility rate). It is a more precise measure than natality because it relates actual births to the sector of the population capable of giving birth.

Formula 2–8

Fertility rate = Number of live births (usually in one year)/Number of females aged 15–44

Migration

Migration refers to the geographic movement of populations between defined geographic units and involves a permanent change of residence. The net migration rate (Formula 2–9) defines the change in the population as a result of ***immigration*** (in migration) and ***emigration*** (out migration) (Dever 1984, 249). The rate is calculated for a specified period, such as one year, two years, five years, and so on.

Formula 2–9

Net migration rate = (Number of immigrants × Number of emigrants)/Total population (during a specific period of time)

Measures of Mental Health

Measurement of mental health is less objective than measurement of mortality and morbidity because mental health often encompasses feelings that cannot be observed. Physical functioning, by contrast, reflected in behaviors and performances can be more readily observed. Hence, measurement of mental health more appropriately refers to assessment rather than measurement. Mental health can be assessed by the presence of certain symptoms, including both psychophysiologic and psychological symptoms. Examples of psychophysiologic symptoms are low energy, headaches, and upset stomach. Examples of psychological symptoms are nervousness, depression, and anxiety.

Self-assessment of one's own psychological state may also be used for mental health assessment. Examples are self-reports of the frequency and intensity of psychological distress, anxiety, depression, and psychological well-being.

Measures of Social Health

Measures of social health extend beyond the individual to encompass the extent of social contacts across various facets of life, such as family life, work life, and community life. Breslow (1972) attempted to measure social health along four dimensions: (1) employability, based on educational achievement, occupational status, and job experience; (2) marital satisfaction; (3) sociability, determined by the number of close friends and relatives; and (4) community involvement, which encompasses attendance at religious services, political activity, and organizational membership.

Social health status is sometimes evaluated in terms of social contacts and social resources. ***Social contacts*** are evaluated in terms of the number of social contacts or social activities a person engages in within a specified period. Examples are visits with friends and relatives and attendance at social events, such as conferences, picnics, or other outings. ***Social resources*** refer to social contacts that can be relied on for support, such as family, relatives, friends, neighbors, and members of a religious congregation. They are indicative of adequacy of social relationships. Social contacts can be observed, and they represent the more objective of the two categories; however, one criticism of social contact measures is their focus on events and activities, with little consideration of how the events are personally experienced. Unlike social contacts, social resources cannot be directly observed. They are best measured by asking the individuals directly. Evaluative questions include whether these individuals can rely on their social contacts to provide tangible support and needed companionship, and whether they feel cared for, loved, and wanted.

Measures of Spiritual Health

Within a person's individual, social, and cultural context, spiritual well-being can have a large variety of connotations. Such variations make it extremely difficult to propose standardized approaches for measuring the spiritual dimension. Attempts to measure this dimension are illustrated in the General Social Survey, which includes people's self-perceptions about happiness, religious experiences, and degree of involvement in activities such as prayer and church attendance. The spiritual well-being scale developed by Vella-Brodrick and Allen (1995) evaluates items such as reaching out for spiritual intervention; duration of meditation or prayer for inner peace; engaging in meditation, yoga, or prayer; frequency of meditation or prayer; reading about religion; and discussions or readings about ethical and moral issues.

Measures of Health Services Utilization

Utilization refers to the consumption of health care services or the extent to which health care services are used. Measures of utilization can be used to determine which individuals, in a population group, receive certain types of medical services, which ones do not receive services, and why. A health care provider, such as a hospital, can find out the extent to which its services are used. Measures of utilization can help managers decide whether certain services should be added or eliminated. Health planners can determine whether programs have been effective in reaching their targeted populations. Measures of utilization therefore play a critical role in the planning of health care delivery capacity, for example, how many hospital beds are required to meet the acute care needs of a given population (Pasley et al. 1995). Measures of utilization are too numerous to be covered here, but some selected common measures are given below (Formulas 2–10 to 2–16).

Crude Measures of Utilization

Formula 2–10

Access to primary care services = Number of persons in a given population who visited a primary care provider in a given year/Size of the population

(This measure is generally expressed as a percentage; i.e., the fraction is multiplied by 100.)

Formula 2–11

Utilization of primary care services = Number of primary care visits by people in a given population in a given year/Size of the population

(This measure is generally expressed as number of visits per person per year.)

Specific Measures of Utilization

Formula 2–12

Utilization of targeted services = Number of people (visits) using special services targeted at a specific population group/Size of the targeted population group

(The fraction obtained is multiplied by 100, 1,000, or a higher multiple of 10 to facilitate interpretation of the result.)

Formula 2–13

Utilization of specific inpatient services = Number of bed (inpatient) days/Size of the population

(The fraction obtained is multiplied by 100, 1,000, or a higher multiple of 10 to facilitate interpretation of the result.)

Measures of Institution-Specific Utilization

Formula 2–14

Average daily census = Total number of inpatient days in a given time period/Number of days in the same time period

Formula 2–15

Occupancy rate = Total number of inpatient days in a given time period/Total number of available beds during the same time period

or

Average daily census/Total number of beds in the facility

(This measure is generally expressed as a percentage; i.e., the fraction is multiplied by 100.)

Formula 2–16

Average length of stay = Total number of inpatient days during a given time period/Total number of patients during the same time period

Summary

The system of health care delivery in the United States is predominantly private. Many of the peculiarities of this system trace back to the beliefs and values underlying the American culture. The delivery of health care is primarily driven by the medical model, which emphasizes illness rather than wellness. Even though major efforts and expenditures have been directed toward the delivery of medical care, they have failed to produce a proportionate impact on the improvement of health status. Holistic concepts of health care, along with integration of medical care with preventive and health promotional efforts, need to be adopted to significantly improve the health of Americans. Such an approach would require a fundamental change in how Americans view health. It would also require individual responsibility for one's own health-oriented behaviors as well as community partnerships to improve both personal and community health. An understanding of the determinants of health, health education, community health assessment, and national initiatives, such as *Healthy People 2010*, are essential to accomplishing these goals. The emphasis on market justice in the US health care delivery system, however, leaves the critical problem of access unaddressed. Commonly used measures of health status and health care utilization provide quantitative means for evaluating health status and measuring progress.

Test Your Understanding

Terminology

activities of daily living (ADL)
acute condition
agent
bioterrorism
cases
chronic condition
community health assessment

crude rates
demand-side rationing
deontology
development
disease
emigration
environment
environmental health
epidemic
fertility
health care
health risk appraisal
holistic health
holistic medicine
host
iatrogenic illnesses
illness
immigration
incidence
instrumental activities of daily living (IADL)
life expectancy
market justice
medical model
migration
morbidity
mortality
natality
planned rationing
population at risk
prevalence
primary prevention
public health
quality of life
risk factor
secondary prevention
social contacts
social justice
social resources
subacute condition
supply-side rationing
tertiary prevention
utilitarianism
utilization
wellness model

Review Questions

1. Distinguish between illness and disease. How are these concepts related to the medical model of health care delivery?
2. What is the role of health risk appraisal in health promotion and disease prevention?
3. Health promotion and disease prevention may require both behavioral modification and therapeutic intervention. Discuss.
4. Discuss the definitions of health presented in this chapter in terms of their implications for the health care delivery system.
5. What implications does early childhood development have for health care delivery?
6. What are the main objectives of public health?
7. Discuss the significance of an individual's quality of life from the health care delivery perspective.
8. The Blum model points to four key determinants of health. Discuss their implications for health care delivery.
9. What has been the main cause of the dichotomy in the way physical and mental health issues have traditionally been addressed by the health care delivery system?
10. Discuss the main cultural beliefs and values in American society that have influenced health care delivery and how they have shaped the health care delivery system.
11. Discuss the main elements of Parsons's sick role model. What implications does the sick role model have for health services delivery?
12. Briefly describe the concepts of market justice and social justice. In what way do the two principles complement each other and in what way are they in conflict in the US system of health care delivery?

13. Describe how health care is rationed in the market justice and social justice systems.
14. To what extent do you think the objectives set forth in Healthy People initiatives can achieve the vision of an integrated approach to health care delivery in the United States?
15. How can health care administrators and policymakers use the various measures of health status and service utilization? Please illustrate your answer.
16. Describe how health care is rationed in the market justice and social justice systems.
From the data given below:
    a. Compute crude birth rates for 1990 and 1995.
    b. Compute crude death rates for 1990 and 1995.
    c. Compute cancer mortality rates for 1990 and 1995.
    d. Answer the following questions:
        (i) Did the infant death rates improve between 1990 and 1995?
        (ii) What conclusions can you draw about the demographic change in this population?
        (iii) Have efforts to prevent death from heart disease been successful in this population?

Population:	1990	1995
Total	248,710	262,755
Male	121,239	128,314
Female	127,471	134,441
Whites	208,704	218,086
Blacks	30,483	33,141
Number of live births	4,250	3,840
Number of infant deaths (birth to one year)	39	35
Number of total deaths	1,294	1,324
Deaths from heart disease	378	363
Deaths from cancer	336	342

REFERENCES

American Institute for Cancer Research. 1996. *Food, nutrition and the prevention of cancer: A global perspective*. Washington, DC.

American Physical Therapy Association. 1997. Religion called valuable health tool. *PT Bulletin*, 10 October, 7.

Appel, L.J. et al. 1997. A clinical trial of the effects of dietary patterns on blood pressure. *New England Journal of Medicine* 336, no. 16: 1117–1124.

Berger, K.S. 1988. *The developing person through the lifespan*. 2nd ed. New York: Worth Publishers.

Blum, H.L. 1981. *Planning for health*. 2nd ed. New York: Human Sciences Press.

Breslow, L. 1972. A quantitative approach to the World Health Organization definition of health: Physical, mental and social well-being. *International Journal of Epidemiology* 1, no. 4: 347–355.

Breslow, L. 1989. Health status measurement in the evaluation of health promotion. *Medical Care* 27, no. 3: S205–S216.

Brown, K. 1992. Death and access: Ethics in cross-cultural health care. In *Choices and conflict: Explorations in health care ethics*, ed. E. Friedman, 85–93. Chicago: American Hospital Publishing.

Centers for Disease Control and Prevention. 1979. *Healthy people: The Surgeon General's report on health promotion and disease prevention*. Washington, DC: US Department of Health and Human Services, Public Health Service.

Centers for Disease Control and Prevention. 1999. *Morbidity and Mortality Weekly Report* 48, no. 29.

Centers for Disease Control and Prevention. 1999. Tobacco use—United States, 1900–1999. *Morbidity and Mortality Weekly Report* 48, no. 43:986–993.

Centers for Disease Control and Prevention. 2007. Avian Influenza (Bird Flu). Available at: *http://www.cdc.gov/flu/avian/*. Accessed January 2007.

Clinton, H.R. 1995. Health care: We can make a difference. In *Leading economic controversies of 1995*, ed. E. Mansfield. New York: W.W. Norton & Company.

Darr, K. 1991. *Ethics in health services management*. Baltimore: Health Professions Press.

Davis, D.L., and P.S. Webster. 2002. The social context of science: cancer and the environment. *The Annals of the American Academy of Political and Social Science* 584 (November): 13–34.

de Leeuw, E. 1989. Concepts in health promotion: The notion of relativism. *Social Science and Medicine* 29, no. 11: 1281–1288.

Department of Health and Human Services. 1998. *Healthy People 2010 objectives: Draft for public comment*. Washington, DC: US Government Printing Office.

Department of Health and Human Services. 2000. *Healthy People 2010: Understanding and improving health*. 2nd ed. Washington, DC: US Government Printing Office.

Department of Health and Human Services. 2001. *Healthy People 2000: Final Review*. Hyattsville, MD: Public Health Service.

Department of Health and Human Services. 2006. Healthy People 2010: Midcourse Review. Available at: *http://www.healthypeople.gov/data/midcourse/default.htm#pubs*. Accessed January 2007.

Dever, G.E. 1984. *Epidemiology in health service management*. Gaithersburg, MD: Aspen Publishers, Inc.

Dye, T.R. 1991. *Politics in states and communities*. 7th ed. Englewood Cliffs, NJ: Prentice-Hall.

Ethics Committee, Society for Academic Emergency Medicine. 1992. An ethical foundation for health care: An emergency medicine perspective. *Annals of Emergency Medicine* 21, no. 11: 1381–1387.

Feldstein, P.J. 1994. *Health policy issues: An economic perspective on health reform*. Ann Arbor, MI: AUPHA/HAP.

Ferguson, C.E., and S.C. Maurice. 1970. *Economic analysis*. Homewood, IL: Richard D. Irwin.

Friedman, G.D. 1980. *Primer of epidemiology*. New York: McGraw-Hill.

Grossman, M. 1972. On the concept of health capital and the demand for health. *Journal of Political Economy* 80, no. 2: 223–255.

Hancock, L.A., and C.L. Mandle. 1994. Overview of growth and development framework. In *Health promotion through the lifespan*, eds. C.L. Edelman and C.L. Mandle. St. Louis, MO: Mosby–Year Book.

Hatch, R.L. et al. 1998. The spiritual involvement and beliefs scale: Development and testing of a new instrument. *Journal of Family Practice* 46: 476–486.

Henry, R.C. 1993. Community partnership model for health professions education. *Journal of the American Podiatric Medical Association* 83, no. 6: 328–331.

Ibrahim, M.A. 1985. *Epidemiology and health policy*. Gaithersburg, MD: Aspen Publishers, Inc.

Institute of Medicine, National Academy of Sciences. 1988. *The future of public health*. Washington, DC: National Academy Press.

Jonsen, A.R. 1986. Bentham in a box: Technology assessment and health care allocation. *Law, Medicine, and Health Care* 14, no. 3–4: 172–174.

Kane, R.L. 1988. Empiric approaches to prevention in the elderly: Are we promoting too much? In *Health promotion and disease prevention in the elderly*, eds. R. Chernoff and D.A. Lipschitz, 127–141. New York: Raven Press.

Kaplan, G.A. et al. 1996. Income inequality and mortality in the United States. *British Medical Journal* 312, no. 7037: 999–1003.

Katz, S., and C.A. Akpom. 1979. A measure of primary sociobiological functions. In *Sociomedical health indicators*, eds. J. Elinson and A.E. Siegman, 127–141. Farmingdale, NY: Baywood Publishing Co.

Kawachi, I. et al. 1997. Social capital, income inequality, and mortality. *American Journal of Public Health* 87: 1491–1498.

Kawachi, I. et al. 1999. Social capital and self-rated health: A contextual analysis. *American Journal of Public Health* 89: 1187–1193.

Kennedy, B.P. et al. 1996. Income distribution and mortality: Cross sectional ecological study of the Robin Hood Index in the United States. *British Medical Journal* 312, no. 7037: 1004–1007.

Kristol, I. 1978. A capitalist conception of justice. In *Ethics, free enterprise, and public policy: Original essays on moral issues in business*, eds. R.T. De George and J.A. Pichler, 57–69. New York: Oxford University Press.

Lasker, R. et al. 1998. *Pocket guide to cases in medicine and public health collaboration*. New York: The New York Academy of Medicine.

Lasker, R.D. 1997. *Medicine and public health: The power of collaboration*. New York: The New York Academy of Medicine.

Levin, J.S. 1994. Religion and health: Is there an association, is it valid, and is it causal? *Social Science and Medicine* 38, no. 11: 1475–1482.

Long, M.J. 1994. *The medical care system: A conceptual model*. Ann Arbor, MI: Health Administration Press.

Macfarlane, G.J., and A.B. Lowenfels. 1994. Physical activity and colon cancer. *European Journal of Cancer Prevention* 3, no. 5: 393–398.

Mackenbach, J.P. et al. 1997. Socioeconomic inequalities in morbidity and mortality in Western Europe. *The Lancet* 349 (June 7): 1655–1660.

Marwick, C. 1995. Should physicians prescribe prayer for health? Spiritual aspects of well-being considered. *Journal of the American Medical Association* 273, no. 20: 1561–1562.

Maugans, T.A. 1996. The SPIRITual history. *Archives of Family Medicine* 5, no. 1:11–16.

May, L.A. 1993. The physiologic and psychological bases of health, disease, and care seeking. In *Introduction to health services,* 4th ed., eds. S.J. Williams and P.R. Torrens, 31–45. New York: Delmar Publishers.

McCullough, M.E., and D.B. Larson. 1999. Religion and depression: A review of the literature. *Twin Research* 2: 126–136.

McCullough, M.E. et al. 2000. Religious involvement and mortality: A meta-analytic review. *Health Psychology* 19, no. 3: 211–222.

McKee, M. 2001. Measuring the efficiency of health systems. *British Medical Journal* 323, no. 7308: 295–296.

National Association of Community Health Centers (NACHC). 2005. *The Safety Net on the Edge.* Washington, DC: NACHC.

National Cancer Institute. 2006. *SEER Cancer Statistics Review, 1975–2003.*

National Center for Health Statistics. 2006. *Health, United States, 2006.* Hyattsville, MD: Department of Health and Human Services.

Navarro, V., and L. Shi. 2001. The political context of social inequalities and health. *Social Science and Medicine* 52, no. 3: 481–491.

Niskanen, W. 1995. Government-managed health care. In *Leading economic controversies of 1995*, ed. E. Mansfield, 15–20. New York: W.W. Norton & Co.

Ostir, G.V. et al. 1999. Disability in older adults 1: Prevalence, causes, and consequences. *Behavioral Medicine* 24, no. 4: 147–156.

Parsons, T. 1972. Definitions of health and illness in the light of American values and social structure. In *Patients, physicians and illness: A sourcebook in behavioral science and health.* 2nd ed., ed. E.G. Jaco. New York: Free Press.

Pasley, B.H. et al. 1995. Excess acute care bed capacity and its causes: The experience of New York State. *Health Services Research* 30, no. 1: 115–131.

Peters, K.E. et al. 2001. *Cooperative actions for health programs: Lessons learned in medicine and public health collaboration.* Chicago: American Medical Association and Washington, DC: American Public Health Association.

Pincus, T. et al. 1998. Social conditions and self-management are more powerful determinants of health than access to care. *Annals of Internal Medicine* 129, no. 5: 406–411.

Plotkin, S.L., and S.A. Plotkin. 1999. A short history of vaccination. In *Vaccines*, 3rd ed., eds. S.A. Plotkin and W.A. Orenstein, Philadelphia: W.B. Saunders: 1.

Post, S.G. et al. 2000. Physicians and patient spirituality: Professional boundaries, competency, and ethics. *Annals of Internal Medicine* 132, no. 7: 578–583.

President's Commission for the Study of Ethical Problems in Medicine and Biomedical and Behavioral Research. 1983. *Securing access to health care: The ethical implications of differences in the availability of health services*. Vol. 1. Washington, DC.

Puchalski, C., and A.L. Romer. 2000. Taking a spiritual history allows clinicians to understand patients more fully. *Journal of Palliative Medicine* 3, no. 1: 129–137.

Reinhardt, U.E. 1994. Providing access to health care and controlling costs: The universal dilemma. In *The nation's health*, 4th ed., eds. P.R. Lee and C.L. Estes, 263–278. Boston: Jones & Bartlett Publishers.

Roberts, J.A. et al. 1997. Factors influencing the views of patients with gynecologic cancer about end-of-life decisions. *American Journal of Obstetrics and Gynecology* 176: 166–172.

Rosen, G. 1993. *A history of public health*. Baltimore, MD: Johns Hopkins University Press.

Ross, L. 1995. The spiritual dimension: Its importance to patients' health, well-being and quality of life and its implications for nursing practice. *International Journal of Nursing Studies* 32, no. 5: 457–468.

Santerre, R.E., and S.P. Neun. 1996. *Health economics: Theories, insights, and industry studies*. Chicago: Irwin.

Saward, E. and A. Sorensen. 1980. The current emphasis on preventive medicine. In *Issues in health services*, ed. S.J. Williams, 17–29. New York: John Wiley & Sons.

Schneider, M.J. 2000. *Introduction to public health*. Gaithersburg, MD: Aspen Publishers, Inc.

Shellenbarger, S. 1997. Good, early care has a huge impact on kids, studies say. *The Wall Street Journal*, 9 April, B1.

Shi, L., and B. Starfield. 2001. Primary care physician supply, income inequality, and racial mortality in US metropolitan areas. *American Journal of Public Health*, 91, no. 8: 1246–1250.

Shi, L. et al. 2002. Primary care, self-rated health, and reduction in social disparities in health. *Health Services Research* 37, no. 3: 529–550.

Shi, L. et al. 1999. Income inequality, primary care, and health indicators. *Journal of Family Practice* 48, no. 4: 275–284.

Shortell, S.M. et al. 1995. Reinventing the American hospital. *The Milbank Quarterly* 73, no. 2: 131–160.

Siegmann, A.E. 1979. A classification of sociomedical health indicators: Perspectives for health administrators and health planners. In *Socio-medical health indicators*, eds. J. Elinson and A.E. Siegmann. Farmingdale, NY: Baywood Publishing Co.

Smith, B.C. 1979. *Community health: An epidemiological approach*, 197–213. New York: Macmillan Publishing Co.

Starfield, B. 1973. Health services research: A working model. *New England Journal of Medicine* 289, no. 2: 132–136.

Starfield, B. 1998. *Primary care and health services*. Oxford: Oxford University Press.

Swanson, C.S. 1995. A spirit-focused conceptual model of nursing for the advanced practice nurse. *Issues in Comprehensive Pediatric Nursing* 18, no. 4: 267–275.

Tamm, M.E. 1993. Models of health and disease. *British Journal of Medical Psychology* 66, no. 3: 213–228.

Tanne, J.H. 2002. Cause of death among Americans differs with race and education. *British Medical Journal* 325, no. 7374: 1192–1196.

Timmreck, T.C. 1994. *An introduction to epidemiology*. Boston: Jones & Bartlett Publishers.

Turnock, B.J. 1997. *Public health: What it is and how it works*. Gaithersburg, MD: Aspen Publishers, Inc.

Vella-Brodrick, D.A., and F.C. Allen. 1995. Development and psychometric validation of the mental, physical, and spiritual well-being scale. *Psychological Reports* 77, no. 2: 659–674.

Ward, B. 1995. Holistic medicine. *Australian Family Physician* 24, no. 5: 761–762, 765.

White, E. et al. 1996. Physical activity in relation to colon cancer in middle-aged men and women. *American Journal of Epidemiology* 144, no. 1: 42–50.

White House. 2006. Statement on U.S. Pledge of $334 Million in Global Fight Against Bird Flu. Available at: *http://www.whitehouse.gov/news/releases/2006/01/20060118-6.html*. Accessed January 2007.

White House. 2007. Strengthening Healthcare. Available at: *http://www.whitehouse.gov/infocus/healthcare/*. Accessed January 2007.

Wilkinson, R.G. 1997. Comment: Income, inequality, and social cohesion. *American Journal of Public Health* 87: 1504–1506.

Wilson, F.A., and D. Neuhauser. 1985. *Health services in the United States*. 2nd ed. Cambridge, MA: Ballinger Publishing Co.

Winslow, C.E.A. 1920. The untilled field of public health. *Modern Medicine* 2, no. 1: 183–191.

Wolinsky, F. 1988. *The sociology of health: Principles, practitioners, and issues*. 2nd ed. Belmont, CA: Wadsworth Publishing.

World Health Organization. 1948. *Preamble to the constitution*. Geneva, Switzerland.

Wynder, E.L., and M.A. Orlandi. 1984. *The American Health Foundation guide to lifespan health: A family program for physical and emotional well-being*. New York: Dodd, Mead & Company.

Chapter 3

The Evolution of Health Services in the United States

Learning Objectives

- To discover historical developments that have shaped the nature of the US health care delivery system
- To evaluate why the system has been resistant to national health insurance reforms
- To explore some of the recent developments and key forces that will likely shape the delivery of health services in the future

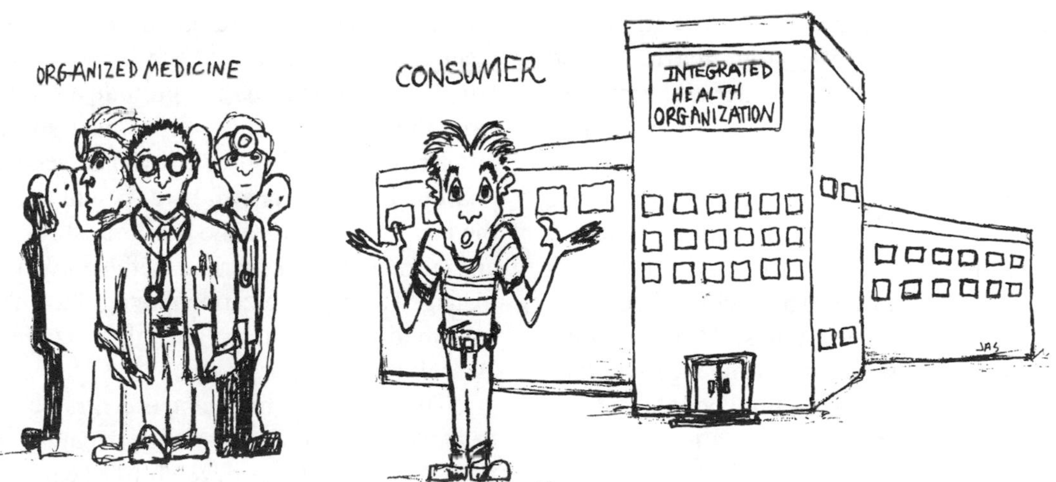

"Where's the market?"

Introduction

The health care delivery system in the United States evolved quite differently than the systems in Europe. American values and the social, political, and economic antecedents on which the US system is based have led to the formation of a unique system of health care delivery, as described in Chapter 1. This chapter discusses how these forces have been instrumental in shaping the current structure of medical services and are likely to shape its future. The evolutionary changes discussed here illustrate the American beliefs and values (discussed in Chapter 2) in action, within the context of broad social, political, and economic exigencies. Because social, political, and economic contexts do not remain static, their shifting influences lend a certain dynamism to the health care delivery system. On the other hand, beliefs and values remain relatively stable over time. Consequently, in the American health care delivery experience, initiatives toward a national health care program have failed to make significant inroads, but social, political, and economic forces have led to certain compromises, as seen in the creation of Medicare and Medicaid and other public programs to extend health insurance to certain defined groups of people. Could major social or economic shifts in the future eventually usher in a national health care program? It is anyone's guess. Although there is always a possibility that, given the right set of conditions, a national health care program could become a reality in the United States, no one seriously thinks that such a drastic change will take place anytime soon. Cultural beliefs and values are strong forces against attempts to initiate fundamental changes in the financing and delivery of health care. Therefore, enactment of major health system reforms would require consensus among Americans on basic values and ethics (C. Everett Koop, US Surgeon General 1982–1989, cited in Kardos and Allen 1993).

The growth of medical science and technology (discussed in Chapter 5) has also played a key role in shaping the system of health services delivery. Stevens (1971, 1) points out that the technological revolution has been primarily responsible for bringing medicine into the public domain. Advancement of technology has influenced other factors, such as medical education, growth of institutions, and urban development. Hence, American medicine did not emerge as a professional entity until the beginning of the 20th century with the progress in biomedical science. Since then, the US health care delivery system has been a growth enterprise. Debates over issues such as methods of financing health care, quality improvement, and the appropriate role of government have also been rooted in the presumed importance of gaining access to ever-rising levels of scientific medicine (Somers and Somers 1977, 1).

This chapter traces the evolution of health care delivery through three major historical phases, each demarcating a major change in the structure of the delivery system. The first phase is the preindustrial era from the middle of the 18th century to the latter part of the 19th century. The second phase is the postindustrial era, beginning in the late 19th century. The third, most recent and current phase is marked by the growth of managed care, organizational integration, the information revolution, and globalization. We call it the corporate era.

The practice of medicine is central to the delivery of health care; therefore, a major portion of this chapter is devoted to tracing the transformations in medical practice from a weak and insecure trade to an independent, highly respected, and lucrative profession. The growing power of managed care and the corporatization of physician practices, however, have made a significant impact on the practice styles and have compromised the autonomy that physicians had historically enjoyed. The medical profession, in turn, has consolidated into larger organizational units, away from the solo practice of medicine that had once prevailed. Compromises have also occurred.

Medical Services in Preindustrial America

From Colonial times to the beginning of the 20th century, American medicine lagged behind the advances in medical science, experimental research, and medical education that were taking place in Britain, France, and Germany. While London, Paris, and Berlin were flourishing as major research centers, Americans had a tendency to neglect research in basic sciences and place more emphasis on applied science (Shryock 1966, 71). In addition, American attitudes about medical treatment placed a strong emphasis on natural history and conservative common sense (Stevens 1971, 13). Consequently, the practice of medicine in the United States had a strong domestic, rather than professional, character. Medical services, when deemed appropriate by the consumer, were purchased out of one's own private funds because there was no health insurance. The health care market was characterized by competition among providers. The consumer decided who the provider would be. Thus, the consumer was sovereign in the health care market, and health care was delivered under free market conditions.

Five main factors explain why the medical profession remained largely an insignificant trade in preindustrial America:

1. Medical practice was in disarray.
2. Medical procedures were primitive.
3. An institutional core was missing.
4. Demand was unstable.
5. Medical education was substandard.

Medical Practice in Disarray

The early practice of medicine could be regarded more as a trade than a profession. It did not require the rigorous course of study, clinical practice, residency training, board exams, and licensing without which it is impossible to practice today. At the close of the Civil War (1861–1865), "anyone who had the inclination to set himself up as a physician could do so, the exigencies of the market alone determining who would prove successful in the field and who would not" (Hamowy 1979). The clergy, for example, often combined medical services and religious duties. The generally well-educated clergyman or government official was more learned in medicine than physicians were (Shryock 1966, 252). Tradesmen, such as tailors, barbers, commodity merchants, and those engaged in numerous other trades, also practiced the healing arts by selling herbal prescriptions, nostrums, elixirs, and cathartics. Midwives, homeopaths, and naturalists could also practice medicine without any restriction. The red-and-white striped poles (symbolizing blood and bandages) outside barber shops today are reminders that barbers also functioned as surgeons at one time, using the same blade to cut hair, shave beards, and bleed the sick. This era of medical pluralism has been referred to as a "war zone" by Kaptchuk and Eisenberg (2001) because it was marked by bitter antagonism among the various practicing sects. Later, in 1847, the American Medical Association (AMA) was founded with the main purpose of erecting a barrier between orthodox practitioners and the "irregulars" (Rothstein 1972).

In the absence of minimum standards of medical training, entry into private practice was relatively easy for both trained and untrained practitioners. Free entry into medical practice created intense competition. Medicine as a profession was weak and unorganized. Hence, physicians did not enjoy the prestige, influence, and incomes that they do today. Many physicians found it necessary to engage in a second occupation because income from medical practice alone was inadequate to support a family. It is estimated that most physicians' incomes in the mid-19th century placed them at the lower end of the middle class (Starr 1982, 84). It is estimated that in 1830 there were 6,800 physicians serving primarily the upper classes (Gabe et al. 1994). It was not until 1870 that medical education was reformed and licensing laws were passed in the United States.

Primitive Medical Procedures

Up until the mid-1800s, medical care was based more on primitive medical traditions than science. In the absence of diagnostic tools, a theory of "intake and outgo" served as an explanation for all diseases (Rosenberg 1979). It was believed that diseases needed to be expelled from the body. Hence, bleeding, use of emetics (to induce vomiting) and diuretics (to increase urination), and purging with enemas and purgatives (to clean the bowels) were the popular forms of clinical therapy.

When George Washington became ill with an inflamed throat in 1799, he too was bled by physicians. One of the attending physicians argued unsuccessfully in favor of making an incision to open the trachea, which today would be considered a more enlightened procedure. The bleeding most likely weakened Washington's resistance although historians have debated whether it played a role in his death (Clark 1998).

Surgeries were limited because anesthesia had not yet been developed, and antiseptic techniques were not known. The stethoscope and X-rays had not been discovered, the clinical thermometer was not in use, and the microscope was not available for medical diagnosis. Physicians relied mainly on their five senses and experience to diagnose and treat medical problems. Hence, in most cases, physicians did not possess technical expertise any greater than mothers and grandparents at home or experienced neighbors in the community.

Missing Institutional Core

In the United States, no widespread development of hospitals occurred before the 1880s. A few isolated hospitals were either built or developed in rented private houses in large cities, such as Philadelphia, New York, Boston, Cincinnati, New Orleans, and St. Louis. In France and Britain, by contrast, general hospital expansion began much before the 1800s (Stevens 1971, 9–10). In Europe, medical professionals were closely associated with hospitals. New advances in medical science were being pioneered, which European hospitals readily adopted. The medical profession came to be supremely regarded because of its close association with an establishment that was scientifically advanced. In contrast, American hospitals played only a small part in medical practice because most hospitals served a social welfare function by taking care of the poor, those without families, and those away from home on travel. Similarly, dispensaries were established to provide free care to those who could not afford to pay. Urban workers and their families often depended on such charity (Rosen 1983, 33). Hence, medical practice in the United States was not legitimized because it lacked organizational affiliation.

Starting with Philadelphia in 1786, dispensaries gradually spread to many other cities. They were private institutions financed by bequests and voluntary subscriptions, and their main function was to provide basic medical care and to dispense drugs to ambulatory patients (Raffel 1980, 239). Dispensaries were independent of hospitals. Generally, young physicians and medical students desiring clinical experience staffed the dispensaries (as well as hospital wards) on a part-time basis for little or no income (Martensen 1996), which served a dual purpose. It provided needed services to the poor and enabled both physicians and medical students to gain experience diagnosing and treating a variety of cases. Later, as the practice of specialized medicine, as well as teaching and research, was transferred to hospital settings, dispensaries gradually became part of the institutional setting. Many dispensaries were absorbed into hospitals as outpatient departments. Indeed, outpatient or ambulatory care departments became an important locale for specialty consultation services in large hospitals (Raffel 1980, 267).

In the United States, the ***almshouse*** was the precursor of hospitals, but it was not a hospital in the true sense. Almshouses (also called poorhouses because they served primarily the poor) existed in almost all cities of moderate size and were run by the local governments. These institutions served primarily general welfare functions by providing food and shelter to the destitute. Therefore, their main function was custodial. Caring for the sick was incidental because some of the residents would inevitably become ill and would usually be cared for in an adjoining infirmary. Almshouses were unspecialized institutions that admitted poor and needy persons of all kinds who were mostly homeless or away from home: the elderly, the orphaned, the insane, the ill, and the disabled. Hence, the early hospital-type institutions emerged mainly to take care of indigent people whose own families could not care for them.

Another type of institution, the ***pesthouse***, was operated by local governments to quarantine people who had contracted a contagious disease such as cholera, smallpox, typhoid, or yellow fever. Located primarily in seaports, the primary function of a pesthouse was to isolate people with contagious diseases in order to contain the spread of disease to the inhabitants of a city. These institutions were the predecessors of contagious-disease and tuberculosis hospitals.

Not until the 1850s were hospitals similar to ones in Europe developed in the United States. These early hospitals generally had deplorable conditions because of a lack of resources. Poor sanitation and inadequate ventilation were their hallmarks. Unhygienic practices prevailed because nurses were generally unskilled and untrained. These early hospitals had an undesirable image as houses of death. The mortality rate among hospital patients both in Europe and America stood around 74 percent in the 1870s (Falk 1999, 116). People went into hospitals only because of dire consequences, not by personal choice. It is not hard to imagine why members of the middle and upper classes, in particular, shunned such establishments.

Unstable Demand

Professional services suffered from low demand in the mainly rural, preindustrial society. Much medical care was provided by people who were not physicians. The most competent physicians were located in more populated communities (Bordley and Harvey 1976, 41–42). In the small communities of rural America, a spirit of strong self-reliance prevailed. Families and communities were accustomed to treating the sick, often using folk remedies that were passed on from one generation to the next. It was also common to consult published books and pamphlets on home remedies (Rosen 1983, 2).

The market for physicians' services was also limited by economic conditions. Many families could not afford to pay for medical services. Two factors contributed to the high cost associated with obtaining professional medical care: (1) The indirect costs of transportation and the "opportunity cost" of travel (i.e., forgone value of time that could have been used for something more productive) could easily outweigh the direct costs of physicians' fees. (2) The costs of travel often doubled because two people, the physician and an emissary, had to make the trip back and forth. For a farmer, a trip of 10 miles into town could mean an entire day's work lost. Physicians passed much of their day traveling along backcountry roads. They had to cover travel costs and the opportunity cost of time spent traveling. Mileage charges typically amounted to four or five times the basic fee for a visit if a physician had to travel 5 to 10 miles. Hence, most families obtained only occasional intervention from physicians, generally for nonroutine and severe conditions (Starr 1982, 66–68).

Personal health services had to be purchased without the help of government or private insurance. Private practice and *fee-for-service*—the practice of billing separately for each individual type of service performed—had been firmly embedded in American medical care. Similar to physicians, dentists were private entrepreneurs who made their living by private fee-for-service dental practice, but their services were not in great demand because there was little public concern about dental health (Anderson 1990, 14–15).

Substandard Medical Education

From about 1800 to 1850, medical training was largely received through individual apprenticeship with a practicing physician, referred to as a preceptor, rather than through university education. Many of the preceptors were themselves poorly trained, especially in the basic medical sciences (Rothstein 1972, 86). By 1800, only four medical schools were operating in the United States: College of Philadelphia (which was established in 1756 and later became the University of Pennsylvania), King's College (which was established in 1768 and later became Columbia University), Harvard University (opened in 1783), and Dartmouth College (started in 1797). These schools were small, graduating only a handful of students each year (Sultz and Young 1997, 115).

American physicians later initiated the establishment of medical schools in large numbers. It was partly to enhance one's professional status and prestige and partly to enhance one's income. Medical schools were inexpensive to operate and often quite profitable. All that was required was a faculty of four or more physicians, a classroom, a back room to conduct dissections, and legal authority to confer degrees. Operating expenses were met totally out of student fees that were paid directly to the physicians (Rothstein 1972, 94). Physicians would affiliate with a local college for the conferral of degrees and use of classroom facilities. Large numbers of men entered medical practice as education in medicine became readily available, and unrestricted entry into the profession was still possible (Hamowy 1979). Gradually, as physicians from medical schools began to outnumber those from the apprenticeship system, the Doctor of Medicine degree became the standard of competence. The number of medical schools tripled between 1800 and 1820, and tripled again between 1820 and 1850, numbering 42 in 1850 (Rothstein 1972, 91). Academic preparation gradually replaced apprenticeship training.

At this point, medical education in the United States was seriously deficient in science-based training, unlike European medical schools. Medical schools in the United States did not have laboratories, and clinical observation and practice were not part of the curriculum. In contrast, European medical schools, particularly those in Germany, were emphasizing laboratory-based medical research. At the University of Berlin, for example, professors were expected to conduct research as well as teach, and were paid by the state. In American medical schools students were taught by local practitioners who were ill-equipped in education and training. Unlike Europe, where medical education was financed and regulated by the government, proprietary medical schools in the United States could set their own standards (Numbers and Warner 1985). A year of medical school in the United States generally lasted only four months and required only two years for graduation. In addition, American medical students customarily repeated the same courses during their second year that they had taken during their first (Numbers and Warner 1985; Rosner 2001). The physicians' desire to keep their schools profitable also contributed to low standards and a lack of rigor. It was feared that higher standards in medical education would drive enrollments down, which could lead the schools into bankruptcy (Starr 1982).

Medical Services in Postindustrial America

In the postindustrial period, American physicians, unlike other physicians in the world, became enormously successful in retaining private practice of medicine and resisting national health care. Consequently, physicians now belong to a well-organized medical profession and deliver scientifically and technically advanced services to insured patients who do not have to bear the bulk of the expenses themselves. Notably, much of this transformation occurred in the aftermath of the Civil War. Social and scientific changes in the period following the war were accompanied by a transition from a rural agricultural economy to a system of industrial capitalism. Mass production techniques used in the war were applied to peacetime industries. Railroads linked the east and west coasts, and small towns became cities (Stevens 1971, 34).

The American system for delivering health care took its current shape during this period. Private practice of medicine became firmly entrenched as physicians grew into a cohesive profession and gained power and prestige. Organized efforts of the medical profession have also been instrumental in blocking attempts to create a national health care program in the United States. The well-defined role of employers in providing workers' compensation for work-related injuries and illnesses, together with other economic considerations, was instrumental in the growth of private health insurance. Rising costs of health care, however, prompted the US Congress to create the publicly financed Medicare and Medicaid programs for the most vulnerable sectors of the population. Cost considerations also motivated the formation of prototypes for modern managed care organizations (MCOs).

Growth of Professional Sovereignty

The 1920s may well mark the consolidation of physicians' professional power. During and after World War I, physicians' incomes grew sharply, and their prominence as a profession finally emerged, although this prestige and power did not materialize overnight. Through the years, several factors interacted in the gradual transformation of medicine from a weak, insecure, and isolated trade into a profession of power and authority. Seven key factors contributed to this transformation:

1. urbanization
2. science and technology
3. institutionalization
4. dependency
5. cohesiveness and organization
6. licensing
7. educational reform

Urbanization

Urbanization created increased reliance on the specialized skills of paid professionals. First, it distanced people from their families and neighborhoods where family-based care was traditionally given. Women entered the workforce and could no longer care for sick members of the family. Second, physicians became less expensive to consult as telephones, automobiles, and paved roads reduced the opportunity cost of time and travel, and medical care became more affordable. Urban development attracted more and more Americans to the growing towns and cities. In 1840, only 11 percent of the US population lived in urban areas; by 1900, it was up to 40 percent (Stevens 1971, 34). The trend away from home visits to office practice also began to develop around this time because of urban growth and shifting residential patterns, which made it more difficult to make house calls (Rosen 1983, 25–26). Physicians moved to cities and towns in large numbers to be closer to their growing markets. Better geographic proximity increased physicians' productivity. Whereas physicians in 1850 averaged only about five to seven patients a day, by the early 1940s the average load of general practitioners had risen to 18 to 22 patients a day (Starr 1982, 71).

Science and Technology

Exhibit 3–1 summarizes some of the groundbreaking scientific discoveries in medicine. Advances in bacteriology, antiseptic surgery, anesthesia, immunology, and diagnostic techniques, along with an expanding repertoire of new drugs, gave medicine an aura of legitimacy and complexity. Also, the therapeutic effectiveness of scientific medicine became widely recognized.

When advanced technical knowledge becomes essential to practice a profession, and the benefits of professional services are widely recognized, it simultaneously creates greater acceptance and a legitimate need for the services of that profession. ***Cultural authority*** refers to the general acceptance of, and reliance on, the judgment of the members of a profession (Starr 1982, 13) because of their superior knowledge and expertise. In a sense, cultural authority legitimizes a profession in the eyes of common people. Advances in medical science and technology bestowed this legitimacy on the medical profession because medical practice could no longer remain within the domain of lay competence.

Scientific and technological change also required improved therapeutic competence

Exhibit 3-1 Groundbreaking Medical Discoveries

- The discovery of anesthesia was instrumental in advancing the practice of surgery. Nitrous oxide (laughing gas) was first employed as an anesthetic around 1846 for tooth extraction by Horace Wells, a dentist. Ether anesthesia for surgery was first successfully used in 1846 at the Massachusetts General Hospital. Before anesthesia was discovered, strong doses of alcohol were used to dull the sensations. A surgeon who could do procedures, such as limb amputations, in the shortest length of time was held in high regard.
- Around 1847, Ignaz Semmelweis, a Hungarian physician practicing in a hospital in Vienna, implemented the policy of handwashing. Thus, an aseptic technique was born. Semmelweis was concerned about the high death rate from puerperal fever among women after childbirth. Even though the germ theory of disease was unknown at this time, Semmelweis surmised that there might be a connection between puerperal fever and the common practice by medical students of not washing their hands before delivering babies and right after doing dissections. Semmelweis' hunch was right.
- Louis Pasteur is generally credited with pioneering the germ theory of disease and microbiology around 1860. Pasteur demonstrated sterilization techniques, such as boiling to kill microorganisms and withholding exposure to air to prevent contamination.
- Joesph Lister is often referred to as the father of antiseptic surgery. Around 1865, Lister used carbolic acid to wash wounds, and popularized the chemical inhibition of infection (antisepsis) during surgery.
- Advances in diagnostics and imaging can be traced to the discovery of X-rays in 1895 by Wilhelm Roentgen, a German professor of physics. Radiology became the first machine-based medical specialty. Some of the first training schools in X-ray therapy and radiography in the United States attracted photographers and electricians to become Doctors in Roentgenology (from the inventor's name).
- Alexander Fleming discovered the antibacterial properties of Penicillin in 1929.

of physicians in the diagnosis and treatment of disease. Developing these skills was no longer possible without specialized training. Science-based medicine created an increased demand for the advanced services that were no longer available through family and neighbors.

Physicians' cultural authority was further bolstered when medical decisions became necessary in various aspects of health care delivery. For example, physicians decide whether a person should be admitted to a medical care institution and for how long; whether surgical or nonsurgical treatments should be used; and which medications should be prescribed. Physicians' decisions have a profound impact on other providers and nonproviders alike. The judgment and opinions of physicians even affect aspects of a person's life beyond the delivery of health care. For example, physicians often evaluate the fitness of persons for jobs during preemployment physicals that many employers demand. Physicians assess the disability of the ill and the injured, as in workers' compensation cases. Granting of medical leave for sickness and release back to work require authorizations from physicians. Payment of medical claims requires physicians' evaluations. Other health care professionals, such as nurses, therapists, and dietitians, are expected to follow physicians' orders for treatment. Thus, during disease and disability, and sometimes even in good health, people's lives have become increasingly governed by decisions made by physicians.

Institutionalization

The evolution of medical technology and the professionalization of medical and nursing staff enabled advanced treatments that necessitated the pooling of resources in a common arena of care (Burns 2004). Rapid urbanization was another factor that necessitated the institutionalization of medical care. As had already occurred in Europe, in the United States the hospital became the core around which the delivery of medical services was organized. Thus, development of the hospital as the center for the practice of scientific medicine and the professionalization of medical practice became closely intertwined. Indeed, the physician and the hospital developed a symbiotic relationship.

For economic reasons, as hospitals expanded, their survival became increasingly dependent on physicians to keep the beds filled because the physicians decided where to hospitalize their patients. Therefore, hospitals had to make every effort to keep the physicians satisfied, which enhanced physicians' professional dominance even though they generally were not employees of the hospitals. It gave physicians enormous influence over hospital policy. Also, for the first time, hospitals began conforming to both physician practice patterns and public expectations about medicine as a modern scientific enterprise. The expansion of surgery, in particular, had profound implications for hospitals, physicians, and the public. As hospitals added specialized facilities and staff, their regular use became indispensable to physicians and surgeons who earlier had been able to manage their practices with little reference to the hospital (Martensen 1996). Affiliation with establishments symbolizing the scientific cutting edge of medicine lent power and prestige to the medical profession.

Hospitals in the United States did not expand and become more directly related to medical care until the late 1890s. However, as late as the 1930s, hospitals incurred frequent deaths due to infections that could not be prevented or cured. Nevertheless, hospital use was on the rise because of the great influx of immigrants into large American cities (Falk 1999, 116). From only a few score in 1875, the number of general hospitals in the United States expanded to 4,000 by 1900 (Anderson 1990, 14), and to 5,000 by 1913 (Wright 1997, 382).

Dependency

Patients depend on the medical profession's judgment and assistance. First, the "sick role" (discussed in Chapter 2) places the patients in a position of dependency because society expects the sick person to seek medical help and try to get well. The person is expected to comply with medical instructions. Second, dependency is created by the profession's cultural authority because its medical judgments must be relied on to (1) legitimize a person's sickness, (2) exempt the individual from social role obligations, and (3) provide competent medical care so the person can get well and resume his or her social role obligations. Third, in conjunction with the physician's cultural authority, the need for hospital services for critical illness and surgery also creates dependency when patients are transferred from their homes to the hospital or to a surgery center.

Once physicians' cultural authority became legitimized, the sphere of their influence expanded into nearly all aspects of health care delivery. For example, laws were passed that prohibited individuals from obtaining certain classes of drugs without a physician's prescription. Health insurance paid for treatments only when they were rendered or prescribed by physicians. Thus, beneficiaries of health insurance became dependent on physicians for reimbursable services. More recently, the referral role (gatekeeping) of primary care physicians in managed care plans has increased patients' dependency on primary care physicians for referral to specialized services.

Cohesiveness and Organization

Toward the end of the 1800s, social and economic changes brought about greater cohesiveness among medical professionals. With the growth of hospitals and specialization, physicians needed support from each other for patient referrals and for access to facilities to admit their patients. Standardization of education also advanced a common core of knowledge among physicians. They no longer remained members of isolated and competing medical sects. Greater cohesiveness, in turn, advanced their professional authority (Starr 1982, 18).

For a long time, physicians' ability to remain free of control from hospitals and insurance companies remained a prominent feature of American medicine. Hospitals and insurance companies could have hired physicians on salary to provide medical services, but individual physicians who took up practice in a corporate setting were castigated by the medical profession and pressured into abandoning such practices. In some states, courts ruled that corporations could not employ licensed physicians without engaging in the unlicensed practice of medicine, a legal doctrine that became known as the "corporate practice doctrine" (Farmer and Douglas 2001). Independence from corporate control enhanced private entrepreneurship and put American physicians in an enviable strategic position in relation to organizations such as hospitals and insurance companies. Later, a formally organized medical profession was in a much better position to resist control from outside entities.

The American Medical Association (AMA) was formed in 1847, but had little strength during its first half-century of existence. Its membership was small, it had no permanent organization, and it had scant resources. The AMA did not attain real strength until it was organized into county and state medical societies, and state societies were incorporated, delegating greater control at the local level. As part of the organizational reform, the AMA also began in 1904 to concentrate attention on medical education (Bordley and Harvey 1976, 364–365). Since then, it has been the chief proponent for the practitioners of conventional medicine in the United States. Although the AMA often stressed the importance of raising the quality of care for patients and protecting the uninformed consumer from "quacks" and "charlatans," its principal goal—like that of other professional associations—was to advance the professionalization, prestige, and financial well-being of its members. The AMA vigorously pursued its objectives by promoting the establishment of state medical licensing laws and the legal requirement that, to be licensed to practice, a physician must be a graduate of an AMA-approved medical school. The concerted activities of physicians through the AMA are collectively referred to as ***organized medicine***, to distinguish them from the uncoordinated actions of individual physicians competing in the marketplace (Goodman and Musgrave 1992, 137, 139).

Licensing

Under the Medical Practice Acts established in the 1870s, medical licensure in the United States became a function of the states (Stevens 1971, 32). By 1896, 26 states had enacted medical licensure laws to license physicians (Anderson 1990, 58). Licensing of physicians and upgrading of medical school standards developed hand in hand. At first, licensing required only a medical school diploma. Later, candidates could be rejected if the school they had attended was judged inadequate. Finally, all candidates were required to present an acceptable diploma and to pass an independent state examination (Starr 1982, 104). Through both licensure and upgrading of medical school standards, physicians obtained a clear monopoly on the practice of medicine (Anderson 1990, 60). Rothstein (1972, 120) suggested that the "irregular" practitioners at the time probably did more good—or less harm—to their patients than did the orthodox ones, because during this period, medical practices such as bloodletting and the use of potent emetics and lethal cathartics, such as mercury, were common. Hence, it can be concluded that the early licensing laws did not so much protect consumers as they protected practitioners from the competitive pressures posed by potential new entrants into the medical profession. Physicians generally led the campaign to restrict the practice of medicine. In 1888, in a landmark Supreme Court decision, *Dent v. West Virginia*, Justice Stephen J. Field wrote that no one had the right to practice "without having the necessary qualifications of learning and skill" (Haber 1974, 260). In the late 1880s and 1890s, many states revised their laws to require all candidates for licensure, including those holding medical degrees, to pass an examination (Kaufman 1980).

Educational Reform

Advanced medical training was made necessary by scientific progress. Reform of medical education started around 1870 with the affiliation of medical schools with universities. In 1871, Harvard Medical School, under the leadership of a new university president, Charles Eliot, completely revolutionized the system of medical education. The academic year was extended from four months to nine, and the length of medical education was increased from two years to three. Following the European model, laboratory instruction and clinical subjects, such as chemistry, physiology, anatomy, and pathology, were added to the curriculum.

Johns Hopkins University took the lead in further reforming medical education when it opened its medical school in 1893 under the leadership of William H. Welch, who trained in Germany. Medical education for the first time became a graduate training course requiring a college degree, not a high school diploma, as an entrance requirement. Johns Hopkins had well-equipped laboratories, a full-time faculty for the basic science courses, and its own teaching hospital (Rothstein 1972, 290). Standards at Johns Hopkins became the model of medical education in other leading institutions around the country. Raising of standards made it difficult for proprietary schools to survive, and in time they were closed.

The Association of American Medical Colleges (AAMC) was founded in 1876 by 22 medical schools (Coggeshall 1965). Later, the AAMC set minimum standards for medical education, including a four-year curriculum, but it was unable to enforce its recommendations. In 1904, the AMA created the Council on Medical Education, which inspected the existing medical schools and found that less than half of them provided acceptable levels of training. The AMA did not publish its own findings, but obtained the help of the Carnegie Foundation for the Advancement of Teaching to provide a rating of medical schools (Goodman and Musgrave 1992, 143). The Foundation appointed Abraham Flexner to investigate medical schools located in both the United States and Canada. The Flexner Report, published in 1910, had a profound effect on medical education reform. The report was widely accepted by both the profession and the public. Schools that did not meet the proposed standards were forced to close. State laws were established requiring graduation from a medical school accredited by the AMA as the basis for a license to practice medicine (Haglund and Dowling 1993).

Once advanced graduate education became an integral part of medical training, it further legitimized the profession's authority and galvanized its sovereignty. Stevens (1971, 55) noted that American medicine moved toward professional maturity between 1890 and 1914 mainly as a direct result of educational reform.

Specialization in Medicine

Specialization has been a key hallmark of American medicine. As a comparison, in 1931, 17 percent of all physicians in the United States were specialists. Today, the proportion of specialists to generalists is approximately 60:40. The growth of allied health care professionals has also diversified, both in medical specialization—such as laboratory and radiological technologists, nurse anesthetists, and physical therapists—as well as in new or expanded specialist fields—such as occupational therapists, psychologists, dietitians, and medical social workers (Stevens 1971, 2–3).

Lack of a rational coordination of medical care in the United States has been one consequence of the preoccupation with specialization. The characteristics of the medical profession in various countries often shape and define the key attributes of their health care delivery systems. The role of the primary care physician (PCP), the relationship between generalists and specialists, the ratio of practicing generalists to specialists, the structure and nature of medical staff appointments in hospitals, and the approach to group practice of medicine have all been molded by the evolving structure and ethos of the medical profession. In Britain, for example, the medical profession has divided itself into general practitioners (GPs) practicing in the community and consultants holding specialist positions in hospitals. This kind of stratification did not develop in American medicine. PCPs in America were not assigned the role that GPs had in Britain, where patients could consult a specialist only by referral from a GP. Unlike Britain, where GPs hold a key intermediary position in relation to the rest of the health care delivery system, the United States has traditionally lacked such a gatekeeping role. Only in the last decade or two, under health maintenance organizations (HMOs), has the ***gatekeeping*** model requiring initial contact with a generalist and the generalist's referral to a specialist gained prominence. The distinctive shaping of medical practice in the United States explains why the structure of medicine did not develop around a nucleus of ***primary care***, in which, apart from delivering routine and basic care, the PCP also ensures the continuity, coordination, and appropriateness of medical services received by a patient. Only in some managed care models, such as HMOs, has the primary care model gained prominence.

The Development of Public Health

Public health practices in the United States have largely concentrated on sanitary regulation, the study of epidemics, and vital statistics. The growth of urban centers for the purpose of commerce and industry, unsanitary living conditions in densely populated areas, inadequate methods of sewage and garbage disposal, limited access to clean water, and long work hours in unsafe and exploitative industries led to periodic epidemics of cholera, smallpox, typhoid, tuberculosis, yellow fever, and other diseases. Such outbreaks sometimes led to arduous efforts to protect the public interest. For example, in 1793, the national capital had to be moved out of Philadelphia because of a devastating outbreak of yellow fever. This epidemic prompted the city to develop its first board of health in that same year. In 1850, Lemuel Shattuck outlined the blueprint for the development of a public health system in Massachusetts. Shattuck also called for the establishment of state and local health departments. A threatening outbreak of cholera in 1873 mobilized the New York City Health Department to alleviate the worst sanitary conditions within the city. Previously, cholera epidemics in 1832 and 1848–1849 had swept through American cities and towns within a few weeks, killing thousands (Duffy 1971).

By 1900, most states had health departments that were responsible for a variety of public health efforts, such as sanitary inspections, communicable disease control, operation of state laboratories, vital statistics, health education, and regulation of food and water (Turnock 1997, 5; Williams 1995, 49). Public health functions were later extended to fill gaps in the medical care system. Such functions, however, were limited mainly to child immunizations, care of mothers and infants, health screening in public schools, and family planning. Federal grants were also made available to state and local governments for programs in substance abuse, mental health, and community prevention services. Thus, public health has a strong social justice orientation (Turnock 1997, 6).

Public health remained separate from the private practice of medicine—as it does even today—because of the skepticism of private physicians that the government could take control of private practice of medicine. Physicians realized that the boards of health could be used to control the supply of physicians and to regulate the practice of medicine (Rothstein 1972, 311). Fear of government intervention, loss of autonomy, and erosion of personal incomes created a wall of separation between public health and private medical practice. Under this dichotomous relationship, medicine has concentrated on the physical health of the individual, whereas public health has focused on the health of whole populations and communities. The extent of collaboration between the two has been largely confined to the requirement by public health departments that private practitioners report cases of contagious diseases such as sexually transmitted diseases, human immunodeficiency virus (HIV) infection, and acquired immune deficiency syndrome (AIDS), and report any outbreaks of cases such as West Nile virus and other types of infections.

The Rise in Chronic Conditions

Until about 1900, infectious diseases posed the greatest health threat to society. The development of public health played a major role in curtailing the spread of infection among populations. Simultaneously, widespread public health measures and better medical care reduced mortality and increased life expectancy. Around 1920, health statisticians noted that chronic illnesses were replacing infectious diseases as the dominant health care challenge (Sydenstricker 1933). Today, chronic conditions are the leading cause of illness, disability, and death in the United States as well as in other developed and developing nations. Almost one-half of all Americans may have one or more chronic conditions (Foundation for Accountability 2001). Chronic conditions may account for three of every four deaths (The Robert Wood Johnson Foundation 1996). It is a paradox that despite a remarkable increase in chronic conditions, the US health care delivery system is still largely designed to treat acute illness and often fails to meet the full needs of persons with chronic conditions (Hoffman et al. 1996).

Health Services for Veterans

Shortly after World War I, the government started to provide hospital services to veterans with service-related disabilities and for nonservice disabilities if the veteran declared an inability to pay for private care. At first, the federal government contracted for services with voluntary hospitals, but over time, the Department of Veterans Affairs (formerly called Veterans Administration) built its own hospitals, outpatient clinics, and nursing homes. Additional details are provided in Chapter 6.

Birth of Workers' Compensation

The first broad-coverage health insurance in the United States emerged in the form of workers' compensation programs initiated in 1914 (Whitted 1993). Workers' compensation was originally concerned with cash payments to workers for wages lost due to job-related injuries and disease. Compensation for medical expenses and death benefits to the survivors were added later (discussed in Chapter 6).

Between 1910 and 1915, workers' compensation laws made rapid progress in the United States (Stevens 1971, 136). Looking at the trend, some reformers believed that since Americans had been persuaded to adopt compulsory insurance against industrial accidents, they could also be persuaded to adopt compulsory insurance against sickness. Workers' compensation served as a trial balloon for the idea of government-sponsored universal health insurance in the United States. However, the growth of private health insurance, along with other key factors that will be discussed later, has prevented any proposals for a national health care program from taking hold.

Rise of Private Health Insurance

Private health insurance was commonly referred to as ***voluntary health insurance*** in contrast to proposals for a publicly organized compulsory health insurance system. The initial role of private health insurance was income protection during sickness and temporary disability. Some private insurance coverage limited to bodily injuries has been available since about 1850. By 1900, health insurance policies became available, but their primary purpose was to protect against loss of income during sickness (Whitted

1993). In the early 20th century, coverage was added for surgical fees, but the emphasis remained on replacing earned income lost due to sickness or injury. Thus, the coverage was in reality disability insurance rather than health insurance as we know it today (Mayer and Mayer 1984, 31).

Technological, social, and economic factors created a general need for health insurance. However, certain economic conditions that prompted private initiatives, self-interests of a well-organized medical profession, and the momentum of a successful health insurance enterprise gave private health insurance a firm footing in the United States. Coverage for hospital and physician services began separately and was later combined under the auspices of Blue Cross and Blue Shield. Later, economic conditions during the World War II period laid the foundations for health insurance to become an employment-based benefit.

Technological, Social, and Economic Factors

The health insurance movement of the early 20th century was the product of three converging developments: the technological, the social, and the economic. From a technological perspective, medicine offered new and better treatments. Because of its well-established healing values, medical care was regarded as socially desirable. The value placed on medical services by individuals and society created a growing demand for medical services. From an economic perspective, people could predict neither their future needs for medical care nor the costs, both of which had been gradually increasing. In short, scientific and technological advances made health care more desirable but less affordable. These developments pointed to the need for some kind of insurance to spread the financial risks over a large number of people.

Early Blanket Insurance Policies

In 1911, insurance companies began to offer blanket policies for large industrial populations, usually covering life insurance, accidents and sickness, and nursing services. A few industrial and railroad companies set up their own medical plans covering specified medical benefits, as did several unions and fraternal orders; however, the total amount of voluntary health insurance was minute (Stevens 1971, 137). Between 1916 and 1918, 16 state legislatures, including New York and California, attempted to enact legislation compelling employers to provide health insurance, but the efforts were unsuccessful (Davis 1996).

Economic Necessity and the Baylor Plan

The Great Depression, which started at the end of 1929, forced hospitals to turn from philanthropic donations to patient fees for support. Patients now faced not only loss of income from illness but also increasing debt from medical care costs when they became sick. People needed protection from the economic consequences of sickness and hospitalization. Hospitals also needed protection from economic instability (Mayer and Mayer 1984, 31). During the Depression, occupancy rates in hospitals fell, income from endowments and contributions dropped sharply, and the charity load almost quadrupled (Richardson 1945).

In 1929, the blueprint for modern health insurance was established when J.F. Kimball began a hospital insurance plan for public school teachers at the Baylor University Hospital in Dallas, Texas. Kimball was able to enroll over 1,200 teachers who paid $0.50 a month for a maximum of 21 days of hospital care. Within a few years, it became the model for Blue Cross plans around the country (Raffel 1980, 394). At first, other independent hospitals copied Baylor and started to offer single-hospital plans. It was not long before communitywide plans offered jointly by more than one hospital became more popular because they provided consumers a choice of hospitals. The underwriting was assumed by the hospitals, which agreed to provide services regardless of the remuneration they would receive. Hence, in essence, these were prepaid plans for hospital services. A ***prepaid plan*** is a contractual arrangement under which a provider must provide all needed services to a group of members (or enrollees) in exchange for a fixed monthly fee paid in advance.

Successful Private Enterprise—The Blue Cross Plans

A hospital plan in Minnesota was the first to use the name Blue Cross in 1933 (Davis 1996). The American Hospital Association (AHA) lent support to the hospital plans and became the coordinating agency to unite these plans into the Blue Cross network (Koch 1993; Raffel 1980, 395). The Blue Cross plans were nonprofit—that is, they had no shareholders who would receive profit distributions—and covered only hospital charges, so as not to infringe on the domain of private physicians (Starr 1982, 296). Later, control of the plans was transferred to a completely independent body, the Blue Cross Commission, which later became the Blue Cross Association (Raffel 1980, 395). In 1946, Blue Cross plans in 43 states served 20 million members. Between 1940 and 1950 alone, the proportion of the population covered by hospital insurance increased from 9 percent to 57 percent (Anderson 1990, 128).

Self Interests of Physicians—Birth of Blue Shield

Voluntary health insurance had received the AMA's endorsement, but the AMA had also made it clear that private health insurance plans should include only hospital care. It is therefore not surprising that the first Blue Shield plan designed to pay for physicians' bills was started by the California Medical Association, which established the California Physicians Service in 1939 (Raffel 1980, 396). By endorsing hospital insurance and by actively developing medical service plans, the medical profession committed itself to private health insurance as the means to spread the financial risk of sickness, and assured that its own interests would not be threatened.

From the medical profession's point of view, voluntary health insurance in conjunction with private fee-for-service practice by physicians was regarded as a desirable feature of the evolving health system (Stevens 1971, 270). Throughout the Blue Shield movement, physicians dominated the boards of directors not only because they underwrote the plans but also because the plans were, in a very real sense, their response to the challenge of national health insurance. In addition, the plans met the AMA's stipulation of keeping medical matters in the hands of physicians (Raffel and Raffel 1994, 213).

Combined Hospital and Physician Coverage

Even though Blue Cross and Blue Shield developed independently, and were financially and organizationally distinct, they often worked together to provide hospital and physician coverage (Law 1974). In 1974, the New York Superintendent of Insurance approved a merger of the Blue Cross and Blue Shield plans of Greater New York (Somers and Somers 1977, 111). Since then, similar mergers have occurred in most states. Now, in nearly every state Blue Cross and Blue Shield plans are joint corporations or have close working relationships (Davis 1996).

The for-profit insurance companies were initially skeptical of the Blue Cross plans and adopted a wait-and-see attitude. Their apprehension was justified because no actuarial information was available to predict losses. But, lured by the success of the Blue Cross plans, within a few years commercial insurance companies also started offering health insurance.

Employment-Based Health Insurance

As a result of wage freezes during the World War II period, group health insurance became an important component of collective bargaining between unions and employers. In 1948, the US Supreme Court ruled that employee benefits, including health insurance, were a legitimate part of the union-management bargaining process. Health insurance then became a permanent part of employee benefits in the postwar era (Health Insurance Association of America 1991, 2). A 1954 revision to the Internal Revenue Code also had a profound influence on the expansion of employer-sponsored health insurance. Now, employer contributions toward the purchase of employee health insurance became exempt from taxable income for the employee. Employment-based health insurance expanded rapidly. The economy was strong during the postwar years of the 1950s, and employers started offering more extensive benefits. This led to the birth of "major medical" expense coverage to protect against prolonged or catastrophic illness or injury (Mayer and Mayer 1984, 31). Thus, private health insurance became the primary vehicle for the delivery of health care services in the United States.

Failure of National Health Care Initiatives

Starting with Germany in 1883, compulsory sickness insurance had spread throughout Europe by about 1912. Health insurance in European countries was viewed as a natural outgrowth of insurance against industrial accidents. Hence, it was considered logical that Americans would also be willing to espouse a national health care program to protect themselves from the high cost of sickness and accidents occurring outside employment.

The American Association of Labor Legislation (AALL) was founded in 1906. Although the AALL took no official position on labor unions, its membership included some prominent labor leaders (Starr 1982, 243), but its relatively small membership was mainly academic, including some leading economists and social scientists, whose all-important agenda was to bring about social reform through government action. The AALL was primarily responsible for leading the successful drive for workers' compensation. It then spearheaded the drive for a government-sponsored health insurance system for the general population (Anderson 1990, 67–68). The AALL supported the Progressive movement headed by former President Theodore Roosevelt, who was again running for the presidency in 1912 on a platform of social reform. Roosevelt, who might have been a national political sponsor for compulsory health insurance, was defeated by Woodrow Wilson. But the Progressive movement for national health insurance did not die.

The AALL continued its efforts toward a model for national health insurance by appealing to both social and economic concerns. The reformers argued that it would relieve poverty because sickness usually brought wage loss and high medical costs to individual families. They also argued that it would contribute to national efficiency by reducing illness, lengthening life, and diminishing the causes of industrial discontent (Starr 1982, 244–246). Leadership of the AMA at the time showed outward support for a national plan, and the AALL and the AMA formed a united front to secure legislation. A standard health insurance bill was introduced in 15 states in 1917 (Stevens 1971, 137).

As long as compulsory health insurance was only under study and discussion, potential opponents paid no heed to it; but once bills were introduced into state legislatures, opponents expressed vehement disapproval. Eventually, it turned out that the AMA's support for social change was only superficial.

Repeated attempts to pass national health insurance legislation in the United States have failed for several reasons, which can be classified under four broad categories: political inexpediency, institutional dissimilarities, ideological differences, and tax aversion.

Political Inexpediency

Before embarking on their national health programs, countries in Western Europe, notably Germany and England, were experiencing labor unrest that threatened political stability. Social insurance was seen as a means to obtain workers' loyalty and ward off political instability. Political conditions in the United States were quite different. There was no threat to political stability. Unlike countries in Europe, the American government was highly decentralized and engaged in little direct regulation of the economy or social welfare. Although Congress had set up a system of compulsory hospital insurance for merchant seamen as far back as 1798, it was an exceptional measure.* Matters related to health and welfare were typically left to state and local governments, and the general rule at these levels of government was to leave as much as possible to private and voluntary action.

The entry of America into World War I in 1917 provided a final political blow to the health insurance movement as anti-German feelings were aroused. The US government denounced German social insurance, and opponents of health insurance called it a Prussian menace inconsistent with American values (Starr 1982, 240, 253).

After attempts to pass compulsory health insurance laws failed at the state levels in California and New York, by 1920 the AALL itself lost interest in an obviously lost cause. Also in 1920, the AMA's House of Delegates approved a resolution condemning compulsory health insurance that would be regulated by any state government or the federal government (Numbers 1985). This AMA resolution opposing national health insurance solidified the profession against "government interference with the practice of medicine."

*Important seaports, such as Boston, were often confronted with many sick and injured seamen who were away from their homes and families. Congress enacted a law requiring that 20 cents a month be withheld from the wages of each seaman on American ships to support merchant marine hospitals (Raffel and Raffel 1994, 115–116).

Institutional Dissimilarities

The preexisting institutions in Europe and America were dissimilar. Germany and England had some mutual benefit funds to provide sickness benefits. These benefits reflected an awareness of the value of insuring against the cost of sickness among a sector of the working population. Voluntary sickness funds were less developed in the United States than in Europe, reflecting less interest in health insurance and less familiarity with it. More important, American hospitals were mainly private, whereas in Europe they were largely government operated (Starr 1982, 238–240).

Dominance of private institutions of health care delivery is generally not consistent with national financing and payment mechanisms. For instance, compulsory health insurance proposals of the AALL were regarded by individual members of the medical profession as a threat to their private practice because it would shift their primary source of income from individual patients to the government (Anderson 1990, 72). Any efforts that would potentially erode the fee-for-service payment system and let private practice of medicine be controlled by a powerful third party—particularly the government—were opposed.

Other institutional forces also were opposed to government-sponsored universal coverage. The insurance industry feared losing the income it derived from disability insurance, some insurance against medical services, and funeral benefits* (Anderson 1990, 73). The pharmaceutical industry feared the government as a monopoly buyer, and retail pharmacists feared that hospitals would establish their own pharmacies under a government-run national health care program (Anderson 1990, 88). Employers also generally saw the proposals as contrary to their interests. Spokespersons for American business rejected the argument that health insurance would add to worker productivity. It may seem ironic, but the labor unions—the American Federation of Labor in particular—also denounced compulsory health insurance at the time. Union leaders were afraid that they would transfer over to the government their own legitimate role of providing social benefits, thus weakening the unions' influence in the workplace. Organized labor was the largest and most powerful interest group at that time. Its lack of support is considered instrumental in the defeat of national health insurance (Anderson 1990, 92).

Ideological Differences

As discussed in Chapter 2, the American value system is based on the principles of market justice. Individualism and self-determination, distrust of government, and reliance on the private sector to address social concerns are typical American ideologies, which seem to stand as a bulwark against anything that is perceived as an onslaught on individual liberties. The cultural and ideological values represent the sentiments of the American middle class, whose support is generally necessary for any broad-based reform. Without such support, a national health care program was unable to withstand the attacks of its well-organized opponents (Anderson 1990, 67). On the other hand, during times of national distress, such as the Great

*Patients admitted to a hospital were required to pay a burial deposit so the hospital would not have to incur a burial expense if they died (Raffel and Raffel 1994, 111). Therefore, many people bought funeral policies from insurance companies.

Depression, pure necessity may have legitimized the advancement of social programs, such as the New Deal programs of the Franklin Roosevelt era (for example, Social Security legislation providing old-age pensions and unemployment compensation).

In the early 1940s, during Roosevelt's presidency, several bills on national health insurance were introduced in Congress, but they all died. Perhaps the most notable bill was the Wagner-Murray-Dingell bill drafted in 1943 and named after the bill's congressional sponsors. However, this time World War II diverted the nation's attention to other issues, and without the president's active support the bill died quietly (Numbers 1985).

In 1946, Harry Truman became the first president to make an appeal for a national health care program (Anderson 1990, 119). Unlike the Progressives, who had proposed a plan for the working class, Truman proposed a single health insurance plan that would include all classes of society. At the president's behest, the Wagner-Murray-Dingell bill was redrafted and reintroduced. The AMA was vehement in opposing the plan. Other health care interest groups, such as the American Hospital Association (AHA), also opposed it. By this time, private health insurance had expanded. Initial public reaction to the Wagner-Murray-Dingell bill was positive; however, when a government-controlled medical plan was compared to private insurance, polls showed that only 12 percent of the public favored extending Social Security to include health insurance (Numbers 1985).

During this era of the Cold War,* any attempts to introduce national health insurance were met with the stigmatizing label of "socialized medicine." The Republicans took control of Congress in 1946, and any interest in enacting national health insurance was put to rest. However, to the surprise of many, Truman was reelected in 1948, promising national health insurance if the Democrats would be returned to power (Starr 1982, 282–284). Fearing the inevitable, the AMA levied a $25 fee on each of its members toward a war chest of $3.5 million (Anderson 1990, 118). It hired the public relations firm of Whitaker and Baxter and spent $1.5 million in 1949 alone to launch one of the most expensive lobbying efforts in American history. The campaign directly linked national health insurance with communism until the idea of "socialized medicine" was firmly implanted in the public's minds. Republicans proposed a few compromises, but neither the Democrats nor the AMA were interested in them. By 1952, the election of a Republican president, Dwight Eisenhower, effectively ended any further debate over national health insurance. Failure of government-sponsored universal health care coverage is often presented as a classic case of the tremendous influence of interest groups in American politics, especially in major health policy outcomes.

Tax Aversion

An aversion to increased taxes to pay for social programs is another reason why middle-class Americans, who are already insured, have opposed national initiatives to expand health insurance coverage. According to polls, Americans have been found to generally support the idea that the government ought to help people who are in financial need to pay for their medical care. Howev-

* Rivalry and hostility after World War II between the United States and the then Soviet Union.

er, most Americans have not favored an increase in their own taxes to pay for such care.

The most recent unsuccessful attempt to bring about a national health care program was initiated by the Clinton administration. While seeking the presidency in 1992, Governor Bill Clinton made health system reform a major campaign issue. Not since Harry Truman's initiatives a few decades earlier had such a bold attempt been made by a presidential candidate. As long as the electorate has remained reasonably satisfied with health care—with the exception of uninsured Americans, who have not been politically strong—elected officials have feared the political clout of big interest groups and have refrained from raising tough reform issues. In the Pennsylvania US Senate election in November 1991, however, the victory of Democrat Harris Wofford over Republican Richard Thornburgh sent a clear signal that the time for a national health care program might be ripe. Wofford's call for national health insurance was widely supported by middle-class Pennsylvanians. Election results in other states were not quite as decisive on the health reform issue, but various public polls seemed to confirm that after the economy (America was in a brief recession at the time), health care was the second most pressing concern on the minds of the American people. One national survey conducted by Louis Harris and Associates reported some disturbing findings about health care delivery. Substantial numbers of insured and relatively affluent people said that they had not received the services they needed. The poll also suggested that the public was looking to the federal government, not the states or private sector, to contain rising health care costs (Smith et al. 1992). In other opinion polls, Americans expressed concerns that they might not be adequately insured in the future (Skocpol 1995). Against this backdrop, both Bill Clinton and the running incumbent, President George (Herbert Walker) Bush, advanced health care reform proposals.

After taking office, President Clinton made health system reform one of his top priorities. Policy experts and public opinion leaders have since debated over what went wrong. Some of the fundamental causes for the failure of the Clinton plan were no doubt historical in nature, as discussed earlier in this chapter. One seasoned political observer, James J. Mongan, however, remarked that reform debates in Congress have never been about the expansion of health care services but about the financing of the proposed services:

> Thus, the most important cause of health care reform's demise was that avoiding tax increases and their thinly veiled cousin, employer mandates, took priority over expanding coverage. . . . There undoubtedly would have been pitched legislative battles over other issues—how to pay doctors and hospitals, the role of health insurers, the structure of (regional health) alliances—but these debates never happened in detail. The first and only battle . . . was how to pay for reform. . . . What explains this unwillingness to pay for expanded coverage, on the part of citizens and government alike? Any answer must take into account the economic, social, and political context of the past two decades. . . . The social context is that people tend to take for granted the progress achieved through social insurance programs such as Medicare and Social Security, and they perceive little progress or achievement from welfare expenditures targeted on low-income people.

> Politically, politicians from the courthouse to the White House have played to an antitax sentiment and have convinced Americans and American businesses that they are staggering under an oppressive burden of taxation that saps most productive effort. Although there is little evidence from other countries to support this belief, it is widely held. This climate fosters a self-centeredness—a focus more on the individual's needs than on the community's needs. Some liberals might use a harsher, more grating word—selfishness—to describe this state of mind. But many conservatives would use the phrase *rugged individualism* to describe the same phenomenon. . . . Somewhere in here is where health reform died. . . . Until we as a nation make the right diagnosis and begin an honest dialogue about our national values, about the balance between self-interest and community interests, we will not see our nation join almost all others in guaranteeing health coverage to all of its citizens (Mongan 1995, 99–101).

When American polls indicated that a fundamental reform was needed, the people did not have in mind more government regulation or any significant redistribution of income through increased taxes. Most important, they did not wish to have a negative effect on their own access to care or the quality of care they would receive (Altman and Reinhardt 1996, xxviii).

For now, employer-based private health insurance is firmly entrenched in the United States. Americans, regardless of gender, race, age, or working status, have indicated that employers would be their preferred source for obtaining health insurance (Duchon et al. 2000). Among both the insured and the uninsured, only a relatively small proportion of adults believe that the government would be the best source for obtaining health coverage (Schoen et al. 2000). The confidence expressed by Americans in their ability to pay for a major illness has also improved over time. The proportion reporting such confidence has risen from 50 percent in 1978 to 67 percent in 2000 (Blendon and Benson 2001). But, the 2006 Health Confidence Survey conducted by the Employee Benefit Research Institute (EBRI) finds that the public is increasingly getting dissatisfied with the US health system primarily because of rising health care costs. On the other hand, despite the costs, Americans are satisfied with the quality of health care, and only a minority of Americans identify health care as the country's most critical issue (EBRI 2006).

Although people's sentiments can change with the ebb and flow of the nation's economic state and other pressing concerns, health care has not been a major political issue in recent years. Health care issues played only a minor role in the 2002 congressional elections and the 2004 presidential election, and concerns about the cost of health care "are not breaking through as a top voting issue in the mid-term election" in 2006 (Blendon and Altman 2006). Americans are more concerned with other social issues, such as crime, education, the war on terrorism, and homeland security. Cost of health care, however, continues to be a major concern. But, direct government involvement to control rising health care expenditures is not the approach with which Americans are most comfortable. Hence, any major health care initiatives between now and the next presidential election in 2008 are highly unlikely even though control of the US Congress passed into the hands of the Democratic Party in January 2007.

Creation of Medicaid and Medicare

Before 1965, private health insurance was the only widely available source of payment for health care, and it was available primarily to middle-class working people and their families. The elderly, the unemployed, and the poor had to rely on their own resources, on limited public programs, or on charity from hospitals and individual physicians. Often, when charity care was provided, private payers were charged more to make up the difference, a practice referred to as ***cost-shifting*** or ***cross-subsidization***. In 1965, Congress passed the amendments to the Social Security Act that created the Medicare and Medicaid programs, and the government assumed direct responsibility to pay for some of the health care on behalf of two vulnerable population groups—the elderly and the poor (Potter and Longest 1994).

Medicaid and Medicare are prime representations of the public sector in the amalgam of private and public approaches for providing access to health care in the United States. Through the debates over how to protect the public from rising costs of health care and the opposition to national health insurance, one thing had become clear: Government intervention was not desired insofar as it pertained to how most Americans would receive health care, with one exception. Less opposition would be encountered if reform initiatives were proposed for the underprivileged classes. In principle, the poor were considered a special class who could be served through a government-sponsored program. The elderly—those 65 years of age and over—were another group that started to receive increased attention in the 1950s. On their own, most of the poor and the elderly could not afford the increasing cost of health care. Also, because the health status of these population groups was significantly worse than that of the general population, they required a higher level of health care services. The elderly, particularly, had higher incidence and prevalence of disease compared to younger groups. It was also estimated that less than half of the elderly were covered by private health insurance. By this time, the growing elderly middle class was also becoming a politically active force.

Government assistance for the poor and the elderly was sought once it became clear that the market alone would not ensure access for these vulnerable population groups. A bill introduced in Congress by Aime Forand in 1957 provided the momentum for including necessary hospital and nursing home care as an extension of Social Security benefits (Stevens 1971, 434). The AMA, however, undertook a massive campaign to portray a government insurance plan as a threat to the physician-patient relationship. The bill was stalled, but public hearings around the country, which were packed by the elderly, produced an intense grassroots support to push the issue onto the national agenda (Starr 1982, 368). A compromised reform, the Medical Assistance Act (Public Law 86–778), also known as the Kerr-Mills Act, went into effect in 1960. Under the act, federal grants were given to the states to extend health services provided by the state welfare programs to those low-income elderly who previously did not qualify (Anderson 1990, 156). Since the program was based on a ***means test*** that confined eligibility to people below a predetermined income level, it was opposed by liberal congressional representatives as a source of humiliation to the elderly (Starr 1982, 369). Within three years, the program was declared ineffective because many states did not even implement it (Stevens 1971, 438). In 1964, health insurance for the aged and the poor became top priorities of President Johnson's Great Society programs.

During the debate over Medicare, the AMA developed its own "Eldercare" proposal, which called for a federal-state program to subsidize private insurance policies for hospital and physician services. Representative John W. Byrnes introduced another proposal, dubbed "Bettercare." It proposed a federal program based on partial premium contributions by the elderly and the remainder subsidized by the government. Other proposals included tax credits and tax deductions for health insurance premiums.

In the end, a three-layered program emerged. The first two layers constituted Part A and Part B of ***Medicare***, or ***Title XVIII*** of the Social Security Amendment of 1965 to provide publicly financed health insurance to the elderly. Based on Forand's initial bill, the administration's proposal to finance hospital insurance for the elderly through Social Security to provide hospital care and limited nursing home coverage became ***Part A*** of Medicare. The Byrnes' proposal to cover physicians' bills through government-subsidized insurance became ***Part B*** of Medicare. An extension of the Kerr-Mills program of federal matching funds to the states based on each state's financial needs became ***Medicaid***, or ***Title XIX*** of the Social Security Amendment of 1965. The Medicaid program was for the indigent, based on means tests established by each state, but it was expanded to include all age groups, not just the poor elderly (Stevens 1971, 439–440).

Although adopted together, Medicare and Medicaid reflected sharply different traditions. Medicare was upheld by broad grassroots support and, being attached to Social Security, had no class distinction. Medicaid, on the other hand, was burdened by the stigma of public welfare. Medicare had uniform national standards for eligibility and benefits; Medicaid varied from state to state in terms of eligibility and benefits. Medicare allowed physicians to ***balance bill***, that is, charge the patient the amount above the program's set fees and recoup the difference. Medicaid prohibited balance billing and, consequently, had limited participation from physicians (Starr 1982, 370). Medicaid, in essence, has created a two-tier system of medical care delivery because some physicians refuse to accept Medicaid patients because of low fees set by the government.

Not long after Medicare and Medicaid were in operation, national spending for health services began to rise. So did public outlays of funds in relation to private spending for health services (Anderson 1990, 209).

Regulatory Role of Public Health Agencies

With the expansion of publicly financed Medicare and Medicaid programs, the regulatory powers of government have increasingly encroached upon the private sector. This is because the government provides financing for the two programs, but services are delivered by the private sector. After the federal government developed the standards for participation in the Medicare program, states developed regulations in conjunction with the Medicaid program. The regulations often overlapped, and the federal government delegated authority to the states to carry out the monitoring of compliance with the regulations. As a result, the regulatory powers assigned to state public health agencies increased dramatically. Thus, most institutions of health care delivery are subject to annual scrutiny by public health agencies under the authority delegated to them by the federal and state governments.

Prototypes of Managed Care

Even though the early practice of medicine in the United States was mainly characterized by private solo practice, three subsequent developments in medical care delivery are noteworthy. All three required some sort of organizational integration, which was a departure from solo practice. These innovative arrangements can also be regarded as early precursors of managed care and integrated organizations (discussed in Chapter 9). The three developments were contract practice, group practice, and prepaid group practice.

Contract Practice

In 1882, Northern Pacific Railroad Beneficial Association was one of the first employers to provide medical care expense coverage (Davis 1996). Between 1850 and 1900, other railroad, mining, and lumber enterprises developed extensive employee medical programs. Such companies conducted operations in isolated areas where physicians were generally unavailable. Inducements, such as a guaranteed salary, were commonly offered to attract physicians. Another common arrangement was to contract with independent physicians and hospitals at a flat rate per worker per month, referred to as ***capitation***. The AMA recognized the necessity of contract practice in remote areas, but elsewhere contract practice was regarded as a form of exploitation because it was assumed that physicians would bid against each other and drive down the price. Offering services at reduced rates was regarded by the AMA as an unethical invasion of private practice. When group health insurance became common in the 1940s through collective bargaining, the medical profession was freed from the threat of direct control by large corporations. Health insurance also enabled workers to go to physicians and hospitals of their choice (Starr 1982, 201–204).

Corporate practice of medicine—that is, provision of medical care by for-profit corporations—was generally prohibited by law. It was labeled as commercialism in medicine. In 1917, however, Oregon passed the Hospital Association Act, which permitted for-profit corporations to provide medical services. Whereas health insurance companies, functioning as insurers and payers, acted as intermediaries between patients and physicians, the hospital associations in Oregon contracted directly with physicians and exercised some control over them. Utilization was managed by requiring second opinions for major surgery and by reviewing the length of hospital stays. The corporations also restricted medical fees, refusing to pay prices they deemed excessive. In short, they acted as a countervailing power in the medical market to limit physicians' professional autonomy. Even though physicians resented controls, they continued to do business with the hospital associations because of guaranteed payments (Starr 1982, 204–205).

Early contract practice arrangements and the Oregon hospital associations can be viewed as prototypes of managed care. With the growth of managed care, the traditional fee-for-service payment arrangements have been largely replaced by capitation and discounted fees. Mechanisms to control excessive utilization are another key feature of managed care.

Group Practice

Group medicine represented another form of corporate organization for medical care. Group practice changed the relationship among physicians by bringing them together with business managers and technical assistants in a more elaborate division of labor (Starr 1982, 209). The Mayo Clinic, started in Rochester, Minnesota, in 1887, is generally regarded as a prototype of the consolidation of specialists into group practice. The concept of a multispecialist group presented a threat to the continuation of general practice. It also presented competition to specialists who remained in solo practice. Hence, the development of group practice met with widespread professional resistance (Stevens 1971, 142). Although specialist group practice did not become a movement, sharing of expenses and incomes, along with other economic advantages, has caused group practices to continue to grow over the years.

Prepaid Group Plans

In time, the efficiencies of group practice led to the formation of prepaid group plans in which an enrolled population received comprehensive services for a capitated fee. The HIP Health Plan of New York (started in 1947) stands as one of the most successful programs providing comprehensive medical services through organized medical groups of family physicians and specialists (Raffel 1980, 415). Similarly, Kaiser-Permanente (started in 1942) has grown on the West Coast. Other examples are the Group Health Cooperative of Puget Sound in Seattle (operating since 1947), a consumer-owned cooperative prepaid group practice (Williams 1993), and the Labor Health Institute in St. Louis (1945), a union-sponsored group practice scheme (Stevens 1971, 423).

The idea of prepaid group practice had limitations. It required the sponsorship of large organizations. HIP, for example, was created by New York's Mayor Fiorello La Guardia for city employees. Industrialist Henry Kaiser initially set up his prepaid plan to provide comprehensive health care services to his own employees. For most employers, it was impractical to have their own health plans; they had to rely on health insurance plans offered by the insurance industry. The Kaiser-Permanente health plan was later extended to other employers.

In 1971, President Nixon singled out prepaid group practice organizations as the model for a rational reorganization in the delivery of health services. They became the prototype of health maintenance organizations, or HMOs (Somers and Somers 1977, 221–222). During the Nixon administration, the use of HMOs in the private sector was encouraged by federal legislation, the Health Maintenance Organization Act (HMO Act) of 1973. The HMO Act required employers to offer an HMO alternative to conventional health insurance (Goodman and Musgrave 1992, 194). MCOs today attempt to combine the efficiencies of contract and group arrangements with the objective of delivering comprehensive health care services at predetermined costs.

Medical Care in the Corporate Era

The latter part of the 20th century and start of the 21st have been marked by the growth and consolidation of large business corporations, and tremendous advances in global communications, transportation, and trade. These developments are starting to change the way health care is delivered in the United States, and, indeed, around the world. The rise of multinational corporations, the information revolution, and globalization have been interdependent phenomena. The General Agreement on Trade in Services (GATS), which came into effect in 1995, aims to gradually remove all barriers to international trade in services. In health care services, GATS may regulate health insurance, hospital services, telemedicine, and acquisition of medical treatment abroad. GATS negotiations, however, have met with controversy as various countries fear that it may shape their domestic health care systems (Belsky et al. 2004), although most analysts predict that GATS is likely to produce future market liberalization (Mutchnick et al. 2005). No one, however, is certain how the increasing corporatization of medicine and exertion of global forces will eventually shape health care delivery.

Corporatization of Health Care Delivery

Corporatization here refers to the ways in which health care delivery in the United States has become the domain of large organizations. These corporations may operate either on a for-profit or nonprofit basis, yet they are driven for the most part by the common goal of maximizing their revenues. At least one benefit of this corporatization has been the ability of these organizations to deliver sophisticated modern health care in comfortable and pleasant surroundings. But, one main expectation of delivering the same quality of health care at lesser cost remains largely unrealized.

On the supply side, until the mid-1980s, physicians and hospitals clearly dominated the medical marketplace. Since then, managed care has emerged as a dominant force by becoming the primary vehicle for insuring and delivering health care to the majority of Americans. The rise of managed care consolidated immense purchasing power on the demand side. It was to counteract this imbalance that providers began to consolidate, and larger, integrated health care organizations began forming (see Chapter 9). A second influential factor behind health care integration was reimbursement cuts for inpatient acute care hospital services in the mid-1980s. To make up for lost revenues in the inpatient sector, hospitals developed various types of outpatient services such as primary care, outpatient surgery, and home health care, and expanded into other differentiated health care services such as long-term care and specialized rehabilitation services. Together, managed care and integrated delivery organizations have in reality corporatized the delivery of health care in the United States.

In a health care landscape that has been increasingly dominated by corporations, individual physicians have struggled to preserve their autonomy. As a matter of survival, many physicians had to consolidate into large clinics, form strategic partnerships with hospitals, or start their own specialty hospitals. A growing number of physicians have become employees of large medical corporations. Proliferation of these new models of health care delivery has made it increasingly difficult for states to maintain outright bans on the employment of physicians (Farmer and Douglas 2001).

Both managed care and corporate delivery of medicine have made the health care system extremely complex from the consumer's standpoint. Managed care was supposedly a market-based reform, but it has stripped the primary consumer, the patient, of practically all marketplace power. Dominance by any entity, whether organized medicine or integrated health organizations, subverts the sovereignty of the health care consumer. In this so-called market-driven integration, the consumer continues to wonder, "Where's the market?"

Information Revolution

The delivery of health care is being transformed in unprecedented and irreversible ways by telecommunication. The use of telemedicine and telehealth is on the rise. In a general sense, the terms ***telemedicine*** and ***telehealth*** are used interchangeably (although strictly speaking there is a difference—see Chapter 5) to refer to the integration of telecommunication systems into the practice of protecting and promoting health in distant caregiving. It may or may not incorporate actual physician-patient interactions. Telemedicine came to the forefront in the 1990s with the technological advances in the distant transmission of image data and the recognition that there was inequitable access to medical care in rural America. Federal dollars were poured into rural telemedicine projects.

Telehealth consultations can occur in real time. Videoconferencing is now replacing telephone consultation as the preferred vehicle for behavioral telehealth or telepsychiatry. ***E-health*** has also become an unstoppable force that is driven by consumer demand for health care information and services offered over the Internet by professionals and nonprofessionals alike (Maheu et al. 2001). The Internet has created a new revolution that is increasingly characterized by patient empowerment. Access to expert information is no longer strictly confined to the physician's domain, which in some ways has led to a dilution of the dependent role of the patient.

Further elaborations on telehealth and e-health are provided in Chapter 5.

Globalization

Although there is no standard definition for ***globalization***, it refers to various forms of cross-border economic activities. Globalization is driven by global exchange of information, production of goods and services more economically in developing countries, and increased interdependence of mature and emerging world economies. It confers many advantages, but also has its downsides.

From the standpoint of cross-border trade in health services, Mutchnick and colleagues (2005) identified four different modes of economic interrelationships: (1) Use of advanced telecommunication infrastructures in telemedicine. For example, teleradiology (the electronic transmission of radiological images over a distance) now enables physicians in the United States to transmit radiological images to Australia where they are interpreted and reported back the next day (McDonnell 2006). On the other hand, innovative telemedicine consulting services in pathology and radiology are being delivered to other parts of the world by cutting-edge US medical institutions such as Johns Hopkins. (2) Consumers travel abroad to receive medical care. Specialty hospitals, such as the Apollo chain in India, offers state-of-the-art technology to foreigners at a fraction of what it would cost to have the same procedures done in the United States or Europe. Physicians and hospitals outside the United States have clear competitive advantages: reasonable malpractice costs, minimum regulation, and lower costs of labor. As a result of these efficiencies, Indian specialty hospitals can do quality liver transplants for one-tenth the cost of US hospitals (Mutchnick et al. 2005). On the other hand, dignitaries and other wealthy foreigners come to multispecialty centers in the United States, such as the Mayo Clinic, to receive highly specialized services. (3) Foreign direct investment in health services enterprises. For example, Chindex International, a US corporation, provides medical equipment, supplies, and clinical care in China. Chindex opened the Beijing United Family Hospital and Clinics in 1997 (Mutchnick et al. 2005). (4) Health professionals move to other countries that present high demand for their services and better economic opportunities than their native countries. For example, nurses from other countries are moving to the United States to relieve the existing personnel shortage. Migration of physicians from developing countries helps alleviate at least some of the shortage in underserved locations in the developed world. On the downside, the developing world pays a price when emigration leaves these countries with shortages of trained professionals. The burden of disease in these countries is often greater than it is in the developed world, and emigration only exacerbates the ability of these countries to provide adequate health care to their own populations (Norcini and Mazmanian 2005).

Globalization produces other negative effects that are indirect. Tobacco use is on the decline in many developed countries, yet economic development and emerging markets provide new targets for the tobacco industry. Today, rapid economic development in China and India offers multinational tobacco companies new markets of potential smokers. In addition, as developing countries become more prosperous, they acquire Western tastes and lifestyles. In some instances, negative health consequences follow. For example, increased use of motorized vehicles results in a lack of physical exercise, which, along with changes in diet, are greatly increasing the prevalence of chronic diseases such as heart disease and diabetes in the developing world. On the other hand, better information about health promotion and disease prevention, and access to gyms and swimming pools in developing countries are making a positive impact on the health and well-being of their middle-class citizens.

Globalization has also posed some new threats, for instance, the threat of diseases that were previously unknown in the United States. Infectious diseases appearing in one country can spread rapidly to other countries. HIV/AIDS, hepatitis B, and hepatitis C infections have spread worldwide. New viral infections such as avian flu and SARS (severe acute respiratory syndrome) have at times threatened to create worldwide pandemics.

Another ill effect of globalization, bioterrorism, is the latest threat gripping the nation since the tragic events of September 11, 2001. Vital resources are being deployed to counteract the fear of possible clandestine warfare through deadly agents, such as smallpox, a disease that was eradicated from the planet by 1977.

Other Developments in US Health Care

Health care delivery in the United States has been driven primarily by economics, but social and political exigencies do call for incremental change from time to time. Two notable examples that fall in the latter category were expansion of social entitlements. The first was the State Children's Health Insurance Program (SCHIP) enacted in 1997, and the second was creation of Part D of Medicare (implemented in 2006) to assist seniors with their prescription drug costs (both are discussed in Chapter 6).

The United States now has an expanding market of self-care products and alternative therapies (discussed in Chapter 7). In a sense, health care delivery to a small degree has reverted to the bygone era of familial medicine and use of products and procedures of questionable scientific validity. This consumer-driven phenomenon has not gone unnoticed by the traditional medical establishment. The private medical establishment and the government have intensified efforts to understand the potential benefits as well as any undesirable consequences of alternative treatments.

Summary

Figure 3–1 provides a snapshot of the historical developments in US health care delivery. The evolution of health care services has been strongly influenced by the advancement of scientific research and technological development. Early scientific discoveries were pioneered in Europe, but they were not readily adopted in the United States; therefore, medicine had a largely domestic, rather than a professional, character in preindustrial America. The absence of standards of practice and licensing requirements allowed the trained and untrained alike to deliver medical care. Hospitals were more akin to places of refuge than centers of medical practice. The demand for professional services was relatively low because they had to be purchased privately, without the help of government or health insurance. Medical education was seriously deficient in providing technical training based on scientific knowledge. The medical profession faced intense competition; it was weak, unorganized, and insecure.

Scientific and technological advances led to the development of sophisticated in-

Figure 3–1 Evolution of the Health Care Delivery System.

Development of science and technology

Mid 18th to late 19th century	Late 19th to late 20th century	Late 20th to 21st century
• Open entry into medical practice • Intense competition • Weak and unorganized profession • Apprenticeship training • Undeveloped hospitals • Private payment for services • Low demand for services • Private medical schools providing only general education	• Scientific basis of medicine • Urbanization • Emergence of the modern hospital • Emergence of organized medicine • Emergence of scientific medical training • Licensing • Development of public health • Specialization in medicine • Emergence of workers' compensation • Emergence of private insurance • Failure of national health insurance • Medicaid and Medicare • Prototypes of managed care	• **Corporatization** Managed care Health care integration Diluted physician autonomy Complexity for the patient • **Information revolution** Telemedicine E-health Patient empowerment • **Globalization** Global telemedicine Medical travel Foreign investment in health care Migration of professionals Exportation of lifestyles Challenge of new diseases Bioterrorism
Consumer sovereignty	Professional dominance	Corporate dominance

Beliefs and values/Social, economic, and political constraints

stitutions where better trained physicians could practice their art. The transformation of America from a mainly rural, sparsely populated country to one with growing centers of urban population created increased reliance on the specialized skills that only trained professionals could offer. Simultaneously, medical professionals banded together into a politically strong organization. The AMA succeeded in controlling the practice of medicine mainly through its influence on medical education, licensing of physicians, and political lobbying.

In Europe, national health insurance has been an outgrowth of generous social programs. In the United States, by contrast, the predominance of private institutions, ideologies founded on the principles of market justice, and an aversion to tax increases have been instrumental in maintaining a health care delivery system that is mainly privately financed and operated. The AMA and other interest groups have also wielded enormous influence in opposing efforts to initiate comprehensive reforms based on national health insurance. Access to health services in the United States is achieved primarily through private health insurance; however, two major social programs, Medicaid and Medicare, were expediently enacted to provide affordable health services to vulnerable populations.

Growth in science and technology engenders greater specialization, but a lack of rational coordination of medical care in the United States has created a surplus of specialists and has relegated primary care to a secondary status. Public health and private medicine also function in a dichotomous and sometimes adversarial relationship.

The corporate era in health care dawned in the latter part of the 20th century. The rise of multinational corporations, the information revolution, and globalization have marked this current era. Managed care represents corporatization of health care delivery on the demand side. On the supply side, providers have integrated into various types of consolidated arrangements. The information revolution is characterized by the growth of telehealth (or telemedicine) and e-health. Globalization has made the mature and the emerging world economies more interdependent, which has both advantages and disadvantages.

Test Your Understanding

Terminology

almshouse
balance bill
capitation
cost-shifting
cross-subsidization
cultural authority
E-health
fee-for-service
gatekeeping
globalization
means test
Medicaid
Medicare
organized medicine
Part A
Part B
pesthouse
prepaid plan
primary care
telehealth
telemedicine
Title XVIII
Title XIX
voluntary health insurance

Review Questions

1. Why did the professionalization of medicine start later in the United States than in some Western European nations?
2. Why did medicine have a domestic rather than a professional character in the preindustrial era? How did urbanization change that?
3. Which factors explain why the demand for the services of a professional physician was inadequate in the preindustrial era? How did scientific medicine and technology change that?
4. How did the emergence of general hospitals strengthen the professional sovereignty of physicians?
5. Discuss the relationship of dependency within the context of the medical profession's cultural and legitimized authority. What role did medical education reform play in galvanizing professional authority?
6. How did the organized medical profession manage to remain free of control by business firms, insurance companies, and hospitals until the latter part of the 20th century?
7. In general, discuss how technological, social, and economic factors created the need for health insurance.
8. Which conditions during the World War II and post war period lent support to private health insurance in the United States?
9. Discuss, with particular reference to the roles of (a) organized medicine, (b) the middle class, and (c) American beliefs and values, why reform efforts to bring in national health insurance have been unsuccessful in the United States.
10. Which particular factors that earlier may have been somewhat weak in bringing about national health insurance later led to the passage of Medicare and Medicaid?
11. On what basis were the elderly and the poor regarded as vulnerable groups for whom special government-sponsored programs needed to be created?
12. Discuss the government's role in the delivery and financing of health care with specific reference to the dichotomy between public health and private medicine.
13. Discuss why the structure of medical care delivery in the United States did not develop around a nucleus of primary care.
14. Explain how contract practice and prepaid group practice were the prototypes of today's managed care plans.
15. Discuss the main ways in which current delivery of health care has become corporatized.
16. How has the information revolution affected the practice of medicine?
17. In the context of globalization in health services, what are the four main economic relationships identified by Mutchnick and colleagues?

REFERENCES

Altman, S.H., and U.E. Reinhardt, eds. 1996. *Strategic choices for a changing health care system*. Chicago: Health Administration Press.

Anderson, O.W. 1990. *Health services as a growth enterprise in the United States since 1875*. Ann Arbor, MI: Health Administration Press.

Belsky, L. et al. 2004. The general agreement on trade in services: Implications for health policymakers. *Health Affairs* 23, no. 3: 137–145.

Blendon, R.J., and D.E. Altman. 2006. Voters and health care in the 2006 election. *The New England Journal of Medicine* 355, no. 18: 1928–1933.

Blendon, R.J., and J.M. Benson. 2001. Americans' views on health policy: A 50-year historical perspective. *Health Affairs* 20, no. 2: 33–46.

Blendon, R.J. et al. 2002. Where was health care in the 2002 election? *Health Affairs Web Exclusive* (December 11). *http://www.healthaffairs.org/WebExclusives/Blendon_Web_Excl_121102.htm.*

Bordley, J., and A.M. Harvey. 1976. *Two centuries of American medicine 1776–1976*. Philadelphia: W.B. Saunders Company.

Burns, J. 2004. Are nonprofit hospitals really charitable? Taking the question to the state and local level. *Journal of Corporate Law* 29, no. 3: 665-683.

Clark, C. 1998. *A bloody evolution: Human error in medicine is as old as the practice itself. The Washington Post*, 20 October, Z10.

Coggeshall, L.T. 1965. *Planning for medical progress through education*. Evanston, IL: Association of American Medical Colleges.

Davis, P. 1996. The fate of Blue Shield and the new Blues. *South Dakota Journal of Medicine* 49, no. 9: 323–330.

Duchon, L. et al. 2000. *Listening to workers: Findings from The Commonwealth Fund 1999 national survey of workers' health insurance*. New York: The Commonwealth Fund.

Duffy, J. 1971. Social impact of disease in the late 19th century. *Bulletin of the New York Academy of Medicine* 47: 797-811.

Employee Benefit Research Institute (EBRI). 2006. *2006 health confidence survey: Dissatisfaction with health care system doubles since 1998. http://www.ebri.org/pdf/notespdf/EBRI_Notes_11-20061.pdf.*

Falk, G. 1999. *Hippocrates assailed: The American health delivery system*. Lanham, MD: University Press of America, Inc.

Farmer, G.O., and J.H. Douglas. 2001. Physician "unionization"—A primer and prescription. *Florida Bar Journal* 75, no. 7: 37-42.

Foundation for Accountability. 2001. *Portrait of the chronically ill in America, 2001*. Portland, OR: The Foundation for Accountability, and Princeton, NJ: The Robert Wood Johnson Foundation.

Gabe, J. et al. 1994. *Challenging medicine*. New York: Routledge.

Goodman, J.C., and G.L. Musgrave. 1992. *Patient power: Solving America's health care crisis*. Washington, DC: CATO Institute.

Haber, S. 1974. The professions and higher education in America: A historical view. In *Higher education and labor markets*, ed. M.S. Gordon. New York: McGraw-Hill Book Co.

Haglund, C.L., and W.L. Dowling. 1993. The hospital. In *Introduction to health services*. 4th ed., eds. S.J. Williams and P.R. Torrens, 135–176. New York: Delmar Publishers.

Hamowy, R. 1979. The early development of medical licensing laws in the United States, 1875–1900. *Journal of Libertarian Studies* 3, no. 1: 73–119.

Health Insurance Association of America. 1991. *Source book of health insurance data*. Washington, DC.

Hoffman, C. et al. 1996. Persons with chronic conditions: Their prevalence and costs. *Journal of the American Medical Association* 276, no. 18: 1473–1479.

Kaptchuk, T.J., and D.M. Eisenberg. 2001. Varieties of healing 1: Medical pluralism in the United States. *Annals of Internal Medicine* 135, no. 3: 189-195.

Kardos, B.C., and A.T. Allen. 1993. Healthy neighbors: Exploring the health care systems of the United States and Canada. *Journal of Post Anesthesia Nursing* 8, no. 1: 48–51.

Kaufman, M. 1980. American medical education. In *The education of American physicians: Historical essays*, ed. R.L. Numbers. Berkeley and Los Angeles: University of California Press.

Koch, A.L. 1993. Financing health services. In *Introduction to health services*. 4th ed., eds. S.J. Williams and P.R. Torrens, 299–331. New York: Delmar Publishers.

Law, S.A. 1974. *Blue Cross: What went wrong?* New Haven, CT: Yale University Press.

Maheu, M.M. et al. 2001. *E-health, telehealth, and telemedicine: A guide to start-up and success*. San Francisco: Jossey-Bass.

Martensen, R.L. 1996. Hospital hotels and the care of the "worthy rich." *Journal of the American Medical Association* 275, no. 4: 325.

Mayer, T.R., and G.G. Mayer. 1984. *The health insurance alternative: A complete guide to health maintenance organizations*. New York: Putnam Publishing Group.

McDonnell, J. 2006. Is the medical world flattening? *Ophthalmology Times* 31, no. 19: 4.

Mongan, J.J. 1995. Anatomy and physiology of health reform's failure. *Health Affairs* 14, no. 1: 99–101.

Mutchnick, I.S. et al. 2005. Trading health services across borders: GATS, markets, and caveats. *Health Affairs—Web Exclusive* 24, suppl. 1: W5-42–W5-51.

Norcini, J.J., and P.E. Mazmanian. 2005. Physician migration, education, and health care. *Journal of Continuing Education in the Health Professions* 25, no. 1: 4–7.

Numbers, R.L. 1985. The third party: Health insurance in America. In *Sickness and health in America: Readings in the history of medicine and public health*, eds. J.W. Leavitt and R.L. Numbers. Madison: The University of Wisconsin Press.

Numbers, R.L., and J.H. Warner. 1985. The maturation of American medical science. In *Sickness and health in America: Readings in the history of medicine and public health*, eds. J.W. Leavitt and R.L. Numbers. Madison: The University of Wisconsin Press.

Potter, M.A., and B.B. Longest. 1994. The divergence of federal and state policies on the charitable tax exemption of nonprofit hospitals. *Journal of Health Politics, Policy and Law* 19, no. 2: 393–419.

Raffel, M.W. 1980. *The US health system: Origins and functions*. New York: John Wiley & Sons.

Raffel, M.W., and N.K. Raffel. 1994. *The US health system: Origins and functions*. 4th ed. Albany, NY: Delmar Publishers.

Richardson, J.T. 1945. *The origin and development of group hospitalization in the United States, 1890–1940* (University of Missouri Studies, Vol. XX, No. 3). Columbia: University of Missouri.

The Robert Wood Johnson Foundation. 1996. *Chronic care in America: A 21st century challenge*. Princeton, New Jersey: The Robert Wood Johnson Foundation.

Rosen, G. 1983. *The structure of American medical practice 1875–1941*. Philadelphia: University of Pennsylvania Press.

Rosenberg, C.E. 1979. The therapeutic revolution: Medicine, meaning, and social change in 19th-century America. In *The therapeutic revolution*, ed. M.J. Vogel. Philadelphia: The University of Pennsylvania Press.

Rosner, L. 2001. The Philadelphia medical marketplace. In *Major problems in the history of American medicine and public health*, eds. J.H. Warner and J.A. Tighe. Boston: Houghton Mifflin Company.

Rothstein, W.G. 1972. *American physicians in the nineteenth century: From sect to science*. Baltimore, MD: Johns Hopkins University Press.

Schoen, C. et al. 2000. A vote of confidence: Attitudes toward employer-sponsored health insurance. *Issue Brief*. New York, NY: The Commonwealth Fund.

Shryock, R.H. 1966. *Medicine in America: Historical essays*. Baltimore: The Johns Hopkins Press.

Skocpol, T. 1995. The rise and resounding demise of the Clinton plan. *Health Affairs* 14, no. 1: 66–85.

Smith, M.D. et al. 1992. Taking the public's pulse on health system reform. *Health Affairs* 11, no. 2: 125–133.

Somers, A.R., and H.M. Somers. 1977. *Health and health care: Policies in perspective*. Germantown, MD: Aspen Systems.

Starr, P. 1982. *The social transformation of American medicine*. Cambridge, MA: Basic Books.

Stevens, R. 1971. *American medicine and the public interest*. New Haven, CT: Yale University Press.

Stevens, R. 1989. *In sickness and in wealth*. New York: Basic Books.

Sultz, H.A., and K.M. Young. 1997. *Health care USA: Understanding its organization and delivery*. Gaithersburg, MD: Aspen Publishers, Inc.

Sydenstricker, E. 1933. *Recent trends in the United States*. New York: McGraw-Hill Co.

Turnock, B.J. 1997. *Public health: What it is and how it works*, 3–38. Gaithersburg, MD: Aspen Publishers, Inc.

Whitted, G. 1993. Private health insurance and employee benefits. In *Introduction to health services*. 4th ed., eds. S.J. Williams and P.R. Torrens, 332–360. New York: Delmar Publishers.

Williams, S.J. 1993. Ambulatory health care services. In *Introduction to health services*. 4th ed., eds. S.J. Williams and P.R. Torrens. New York: Delmar Publishers.

Williams, S.J. 1995. *Essentials of health services*, 108–134. Albany, NY: Delmar Publishers.

Wright, J.W. 1997. *The New York Times almanac*. New York: Penguin Putnam, Inc.

PART II

System Resources

Chapter 4

Health Services Professionals

Learning Objectives

- To recognize the various types of health services professionals and their training, practice requirements, and practice settings
- To differentiate between primary care and specialty care and find the causes for an imbalance between primary care and specialty care in the United States
- To learn about the extent of maldistribution in the physician labor force and to comprehend the reasons for such maldistribution
- To discover various remedies to help overcome the problems of physician imbalance and maldistribution
- To understand the role of nonphysician providers in health care delivery
- To identify allied health professionals and their role in health care delivery
- To discuss the functions and qualifications of health services administrators

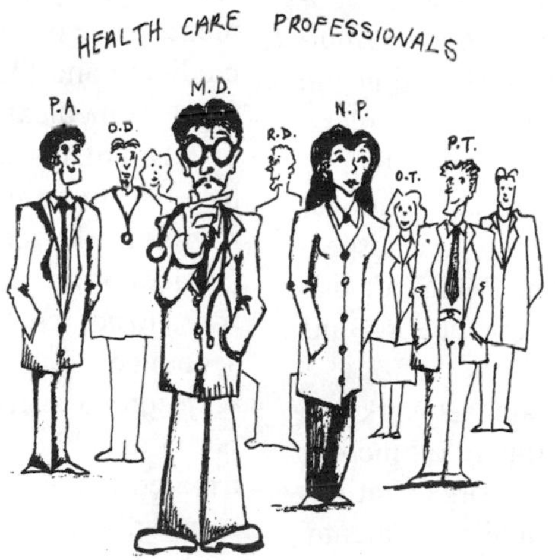

"Hmm, they're all beginning to look like me."

Introduction

The US health care industry is the largest and most powerful employer in the nation. It constitutes more than 3 percent of the total labor force in the United States. In terms of total economic output, in 2005, the health care sector in the United States contributed 16 percent to the gross domestic product (Catlin et al. 2007). The US Bureau of Labor Statistics projects seven of the 10 fastest-growing occupations for 2004–2014 are health related (2005). The health care sector of the US economy will continue to grow for two main reasons: (1) growth in population mainly due to immigration, and (2) aging of the population, especially as the baby boom generation starts to hit retirement age in 2011 and beyond. Consequently, the rate of growth in new jobs in health care occupations is projected to be around 29 percent between 2000 and 2010 (Mertz and O'Neil 2002).

Health services professionals include physicians, nurses, dentists, pharmacists, optometrists, psychologists, podiatrists, chiropractors, nonphysician practitioners (NPPs), health services administrators, and allied health professionals. The latter category incorporates therapists, laboratory and radiology technicians, social workers, and health educators. Health professionals are among the most well-educated and diverse of all labor groups. Almost all of these practitioner groups are now represented by their respective professional associations, which are listed in Appendix 4–A at the end of this chapter.

Health services professionals work in a variety of health care settings that include hospitals, managed care organizations (MCOs), nursing care facilities, mental health institutions, insurance firms, pharmaceutical companies, outpatient facilities, community health centers, migrant health centers, mental health centers, school clinics, physicians' offices, laboratories, voluntary health agencies, professional health associations, colleges of medicine and allied health professions, and research institutions. According to 2005 data (Table 4–1), most health professionals were employed by hospitals (42.6%), followed by nursing and personal care facilities (13%), and physicians' offices and clinics (11.4%).

Growth of health care services is closely linked to the demand for health services professionals. The expansion of the number and types of health services professionals closely follows population trends, advances in research and technology, disease and illness trends, and changes in health care financing and delivery of services. Population growth and the aging of the population enhance the demand for health services. Advances in scientific research contribute to new methods of preventing, diagnosing, and treating illness. New and complex medical techniques and machines are constantly introduced. Health services professionals must then learn how to use these innovations. Scientific research and technological development have contributed to specialization in medicine and the proliferation of different types of medical technicians. The changing patterns of disease from acute to chronic have led to an increasing emphasis on behavioral risk factors and the need for health services professionals who are formally prepared to address these health risks, their consequences, and their prevention. The widespread availability of insurance from both the public and private sectors has contributed to the increase in medical care utilization, which has created a greater demand for health services providers. Changes in reimbursement from retrospective to prospec-

Table 4–1 Persons Employed in Health Service Sites (141,730 employed civilians in 2005)

	2000		2005	
Site	Number of Persons (in thousands)	Percentage Distribution	Number of Persons (in thousands)	Percentage Distribution
All employed civilians	136,891	100.0	141,730	100.0
All health service sites	12,211	100.0	14,052	100.0
Offices and clinics of physicians	1,387	11.4	1,801	12.8
Offices and clinics of dentists	672	5.5	792	5.6
Offices and clinics of chiropractors	120	1.0	163	1.2
Offices and clinics of optomerists	95	0.8	98	0.7
Offices and clinics of other health practitioners	143	1.2	275	3.0
Outpatient care centers	772	6.3	901	6.4
Home health care services	548	4.5	795	5.7
Other health care services	1,027	8.4	1,045	7.4
Hospitals	5,202	42.6	5,719	40.7
Nursing care facilities	1,593	13.0	1,848	13.2
Residential care facilities, without nursing	652	5.3	615	4.4

Sources: Data from *Health, United States, 2006,* p. 353.

tive payment methods (see Chapter 6) and increased enrollment in managed care have contributed to a slowdown in cost escalation, a shift from inpatient to outpatient care, and an emphasis on the role of primary care providers.

This chapter provides an overview of the large array of health services professionals employed in a vast assortment of health delivery settings. It briefly discusses the training and practice requirements for the various health professionals, their major roles, the practice settings in which they are generally employed, and some critical issues concerning their professions. Emphasis is placed on physicians because they play a leading role in the delivery of health care. There has been increased recognition of the role NPPs play in the delivery of primary care services. Notably, now performed by other trained professionals are some basic medical functions that were traditionally performed by physicians alone.

The US health care delivery system is characterized by an imbalance between primary and specialty care services, which has contributed to an imbalance in the ratio of generalists to specialists. There is also a geographic maldistribution of practitioners. This chapter discusses the main causes for these disparities, and possible solutions are explored. Although a detailed discussion of primary care is provided in Chapter 7, this chapter highlights some of the main differences between primary and specialty care.

Physicians

In the delivery of health services, physicians play a central role by evaluating a patient's health condition, diagnosing abnormalities, and prescribing treatment. Some physicians are engaged in medical education and research to find new and better ways to control and cure health problems. A growing number are involved in the prevention of illness.

All states require physicians to be licensed in order to practice. The licensure requirements include graduation from an accredited medical school that awards a Doctor of Medicine (MD) or Doctor of Osteopathic Medicine (DO) degree, successful completion of a licensing examination governed by either the National Board of Medical Examiners or the National Board of Osteopathic Medical Examiners, and completion of a supervised internship/residency program (Stanfield 1995, 102–104). The term ***residency*** refers to graduate medical education in a specialty that takes the form of paid on-the-job training, usually in a hospital. Before entering a residency, which may last two to six years, most DOs serve a 12-month rotating internship after graduation.

The number of active physicians, both MDs and DOs, has steadily increased from 14.1 physicians per 10,000 population in 1950 to 27.4 per 10,000 population in 2001 (Table 4–2). Of the 144 medical schools in the United States, 125 teach allopathic medicine and award a Doctor of Medicine (MD) degree; 19 teach osteopathic medicine and award the Doctor of Osteopathic Medicine (DO) degree (US Bureau of Labor Statistics 2007).

Similarities and Differences between MDs and DOs

Both MDs and DOs use accepted methods of treatment, including drugs and surgery.

Table 4–2 Active Physicians, According to Type of Physician and Number per 10,000 Population

Year	All Active Physicians	Doctors of Medicine	Doctors of Osteopathy	Active Physicians per 10,000 Population
1950	219,900	209,000	10,900	14.1
1960	259,500	247,300	12,200	14.0
1970	326,500	314,200	12,300	15.6
1980	427,122	409,992	17,130	19.0
1990	567,610	539,616	27,994	22.4
1995	672,859	637,192	35,667	25.0
2000	772,296	727,573	44,723	27.0
2001	793,263	751,689	41,574	

Sources: Data from *Health, United States,* 1995, p. 220; *Health, United States,* 2002, p. 274; and *Health, United States, 2006*, p. 358.

The two differ mainly in their philosophies and approaches to medical treatment. ***Osteopathic medicine***, practiced by DOs, emphasizes the musculoskeletal system of the body, such as correction of joints or tissues. In their treatment plans, DOs stress preventive medicine, such as diet and the environment, as factors that might influence natural resistance. They take a holistic approach to patient care. MDs are trained in ***allopathic medicine***, which views medical treatment as active intervention to produce a counteracting reaction in an attempt to neutralize the effects of disease. MDs, particularly generalists, may also use preventive medicine along with allopathic treatments. About 5 percent of all active physicians are osteopaths (American Association of Colleges of Osteopathic Medicine 2007). About 40 percent of MDs and more than half of DOs work in primary care (US Bureau of Labor Statistics 2007).

Generalists and Specialists

Most DOs are generalists and most MDs are specialists. In the United States, physicians trained in family medicine/general practice, general internal medicine, and general pediatrics are considered primary care physicians (PCPs) or ***generalists*** (Rich et al. 1994). In general, PCPs provide preventive services (e.g., health examinations, immunizations, mammograms, Papanicolaou smears) and treat frequently occurring and less severe problems. Problems that occur less frequently, or that require complex diagnostic or therapeutic approaches, may be referred to specialists.

Physicians in nonprimary care specialties are referred to as ***specialists***. Specialists must seek certification in an area of medical specialization, which commonly requires additional years of advanced residency training followed by several years of practice in the specialty. A specialty board examination is often required as the final step in becoming a board certified specialist. The common medical specialties include anesthesiology, cardiology, dermatology, family medicine, internal medicine, neurology, obstetrics and gynecology, ophthalmology, pathology, pediatrics, psychiatry, radiology, and surgery. These specialties may be divided into six major functional groups: (1) the subspecialties of internal medicine; (2) a broad group of medical specialties; (3) obstetrics and gynecology; (4) surgery of all types; (5) hospital-based radiology, anesthesiology, and pathology; and (6) psychiatry (Cooper 1994). Exhibit 4–1 briefly explains these main specialties and some of the subspecialties. The distribution of physicians by specialty appears in Table 4–3. PCPs often coordinate referrals with members of these specialty groups based on an initial evaluation of the patient's medical needs.

Work Settings and Practice Patterns

Physicians practice in a variety of settings and arrangements. Some work in hospitals as medical residents or staff physicians. Others work in the public sector, such as federal government agencies, public health clinics, community and migrant health centers, schools, and prisons. Most physicians, however, are office-based practitioners and most physician contacts occur in physician offices. An increasing number of physicians are partners or salaried employees under contractual arrangements working in various outpatient settings, such as group practices, freestanding ambulatory care clinics, diagnostic imaging centers, and MCOs.

Exhibit 4–1 Definitions of Medical Specialties and Subspecialties

Allergists	Treat conditions and illnesses caused by allergies or related to the immune system
Anesthesiologists	Use drugs and gases to render patients unconscious during surgery
Cardiologists	Treat heart diseases
Dermatologists	Treat infections, growths, and injuries related to the skin
Emergency Medicine	Work specifically in emergency departments where they treat acute illnesses and emergency situations, e.g., trauma
Family Physicians	Involved with the care of the total patient and are prepared to handle most types of illnesses
General Practitioners	Similar to family physicians—examine patients or order tests and have X-rays done to diagnose illness and treat the patient
Geriatrician	Specializes in problems and diseases that accompany aging
Gynecologists	Involved in the health care and maintenance of the reproductive system of women
Internists	Treat diseases related to the internal organs of the body, e.g., conditions of the lungs, blood, kidneys, and heart
Neurologists	Treat disorders of the central nervous system and order tests necessary to detect diseases
Obstetricians	Work with women throughout their pregnancy, deliver infants, and care for the mother after the delivery
Oncologist	Specializes in the diagnosis and treatment of cancers and tumors
Ophthalmologists	Treat diseases and injuries of the eye
Otolaryngologists	Specialize in the treatment of conditions or diseases of the ear, nose, and throat
Pathologists	Study the characteristics, causes, and progression of diseases
Pediatricians	Provide care for children from birth to adolescence
Preventive Medicine	A specialty that includes occupational medicine, public health, and general preventive treatments
Psychiatrists	Help patients recover from mental illness and regain their mental health
Radiologists	Perform diagnosis and treatment by the use of X-rays and radioactive materials
Surgeons	Operate on patients to treat disease, repair injury, correct deformities, and improve the health of patients
General Surgeons	Perform many different types of surgery, usually of relatively low degree of difficulty
Neurologic Surgeons	Specialize in surgery of the brain, spinal cord, and nervous system
Orthopaedic Surgeons	Specialize in the repair of bones and joints
Plastic Surgeons	Repair malformed or injured parts of the body
Thoracic Surgeons	Perform surgery in the chest cavity, e.g., lung and heart surgery
Urologists	Specialize in conditions of the urinary tract in both sexes and of the sexual/reproductive system in males

Source: Adapted from P.S. Stanfield, *Introduction to the Health Professions,* 2nd ed., 1995, Jones and Bartlett Publishers, Boston, MA. www.jbpub.com. Reprinted with permission.

Table 4–3 Physicians, According to Activity and Place of Medical Education, 2004

Activity and Place of Medical Education	Numbers	Percentage	Distribution
Doctors of medicine (professionally active)*	744,143	100.0	
Place of medical education:			
US medical graduates	563,118	76.2	
International medical graduates	181,025	24.3	
Activity			
Patient care	700,287	100.0	
Office-based practice	538,538	76.9	100.0
General and family practice	73,234		13.6
Cardiovascular diseases	17,252		3.2
Dermatology	8,651		1.6
Gastroenterology	9,430		1.8
Internal medicine	101,776		18.9
Pediatrics	49,356		9.2
Pulmonary diseases	7,072		1.3
General surgery	25,229		4.7
Obstetrics and gynecology	33,811		6.3
Ophthalmology	16,304		3.0
Orthopaedic surgery	18,632		3.5
Otolaryngology	8,160		1.5
Plastic surgery	5,845		1.1
Urological surgery	8,793		1.6
Anesthesiology	29,984		5.6
Diagnostic radiology	16,828		3.1
Emergency medicine	18,961		3.5
Neurology	9,632		1.8
Pathology, anatomical/clinical	10,653		2.0
Psychiatry	25,998		4.8
Radiology	6,900		1.3
Other specialty	36,037		6.7
Hospital-based practice	161,749	23.1	100.0
Residents and interns	102,563		63.4
Full-time hospital staff	59,186		36.6

*Excludes inactive, not classified, and address unknown.

Source: Data from *Health, United States, 2006,* p. 356.

Figure 4–1 Ambulatory Care Visits to Physicians According to Physician Specialty, 2000.

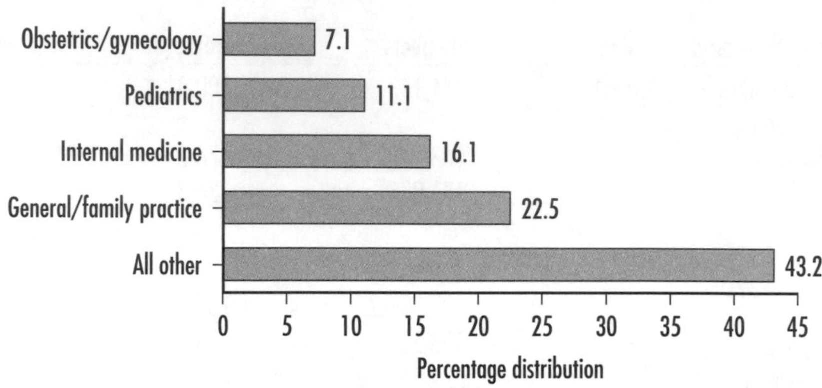

Source: Data from *Health, United States, 2002,* p. 244–245; 2006, pp. 327–328.

Figure 4–1 shows that, in 2004, physicians in general/family practice accounted for the greatest proportion of ambulatory care visits, followed by those in internal medicine and pediatrics.

Other medical practice characteristics appear in Table 4–4. For example, physicians in obstetrics and gynecology spent the most hours in patient care per week, even exceeding those in surgery. Surgeons, however, had the highest average annual net income ($269,400). Operating expenses and malpractice insurance premiums were the highest in obstetrics/gynecology.

Table 4–4 Medical Practice Characteristics by Selected Specialty, 1999

Characteristics	All Physicians	General/ Family Practice	Internal Medicine	Surgery	Pediatrics	Obstetrics/ Gynecology
Mean patient visits per week	106.7	122.9	103.0	95.8	120.5	101.8
Mean hours in patient care per week	51.6	50.6	54.2	53.3	49.5	59.0
Mean net income ($1,000) 1998	194.4	142.5	182.1	268.2	139.6	214.4
Mean liability premium ($1,000) 1998	16.8	10.9	16.5	22.8	9.0	35.8

Source: Data from *Statistical Abstracts of the United States: 2002,* p. 108.

Differences Between Primary and Specialty Care

Primary care may be distinguished from ***specialty care*** according to the time, focus, and scope of the services provided to patients. The five main areas of distinction are as follows:

1. In linear time sequence, primary care is first-contact care and is regarded as the portal to the health care system (Kahn et al. 1994). Specialty care, when needed, generally follows primary care.
2. In a managed care environment in which health services functions are integrated, primary care physicians serve as gatekeepers, an important role in controlling cost, utilization, and the rational allocation of resources. In the gatekeeping model, specialty care requires referral from a primary care physician.
3. Primary care is longitudinal (Starfield and Simpson 1993). In other words, primary care providers follow through the course of treatment and coordinate various activities, including initial diagnosis, treatment, referral, consultation, monitoring, and follow-up. Primary care providers serve as patient advisors and advocates (Williams 1994). Their coordinating role is especially important in the provision of continuing care for chronic conditions. Specialty care is episodic and thus more focused and intense.
4. Primary care focuses on the person as a whole, whereas specialty care centers on particular diseases or organ systems of the body. Primary care is holistic in nature and provides an integrating function. Patients often have multiple problems, a condition referred to as ***comorbidity***. In such cases, attention from a specialist focusing on one problem may make another problem worse. Primary care, in essence, seeks to balance the multiple requirements a patient's condition may call for, and refers patients to appropriate specialty care when needed. Specialty care, by contrast, tends to be limited to illness episodes, the organ system, or the disease process involved. Consequently, specialists such as oncologists and cardiologists deal only with specific diseases and body organs (Hibbard and Nutting 1991). Specialty care is also associated with secondary and tertiary levels of services (see *secondary care* and *tertiary care* in the Glossary).
5. The difference in scope is reflected in how primary and specialty care providers are trained. Primary care students spend a significant amount of time in ambulatory care settings, familiarizing themselves with a variety of patient conditions and problems. Students in medical subspecialties spend significant time in inpatient hospitals, where they are exposed to state-of-the-art medical technology.

The Expanding Role of Hospitalists

An increasing amount of inpatient medical care in the United States has been delivered by hospitalists, physicians who specialize in the care of hospitalized patients, since the mid-1990s (Schneller 2006). Hospitalists usually do not have a relationship with the patient prior to hospitalization. Essentially, the patient's primary care provider entrusts the oversight of the patient's care to a hospitalist upon admission, and patients return to their regular physicians after discharge (Freed 2004). Approximately 12,000 hospitalists currently practice in the United States, and it is estimated the field will soon grow to 30,000, exceeding the number of cardiologists (Sehgal 2006).

The initial shift toward hospitalist care was influenced by the desire of hospital leaders, HMOs, and medical groups to reduce inpatient costs without compromising quality or patient satisfaction. Later, published data provided evidence that using hospitalists was, in fact, achieving these goals (Wachter 2004). Initially, many primary care physicians, accustomed to the traditional method of rounding on their hospitalized patients, were skeptical about the role of hospitalists. PCPs voiced concerns about discontinuity of care and acceptance of the new practice by patients (Wachter 2004). However, these concerns were allayed by the late 1990s, when evidence had mounted in support of the quality and efficiency of care delivered by hospitalists (Wachter 2004). Recently, the debate over hospitalists has largely shifted from quality and efficiency to optimizing hospitalists' skills and expanding their roles (Sehgal 2006). Hospitalists are not yet certified as a distinct subspecialty of hospital medicine. However, hospitalists convene for large annual meetings, have their own textbook, their own journal (the *Journal of Hospital Medicine*), and their own specialty society (Sehgal 2006). It is expected their role in the American medical system will continue to increase in importance.

Some Key Issues in Medical Practice

Involvement in the Development of Clinical Practice Guidelines

Research has shown that the way physicians practice medicine and prescribe treatments for similar conditions varies significantly because clinical decisions made by physicians are not always based on strong evidence founded on clinical research (Field and Lohr 1992). Physicians have at their disposal an increasing number of therapeutic options because of the exponential growth in medical science and technology. On the other hand, increasing health care costs continue to threaten the viability of the health care delivery system. The responsibilities placed on physicians to perform difficult balancing acts between the availability of the most advanced treatment plans, uncertainties about their potential benefits, and whether the higher costs of treatment are justified have created a confusing environment. Hence, there is growing support for the development and refinement of standardized clinical guidelines to streamline clinical decision-making and improve quality of care (discussed in Chapter 12).

Involving physicians in the development of standardized practice guidelines will reduce the gap between methodological research and the implementation of research findings in actual practice (Deyo and Patrick 1995; Greenfield and Nelson 1992). Experiences in cost containment indicate that information, especially information not tailored to a specific practice environment, will not by itself change physician behavior and thereby improve the practice of health care or the people's health (Eisenberg 1986). It is also a mistake to expect clinical guidelines developed by nonpracticing "experts" to be implemented by practicing physicians.

Threat of Compromise

The development of managed care is likely to subject physicians to greater constraints in exercising their professional judgment than has traditionally been the case (Rodwin 1995). Managed care arrangements generally limit payments to participating physicians through capitation or discounted fees. Access to specialists is controlled by generalist gatekeepers, who are provided incentives to reduce inpatient care, X-rays, laboratory services, and specialist consultations (Foreman 1996). Increasingly, specialists are offered a single price for providing bundled services, such as cardiac diagnostics, surgeries, hospital services, and psychiatric care. With strong financial incentives pointing toward low and inexpensive utilization, some concerns exist that physicians' professional judgment and service quality may be compromised.

Lopsided Medical Training

The principal source of funding for graduate medical education is the Medicare program, which provides explicit payments to teaching hospitals for each resident in training. These payments exceed $7 billion per year, or more than $70,000 per resident per year (Council on Graduate Medical Education 2001). The government, however, does not mandate how these physicians should be trained. By contrast, in Great Britain, the government finances all residency slots and controls the number of positions by specialty. In Canada, the number of positions funded by the provincial ministries of health care is determined in negotiations between the medical schools, provincial governments, and physician associations.

Emphasis on hospital-based training in the United States has produced too many specialists. Also, research fellowships offered by the National Institutes of Health attract some physicians to medical research. Most of these physicians eventually become clinical specialists (Friedenberg 1996). In the meanwhile, the health care delivery system is evolving toward a primary care orientation. The result is that many physicians in the workforce today are ill-prepared to practice in the wellness-oriented, ambulatory-based environment (American Physical Therapy Association 1998).

Aggregate Physician Oversupply

Aided by tax-financed subsidies, the United States has experienced a sharp increase in its physician labor force. Between 1950 and 1990, the supply of physicians increased by 173 percent (Health Resources and Services Administration 1996), and has steadily increased since then (Figure 4–2). In 1950, there were 142 physicians per 100,000 population. By 2000, this number had increased to more than 270 per 100,000 population (Cooper et al. 2002). According to the Health Resources and Services Administration's Bureau of Health Professions, the number of active physicians under age 75 grew from approximately 756,000 in 2000 to approximately 817,500 in 2005. This number is expected to grow to 951,700 by 2020, if current trends continue (HRSA/BHP 2006). Current numbers far surpass the estimated 145 to 185 physicians per 100,000 population that the United States actually needs, according to the Council on Graduate Medical Education.

Figure 4–2 Supply of Physicians Including International Medical Graduates (IMGs) Per 100,000 Population, 1980–2000.

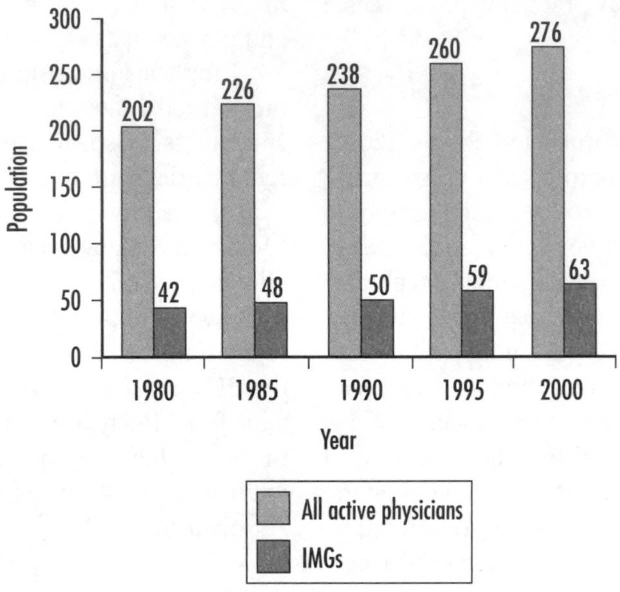

Source: Data from E.S. Salsberg and G.J. Forte, Trends in the physician workforce, 1980–2000, *Health Affairs* (September/October 2002), pp. 166, 168.

Current physician supply also exceeds future growth projections at least through 2010 (Institute for the Future 2000). The increasing participation of NPPs in delivering medical care will make the projected surpluses even greater.

The Balanced Budget Act of 1997 capped the number of residency positions for which Medicare would pay, and it required reductions in expenditures for medical residency training. The Pew Health Professions Commission (based at the Center for Health Professions at the University of California in San Francisco) has recommended a reduction of 25 percent in the number of residency positions (American Physical Therapy Association 1998).

A surplus of physicians leads to unnecessary increases in health care expenditures. A shortage, on the other hand, adversely affects the delivery of health services. The irony is that despite sharp increases in the aggregate surplus of physicians, physician shortages still exist in certain parts of the country. The shortages are caused by a maldistribution of physicians in terms of both geography and specialty. ***Maldistribution*** refers to either a surplus or a shortage of the type of physicians needed to maintain the health status of a given population at an optimum level.

Geographic Maldistribution

One of the ironies of excess physician supply is that localities outside metropolitan areas (that is, counties with <50,000 residents) continue to have a shortage of physicians. In the past two decades, diffusion of physicians from high- to low-supply regions has improved access to physicians in rural areas; however, the majority of additional physicians have located in areas with an already large supply of physicians (Goodman 2004). Between 1980 and 2000, the number of active allopathic nonfederal physicians in metropolitan areas increased by 260,000, or 74 percent. By contrast, the increase in physicians in nonmetropolitan areas was only 30,000, or 61 percent (Salsberg and Forte 2002). Of even greater concern, however, is the fact that in spite of the overall increase in the number of physicians, the ratio of generalists to population in nonmetropolitan areas has remained at about 5 per 10,000 (Colwill and Cultice 2003). Hence, access to primary care services in rural counties remains a major concern.

Physicians are more likely to concentrate in metropolitan and suburban areas than in rural and inner city areas because the former generally offer greater prospects for high income, professional interaction, access to modern facilities and technology, continuing education and professional growth, higher standards of living, and such social amenities as cultural diversity, recreational activities, and quality of education for children. Problems contributing to the difficulties in recruiting physicians in rural areas include long working hours, requirements to frequently be on call, smaller financial rewards, and a greater degree of professional isolation, such as limited access to high technology, which is more commonly available in large medical centers (Kohler 1994).

The basic source of the physician distribution problem in the United States, however, is a system that does not extend health care coverage to all Americans. The need for additional physicians is determined primarily based on the population's health care needs. Medical services, on the other hand, are delivered in a market that links delivery of services to people's ability to pay for them, mainly through health insurance. The need-based model assumes an even distribution of physicians in the projection of labor force requirements, but the market model is based on consumer demand factors. The inconsistency between the two models largely contributes to provider surpluses in metropolitan and suburban areas and to shortages in rural areas and inner cities. The problem of obtaining medical care in the underserved areas is further exacerbated by low rates of health insurance coverage, because of which many such areas lack the economic capacity to support additional physicians.

A variety of federal programs have demonstrated success in increasing the supply of primary care services available to underserved populations. Some of these programs are discussed in Chapter 11. They include the National Health Service Corps (which makes scholarship support conditional on a commitment to future service in an underserved area), the Migrant and Community Health Center Programs (designated to provide primary care services to the poor and underserved using federal grants), and the support of primary care training programs and Area Health Education Centers.

Other policy options include regulation of health care professions, reimbursement policies, targeted programs for underserved areas, and health professional schools (Cohen 1993; Kindig and Yan 1993; Weiner 1993; Wennberg et al. 1993). Regulations governing the health professions specify the types of tasks different practitioners are permitted to perform and the forms of supervision required for these tasks. Of particular significance is the expansion of the scope of practice for advanced nurses, such as nurse practitioners, physician assistants, and pharmacists. Such scope can include the right to prescribe drugs. The expanded role of nursing emerged as a viable option to remedy the many facets of the health labor force problem after research showed that the clinical skills of NPs were comparable to those of physicians when employed for conditions cared for by both. Patients also seemed to be more satisfied with the care received from NPs than with care received from physicians (Office of Technology Assessment 1986, 1991).

Reimbursement policies affect practice-related choices of current and future physicians. Typically, financial rewards in rural settings are lower, compared to more affluent urban areas. Hence, positive incentives are needed to attract professionals to underserved locations. Differential rewards to providers who choose to practice in less desirable areas or care for socially disadvantaged populations can be attractive to some physicians. Reimbursement is also crucial to nonphysician health professionals. A powerful incentive for attracting and retaining nurses with advanced training would be reimbursement rates that are comparable to those paid to physicians for the same procedures.

Research indicates that physicians' personal characteristics play a significant role in their practice location decision (Crandall et al. 1990; Eisenberg 1985; Samuels and Shi 1993). Physicians are more likely to be attracted to rural practice if they have a rural background or exposure to rural practice settings in their clinical training. To ensure a sufficient supply of rural physicians, a comprehensive approach is recommended. Such an approach would facilitate admission to medical schools for students from rural communities, foster premedical training in rural settings, and use rural preceptorships or externships by medical schools and rural residency training programs to expose students to medical practice in small towns and rural areas.

Targeted programs for underserved areas include setting up task forces or commissions, offices of rural health, and incentive programs to encourage health professionals to choose primary care and to practice in rural and underserved areas. Schools that train health professionals can promote rural-focused training programs, allocate more funds for family practice physician training, and incorporate the concerns of practicing in underserved areas into medical curricula. Appropriate training can help alleviate some of the preconceived deterrents to rural and inner city practice. Specific training can be directed at practice management, cost-effective care, preventive care, and the coordination of community resources and services. Continued efforts are needed for medical schools to find ways to recruit underserved minority groups, such as African Americans and Hispanics (see Table 4–5 for the racial distribution of medical school enrollment). Although various steps can be taken to address the issue, unfortunately, distributional shortages of physicians are likely to persist in many rural and selected inner city areas.

Specialty Maldistribution

Besides geographic maldistribution of physicians, a considerable imbalance exists between primary and specialty care in the United States. From 1979 to 1999, the supply of family practitioners per 100,000 people in the United States increased only 18 percent, whereas the supply of medical specialists increased by 118 percent (Goodman 2004). The supply of primary care physicians

Table 4–5 Percentage of Total Enrollment of Students for Selected Health Occupations, 2003–2004*

Race	Allopathic	Osteopathic	Dentistry	Pharmacy	Registered Nurses*
All races	100.0	100.0	100.0	100.0	100.0
White, non-Hispanic	63.0	73.8	65.6	58.4	81.0
Black, non-Hispanic	7.4	3.6	5.4	9.7	9.9
Hispanic	6.7	3.5	5.9	3.7	3.9
American Indian	0.9	0.7	0.4	0.4	0.8
Asian	20.3	15.4	22.7	20.9	4.4

*Registered nurses figures are for 1999–2000.

Source: Data from *Health, United States, 2006*, p. 361, and 2002, p. 276.

dropped sharply between 1949 and 1970, then experienced a slow decline until the early 1990s; it has been relatively stable since then (Figure 4–3). The number of positions filled in family practice residency programs showed an increase during the first few years of the 1990s, but there has been a slow decline since 1998 (Pugno et al. 2001). Other areas in primary care training show similar trends. The trends portray a declining interest in primary care among current medical graduates.

In the United States, approximately 40.8 percent of the physicians work in primary care and the remaining 59.2 percent are specialists, according to 2003 data from the American Medical Association (US Bureau of Labor Statistics 2007). In other industrialized countries, only 25 to 50 percent of physicians are specialists (Schroeder 1992). The delivery of health care in the United States has been moving toward the managed care model. HMOs reduce the demand for physician services, particularly for specialists' services. Escarce and colleagues (2000) concluded that faster HMO growth led to increases in the proportion of physicians who were generalists. They estimated that an increase in HMO penetration of 0.10 between 1986 and 1996 reduced the rate of increase in medical/surgical specialists by 10.3 percent and reduced the rate of increase in total physicians by 7.2 percent.

Specialty maldistribution has become ingrained in the US health care delivery system for three main reasons: medical technology, reimbursement methods and remuneration, and specialty-oriented medical education. On the other hand, the need for primary care physicians is determined mainly by the demographics of the general population.

The major driving force behind the increasing number of specialists is the development of medical technology. The rapid advances in medical technology have continuously expanded the diagnostic and therapeutic options at the disposal of specialists. Most hospitals with more than 100 beds try to become clinical centers offering medical services in all major specialty fields and, consequently, employ specialists in these

Figure 4–3 Trend of Primary Care Generalists of Medicine.

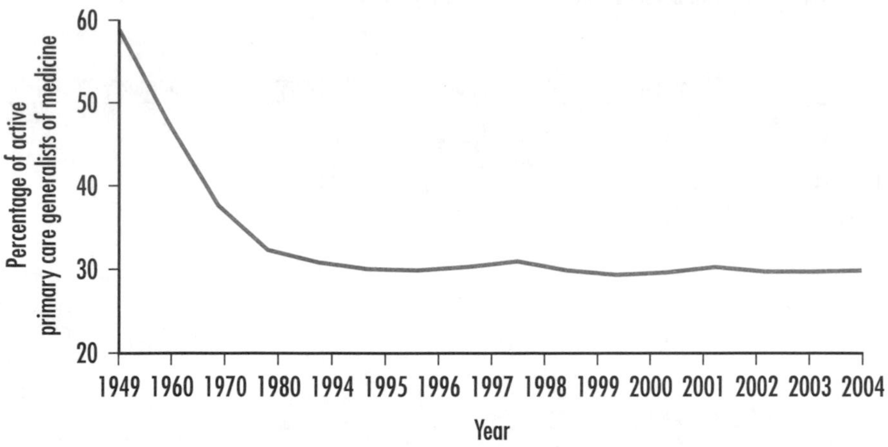

Sources: Data from National Center for Health Statistics, *Health, United States, 1995*. Hyattsville, MD: Public Health Service, 1996, p. 222; and *Health, United States, 2002*, Hyattsville, MD: Public Health Services, 1999, p. 273.

fields (Friedenberg 1996). Most patients, because they are shielded from the financial burden of health care, have the tendency to turn to physicians who provide them with the most up-to-date, sophisticated treatment. Because the population increases at a significantly slower rate than technological advancements, the gap between primary and specialty care workforces continues to expand.

Higher incomes of specialists relative to primary care physicians have also contributed to an oversupply of specialists. Traditionally, physician payments by Medicare have been based on historically determined practice costs (Hsiao et al. 1993; Physician Payment Review Commission 1993), which have been higher in specialist practice. In the last few years, reimbursement systems designed to increase payments to primary care physicians have been implemented. In the past, insurance companies also have more readily paid for hospital-based complex diagnostic and invasive procedures, whereas routine preventive visits and consultations have not been covered to the same extent. Although incomes for primary care physicians have increased in recent years, wide disparities between the incomes of generalists and specialists continue (Table 4–6).

Specialists not only earn higher incomes, but they also have more predictable work hours and enjoy higher prestige among their colleagues and the public at large (Rosenblatt and Lishner 1991; Samuels and Shi 1993). High status and prestige are accorded to tertiary care and specialties employing high technology. Such considerations have influenced career decisions of medical students. Other factors affecting their career choices are society's perception of value, intellectual challenge, and future financial rewards (Kassebaum 1994; Rosenthal et al. 1994; Steinbrook 1994). The medical education environment in the United States is organized according to specialties

Table 4–6 Median Total Compensation of Physicians by Specialty, 2004*

All physicians	$160,000
Anesthesiology	321,686
Surgery	282,504
Obstetrics/gynecology	247,348
Psychiatry	180,000
General internal medicine	166,420
Pediatrics	161,331
General/family practice	156,010

*Compensation is for physicians with over one year in specialty.

Source: Data from Occupational Outlook Handbook 2006–2007. *http://www.bls.gov/oco/ocos074.htm.* US Department of Labor, Bureau of Labor Statistics.

and controlled by those who have achieved leadership positions by demonstrating their abilities in narrow scientific or clinical areas. Medical education in the United States emphasizes technology, intensive procedures, and tertiary care settings, which are generally more appealing to medical students than more rudimentary primary care (Anonymous 1990; Verby et al. 1991).

The imbalance between generalists and specialists has several undesirable consequences. Having too many specialists has contributed to the high volume of intensive, expensive, and invasive medical services, and to the rise in health care costs (Greenfield et al. 1992; Rosenblatt 1992; Schroeder and Sandy 1993; Wennberg et al. 1993). A greater supply of surgeons increases the demand for initial contacts with surgeons (Escarce 1992). In fact, the rate of surgery in the United States grew at twice the rate of the population from 1979 to 1986 (Kramon 1991). Seeking care directly from specialists is often less effective than using primary care because the latter attempts to provide early intervention before complications develop (Starfield 1992; Starfield and Simpson 1993). Higher levels of primary care professionals are associated with lower overall mortality and lower death rates due to diseases of the heart and cancer (Shi 1992; 1994). PCPs have been the major providers of care to minorities, the poor, and people living in underserved areas (Ginzberg 1994; Starr 1982). Hence, the underserved populations suffer the most from shortages of PCPs.

The need to achieve a better balance in the distribution of primary care physicians and specialists is clear. Medical schools need to develop students' competencies in skills, values, and attitudes relevant to the practice of primary care. Their curricula can be oriented toward issues of special concern to generalists, such as outpatient experience; public health concepts; disease prevention; and cultural, ethnic, and population-specific knowledge. They must also provide students with opportunities to work with the poor, minorities, and the uninsured, and make such opportunities available in rural and other underserved areas (Verby et al. 1991).

The means of financing medical training and physician services could be improved. The system of graduate medical education payments through Medicare is based on the number of trainees. Such a payment system contributes to specialty-oriented training and creates disincentives for primary care training (Institute of Medicine 1989; Wennberg et al. 1993). Much of the clinical research, funded by the National Institutes of Health, is carried out under the auspices of specialty departments of medical schools (Ginzberg and Dutka 1989).

A possible solution is to provide priority funding for primary care residency slots and to encourage primary care–related research. Hospitals whose graduates enter primary care in underserved areas should be rewarded.

In the past, the predominance of fee-for-service reimbursement has favored the practice of specialists. Even though the growth of managed care has drastically curtailed the use of fee-for-service reimbursement, current payment structures still lack appropriate financial incentives aimed at advancing health promotion, disease prevention, and other primary care services. Financing of health care delivery also needs built-in incentives that stress primary care seeking behavior among patients. For example, primary care services should be exempt from deductibles and copayments. Such out-of-pocket costs discourage primary care seeking behavior and eventually lead to higher health care expenditures and poorer health outcomes (Lurie et al. 1986). Managed care has been successful in implementing disincentives for nonreferred specialist care; however, enrollees and physicians alike have increasingly protested such constraints.

A more rational referral system that achieves a reasonable division of work based on the frequency and severity of health problems in the served populations needs to be established (Starfield and Simpson 1993). The medical team that comprises both primary care physicians and specialists should discuss and decide on the specific division of labor.

International Medical Graduates

The ratio of international medical graduates (IMGs) to population has steadily grown (Figure 4–2), and so has the proportion of IMGs to total active physicians practicing in the United States (Figure 4–4). About 25 percent of professionally active physicians in the United States are IMGs, also known as foreign medical graduates (Cohen 2006).

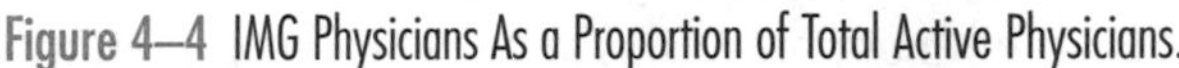

Figure 4–4 IMG Physicians As a Proportion of Total Active Physicians.

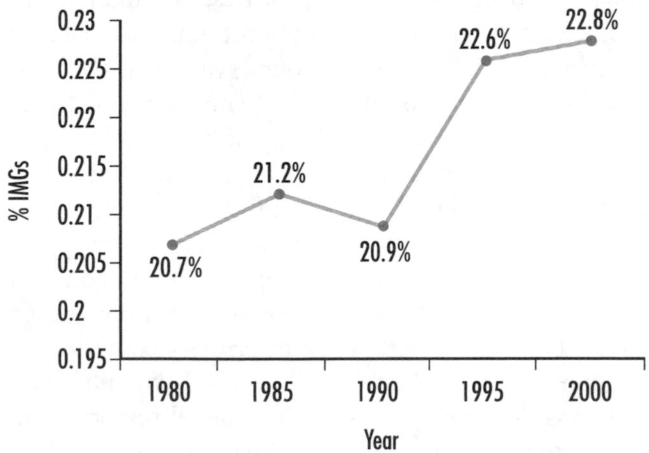

Source: Data from E.S. Salsberg and G.J. Forte, Trends in the physician workforce, 1980–2000, *Health Affairs* (September/October 2002), pp. 166, 168.

This translates to more than 150,000 active IMGs in the United States physician workforce (Gastel 2006). An estimated one-fourth of all residency positions are filled by IMGs (Mullan 1999), and an increasing number of IMGs are filling family practice residency slots (Koehn et al. 2002). In 1995 only 6.3 percent of IMGs entered family practice residencies; by 2003, the number increased to 15.8 percent (Boulet 2006). A review of research to date yields ambiguous conclusions as to whether IMGs provide medical care equal in quality (or of a lesser quality) to that given by US graduates (Mick and Comfort 1997; Rao et al. 2007). It has been commonly thought that many IMGs establish their practices in localities generally shunned by US medical graduates, and thus help reduce geographic maldistribution of physician supply. In recent years, reliance of hospitals on IMGs has reached unprecedented levels, but there are indications that although many IMGs may train in hospitals located in underserved areas, they ultimately relocate their practices to more lucrative areas (Mullan et al. 1995). More recent evidence confirms that primary care IMGs are no more likely than primary care US medical graduates to practice in rural underserved areas (Fink et al. 2003). There are also indications that the ratio of specialists to generalists is more imbalanced among IMGs than it is among US graduates (Politzer 1998). Hence, under current policies, IMGs are not the solution to the problems of specialty and geographic maldistribution of physicians. Pointing to the physician surplus, specialty imbalance, and growing costs of graduate medical education in the United States, organizations such as the Institute of Medicine, the Pew Health Professions Commission, the Council on Graduate Medical Education, and a consortium of professional medical groups led by the Association of American Medical Colleges have all called for reductions in the number of IMGs in residency training (Mick and Comfort 1997).

Dentists

Dentists are the major providers of dental care. All dentists must be licensed to practice. The licensure requirements include graduation from an accredited dental school that awards a Doctor of Dental Surgery (DDS) or Doctor of Dental Medicine (DMD) degree and successful completion of both written and practical examinations. Some states require dentists to obtain a specialty license before practicing as a specialist in that state (Stanfield 1995, 110–113). Nine specialty areas are recognized by the American Dental Association: orthodontics (straightening teeth), oral and maxillofacial surgery (operating on the mouth and jaws), oral and maxillofacial radiology (producing and interpreting images of the mouth and jaws), pediatric dentistry (dental care for children), periodontics (treating gums), prosthodontics (making artificial teeth or dentures), endodontics (root canal therapy), public health dentistry (community dental health), and oral pathology (diseases of the mouth). The growth of dental specialties is influenced by technological advances including: implant dentistry, laser-guided surgery, orthognathic surgery for the restoration of facial form and function, new metal combinations for use in prosthetic devices, new bone graft materials in "tissue-guided regeneration" techniques, and new materials and instruments.

The major roles of dentists are to diagnose and treat dental problems related to the teeth, gums, and tissues of the mouth. Many dentists are involved in the prevention of dental decay and gum disease. Dental prevention includes regular cleaning of teeth and educating patients on proper dental hygiene. Water fluoridation programs have significantly reduced the rate of caries in children. Dentists also spot symptoms that require treatment by a physician. Dentists employ dental hygienists and assistants to perform many of the preventive and routine care services.

Dental hygienists provide preventive dental care, including cleaning teeth and educating patients on proper dental care. Dental hygienists must be licensed to practice. The licensure requirements include graduation from an accredited school of dental hygiene and successful completion of both a national board written examination and a state or regional clinical examination. Many states require further examination on legal aspects of dental hygiene practice. Dental hygienists usually work in dental offices.

Dental assistants work for dentists in the preparation, examination, and treatment of patients. Dental assistants do not have to be licensed to work; however, formal training programs that offer a certificate or diploma are available. Dental assistants typically work alongside dentists.

Most dentists practice in private offices as solo or group practitioners. As such, dental offices are operated as private businesses, and dentists often perform business tasks, such as staffing, financing, purchasing, leasing, and work scheduling. Some dentists work in dental clinics in private companies, retail stores, franchised dental outlets, or MCOs. Group dental practices, offering lower overhead and increased productivity, have slowly grown. The federal government also employs dentists mainly in the hospitals and clinics of the Department of Veterans Affairs and the US Public Health Service. Median annual earnings of salaried dentists were $129,920 in 2004 (US Bureau of Labor Statistics 2007).

The emergence of employer-sponsored dental insurance caused an increased demand for dental care because it enabled a greater segment of the population to afford dental care. The demand for dentists will continue to grow with an increase in populations having high dental needs, such as the elderly, the handicapped, the homebound, and patients with HIV (human immunodeficiency virus), and an increase in public awareness of the importance of dental care toward general health status. Demand will also be affected by the fairly widespread appeal of cosmetic and esthetic dentistry, the prevalence of dental insurance plans, and the inclusion of dental care as part of many public-funded programs, such as Head Start, Medicaid, community and migrant health centers, and maternal and infant care.

Pharmacists

The traditional role of ***pharmacists*** has been to dispense medicines prescribed by physicians, dentists, and podiatrists, and to provide consultation on the proper selection and use of medicines. All states require a license to practice pharmacy. The licensure requirements include graduation from an accredited pharmacy program that awards a Bachelor of Pharmacy or Doctor of Pharmacy (PharmD) degree, successful completion of a state board examination, and practical experience or completion of a supervised internship (Stanfield 1995, 142–147). After 2005, the bachelor's degree was phased out, and a PharmD requiring six years of postsecondary education became the standard. The median annual earnings of pharmacists in 2004 were $84,900 (US Bureau of Labor Statistics, 2007).

Although most pharmacists are generalists, dispensing drugs and advising providers and patients, some become specialists. Pharmacotherapists specialize in drug therapy and work closely with physicians. Nutrition-support pharmacists determine and prepare drugs needed for nutritional therapy. Radiopharmacists or nuclear pharmacists produce radioactive drugs used for patient diagnosis and therapy.

Most pharmacists hold salaried positions and work in community pharmacies that are independently owned or are part of a national drugstore, grocery store, or department store chain. Pharmacists are also employed by hospitals, MCOs, home health agencies, clinics, government health services organizations, and pharmaceutical manufacturers.

The role of pharmacists has expanded over the last two decades from primarily preparing and dispensing prescriptions to include drug product education and serving as experts on specific drugs, drug interactions, and generic drug substitution. Pharmacists play a critical role in promoting rational drug use and effective drug management (Passmore and Kailis 1994). Under the Omnibus Budget Reconciliation Act of 1990, pharmacists are required to give consumers information about drugs and their potential misuse. This educating and counseling role of pharmacists is broadly referred to as pharmaceutical care. The American Council on Pharmaceutical Education (ACPE) (1992) defined ***pharmaceutical care*** as, "a mode of pharmacy practice in which the pharmacist takes an active role on behalf of patients, by assisting prescribers in appropriate drug choices, by effecting distribution of medications to patients, and by assuming direct responsibilities collaboratively with other health care professionals and with patients to achieve the desired therapeutic outcome." This concept entails a high level of drug knowledge, clinical skill, and independent judgment, and requires that pharmacists share with other health professionals the responsibility for optimizing the outcome of patients' drug therapy, including health status, quality of life, and satisfaction (Helper and Strand 1990; Schwartz 1994; Strand et al. 1991). Pharmacists inform physicians of patient compliance, achievement of therapeutic outcome, and potential drug interactions (Marcrom et al. 1992, 50). Pharmacists identify and prevent potential drug-related problems and resolve actual drug-related problems (Morley and Strand 1989, 328).

Another area in which pharmacists are receiving broadened clinical involvement is referred to as "disease management." In about half the states, pharmacists now have the authority to initiate or modify drug treatment, as long as they have collaborative agreements with physicians. For example, a stroke patient who needs blood thinning medication might walk into the drugstore for an assessment and walk out with a different dosage. Most other states are weighing giving pharmacists similar authority. Other areas in which pharmacists are expected to play an expanded role include management of diabetes, asthma, high cholesterol, and hypertension (Berner 1999).

Other Doctoral-Level Health Professionals

In addition to physicians, dentists, and some pharmacists, other health professionals have doctoral education, including optometrists, psychologists, podiatrists, and chiropractors.

Optometrists provide vision care, such as examination, diagnosis, and correction of vision problems. They must be licensed to practice. The licensure requirements include the possession of a Doctor of Optometry (OD) degree and passing a written and clinical state board examination. Most optometrists work in solo or group practices. Some work for the government, MCOs, optical stores, or vision care centers as salaried employees.

Psychologists provide patients with mental health care. They must be licensed or certified to practice. The ultimate recognition is the diplomate in psychology, which requires a Doctor of Philosophy (PhD) or Doctor of Psychology (PsyD) degree, a minimum of five years' postdoctoral experience, and the successful completion of an examination by the American Board of Examiners in Professional Psychology. Psychologists may specialize in several areas, such as clinical, counseling, developmental, educational, engineering, personnel, experimental, industrial, psychometric, rehabilitation, school, and social domains (Stanfield 1995, 280–282).

Podiatrists treat patients with diseases or deformities of the feet, including performing surgical operations, prescribing medications and corrective devices, and administering physiotherapy. They must be licensed to practice. Requirements for licensure include completion of an accredited program that awards a Doctor of Podiatric Medicine (DPM) degree and passing a national examination by the National Board of Podiatry. Most podiatrists work in private practice. Some are salaried employees of health service organizations.

Chiropractors provide treatment to patients through chiropractic (done by hand) manipulation, physiotherapy, and dietary counseling. They typically help patients with neurological, muscular, and vascular disturbances. Chiropractic care is based on the belief that the body is a self-healing organism. Chiropractors do not prescribe drugs or perform surgery. Chiropractors must be licensed to practice. Requirements for licensure include completion of an accredited program that awards a four-year Doctor of Chiropractic (DC) degree and passing an examination by the state chiropractic board. Most chiropractors work in private solo or group practice.

Nurses

Nurses constitute the largest group of health care professionals. The nursing profession developed around hospitals after World War I, and it primarily attracted women. Before World War I, more than 70 percent of nurses worked in private duty, either in patients' homes or for private pay patients in hospitals. Hospital-based nursing flourished after the war as the effectiveness of nursing care became apparent. Federal support of nursing education increased after World War II, represented by the Nursing Training Act of 1964, the Health Manpower Act of 1968, and the Nursing Training Act of 1971, but state funding remains the primary source of financial support for nursing schools.

Nurses are the major caregivers of sick and injured patients, addressing their physical, mental, and emotional needs. All states require nurses to be licensed to practice. Nurses can be licensed in more than one state through examination or endorsement of a license issued by another state. The licensure requirements include graduation from an approved nursing program and successful completion of a national examination. Educational preparation distinguishes between two levels of nurses. ***Registered nurses*** (RNs) must complete an associate's degree

(ADN), a diploma program, or a baccalaureate degree (BSN). ADN programs take about two to three years and are offered by community and junior colleges. Diploma programs take two to three years and are offered by hospitals. BSN programs take four to five years and are offered by colleges and universities (Stanfield 1995, 126–199). ***Licensed practical nurses*** (LPNs)—called licensed vocational nurses (LVNs) in some states—must complete a state-approved program in practical nursing and a national written examination. Most practical nursing programs last about one year and include classroom study as well as supervised clinical practice.

Nurses work in a variety of settings, including hospitals, nursing homes, private practice, ambulatory care centers, community and migrant health centers, emergency medical centers, MCOs, work sites, government and private agencies, clinics, schools, retirement communities, rehabilitation centers, and as private-duty nurses in patients' homes. Nurses are often classified according to the settings in which they work: hospital nurses, long-term care nurses, public health nurses, private duty nurses, office nurses, and occupational health or industrial nurses. Head nurses act as supervisors of other nurses. RNs supervise LPNs.

Since the mid-1980s, minimizing inpatient hospital stays has been increasingly emphasized. Reduction in hospital length of stay and continued hospital downsizing had temporarily reduced the demand for nurses. However, since hospitals now treat much sicker patients than before, more nurses are needed per unit, and their work has become more intensive. In addition, the remarkable growth in alternative settings has created new opportunities for nursing employment. Patients discharged from hospitals earlier than usual need to receive extended treatments in various settings, including long-term care, home care, and outpatient care. The growing opportunities for RNs in supportive roles, such as case management, utilization review, quality assurance, and prevention counseling, have also expanded the demand for their services. Estimates show a current national shortfall of 110,700 RNs, and roughly 120,000 trained RNs are not working in nursing (Sochalski 2002). Projections of the future nursing shortage indicate there will be a deficit of 340,000 nurses in 2020 (Auerbach 2007). Based on these projections of future demand coupled with falling enrollments in nursing schools, some have painted a dire picture. Sluggish wages, low levels of job satisfaction, and inadequate career mobility are believed to pose some major impediments to attracting and retaining nurses (Sochalski 2002). The Institute for the Future (2000), however, predicts that the future supply of RNs would be sufficient to respond to increased demands. Employment for RNs as well as licensed practical nurses is expected to grow in nonhospital settings, such as nursing homes, outpatient clinics, and home health care. The US Bureau of Labor Statistics reports registered nurses are projected to create the second largest number of new jobs among all occupations through 2014 (2007).

Recognizing the looming nursing shortage, President Bush signed the Nurse Reinvestment Act of 2002 (PL 107–205), commonly referred to as the NRA. The law authorizes a variety of grants and scholarships to attract and keep nurses in the field. Most of the funding will go to nursing schools, but hospitals will benefit directly from grants that will encourage nurses to advance their careers through further education and training, nurse internships, and retention programs that enhance the role of nurses in the workplace (Duff 2002). Nurses have been active in lobbying members of Congress to appropriate sufficient funding for the NRA, which has proven challenging in the face of many competing budget priorities. For FY 2007, the American Nursing Association called for $175 million for NRA programs, an increase of $25 million from FY 2006. However, the funding bill approved by the House Appropriations Committee contained no increase for the NRA in FY 2007 (McKeon 2006).

To make the nursing profession more attractive, health services organizations need to initiate measures such as creating incentive packages to attract new nurses, increasing pay and benefits of current nurses, introducing more flexible work schedules, awarding tuition reimbursement for continuing education, and providing on-site day care assistance. The role of nurses has undergone a significant change. To reduce their subservience to physicians, nurses are clarifying their relationship to physicians within the context of clinical decision-making. The growing opportunities for RNs in supportive roles, such as case management, utilization review, quality assurance, and prevention counseling, have not only expanded the demand for their services but also given them greater autonomy.

Advanced Practice Nurses

The term ***advanced practice nurse*** (APN) is a general name for nurses who have education and clinical experience beyond that required of an RN. APNs include four areas of specialization in nursing (Cooper et al. 1998): clinical nurse specialists (CNSs), certified registered nurse anesthetists (CRNAs), nurse practitioners (NPs), and certified nurse midwives (CNMs). NPs and CNMs are also categorized as NPPs and will be discussed in the next section. Besides being direct caregivers, APNs perform other professional activities, such as collaborating and consulting with other health care professionals; educating patients and other nurses; collecting data for clinical research projects; and participating in the development and implementation of total quality management programs, critical pathways, case management, and standards of care (Grossman 1995).

The main difference between CNSs and NPs is that CNSs work in hospitals, whereas NPs work mainly in primary care settings. CNSs can specialize in specific fields, such as oncology, neonatal health, cardiac care, or psychiatric care. Examples of their functions in an acute care hospital include admission histories and physical assessments, adjusting IV infusion rates, pain management, managing resuscitation orders, removing intracardiac catheters, and ordering routine laboratory tests and radiographic examinations. They generally do not have the legal authority to prescribe drugs. NPs, on the other hand, may prescribe drugs in most states. CRNAs are trained to manage anesthesia care during surgery, and CNMs deliver babies and manage the care of mothers and healthy newborns before, during, and after delivery.

The requirements for becoming an APN vary greatly from state to state. In general, the designation requires a graduate degree in nursing or certification in an advanced practice specialty area.

Nonphysician Practitioners

The terms ***nonphysician practitioners*** (NPPs), nonphysician clinicians (NPCs), and midlevel providers (MLPs) refer to clinical professionals who practice in many of the areas similar to those in which physicians practice, but who do not have an MD or a DO degree. NPPs receive less advanced training than physicians but more training than RNs. They are also referred to as ***physician extenders*** because in the delivery of primary care they can, in many instances, substitute for physicians. However, they do not engage in the entire range of primary care or deal with complex cases requiring the expertise of a physician (Cooper et al. 1998). Hence, NPPs often work in close consultation with physicians. NPPs typically include physician assistants (PAs), NPs, and CNMs. NPs work predominantly in primary care, whereas PAs are evenly divided between primary care and specialty care. In 2004, there were about 62,000 jobs that employed PAs in the United States (US Bureau of Labor Statistics 2007). The number of PA jobs is greater than the number of PAs, because about 15 percent of PAs work several jobs. As of 2006, there were approximately 115,000 NPs in the United States (American Association of Nurse Practitioners 2007). In addition, there are roughly 8,000 CNMs in the United States.

The American Academy of Physician Assistants (1986) defines ***physician assistants*** "as part of the healthcare team . . . [who] work in a dependent relationship with a supervising physician to provide comprehensive care" (p. 3). PAs are licensed to perform medical procedures only under the supervision of a physician. PAs assist physicians in the provision of care to patients. The supervising physician may be either on-site or off-site. The major services provided by PAs include evaluation, monitoring, diagnostics, therapeutics, counseling, and referral (Fizgerald et al. 1995). They practice in offices, hospitals, MCOs, clinics, nursing homes, mental health facilities, rehabilitation centers, community and migrant health centers, and government institutions. As of 2005, 135 accredited PA training programs were operating in the United States, with a steady growth in enrollment (US Bureau of Labor Statistics 2007). PA programs award bachelor's degrees, certificates, associate degrees, or master's degrees. The mean length of the program is 26 months (Hooker and Berlin 2002). PAs are certified by the National Commission on Certification of Physician Assistants. In most states, PAs have the authority to prescribe medications.

NPs constitute the largest group of NPPs and the group that has undergone the most growth (Cooper et al. 1998). Close to 6,000 new NPs are trained every year in 325 colleges and universities (American Association of Nurse Practitioners 2007). The American Nurses' Association defines ***nurse practitioners*** as individuals who have completed a program of study leading to competence as RNs in an expanded role. The training of NPs may be a certificate program (at least nine months in duration) or a master's degree program (two years of full-time study). States vary with regard to licensure and accreditation requirements. Most NPs are now trained in master's or postmaster's nursing programs. In addition, NPs must complete clinical training in direct patient care. Certification examinations are offered by the American Nurses Credentialing Center, the American Academy of Nurse Practitioners, and specialty nursing organizations. One of the main differences between the practice orientation of NPs and PAs is that NPs are oriented toward a nursing paradigm that emphasizes health promotion and education. PAs, on the other hand, are more directed toward a medical model of practice that focuses on disease (Hooker and McCaig 2001). NPs spend extra time with patients to make them understand the need to take responsibility for their own health. Their traditional nursing role has expanded to include taking patients' comprehensive health histories, assessing health status, performing physical examinations, and formulating and managing a care regimen for acute and chronically ill patients. NPs are prepared to practice independently of physicians; however, physicians are consulted when patients' conditions require treatment beyond NPs' expertise. NP specialties include pediatric, family, adult, psychiatric, and geriatric programs. NPs are particularly valuable in the outpatient settings where, for many patients, they are the first point of contact with the health care system. Another area where they provide service is nursing homes (Brody et al. 1976). They ensure the delivery of continuous comprehensive health care, and they enhance compliance with the treatment regimen. NPs have statutory prescribing authority in almost all states. NPs can also receive direct reimbursement as providers under the Medicaid and Medicare programs.

Certified nurse midwives are RNs with additional training from a nurse-midwifery program in areas such as maternal and fetal procedures, maternity and child nursing, and patient assessment (Endicott 1976). CNMs deliver babies, provide family planning education, manage gynecological and obstetric care, and can be used as substitutes for obstetricians/gynecologists in prenatal and postnatal care. They are certified by the American College of Nurse-Midwives (ACNM) to provide care for normal expectant mothers. They refer abnormal or high-risk patients to obstetricians or jointly manage the care of such patients. There are approximately 45 ACNM accredited nurse-midwifery education programs in the United States (US Bureau of Labor Statistics 2007). Midwifery has never assumed the central role in the management of pregnancies in the United States that it has in Europe (Wagner 1991). Physicians, mainly specialist obstetricians, attend most deliveries in the United States, but some evidence indicates that for low-risk pregnancies, CNMs are much less likely to use a variety of technical tools to monitor or modify the course of labor. Patients of CNMs are less likely to be continuously electronically monitored, to have induced labor, or to receive epidural anesthesia. These differences are associated with lower Caesarean section rates and less resource use, such as hospital stay, operating room costs, and use of anesthesia staff (Rosenblatt et al. 1997).

Value of NPP Services

Efforts to formally establish the roles of NPs, PAs, and CNMs as nonphysician health care providers began in the late 1960s in recognition of the fact that they could improve access to primary care, especially in rural areas. Studies have confirmed the efficacy of NPPs as health care providers. According to a report generated by the Office of Technology Assessment (1986), NPs and PAs often render care equivalent in quality to that provided by physicians. Many other studies have demonstrated that NPPs can provide both high-quality and cost-effective medical care (Hooker 2006; Abdellah 1982; Bessman 1974; Garrard et al. 1990; Lawrence 1978; Ostwald and Abanobi 1986; Sox 1979) because they show greater personal interest in patients and cost significantly less (Sellards and Mills 1995). Moreover, NPs have been noted to have better communication and interviewing skills than physicians do. These skills are considered particularly important in community and migrant health centers in assessing patients who are predominantly of minority origin and often have little education (Brody et al. 1976). Clients are more satisfied with NPs than with physicians because NPs are more likely to do comprehensive examinations. NPPs are also more likely to be employed in rural and medically underserved areas than in urban areas (Hooker 2006; Moscovice and Rosenblatt 1979), which alleviates some of the problems created by the geographic maldistribution of physicians. NPs are essential primary care providers to vulnerable populations served in community health centers and in nurse-managed health centers. CNMs are considered effective in providing access to obstetrical and prenatal services in rural and poor communities (Institute of Medicine 1985; Rosenbaum 1995). The Office of Technology Assessment (1986) report concluded that CNMs manage routine pregnancies as competently as, if not better than, physicians. Patients cared for by CNMs have shorter waiting times for visits, have shorter hospitalizations, and are more likely to express satisfaction with their care. Community Health Plan, an MCO, gave credit to its CNMs for bringing the plan's Caesarean section rate down to 15 percent, which is almost 10 percent lower than the national average (Neimark 1997).

The role of NPPs has grown along with the growth of managed care. Especially repetitive technical tasks, such as the use of flexible sigmoidoscopy to screen for colon cancer, can be performed effectively and less expensively by specially trained nonphysicians. Nonphysicians could also probably manage quick turnover cases in emergency departments, especially when a patient's life is not in jeopardy. In occupational medicine, such as preemployment physicals, drug testing, and disability and workers' compensation evaluations, an NP can probably handle 80 to 90 percent of the tasks performed by physicians. Moreover, NPs and PAs cost about 40 percent of what physicians cost. Hence, utilization of nonphysician providers adds value to the delivery system. MCOs are particularly keen on adopting such a strategy. Some physicians are understandably concerned about their job security and resist the trend, but at this stage, physicians are unable to block the move toward using midlevel practitioners in expanded roles (Appleby 1995). On the other hand, group practices with significant managed care contracts can trim their operating costs by employing NPPs and retain as profit a larger slice of the capitated fees paid to them by MCOs.

NPPs are particularly needed to serve the growing number of medically disadvantaged Americans. Expansion of insurance to children through the State Children's Health Insurance Program (SCHIP) and the growth of community health centers have created an increased demand for primary care providers to serve vulnerable populations. In underserved communities, NPPs fill a significant void in the delivery of quality primary care.

Among the issues that need to be resolved before NPPs can be used to their full potential are legal restrictions to practice, reimbursement policies, and relationships with physicians (Samuels and Shi 1993). The lack of autonomy to practice is a great legislative barrier facing midlevel providers. Most states require physician supervision as a condition for practice. In some states, midlevel providers lack prescriptive authority. NPPs also face reimbursement barriers. Reimbursement for their services is generally indirect; that is, payments are made to the physicians with whom they practice. Also, NPPs' opinions are not actively sought in making medical policies and decisions.

With some caution, the American Medical Association has supported the expanded role of NPPs. As NPPs and certain allied health professionals assume greater roles and perform more specialized tasks, replacing better-trained physicians in some instances, necessary safeguards must be implemented to ensure that the quality of care is not compromised (Appleby 1995).

Allied Health Professionals

In the early part of the 20th century, the health care provider workforce consisted of physicians, nurses, pharmacists, and optometrists. As knowledge in health sciences expanded, technology began to play a major role in the diagnosis and treatment of illness. The growth in technology and specialized interventions subsequently placed greater demands on the time physicians and nurses spent with their patients. Such time constraints, as well as the limitations in learning new skills, created a need to train other professionals who could serve as adjuncts to, or as substitutes for, physicians and nurses. These professionals received specialized training, and their clinical interventions were meant to complement the work of physicians and nurses. Thus, physicians and nurses were relieved of time pressures so they could attend to functions that only they had the expertise to perform. The extra time also allowed them to keep abreast of the latest advances in their disciplines.

As noted in Section 701 of the Public Health Service Act, an allied health professional is someone who has received a certificate; associate's, bachelor's, or master's degree; doctoral level preparation; or post-baccalaureate training in a science related to health care and has responsibility for the delivery of health or related services. These services may include those associated with the identification, evaluation, and prevention of diseases and disorders, dietary and nutritional services, rehabilitation, or health system management. Further, these professionals are other than those who have received a degree of MD, DO, dentistry, veterinary medicine, optometry, podiatry, DC, or pharmacy; a graduate degree in health administration; a degree in clinical psychology; or a degree equivalent to one of these. In broad terms, ***allied health*** includes many health-related areas.

Allied health professionals constitute approximately 60 percent of the US health care workforce. Allied health professionals can be divided into two broad categories: technicians/assistants and therapists/technologists. The main allied health professions in the United States are listed in Exhibit 4–2. Formal requirements for allied health professionals range from certificates gained in postsecondary educational programs to postgraduate degrees for some professions. Typically, technicians and assistants receive less than two years of postsecondary education and are trained to perform procedures. Assistants and technicians require supervision from therapists or technologists to ensure that care plan evaluation occurs as part of the treatment process. This group includes physical therapy assistants (PTAs), certified occupational therapy assistants (COTAs), medical laboratory technicians, radiologic technicians, and respiratory therapy technicians. Technologists and therapists receive more advanced training. They learn how to evaluate patients, diagnose problems, and develop treatment plans. They must also have the training to evaluate the appropriateness and the potential side effects of therapy treatments. Education at the technologist

Exhibit 4–2 Examples of Allied Health Professionals

Activities Coordinator
Audiology Technician
Cardiovascular Technician
Cytotechnologist
Dental Assistant
Dietary Food Service Manager
Exercise Physiologist
Histologic Technician
Laboratory Technician
Legal Services
Medical Records Technician
Medical Technologist
Mental Health Worker
Nuclear Medicine
Occupational Therapist
Occupational Therapy Assistant
Optician
Pharmacist
Physical Therapist
Physical Therapy Assistant
Physician Assistant
Radiology Technician
Recreation Therapist
Registered Dietitian
Registered Records Administrator
Respiratory Therapist
Respiratory Therapy Technician
Social Services Coordinator
Social Worker
Speech Therapist
Speech Therapy Assistant

or therapist level includes skill development in teaching procedural skills to technicians.

Some key allied health professionals are graduates of programs accredited by their respective professional bodies. These programs train ***physical therapists*** (PTs), whose role is to provide care for patients with movement dysfunction. Required education for licensure is a bachelor's or a professional master's degree in physical therapy and licensure examination administered by the American Physical Therapy Association. Certification, registration, or licensure is required based on state requirements. ***Occupational therapists*** (OTs) help people of all ages improve their ability to perform tasks in their daily living and working environments. They work with individuals who have conditions that are mentally, physically, developmentally, or emotionally disabling. Patients requiring OT services need specialized assistance to lead independent, productive, and satisfying lives. The basic education required is either a bachelor's or a professional master's degree in occupational therapy and a certification examination, which is administered by the National Board for Certification in Occupational Therapy.

Medical dietetics includes dietitians or nutritionists and dietetic technicians who ensure that institutional foods and diets are prepared in accordance with acceptable nutritional standards. Dietitians are registered by the Commission on Dietetic Registration of the American Dietetic Association. Dispensing opticians fit eyeglasses and contact lenses. They are certified by the American Board of Opticianry and the National Contact Lens Examiners. Speech-language pathologists treat patients with speech and language problems. Audiologists treat patients with hearing problems. The American Speech-Language-Hearing Association is the credentialing association for audiologists and speech-language pathologists. Social workers help patients and families cope with the problems resulting from long-term illness, injury, and rehabilitation. The Council on

Social Work Education accredits baccalaureate and master's degree programs in social work in the United States.

Many programs are accredited by the Committee on Allied Health Education and Accreditation under the American Medical Association, including: anesthesiologist assistants, cardiovascular technologists, cytotechnologists (study changes in body cells under a microscope), diagnostic medical sonographers (work with ultrasound diagnostic procedures), electroneurodiagnostic technologists (work with procedures related to the electrical activity of the brain and nervous system), emergency medical technician-paramedics (provide medical emergent care to acutely ill or injured persons in prehospital settings), histologic technicians/technologists (analyze blood, tissue, and fluids), medical assistants (perform a number of administrative and clinical duties in physicians' offices), medical illustrators, medical laboratory technicians, medical record administrators (direct the medical records department), medical record technicians (organize and file medical records), medical technologists (perform clinical laboratory testing), nuclear medicine technologists (operate diagnostic imaging equipment and use radioactive drugs to assist in the diagnosis of illness), ophthalmic medical technicians, perfusionists (operate life support respiratory and circulatory equipment), radiation therapy technologists (monitor radiation equipment in assisting a radiologist in patient examination), radiographers (produce X-ray films of the human body), respiratory therapists and technicians (treat patients with breathing disorders), specialists in blood bank technology, surgeon's assistants, and surgical technologists (prepare operating rooms and patients for surgery).

Certain health care workers are not required to be licensed, and they usually learn their skills on the job; however, their roles are generally limited to assisting other professionals in the provision of services. Examples include dietetic assistants, who assist dietitians or dietetic technicians in the provision of nutritional care; electroencephalogram technologists or technicians, who operate electroencephalographs; electrocardiogram technicians, who operate electrocardiographs; paraoptometrics, including optometric technicians and assistants, who perform basic tasks related to vision care; health educators, who provide individuals and groups with facts on health, illness, and prevention to improve individual and community health behaviors; psychiatric/mental health technicians, who provide care to patients with mental illness or developmental disabilities; and sanitarians, who collect samples for laboratory analysis and inspect facilities for compliance with public health laws and regulations. Increasingly, these practitioners seek their credentials through certifications, registrations, and training programs.

Health Services Administrators

Health services administrators are employed at the top, middle, and entry levels of various types of organizations that deliver health services. Top-level administrators provide leadership and strategic direction, work closely with the governing board (see Chapter 8), and are responsible for an organization's long-term success. They are responsible for operational, clinical, and financial outcomes of the entire organization. Middle-level administrators may have leadership roles for major service centers, such as outpatient, surgical services, nursing services, etc., or they may be departmental managers in charge of single departments, such as diagnostics, dietary, rehabilitation, social services, environmental services, or medical records. Their jobs involve major planning and coordinating functions, organizing human and physical resources, directing and supervising, operational and financial controls, and decision-making. They often have direct responsibility for implementing changes, creating efficiencies, and developing new procedures with respect to changes in the health care delivery system. Entry-level administrators may function as assistants to midlevel managers. They may supervise a small number of operatives. Their main function may be to oversee and assist with operations critical to the efficient operation of a departmental unit.

Today's medical centers and integrated delivery organizations are among the most complex organizations to manage. Leaders in health care delivery face some unique challenges, including changes in the financing and payment structures and having to work with reduced levels of reimbursement. Other challenges include pressures to provide uncompensated care, greater responsibility for quality, accountability for community health, separate contingencies imposed by the public and private payers, uncertainties created by new policy developments, changing configurations in the competitive environment, and maintaining the integrity of an organization through the highest level of ethical standards.

Health services administration is taught at the bachelor's and master's level in a variety of settings, and the programs lead to several different degrees. The settings for such academic programs include schools of medicine, public health, public administration, business administration, and allied health sciences. Bachelor's degrees prepare students for entry-level positions. Mid- and senior-level positions require a graduate degree. The most common degrees are the Master of Health Administration (MHA) or Master of Health Services Administration (MHSA), Master of Business Administration (MBA, with a health care management emphasis), Master of Public Health (MPH), or Master of Public Administration (or Affairs) (MPA) (Pew Health Professions Commission 1993). The 38 graduate schools of public health in the United States, which are accredited by the Council on Education for Public Health (CEPH), play a key role in training health services administrators in their MHA (or MHSA) and MPH programs (CEPH 2007). The MHA programs, however, compared to the MPH programs, have more course requirements to furnish skills in business management (both theory and applied management) and quantitative/analytical areas considered crucial for managing today's health services organizations. This disparity has been viewed as a concern that the schools of public health need to address (Singh et al. 1996).

Educational preparation of nursing home administrators is a notable exception to the MHA model. The training of nursing home administrators has been influenced largely by government licensing regulations. Even though licensure of nursing home administrators dates back to the mid-1960s, regulations favoring a formal postsecondary academic degree are more recent. Passing a national examination administered by the National Association of Boards of Examiners of Long-Term Care Administrators (NAB) is a standard requirement; however, educational qualifications needed to obtain a license vary significantly from one state to another. Although about a third of the states still require less than a bachelor's degree as the minimum academic preparation, an increasing number of practicing nursing home administrators have at least a bachelor's degree. The problem is that most state regulations call for only general levels of education rather than specialized preparation in long-term care administration. General education does not furnish adequate skills in all the domains of practice relevant to nursing home management (Singh et al. 1997). However, various colleges and universities offer specialized programs in nursing home administration.

Summary

Health services professionals in the United States constitute the largest labor force. Their development is influenced by demographic trends, advances in research and technology, disease and illness trends, and the changing environment of health care financing and delivery. Physicians play a leading role in the delivery of health services. The United States has an overall surplus of physicians and a maldistribution of physicians both by specialty and by geography. The basic physician labor force problem emanates from the fact that the supply of physicians is largely determined by population need, but medical services are actually delivered according to ability to pay. The inconsistency between supply and demand largely contributes to provider surplus in certain metropolitan and suburban areas and to shortages in rural and inner city areas. Various policies and programs have been used or proposed to address both physician imbalance and maldistribution, including regulation of health care professions, reimbursement initiatives targeting suitable incentives, targeted programs for underserved areas, changes in medical school curricula, changes in the financing of medical training, and a more rational referral system.

In addition to physicians, many other health services professionals also contribute significantly to the delivery of health care, including nurses, dentists, pharmacists, optometrists, psychologists, podiatrists, chiropractors, NPPs, and other allied health professionals. These professionals require different levels of training and work in a variety of health care settings as complements to, or substitutes for, physicians. Health services administrators face new challenges in the leadership of health care organizations. These challenges call for some reforms in the educational programs designed to prepare adequately trained managers for the various sectors of the health care industry.

Test Your Understanding

Terminology

advanced practice nurse
allied health
allopathic medicine
certified nurse midwives
chiropractors
comorbidity
dental assistants
dental hygienists
dentists
generalist
licensed practical nurses
maldistribution
nonphysician practitioners
nurse practitioners
occupational therapists

optometrists
osteopathic medicine
pharmaceutical care
pharmacists
physical therapists
physician assistants
physician extenders
podiatrists
primary care
psychologists
registered nurses
residency
specialist
specialty care

Review Questions

1. Describe the major types of health services professionals (physicians, nurses, dentists, pharmacists, physician assistants, nurse practitioners, certified nurse midwives), including their roles, training, practice requirements, and practice settings.
2. What factors are associated with the development of health services professionals in the United States?
3. What are the major distinctions between primary care and specialty care?
4. Why is there a geographic maldistribution of the physician labor force in the United States?
5. Why is there an imbalance between primary care and specialty care in the United States?
6. What measures have been, or can be, employed to overcome problems related to physician maldistribution and imbalance?
7. Who are nonphysician primary care providers? What are their roles in the delivery of health care?
8. In general, who are allied health professionals? What general role do they play in the delivery of health services?
9. Provide a brief description of the roles and responsibilities of health services administrators.

Appendix 4–A

List of Professional Associations

American Academy of Nurse Practitioners
American Academy of Physician Assistants
American Art Therapy Association, Inc.
American Association for Practical Nurse Education and Service
American Association for Rehabilitation Therapy
American Association for Respiratory Care
American Association of Colleges of Nursing
American Association of Colleges of Osteopathic Medicine
American Association of Colleges of Pharmacy
American Association of Dental Schools
American Association of Homes and Services for the Aging
American Association of Medical Assistants
American Chiropractic Association
American College of Emergency Physicians
American College of Health Care Administrators
American College of Healthcare Executives
American College of Nurse Midwives
American Corrective Therapy Association
American Council on Pharmaceutical Education
American Dance Therapy Association
American Dental Assistants Association
American Dental Association
American Dental Association SELECT Program
American Dental Hygienists' Association
American Dietetic Association
American Health Care Association
American Hospital Association
American Medical Association
American Medical Technologists
American Nurses' Association
American Occupational Therapy Association
American Organization of Nurse Executives
American Optometry Association
American Osteopathic Association
American Pharmaceutical Association
American Physical Therapy Association
American Psychiatric Association
American Psychological Association
American Public Health Association
American Registry of Radiologic Technologists
American School Health Association
American Society of Clinical Pathologists
American Society of Hospital Pharmacists
American Society of Radiologic Technologists
American Speech-Language-Hearing Association
American Therapeutic Recreation Association
Association of American Medical Colleges
Association of Physician Assistant Programs

Association of Schools and Colleges of Optometry
Association of Schools of Public Health
Association of Surgical Technologists
Association of University Programs in Health Administration
Council on Podiatry Education
Council on Social Work Education
Dental Assisting National Board, Inc.
Environmental Management Association
Healthcare Financial Management Association
International Society for Clinical Laboratory Technology
National Academy of Opticianry
National Association for Music Therapy
National Association of Boards of Pharmacy
National Association of Chain Drug Stores, Inc.
National Association of Emergency Medical Technicians
National Association of Social Workers
National Board for Respiratory Care, Inc.
National Board of Podiatry
National Certification Agency for Medical Laboratory Personnel
National Commission for Health Certifying Agencies
National Council for Therapeutic Recreational Certification
National Council for Therapy and Rehabilitation through Horticulture
National Environmental Health Association
National League for Nursing
National Nursing Centers' Consortium
National Registry of Emergency Medical Technicians
National Society of Cardiovascular Technology
National Society of Pulmonary Technology
National Therapeutic Recreation Association
Opticians' Association of America
Society of Nuclear Medicine

REFERENCES

Abdellah, F.G. 1982. The nurse practitioner 17 years later: Present and emerging issues. *Inquiry* 19, no. 1: 105–116.

American Academy of Physician Assistants. 1986. *PA fact sheet*. Arlington, VA.

American Association of Colleges of Osteopathic Medicine. 2007. Available at: *http://www.aacom.org/om.html*. Accessed January 2007.

American Association of Nurse Practitioners. 2007. Available at: *http://www.aanp.org/default.asp*. Accessed February 2007.

American College of Certified Nurse Midwives. 1988. *The scarcity and high cost of insurance*. Testimony before the US Congress Committee on Energy and Commerce, Subcommittee on Commerce, Transportation, and Tourism. September 19, 1988.

American Council on Pharmaceutical Education. 1992. *The proposed revision of accreditation standards and guidelines*. Chicago: National Association of Boards on Pharmacy.

American Physical Therapy Association. 1998. Pew Commission urges increased action to cut US physician supply. *PT Bulletin*, November 10, 10.

Anonymous. 1990. Medical education may deter grads from choosing primary care careers. *AAMC Weekly Rep*, 15 March: 1.

Appleby, C. 1995. Boxed in? *Hospitals and Health Networks* 69, no. 18: 28–34.

Auerbach, D.I., P. Buerhaus, and D.O. Staiger. 2007. Better late than never: Workforce supply implications of later entry into nursing. *Health Affairs* 26, no. 1: 178–85.

Berner, R. 1999. Pharmacists start to vie for a broader range of powers. *The Wall Street Journal*, 28 January: B1.

Bessman, A.N. 1974. Comparison of medical care in nurse clinician and physician clinics in medical school affiliated hospitals. *Journal of Chronic Diseases* 27, no. 3: 115–125.

Boulet, J.R. et al. 2006. The international medical graduate pipeline: Recent trends in certification and residency training. *Health Affairs* 25, no. 6: 469–77.

Brody, S.J. et al. 1976. The geriatric nurse practitioner: A new medical resource in the skilled nursing home. *Journal of Chronic Diseases* 29, no. 8: 537–543.

Catlin, A., C. Cowan, S. Heffler, and B. Washington; National Health Expenditure Accounts Team. 2007. National health spending in 2005: The slowdown continues. *Health Affairs* 26, no. 1: 142–53.

Cohen, J.J. 2006. The role and contribution of IMGs: A US perspective. *Acad Med* 81, no. 12 (suppl): S17–21.

Cohen, J.J. 1993. Transforming the size and composition of the physician work force to meet the demands of health care reform. *New England Journal of Medicine* 329, no. 24: 1810–1812.

Colwill, J.M., and J.M. Cultice. 2003. The future supply of family physicians: Implications for rural America. *Health Affairs* 22, no. 1: 190–198.

Cooper, R.A. 1994. Seeking a balanced physician workforce for the 21st century. *Journal of the American Medical Association* 272, no. 9: 680–687.

Cooper, R.A. et al. 1998. Current and projected workforce of nonphysician clinicians. *Journal of the American Medical Association* 280, no. 9: 788–794.

Cooper, R.A. et al. 2002. Economic and demographic trends signal an impending physician shortage. *Health Affairs* 21, no. 1: 140–154.

Council on Education for Public Health (CEPH). 2007. Available at: *http://www.ceph.org/i4a/pages/Index.cfm?pageid=3275*. Accessed February 2007.

Crandall, L.A. et al. 1990. Recruitment and retention of rural physicians: Issues from the 1990s. *Journal of Rural Health* 6, no. 1: 19–38.

Council on Graduate Medical Education. 2001. *Fifteenth report: Financing graduate medical education in a changing health care environment*. Washington, DC: Health Resources and Services Administration.

Deyo, R.A., and D.L. Patrick. 1995. The significance of treatment effects: The clinical perspective. *Medical Care* 33, no. 4: AS286–AS291.

Duff, S. 2002. Too little too late or enough? *Modern Healthcare* 32, no. 31: 6–8.

Eisenberg, J.M. 1985. Physician utilization: The state of research about physician's practice patterns. *Medical Care* 23, no. 5: 461–483.

Eisenberg, J.M. 1986. *Doctors' decisions and the cost of medical care*. Ann Arbor, MI: Health Administration Press Perspectives.

Endicott, K.M. 1976. Health and health manpower. In *Health in America: 1776–1976*. Health Resources Administration, US Public Health Service. DHEW Pub. No. 76616. Washington, DC: US Department of Health, Education, and Welfare: 138–165.

Escarce, J.J. 1992. Explaining the association between surgeon supply and utilization. *Inquiry* 29, no. 4: 403–415.

Escarce, J.J. et al. 2002. HMO growth and the geographical redistribution of generalist and specialist physicians, 1987–1997. *Health Services Research* 35, no. 4: 825–848.

Field, M.J., and K.N. Lohr. 1992. *Guidelines for clinical practice. Institute of Medicine*. Washington, DC: National Academy Press.

Fink, K.S. et al. 2003. International medical graduates and the primary care workforce for rural underserved areas. *Health Affairs* 22, no. 2: 255–262.

Fizgerald, M.A. et al. 1995. The midlevel provider: Colleague or competitor? *Patient Care* 29, no. 1: 20.

Foreman, S. 1996. Managing the physician workforce: Hands off, the market is working. *Health Affairs* 15, no. 5: 243–249.

Freed D.H. 2004. Hospitalists: Evolution, evidence, and eventualities. *The Health Care Manager* 23, no. 3: 238–56.

Friedenberg, R.M. 1996. Future physician requirements: Generalists and specialists, shortage or surplus. *Radiology* 200, no. 1: 45A–47A.

Garrard, J.L. et al. 1990. Impact of geriatric nurse practitioners on nursing home residents' functional status, satisfaction, and discharge outcome. *Medical Care* 28, no. 3: 271–283.

Gastel, B. 2006. Concurrent sessions: Exploring issues relating to international medical graduates. *Academic Medicine* 81, no. 12 (supplement): S63–8.

Ginzberg, E. 1994. Improving health care for the poor. *Journal of the American Medical Association* 271, no. 6: 464–467.

Ginzberg, E., and A.L. Dutka. 1989. *The financing of biomedical research*. Baltimore, MD: Johns Hopkins University.

Goodman D.C. 7 October 2004. Twenty-year trends in regional variations in the US physician workforce. *Health Affairs Web Exclusive*.

Greenfield, S., and E.C. Nelson. 1992. Recent developments and future issues in the use of health status assessment measures in clinical settings. *Medical Care* 30, no. 5 (Supplement): MS23–MS41.

Greenfield, S. et al. 1992. Variation in resource utilization among medical specialties and systems of care. *Journal of the American Medical Association* 267, no. 12: 1624–1630.

Grossman, D. 1995. APNs: Pioneers in patient care. *American Journal of Nursing* 95, no. 8: 54–56.

Helper, C., and L. Strand. 1990. Opportunities and responsibilities in pharmaceutical care. *American Journal of Hospital Pharmacy* 47, no. 3: 533–543.

Health Resources and Services Administration. 1996. Council on Graduate Medical Education: *Patient care supply and requirements: Testing CHGME recommendations*. 8th report to Congress and the Health and Human Services Secretary. Rockville, MD: Health Resources and Services Administration.

Health Resources and Services Administration, Bureau of Health Professions. October 2006. Physician Supply and Demand: Projections to 2020. Available at: *ftp://ftp.hrsa.gov/bhpr/workforce/PhysicianForecastingPaperfinal.pdf*. Accessed January 2007.

Hibbard, H., and P.A. Nutting. 1991. Research in primary care: A national priority. In *AHCPR conference proceedings: Primary care research: Theory and methods*, ed. M.L. Grady, 1–4. Washington, DC: Department of Health and Human Services.

Hooker, R.S. 2006. Physician assistants and nurse practitioners: The US experience. *Medical Journal of Australia* 185, no. 1: 4–7.

Hooker, R.S., and L.E. Berlin. 2002. Trends in the supply of physician assistants and nurse practitioners in the United States. *Health Affairs* 21, no. 5: 174–181.

Hooker, R.S., and L.F. McCaig. 2001. Use of physician assistants and nurse practitioners in primary care, 1995–1999. *Health Affairs* 20, no. 4: 231–238.

Hsiao, W. et al. 1993. Assessing the implementation of physician-payment reform. *New England Journal of Medicine* 328, no. 13: 928–933.

Institute for the Future. 2000. *Health and Health Care 2010: The forecast, the challenge*. San Francisco: Jossey-Bass Publishers.

Institute of Medicine. 1985. *Preventing low birthweight: Summary*. Washington, DC: National Academy Press.

Institute of Medicine. 1989. *Primary care physicians: Financing their GME in ambulatory settings*. Washington, DC: National Academy Press.

Kahn, N.B. et al. 1994. AAFP constructs definitions related to primary care. *American Family Physician* 50, no. 6: 1211–1215.

Kassebaum, D. 1994. Factors influencing the specialty choices of 1993 medical school graduates. *Academic Medicine* 69, no. 2: 164–170.

Kindig, D., and G. Yan. 1993. Physician supply in rural areas with large minority populations. *Health Affairs* (Summer): 177–184.

Koehn, N.N. et al. 2002. The increase in international medical graduates in family practice residency programs. *Family Medicine* 34, no. 6: 429–435.

Kohler, P.O. 1994. Specialists/primary care professionals: Striking a balance. *Inquiry* 31, no. 3: 289–295.

Kramon, G. 1991. Medical second-guessing—In advance. *New York Times*, 24 February: 12.

Lawrence, D. 1978. Physician assistants and nurse practitioners: Their impact on health care, access, cost, and quality. *Health and Medical Care Services Review* 1, no. 2: 2–12.

Lurie, N. et al. 1986. Termination of medical benefits: A follow-up study one year later. *New England Journal of Medicine* 314, no. 9: 1266–1268.

Marcrom, R. et al. 1992. Create value-added services to meet patient needs. *American Pharmacy* S32, no. 7: 48–57.

Mertz, E., and E. O'Neil. 2002. The growing challenge of providing oral health care services to all Americans. *Health Affairs* 21, no. 5: 65–77.

McKeon, E. 2006. Where is the funding? Several proposed bills merit your voice and attention. *American Journal of Nursing* 106, no. 8, 2006.

Mick, S.S., and M.E. Comfort. 1997. The quality of care of international medical graduates: How does it compare to that of the US medical graduates? *Medical Care Research and Review* 54, no. 4: 379–413.

Morley, P., and L. Strand. 1989. Critical reflections of therapeutic drug monitoring. *Journal of Clinical Pharmacy* 2, no. 3: 327–334.

Moscovice, I., and R. Rosenblatt. 1979. The viability of midlevel practitioners in isolated rural areas. *American Journal of Public Health* 69, no. 5: 503–505.

Mullan, F. 1999. The muscular Samaritan: The National Health Service Corps in the new century. *Health Affairs* 18, no. 2: 168–175.

Mullan, F. et al. 1995. Medical migration and the physician workforce: International medical graduates and American Medicine. *Journal of the American Medical Association* 273, no. 19: 1521–1527.

National Center for Health Statistics. 2006. *Health, United States, 2006*. Hyattsville, MD: Department of Health and Human Services.

Neimark, J. 1997. On the front lines of alternative medicine. *Psychology Today* 30, no. 1: 52–57, 67–68.

Office of Technology Assessment. 1986. *Nurse practitioners, physician assistants, and certified nurse midwives: A policy analysis*. Health technology case study 37. Washington, DC: US Government Printing Office.

Office of Technology Assessment. 1991. *Health care in rural America*. OTA-H-434. Washington, DC: US Government Printing Office.

Ostwald, S.K., and O.C. Abanobi. 1986. Nurse practitioners in a crowded marketplace: 1965–1985. *Journal of Community Health Nursing* 3, no. 3: 145–156.

Passmore, P., and S. Kailis. 1994. In pursuit of rational drug use and effective drug management: Clinic and public health viewpoint. *Asia-Pacific Journal of Public Health* 7, no. 4: 236–241.

Pew Health Professions Commission. 1993. *Health professions education for the future: Schools in service to the nation*. San Francisco.

Physician Payment Review Commission. 1993. *Annual report to Congress*. Washington, DC.

Politzer, R.M. et al. 1998. The geographic distribution of physicians in the United States and the contribution of international medical graduates. *Medical Care Research and Review* 55, no. 1: 116–130.

Pugno, P.A. et al. 2001. Results of the 2001 national resident matching program: Family practice. *Family Medicine* 33, no. 8: 594–601.

Rao, N.R. et al. 2007. An annotated bibliography of professional literature on international medical graduates. *Academic Psychiatry* 31, no. 1: 68–83.

Rich, E.C. et al. 1994. Preparing generalist physicians: The organizational and policy context. *Journal of General Internal Medicine* 9 (suppl 1): S115–S122.

Rodwin, M.A. 1995. Conflicts in managed care. *New England Journal of Medicine* 332, no. 9: 313–321.

Rosenbaum, S. 1995. *The Children's Defense Fund's adolescent pregnancy prevention/prenatal care campaign*. Washington, DC: The Children's Defense Fund.

Rosenblatt, R.A. 1992. Specialists or generalists: On whom should we base the American health care system? *Journal of the American Medical Association* 267, no. 12: 1665–1666.

Rosenblatt, R.A., and D.M. Lishner. 1991. Surplus or shortage? Unraveling the physician supply conundrum. *Western Journal of Medicine* 154, no. 1: 43–50.

Rosenblatt, R.A. et al. 1997. Interspecialty differences in the obstetric care of low-risk women. *American Journal of Public Health* 87, no. 3: 344–351.

Rosenthal, M.P. et al. 1994. Influence of income, hours worked, and loan repayment on medical students' decision to pursue a primary care career. *Journal of the American Medical Association* 271, no. 12: 914–947.

Salsberg, E.S., and G.J. Forte. 2002. Trends in the physician workforce, 1980–2000. *Health Affairs* 21, no. 5: 165–173.

Samuels, M.E., and L. Shi. 1993. *Physician recruitment and retention: A guide for rural medical group practice*. Englewood, CO: Medical Group Management Press.

Schneller E.S. 2006. The hospitalist movement in the United States: Agency and common agency issues. *Health Care Management Review* 31, no. 4: 308–16.

Schroeder, S.A. 1992. Physician supply and the US medical marketplace. *Health Affairs* (Spring): 235–243.

Schroeder, S., and L.G. Sandy. 1993. Specialty distribution of US physicians: The invisible driver of health care costs. *New England Journal of Medicine* 328, no. 13: 961–963.

Schwartz, M. 1994. Creating pharmacy's future. *American Pharmacy* NS34: 44–45, 59.

Sehgal, N.J., and R.M. Wachter. 2006. The expanding role of hospitalists in the United States. *Swiss Medical Weekly* 136: 591–6.

Sellards, S., and M.E. Mills. 1995. Administrative issues for use of nurse practitioners. *Journal of Nursing Administration* 25, no. 5: 64–70.

Shi, L. 1992. The relation between primary care and life chances. *Journal of Health Care for the Poor and Underserved* 3, no. 2: 321–335.

Shi, L. 1994. Primary care, specialty care, and life chances. *International Journal of Health Services* 24, no. 3: 431–458.

Singh, D.A. et al. 1996. A comparison of academic curricula in the MPH and the MHA-type degrees in health administration at the accredited schools of public health. *The Journal of Health Administration Education* 14, no. 4: 401–414.

Singh, D.A. et al. 1997. How well trained are nursing home administrators? *Hospital and Health Services Administration* 42, no. 1: 101–115.

Sochalski, J. 2002. Nursing shortage redux: Turning the corner on an enduring problem. *Health Affairs* 21, no. 5: 157–164.

Sox, H.C. 1979. Quality of patient care by nurse practitioners and physician assistants: A 10-year perspective. *Annals of Internal Medicine* 91, no. 3: 459–468.

Stanfield, P.S. 1995. *Introduction to the health professions*. 2nd ed. Boston: Jones & Bartlett Publishers.

Starfield, B. 1992. *Primary care: Concepts, evaluation, and policy*. New York: Oxford University Press.

Starfield, B., and L. Simpson. 1993. Primary care as part of US health services reform. *Journal of the American Medical Association* 269, no. 24: 3136–3139.

Starr, P. 1982. *The social transformation of American medicine: The rise of a sovereign profession and the making of a vast industry*. New York: Basic Books.

Steinbrook, R. 1994. Money and career choice. *New England Journal of Medicine* 330: 1311–1312.

Strand, L.R. et al. 1991. Levels of pharmaceutical care: A needs-based approach. *American Journal of Hospital Pharmacy* 48, no. 3: 547–550.

US Bureau of Labor Statistics. 2005. Charting the US Labor Market in 2005. Available at: *http://www.bls.gov/cps/labor2005/chart1-19.pdf*. Accessed January 2007.

US Bureau of Labor Statistics. 2007. Occupational Outlook Handbook, 2006–2007. Available at: *http://www.bls.gov/oco/home.htm*. Accessed January 2007.

Verby, J.E. et al. 1991. Changing the medical school curriculum to improve patient access to primary care. *Journal of the American Medical Association* 266, no. 1: 110–113.

Wachter, R.M. 2004. Hospitalists in the United States—Mission accomplished or work in progress? *New England Journal of Medicine* 350, no. 19: 1935–6.

Wagner, M. 1991. Maternal and child health services in the United States. *Journal of Public Health Policy* 12, no. 4: 443–449.

Weiner, J.P. 1993. The demand for physician services in a changing health care system: A synthesis. *Medical Care Review* 50, no. 4: 411–449.

Wennberg, J.E. et al. 1993. Finding equilibrium in US physician supply. *Health Affairs* (Summer): 89–103.

Williams, S.J. 1994. Ambulatory health care services. In *Introduction to health services*, 4th ed., eds. S.J. Williams and P.R. Torrens, 108–133. Albany, NY: Delmar Publishers.

Chapter 5

Medical Technology

Learning Objectives

- To understand the meaning and role of medical technology in health care delivery
- To appreciate the growing role of information technology and informatics in the delivery of health care
- To survey the factors influencing the creation, dissemination, and utilization of technology
- To discuss the government's role in the regulation and assessment of technological innovations
- To examine the impact of technology on various aspects of domestic and global delivery of health care
- To study the various facets of technology assessment
- To discuss the current and future directions in health technology assessment

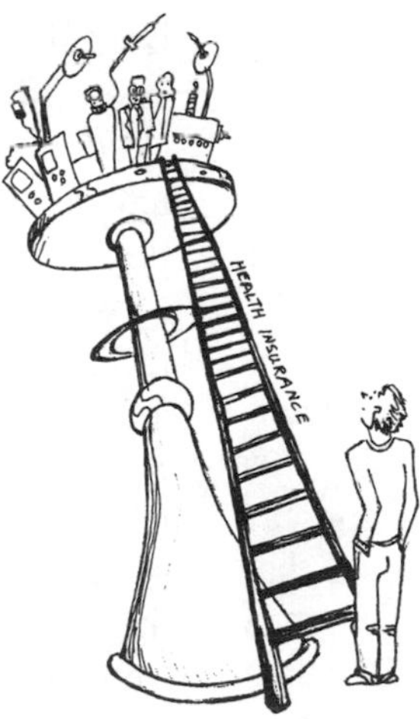

"This must be high technology."

Introduction

Drake and colleagues (1993, 79) labeled technology as "the boon and bane of medicine." In one respect, medical technology has been a great blessing to modern civilization. Sophisticated diagnostic procedures have reduced complications and disability. New medical cures have increased longevity. New drugs have helped stabilize chronic conditions. However, most new technology comes at a price that society must ultimately pay. A tremendous amount of costly research is necessary to produce most modern breakthroughs. Once technology is developed and put into use, even more costs are generated by staff training, increased need for skilled professionals, facility upgrading, and demand from both consumers and providers for the utilization of new technology. As total health care spending continues to rise, debates have emerged as to whether unrestrained development and use of new technology is worth the cost.

In Chapter 3, it was pointed out that developments in science and technology were instrumental in drastically changing the nature of health care delivery during the postindustrial era. Since then, the ever-increasing proliferation of new technology has continued to profoundly alter many facets of health care delivery. Technology has triggered several main changes. (1) It has raised consumer expectations that the latest may also be the best. These expectations have led to increased demand and utilization of new technology once it becomes available. (2) Technology has changed the organization of medical services. Specialized services that previously could be offered only in hospitals are now available in outpatient settings. (3) Technology has driven the scope and content of medical training and the practice of medicine, fueling specialization in medicine. (4) It has influenced the way status is imputed to various medical workers. Specialization is held in higher regard than primary care and public health. (5) Technology has contributed to health care cost inflation. From the consumer's standpoint, the cost of excessive treatment is generally of no concern as long as a third party—either an insurance plan or the government—pays for it. (6) Technology assessment is becoming a growing activity because new drugs, devices, and procedures are not always useful or safe. Their effectiveness and potential negative consequences must be evaluated using scientific methods. (7) Technology has raised complex social and ethical concerns that defy straightforward solutions. Some perplexing social and ethical controversies raised by modern innovations and promises of "miracle cures" include such questions as: Who should be subjected to the experimental evaluations of technological breakthroughs to determine their safety? Who should and who should not receive high-tech interventions? To what extent should life-supporting procedures be continued? Is it moral to use human embryos in biomedical research?

The phenomenon of economic globalization has also enveloped biomedical knowledge and technology. In both developed and developing nations, physicians have access to the same scientific knowledge through medical journals and the Internet. Most drugs and medical devices available in the United States are also available in almost all parts of the world. However, depending on the extent of supply-side rationing (see Chapter 2), the timing of adoption and subsequent diffusion of new technology often differs widely from one country to another. Thus, people even in developed nations do not necessarily have adequate access to the latest high-tech therapies. On the other hand, in almost all parts of the world, people who possess adequate means can gain access to the latest and best in medicine, regardless of the type of health care delivery system in their country.

From an economic standpoint, technology includes all inputs, both human and nonhuman, used in the production and management of medical goods and services (Warner 1982). This chapter discusses technology and related issues within this broad context.

What Is Medical Technology?

At a fundamental level, medical technology is the practical application of the scientific body of knowledge produced by biomedical research. Medical science, in turn, has benefited from rapid developments in other applied sciences, such as chemistry, physics, engineering, and pharmacology. For example, advances in organic chemistry made it possible to identify and extract the active ingredients in plants to produce drugs and anesthetics, which then became available in purer forms that were better adapted to controlled dosages than their earlier botanical forms. Developments in electrical and mechanical engineering led to such medical advances as radiology, cardiology, and encephalography (Bronzino et al. 1990, 11). Magnetic resonance imaging (MRI), a technology that had its origins in basic research on the structure of the atom, was later transformed into a major diagnostic tool (Gelijns and Rosenberg 1994). The disciplines of computer science and communication systems find their application in information technology and telemedicine (Tan 1995, 4).

When growth in scientific knowledge is deployed for the purpose of improving medical care, it leads to advanced techniques for a more precise medical diagnosis than those possible earlier; more effective and less invasive therapeutic and preventive medical procedures; and more advanced equipment, care delivery settings, and programs to facilitate the delivery of health services. It also requires higher skill levels of medical and administrative personnel to achieve the aforementioned objectives. A broad concept of technology thus includes not just sophisticated machines and ultramodern facilities with enhanced designs but also pharmaceuticals and biologicals, medical and surgical procedures used in rendering medical care, organizational and support systems through which care is delivered (Riley and Brehm 1989), and the use of computer-supported information systems. For example, computers used to facilitate billing and other systems used to operate and manage health services organizations are part of health care technology (Rakich et al. 1992, 179). Table 5–1 shows some of the main categories of medical technologies.

Information Technology and Informatics

Information technology (IT) deals with the transformation of data into useful information. IT involves determining data needs, gathering appropriate data, storing and analyzing the data, and reporting the information generated in a user-friendly format. Different types of information are made available for specific uses by health care professionals, managers, payers, and patients. Today, many health care organizations have information systems (IS) departments and managers to handle the continuously increasing flow of information (Tan 1995, xiii). The IS departments play a critical role in decisions to adopt new information technologies that would improve health care delivery and organizational efficiency. These technologies may include medical records

Table 5–1 Types of Medical Technologies

Type	Examples
Diagnostic	CAT scanner Fetal monitor Computerized electrocardiography Automated clinical laboratories Magnetic resonance imaging Ambulatory blood pressure monitor
Survival (life saving)	Intensive care unit (ICU) Cardiopulmonary resuscitation (CPR) Bone marrow transplant Liver transplant Autologous bone marrow transplant
Illness management	Renal dialysis Pacemaker PTCA (angioplasty) Stereotactic cingulotomy (pyschosurgery)
Cure	Hip joint replacement Organ transplant Lithotripter
Prevention	Implantable automatic cardioverter-defibrillator Pediatric orthopaedic repair Diet control for phenylketonuria Vaccines for immunization
System management	Medical information systems Telemedicine
Facilities and clinical settings	Hospitals Satellite centers Clinical laboratories Subacute care units Modern home health
Organizational delivery structure	Managed care Integrated delivery networks

Source: Adapted from Rosenthal, G. Anticipating the costs and benefits of new technology: A typology for policy. Medical technology: The culprit behind health care costs? Washington, DC: Department of Health and Human Services, 1979.

systems (to collect, transcribe, and store clinical data); radiology and clinical laboratory reporting systems; pharmacy data systems (to monitor medication use; and to avoid errors, adverse reactions, and drug interactions); scheduling systems for patients, space (such as surgery suites), and personnel; and financial systems for billing and collections, materials management, and many other aspects of organizational management (Cohen 2004a).

In health care organizations, applications of IT fall into three general categories (Austin 1992, 215):

1. ***Clinical information systems*** involve the organized processing, storage, and retrieval of information to support patient care delivery. Electronic medical records, for example, can provide quick and reliable information necessary to guide clinical decision-making and to produce timely reports on quality of care delivered. Computerized physician order entry (CPOE) enables physicians to transmit orders electronically right from the bedside. The system is designed to increase efficiency and reduce medical errors. However, because of the high costs, only about 5 percent of hospitals are using this technology (Jha et al. 2006).
2. ***Administrative information systems*** are designed to assist in carrying out financial and administrative support activities, such as payroll, patient accounting, billing, materials management, budgeting and cost control, and office automation. For medical clinics, CPOE technology can be designed to interface with the billing system to minimize rejected claims by pinpointing errors in billing codes. Administrative information systems

are also being increasingly used in predictive modeling applications that use health care claims data to identify patients who are likely to generate significant health care costs and therefore would benefit from newer utilization management programs such as case management (see Chapter 9) (Short et al. 2003).

3. ***Decision support systems*** provide information and analytical tools to support managerial decision-making. Such tools are used to forecast patient volume, project staffing requirements, and schedule patients to optimize utilization of patient care and surgical facilities.

Managers, boards of directors, and medical staff increasingly depend on information systems for timely IT outputs in several areas: financial performance, utilization of services, clinical quality, and trends in health care delivery. Such information is used for cost control and productivity enhancement, strategic planning, utilization analysis and demand assessment, program planning and evaluation, simplification of external reporting, clinical research, and quality assessment and improvement (Austin 1992, 7, 11).

The field of ***health informatics*** can be broadly defined as the science that addresses how best to use information to improve health care (Muilner and Chung 2006). Health informatics requires the use of IT, but goes beyond IT by emphasizing the improvement of health care delivery. For example, the use of IT is necessary for designing clinical decision support systems for practitioners, such as those used to improve decision-making in cancer treatment. Health informatics is a wide and growing field. It includes, for example, nursing informatics, imaging informatics, consumer health informatics, public health informatics, clinical research informatics, bioinformatics, and pharmacy informatics. Applications of informatics are also found in electronic health records and telemedicine.

Electronic Health Records and Systems

Electronic health records (EHRs) replace the traditional paper medical records that include a patient's demographic information, problems and diagnoses, plan of care, progress notes, medications, vital signs, past medical history, immunizations, laboratory data, and radiology reports. Medical records stored on paper cannot be used to coordinate care, routinely measure quality, or reduce medical errors (Hillestad et al. 2005).

EHR systems make it possible to access individual records online from many separate, interoperable automated systems within an electronic network. Since the overwhelming majority of Americans receive their care from more than one caregiver, interoperability makes a patient's medical record portable and available to the different clinicians (Brailer 2005). For example, interoperability makes it possible to share EHRs between physicians, pharmacists, and hospitals. More importantly, however, EHR systems integrate individual records with evidence-based clinical decision support, which provides reminders and best-practice guidelines for treatment (Hillestad et al. 2005). The system can also interface with quality management and outcomes reporting. According to the Institute of Medicine (2003), a fully-developed EHR system includes four key components: (1) collection and storage of health information on individual patients over time, where health information is defined as information pertaining to the health of an individual or health care provided to an individual; (2) immediate electronic access to person and population level information by authorized users; (3) provision of knowledge and decision support that enhance the quality, safety, and efficiency of patient care; and (4) support of efficient processes for health care delivery.

It is widely believed that widespread adoption of EHR systems will lead to major savings in health care costs, reduced medical errors, and improved health (Hillestad et al. 2005). However, only 15–20 percent of physicians' offices and 20–25 percent of hospitals have adopted such systems (Fonkych and Taylor 2005). Although adoption of EHRs in the United States has been slow, organizations that have introduced them have often instituted local approaches to facilitate information exchange among their organizational components—physicians' offices, nursing units, labs, and pharmacies (Halamka et al. 2005).

EHR systems require a sizable investment to purchase and implement the technology, which is one major hurdle that many smaller organizations face. For example, group practices with 50 or more physicians are more likely to use EHR technology (Reed and Grossman 2004). Initial acquisition and set-up costs range between $37,000 and $64,000 per physician or nurse practitioner, and annual operating costs average $8,400 per physician or nurse practitioner; however, improved billing and decreased personnel costs do result in savings that may help recoup the investment in less than three years (Miller et al. 2005). On the bright side, however, one study found that 80 percent of young family practice physicians, especially those starting new practices, are adopting EHR systems, and more established physicians are acquiring the systems when they upgrade their in-office computers (Wright 2006).

In the minds of many providers and patients alike, confidentiality of patient information has been a major concern. The Health Insurance Portability and Accountability Act (HIPAA) of 1996 made it illegal to gain access to personal medical information for any reasons other than health care delivery, operations, and reimbursement. HIPAA legislation mandated strict controls on the transfer of personally identifiable health data between two entities, provisions for disclosure of protected information, and criminal penalties for violation (Clayton 2001). The American public, however, has shown much skepticism about public and private institutions' ability to prevent their health information's disclosure to employers, the courts, and law-enforcement agencies (Goldsmith 2000).

The Internet and E-Health

The Internet has continued to revolutionize certain aspects of health care delivery, and its use will continue to grow. "***E-health*** refers to all forms of electronic health care delivered over the Internet, ranging from informational, educational, and commercial 'products' to direct services offered by professionals, nonprofessionals, businesses, or consumers themselves" (Maheu et al. 2001). An increasing number of Americans reported going online to look for health care information, and about half indicated that the information affected their decisions about treatment and care (Blumenthal 2002). Among physicians, at least 80 percent are using the Internet, which is quite a leap from just 3 percent in 1995 (Mullan and Lundberg 2000). Of these physicians, 90 percent indicated they were using the Internet to find clinical information (Blumenthal 2002).

Patients are also forming online communities to help themselves through e-mail discussion groups and bulletin boards. Increasingly, patients are interacting with their health care providers through secured specialty websites that cover disease management, personal health records, self-monitoring, and communication (Maheu et al. 2001). E-therapy has also emerged as an apparently popular alternative to face-to-face therapy for behavioral health support and counseling (Skinner and Latchford 2006). Although at this point e-therapy is not widely used, many Internet mental health interventions have reported early results that are promising. Both therapist-led as well as self-directed online therapies indicate significant alleviation of disorder-related symptomatology (Ybarra and Eaton 2005).

Using the Internet, patients have instant access to a barrage of information on virtually every topic associated with health and medicine. Consequently, patients have become more active participants in their own health care. In many instances, using the right source can provide valid and up-to-date information to both consumers and practitioners. Information empowers patients, which leads to changes in the traditional patient–physician dynamics.

Consumers, however, need to use caution because the Internet, at present, has little oversight. Websites sponsored by the agencies of the US government, professional organizations, and some private companies generally offer reliable information (a list of websites for selected government and private agencies is provided at the end of the book). In many other instances, however, people without formal training and qualifications are dispensing medical advice, which is sometimes free and sometimes paid. Just because a website provides information for a fee does not ensure its validity. Inaccurate and misleading information on the Internet is not uncommon.

To some extent, care providers use the Internet to register patients, direct them to alternative care sites, and order pharmaceuticals and other products. Using Web-based access to patient information from their homes or from hospital lounges, physicians can get a head start on their hospital rounds (Morrissey 2002). The effectiveness of online physician "visits" to assist patients with the monitoring of certain health conditions and treatment follow-up is being investigated. If proved successful, it can reduce the number of actual visits patients would otherwise have to make to physicians' offices. However, reimbursement issues for such virtual visits would be the main hurdle in their widespread use by physicians.

Applications of Internet2, a superfast Web update, are currently being researched. Among its possibilities are three-dimensional virtual meetings and video consults between patients and their physicians.

Telemedicine and Telehealth

Telemedicine, or distance medicine, employs the use of telecommunications technology for medical diagnosis and patient care when the provider and client are separated by distance. It eliminates the requirement for face-to-face contact between the examining physician and the patient. It also enables a generalist to consult a specialist when a patient's illness and diagnosis are complex. Sometimes the term ***telehealth*** is used to encompass educational, research, and administrative uses as well as clinical applications that involve nurses, psychologists, administrators, and other nonphysicians (Field and Grigsby 2002).

Telemedicine can be synchronous or asynchronous. Synchronous technology allows real-time interactive videoconferencing in which two or more professionals can see and hear each other and even share documents in real time. The technology allows a specialist located at a distance to directly interview and examine a patient. Asynchronous technology provides greater flexibility because it does not depend on the simultaneous presence of parties at the sending and receiving ends (Maheu et al. 2001). Asynchronous transmission uses store-and-forward technology, which allows a distant provider to review the information at a later time. Examples of telemedicine services include teleradiology (the transmission of radiographic images and scans), telepathology (viewing of tissue specimens via videomicroscopy), telesurgery (controlling robots from a distance to perform surgical procedures), and clinical consultation provided by a wide range of specialists.

With the exception of teleradiology, in which it is easier and faster to transmit images using asynchronous technology, the adoption of telemedicine in general has been slow. Some of the main barriers have been licensure of physicians and other providers across state lines, concerns about legal liability, and lack of reimbursement for services provided via telemedicine. Also, the cost-effectiveness of most telemedicine applications remains unsubstantiated. Diagnostic and consultative teleradiology, on the other hand, is almost universally reimbursed, and has been proven to be cost-effective (Field and Grigsby 2002). Despite the obstacles, several new applications are being studied. Remote in-home patient monitoring programs that monitor vital signs, blood pressure, and blood glucose levels are proving to be cost-effective. For example, remote video technology in the home health care setting has been shown to be effective, well received by patients, capable of maintaining quality of care, and to have the potential for cost savings (Johnston et al. 2000).

Innovation, Diffusion, and Utilization of Medical Technology

In the context of medical technology, innovation is the creation of a product, technique, or service that is perceived to be new by members of a society. The spread of technology into society once it is developed is referred to as ***technology diffusion*** (Luce 1993). Rapid diffusion of a technology occurs when the innovation is beneficial and the benefit can be evaluated or measured, is compatible with the adopter's values and needs, and is covered through third-party payment. Once technology is acquired, its use is almost ensured. Hence, the diffusion and utilization of technology are closely intertwined. The desire to have state-of-the-art technology available, and to use it, despite the cost, is called the ***technological imperative***.

High-tech procedures are more readily available in the United States than in most other countries, and little is done to limit the expansion of new medical technology. Compared to most European hospitals, American hospitals perform a far greater number of catheterizations, angioplasties, and bypass heart surgeries. The United States also has more high-tech equipment, such as magnetic resonance imaging (MRI) and computed tomography (CT) scanners available for its population than most countries (Kim et al. 2001). By contrast, almost all other nations have tried to limit, mainly through central planning, the diffusion and utilization of high-tech procedures to control medical costs. The British government, for instance, established the National Institute for Health and Clinical Excellence (NICE) in 1999 to decide whether select health technologies should be made available by the National Health Service (Milewa 2006). Thanks to central control, compared to the United States, Canada had 76 percent fewer MRI machines and performed 72 percent fewer coronary bypass procedures per 100,000 population; Great Britain too had 55 percent fewer MRIs and performed 82 percent fewer coronary bypass surgeries (data from Anderson and Hussey 2001). Only Japan and Switzerland were estimated to have more MRI machines per 100,000 population than the United States.

Even though the United States has made tremendous strides in medical innovation, making health care increasingly more complex, corresponding innovations in the health care delivery system have lagged behind. Investments in information technology have particularly lagged behind (Institute of Medicine 2002). For example, smart cards—credit card-like devices with an embedded computer chip and memory are already in use in Europe for health care services. ***Smart cards*** hold personal medical information that can be accessed and updated at the hospital or physician's office (Ellis 2000). Mainly because of privacy concerns, the United States is behind in using this technology

Factors That Drive Innovation and Diffusion

The rate and pattern by which a technology may diffuse is often governed by multiple forces (Cohen 2004b). For example, public and private financing for research and development (R&D) may promote or inhibit innovation; government regulations such as the Food and Drug Administration (FDA) approval process may promote or hinder the availability of new drugs and devices; marketing and promotion by the manufacturers may have an impact on the decisions of both providers and consumers about the adoption and use of technology.

Some of the main forces that have shaped the innovation, diffusion, and utilization of technology in the United States are:

- Cultural beliefs and values
- Medical specialization
- Financing and payment
- Competition
- Expenditures on R&D
- Supply-side controls
- Government policy

Cultural Beliefs and Values

Studies have shown that when technology becomes available for a particular indication, it is used at significantly different intensities in various countries and among regions within countries (Wennberg 1988). American beliefs and values have been instrumental in determining the nature of health care delivery in the United States (discussed in Chapter 2). Based on these beliefs and values, Americans have much higher expectations of what medical technology can do to cure illness than, for instance, Canadians and Germans. Also, in an opinion survey, a significantly higher number of Americans (35 percent) than Germans (21 percent) indicated that it was absolutely essential for them to be able to get the most advanced tests, drugs, medical procedures, and equipment (Kim et al. 2001). In a national, random telephone poll, 58 percent of Americans indicated that increased funding for medical and health research was essential for their future health and economic prosperity, and 63 percent expressed their willingness to pay a modest amount of additional taxes to fund medical research (Research America 2006).

The primacy of technology can also be traced to the medical model that has dominated medical practice in the United States (see Chapter 2). American beliefs and values reinforce delivery of health care according to the medical model. Consequently, the emphasis on specialty care, rather than primary care and preventive services, raises the expectations of both physicians and patients for the use of all available technology. Similarly, cultural beliefs and values have influenced the training of health care providers, the financing of services, and the structure of medical care delivery in the United States. Each of these domains reflects the premium that US society places on high technology, and consequently, the United States leads the world in the development of new technology.

Medical Specialization

Evidence of the technological imperative is most apparent in acute care hospitals, especially the ones affiliated with medical schools, because they are the main centers for specialty residency training programs in which physicians are trained to use the latest medical advances. Broad exposure to technology early in training affects not only clinical preferences but also future professional behavior and practice patterns (Cohen 2004c). Also, both patients and practitioners equate high-quality care with high-intensity care. Patient demand for direct access to specialists is growing in the United States, which reflects the population's insatiable appetite for high-technology medicine (Spann 2001). Specialty training and the inclination of specialists to use the technology they have been trained to use fuel the demand for new technology. Since medical specialization revolves around technology, an oversupply of specialists in the United States (discussed in Chapter 4) has compounded the rate of technology diffusion.

Financing and Payment

Evidence from several countries suggests that fixed provider payments (such as salaried physicians) and strong limits on payments to hospitals (such as stringent use of global budgets) curtail the incentive to use high-tech procedures. Hence, payment incentives can be used to place limitations on how quickly and widely new treatments are diffused into medical practice (McClellan and Kessler 1999).

Traditionally, the US health care delivery system has lacked internal checks and balances to determine when high-cost services are appropriate. Financing of health care through private insurance insulates both patients and providers from any personal accountability for the utilization of high-cost services. As long as out of pocket costs are of little concern, patients expect their physicians to provide all that medical science has to offer. Knowing that the services demanded by their patients are covered by insurance, providers also show little hesitation to provide the services.

There is likely a two-way relationship between technology diffusion and insurance coverage. Increasingly generous insurance coverage causes increases in spending for new products. On the other hand, the development of beneficial but costly new technology puts pressure on insurers to cover those costs (Danzon and Pauly 2001).

The rate of innovation is sensitive to changes in the level of reimbursement set for new interventions. Under the Medicare prospective payment system (discussed in Chapter 6), a higher level of reimbursement than the cost of the procedure itself stimulated rapid adoption of percutaneous transluminal coronary angioplasty (PTCA) and a high degree of innovation in PTCA catheters. By contrast, only a fraction of the cost of cochlear implants was covered. The result was not only underdiffusion but also a markedly reduced subsequent investment in research and development by the manufacturers of cochlear implants (Gelijns and Rosenberg 1994).

Competition

As discussed in earlier chapters, the health care delivery system in the United States is not characterized by true market conditions in which competition is prompted by patients who shop around for the best ***value***, that is, the most benefits possible for the price they are willing to pay. Providers of health care services do compete. Paradoxically, however, competition in health care often increases costs. Hospitals as well as outpatient centers compete to attract insured patients. Well-insured patients look for quality, and institutions create perceptions of higher quality by acquiring and advertising state-of-the-art technology. Specialists have also been responsible for stimulating competition. Many physicians, for example, have opened highly specialized hospitals, diagnostic imaging facilities stocked with next-generation scanners, and same-day surgery centers that have hotel-like touches—these developments have fueled a de facto medical arms race. In response, hospitals are adding new service lines—like cancer, heart, and brain centers—and are acquiring costly CT scanners and high-field MRI machines (Kher 2006). To recruit specialists, medical care centers often have to obtain new technology and offer high-tech procedures. When hospitals develop new services and invest heavily in modernization programs, other hospitals in the area are generally forced to do the same. Such practices result in a tremendous amount of duplication of services and equipment.

Investment interests by physicians in various types of facilities prompted Congress to pass regulations against ***self-referrals***. These laws prohibit physicians from sending patients to facilities in which they have an ownership interest. The Ethics in Patient Referrals Act of 1989 (commonly known as Stark I after Representative Pete Stark, author of the original bill) prohibited the referral of Medicare patients to laboratories in which the referring physician had an ownership interest. Provisions of this law were expanded under the Omnibus Budget Reconciliation Act of 1993 (OBRA-93). Commonly referred to as Stark II, the statute covers both Medicare and Medicaid referrals and substantially expands the types of services to which physicians may not make referrals if they have a financial interest in any of the services (Hudson 1993).

Expenditures on Research and Development

Research and development are essential for innovation. Since the early 1980s, total expenditures in biomedical sciences have exceeded those in engineering and the physical sciences (US Census Bureau 1999). It is estimated that in 2003, the United States spent \$94.3 billion, or approximately 5.5 percent of the total health care expenditures, on biomedical research. After adjusting for inflation, total biomedical research funding almost doubled between 1994 and 2003 (Moses et al. 2005). Figure 5–1 illustrates the sources for this funding. The ratio of private: government spending is 60:40. It is safe to assume that compared to other countries the United States spends the most on medical research.

Figure 5–1 Sources of Funding for Biomedical Research, 2003.

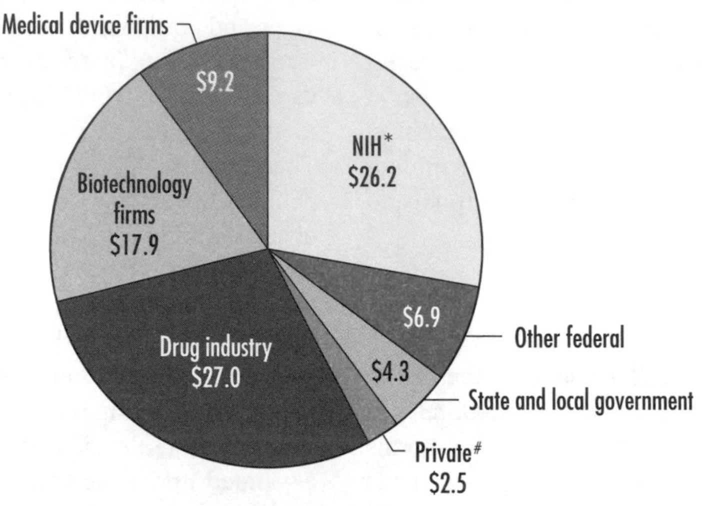

Source: Data from Moses, H. et al. 2005. Financial anatomy of biomedical research. *Journal of the American Medical Association* 294, no. 11: 1333–1342.

Supply-Side Controls

Americans resist supply-side controls. Most countries employ supply-side rationing (discussed in Chapter 2, and also referred to as central planning) to limit the diffusion of medical technology. It curtails costs, but it also restricts access to care that is critically needed. Canada, which restricts specialist services and limits expensive medical equipment to control health care spending, is a case in point. According to a 2006 study by the Fraser Institute, Canadians have to wait on average 8.8 weeks to see a specialist and another 9.0 weeks to obtain specialty treatment. The same study also found that median waiting times across Canada were 4.3 weeks for a CT scan, 10.3 weeks for an MRI, and 3.8 weeks for an ultrasound (Esmail and Walker 2006). Access to care in Canada actually has been deteriorating. The total average waiting time for specialty care increased from 13.1 weeks in 1999 to 17.8 weeks in 2006. Because of unreasonable waits for non-emergency services, as many as 72 percent of Canadians expressed that they experienced worry, stress, or anxiety, and half reported experiencing pain while waiting for specialized services (Statistics Canada 2004). Waiting lists for health care in Canada have even resulted in deaths, for example due to delayed heart surgery (Tuffnell and Kirby 1994; Steinbrook 2006).

Government Policy

Unlike most other developed countries, in the United States, direct controls over the innovation, diffusion, and utilization of technology through government policy have not been possible. Nevertheless, public policy does play a significant role in deciding which drugs and devices will be made available to Americans. The US government is also one of the largest sources of funding for biomedical research. By controlling the amount of funding, public policy indirectly influences medical innovation. A more extensive discussion of the government's role is covered in the upcoming section, "The Government's Role in Technology Diffusion."

Managed Care and Technology Diffusion

The growth of managed care has drawn considerable attention to the question of how managed care may have affected the services delivered to patients enrolled in these plans. An essential aspect of this question relates to the effects of managed care on the availability and use of medical technologies. Research literature that addresses the issue of managed care's impact on technology adoption is relatively small, and it generally supports the view that managed care has contributed to slowing the adoption of high-cost technologies (Baker 2002). For example, a study based on all 3,705 MRI sites across the United States provided some preliminary evidence that high levels of market penetration by health maintenance organizations (HMOs) were associated with reduced levels of availability and use of MRI (Baker and Wheeler 1998). In another study that examined the relationship between managed care penetration and the adoption of neonatal intensive care units (hospital units that organize a range of equipment and personnel to care for newborns with low birth-weight and other serious health problems), it was observed that managed care did not affect the diffusion of the most advanced high-level units although a slower adoption of midlevel units was observed (Baker and Phibbs 2002). The authors of this study concluded that health outcomes for seriously ill newborns are better in higher level units, and that slower growth of midlevel units could actually be beneficial because of a greater likelihood that seriously ill newborns would receive care in higher level units.

Earlier, it was believed that not only managed care was slowing the rate of technology diffusion, but that there could also be potentially harmful effects for patients. Extant literature, however, does not find any negative effects on patient care and outcomes because of slower rates of technology diffusion. On the other hand, there was clear evidence that excessive technology use had occurred during the fee-for-service era before managed care (Brook 1989). Overuse of technology, in fact, needs to be curtailed, because it not only wastes economic resources but can also result in adverse health outcomes. Limitations on the adoption and use of technology do not necessarily correlate with negative health status of a population, as evidence from other industrialized countries demonstrates. Despite the intensive use of high technology in the United States, Americans actually trail behind people in other industrialized nations on broad measures of health. The critical issue is not whether the use of technology is being curtailed, but whether its appropriate use is being curtailed. Future research needs to zero in on this difference. The issue of appropriateness is discussed later in this chapter (see "The Assessment of Medical Technology").

The Government's Role in Technology Diffusion

The growth of technology has been accompanied by issues of cost, safety, benefits, and risks. Federal legislation has been primarily aimed at addressing these concerns. Acquisition of new technology and building construction programs (both construction of new facilities and expansion of existing ones) used to be regulated under the certificate-of-need (CON) legislation, but have more recently been left to the discipline of the marketplace. The government is also a major source of funding for biomedical research, and may be spending as much as 40 percent of all health care research in the United States.

Regulation of Drugs and Devices

The Food and Drug Administration (FDA) is an agency of the DHHS that is responsible for ensuring that drugs and medical devices are safe and effective for their intended use. It also controls access to drugs by deciding whether a certain drug will be available by prescription only or as an over-the-counter purchase. The FDA may also stipulate standards on how certain over-the-counter products may be purchased and sold. For example, under the Patriot Act signed by President Bush in March 2006, certain cold and allergy medicines containing pseudoephedrine were required to be kept behind pharmacy counters and sold in only limited quantities to consumers who must show identification and sign a logbook. The action was taken because pseudoephedrine was used in making methamphetamine—a highly addictive drug—in home laboratories.

The FDA's regulatory functions have evolved over time (Table 5–2). According to the Food and Drugs Act of 1906, the FDA was authorized to take action only after drugs had been marketed to consumers. It was assumed that the manufacturer would conduct safety tests before marketing the product. If innocent consumers were harmed, however, the FDA could act only after such harm had already been done (Bronzino et al. 1990, 198). The drug law was strengthened by the passage of the Federal Food, Drug, and Cosmetic Act of 1938 (FD&C Act) in response to the infamous elixir Sulfanilamide disaster, which caused almost 100 deaths in Tennessee due to poisoning from a toxic solvent used in the liquid preparation (Flannery 1986). According to the revised law, a new drug could not be marketed without first notifying the FDA and allowing the agency time to assess its safety (Merrill 1994).

The drug approval system was further transformed by the drug amendments of 1962 after Thalidomide (a sleeping pill that was distributed in the United States as an experimental drug but had been widely marketed in Europe) was shown to cause birth defects (Flannery 1986). The 1962 amendments (Kefauver-Harris Drug Amendments) essentially stated that premarket notification was inadequate. The amendments put in force a premarket approval system, giving the FDA authority to review the effectiveness and safety of a new drug before it could be marketed. Its consumer protection role now enabled the FDA to prevent harm before it occurred. However, the drug approval process was criticized for slowing down the introduction of new drugs and, consequently, denying patients early benefit of the latest treatments. Drug manufacturers now essentially "became prisoners of the agency's [FDA's] indecision, its preoccupation with other issues, or its lack of resources" (Merrill 1994).

The Orphan Drug Act of 1983 and subsequent amendments were passed to provide incentives for pharmaceutical firms to develop new drugs for rare diseases and conditions. Incentives, such as grant funding to defray the expenses of clinical testing and exclusive marketing rights for seven years, were necessary because a relatively small number of people are afflicted by rare conditions, creating a relatively small market.

Table 5-2 Summary of FDA Legislation

Year	Legislation
1906	**Food and Drugs Act** The FDA was authorized to take action only after drugs sold to consumers caused harm.
1938	**Food, Drug, and Cosmetic Act** Required premarket notification to the FDA so the agency could assess the safety of a new drug or device.
1962	**Kefauver-Harris Amendments** Premarket notification was inadequate. The FDA took charge of reviewing the efficacy and safety of new drugs which could be marketed only once approval was granted.
1976	**Medical Devices Amendments** Authorized premarket review of medical devices, and classified devices into three classes.
1983	**Orphan Drug Act** Drug manufacturers were given incentives to produce new drugs for rare diseases.
1990	**Safe Medical Devices Act** Health care facilities must report serious or potentially serious device-related injuries, illness, or death of patients and/or employees.
1992	**Prescription Drug User Fee Act** The FDA received authority to collect application fees from drug companies to provide addition resources to shorten the drug approval process.
1997	**Food and Drug Administration Modernization Act** Provides for fast-track approvals for life saving drugs when expected benefits exceed those of current therapies.

As a result of the Orphan Drug Act, certain new drug therapies, called ***orphan drugs***, have become available for conditions that affect fewer than 200,000 people in the United States.

In the late 1980s, pressure on the FDA from those wanting rapid access to new drugs for the treatment of the human immunodeficiency virus (HIV) infection called for a reconsideration of the drug review process (Rakich et al. 1992, 186). For example, Saquinavir, a protease inhibitor indicated for patients with advanced HIV infection, received accelerated approval in late 1995; however, its manufacturer, Roche Laboratories, was required to subsequently show that the drug prolonged survival or slowed clinical progression of HIV.

In 1992, Congress passed the Prescription Drug User Fee Act, which authorized the FDA to collect fees from biotechnical and pharmaceutical companies to review their drug applications. The additional funds provided needed resources, and according to the General Accounting Office (GAO), the fees have allowed the FDA to make new drugs available more quickly. From 1993 to 2001, approval times for standard drugs have dropped by nearly half, from a median of 27 months to 14 months. Approval for new drugs has dropped more than two-thirds, from 21 months to about 6 months. At the same time, the percentage of drugs withdrawn from the market after approval has increased, for safety-related reasons (New Leadership for the FDA 2002). A tradeoff clearly exists between accelerating the review process and potential safety risks.

In 1997, Congress passed the Food and Drug Administration Modernization Act. The law provides for increased patient access to experimental drugs and medical devices. It provides for "fast-track" approvals when the potential benefits of new drugs for serious or life-threatening conditions are considered significantly greater than those for current therapies. In 1997, the FDA approved Prandin and Rezulin for Type II diabetes, Evista for the prevention of osteoporosis, and Plavix for atherosclerosis—all within seven months (Neumann and Sandberg 1998). In addition, the law provides for an expanded database on clinical trials, which is accessible to the public. Under a separate provision, when a manufacturer plans to discontinue a drug, patients who are heavily dependent on the drug will receive advance notice.

The FDA first received jurisdiction over medical devices under the FD&C Act of 1938. However, such jurisdiction was confined to the sale of products believed to be unsafe or that made misleading claims of effectiveness (Merrill 1994). In the 1970s, several deaths and miscarriages were attributed to the Dalkon Shield, which had been marketed as a safe and effective contraceptive device (Flannery 1986). In 1976, the Medical Device Amendments extended the FDA's authority to include premarket review of medical devices divided into three classes. Devices in Class I are subject to general controls regarding misbranding, that is, fraudulent claims regarding the therapeutic effects of certain devices. Class II devices are subject to special requirements for labeling, performance standards, and postmarket surveillance. The most stringent requirements of premarket approval regarding safety and effectiveness apply to Class III devices that support life, prevent health impairment, or present an unreasonable risk of illness or injury. For most Class III devices, premarket approval is required to ensure their safety and effectiveness. The Safe Medical Devices Act of 1990 strengthened the FDA's hand in controlling entry of new products and in monitoring use of marketed products (Merrill 1994). Under this Act, health care facilities must report serious or potentially serious device-related injuries or illness of patients and/or employees to the manufacturer of the device, and if death is involved, to the FDA as well. In essence, the Act is intended to serve as an "early warning" system through which the FDA can obtain important information on device problems.

Certificate of Need

The National Health Planning and Resources Development Act of 1974 designated a regional network of health systems agencies (HSAs) for the planning and allocation of health resources, including technology. States were required to enact CON laws to obtain federal funds for planning functions under this act. These activities were intended to influence the diffusion of technology by requiring hospitals to seek state approval before acquiring major equipment or embarking on new construction or modernization projects (Iglehart 1982). In 1986, the federal government terminated funding for HSAs. Although some states have abandoned CON requirements, most states retain some control over planning and construction of new health care facilities.

Various reasons have been cited for the federal government's relinquished support of health planning:

- The assumption that providing quality health care did not require extensive use of technology conflicted with societal expectations that all available technology should be used (Rakich et al. 1992, 188).

- The CON emphasis on high-cost technologies was considered misdirected because high-volume utilization of low-cost technologies could also have a significant effect on health care costs (Rakich et al. 1992, 188).
- The CON regulations fell victim to the shift away from regulatory controls over health care providers in favor of a competitive market approach to cost containment (Haglund and Dowling 1993). In fact, the CON regulations were blamed for unfair interference with the ability of hospitals to compete based on which services they could offer.
- As technology became increasingly portable, freestanding facilities could acquire the same technology that hospitals had been prohibited from acquiring. Because these freestanding facilities were not subject to CON review (Rakich et al. 1992, 188), the state approval process was regarded as unfair toward hospitals.

As noted earlier in this chapter, the proliferation of specialty hospitals and duplication of services have perhaps resulted in unnecessary and costly diffusion of technology. It has been noted that virtually all of the specialty hospitals that opened since 1990 are located in states that have no or minimal CON requirements (Zimmerman 2006).

Research on Technology

The Agency for Healthcare Research and Quality (AHRQ) was established in 1989 under the Omnibus Budget Reconciliation Act of 1989 (Public Law 101–239) and was originally the Agency for Health Care Policy and Research. AHRQ, a division of the DHHS, is the lead federal agency charged with supporting research that would focus on improving the quality of health care, reducing health care cost, and improving access to essential services. For instance, the agency's Center for Outcomes and Effectiveness Research conducts and supports studies of the outcomes and effectiveness of diagnostic, therapeutic, and preventive health services and procedures. The agency's technology assessments are made available to medical practitioners, consumers, and other health care purchasers.

Funding for Research

The federal government is a major provider of financial support for biomedical research. The National Institutes of Health (NIH)—a division of the DHHS—both conducts and supports basic and applied biomedical research in the United States. Funding through NIH provided much of the impetus for medical schools to undertake research in the medical subspecialties, which led to the growth of specialty departments within academic medical centers (Rakich et al. 1992, 183). These institutions have produced many specialists, which is reflected in the sustained imbalance between the number of general practitioners compared to specialists. Adjusted for inflation, NIH obligations nearly doubled from $13.4 billion in 1994 to $26.4 billion in 2003 (Moses et al. 2005).

The Impact of Medical Technology

Health care technology involves the practical application of scientific discoveries in many disciplines. The deployment of scientific knowledge has had far-reaching and pervasive effects, as the various categories in Table 5–1 indicate. The effects of technology often overlap, making it difficult to pinpoint technology's impact on the delivery of health care.

Impact on Quality of Care

Enhancement of quality occurs when new procedures can provide better diagnoses, quicker and more complete cures, or risk reduction in a cost-effective manner. Technology can provide new remedies where none existed. Improvements in diagnostic capabilities increase the likelihood that timely and more appropriate treatments will be provided. Technology continuously offers improved remedies that are more effective, less invasive, or safer. Outcomes can be increased longevity and decreased morbidity, indicating better quality medical care.

Numerous examples illustrate the role of technology in enhancing the quality of care. Laser technology permits surgery with less trauma; it also shortens the period for post-surgical recovery. Laser applications are widely used in most medical specialties for both medical and cosmetic procedures. For example, advanced laser procedures are now available for high-precision eye surgery. In the cosmetic arena, facial resurfacing, wrinkle removal, and many other treatments are now performed using lasers, which deliver a specific wavelength of light to the area to be treated. Discovery of the "beta secretase" enzyme, responsible for the plaques and tangles that disrupt brain activity and cause Alzheimer's disease, can possibly lead to the development of medical technology to detect Alzheimer's before its onset (The Oklahoma Medical Research Foundation 2000). The FDA has recently approved the vaccine, Gardasil, to prevent cervical cancer and other diseases caused by the human papillomavirus (HPV) in females. In 2005, the FDA approved the total artificial heart (TAH) for implantation in desperately ill patients who may be at risk of imminent death. The device is considered appropriate for patients with congestive heart failure awaiting transplantation.

Advanced bioimaging methods have opened new ways to see the body's inner workings while minimizing invasive procedures. Modern imaging technologies include MRI, positron emission tomography (PET), single-photon emission computed tomography (SPECT), CT, and fluorescence imaging. PET has important applications both for research and for clinical purposes in cardiology, neurology, and oncology. PET can show abnormal processes, such as those associated with cancers and metabolic dysfunction. It can spot tumors and other problems that may not be detectable with traditional MRI or CT scans. SPECT is of great value in imaging the brain. SPECT imaging could also reduce inappropriate use of invasive procedures through a more accurate diagnosis of coronary artery disease (Shaw et al. 2000). Integrated PET/CT is increasingly becoming an established imaging technique in the management of many cancers (Devaraj et al. 2007).

Molecular and cell biology has opened a new era in clinical medicine. Screening for genetic disorders, gene therapy, and powerful new drugs for cancer and heart disease promise to radically improve the quality of medical care. Genetic research may even help overcome the critical shortage of transplantable organs. Certain farm animals have now been successfully cloned, which holds the promise of transplanting animal organs into humans, technically referred to as ***xenografting***. On a parallel track, regenerative medicine and tissue engineering hold the promise of creating other biological and bioartificial substitutes that will restore and maintain normal function in a variety of diseased and injured tissues. Products such as bioartificial kidneys, artificial implantable livers, and insulin-producing cells to replace damaged pancreatic cells are some examples of what biomedical science may be able to accomplish in the near future. Treatment of disease using stem cells that can be derived from discarded human embryos (human embryonic stem cells), from fetal tissue, or from adult sources (bone marrow, fat, or skin) is another example of regenerative medicine.

Amid all the enthusiasm that emerging technologies might generate, some degree of caution must prevail. Experience shows that greater proliferation of technology may not necessarily equal higher quality. Unless the effect of each individual technology is appropriately assessed, some innovations may be wasteful and others may be harmful.

Impact on Quality of Life

For the most part, technology has touched people's lives in a positive way. Thanks to new scientific developments, thousands of people are able to live normal lives, which otherwise would not be possible. People with disabling conditions have been able to overcome their limitations in speech, hearing, vision, and movement with the use of prosthetic devices. Major advances have furnished the clinical ability to treat, although not cure, previously untreatable terminal conditions, such as diabetes, end-stage renal disease, and acquired immune deficiency syndrome (AIDS). Thanks to long-term maintenance therapies, people suffering from these conditions can now engage in activities that they otherwise would not be able to do. Major pharmaceutical breakthroughs now enable Americans suffering from heart disease, cancer, AIDS, and preterm birth to have a much longer life expectancy and improved health (Kleinke 2001).

Modern technology has also been instrumental in relieving pain and suffering, and pain management is being recognized as a new subspecialty in medicine. For example, for cancer pain management, new opioids have been developed for transdermal, nasal, and nebulized administration, which allow needleless means of controlling pain (Davis 2006). Apart from new drugs, patient-controlled analgesia allows the patients to determine when and how much medication they receive, which gives patients more independence and control. HIV/AIDS was recognized as a killer disease in the early 1980s. Within 25 years, modern treatments such as protease inhibitors and nonnucleoside reverse transcriptase inhibitors (known as antiretroviral agents) have suppressed HIV's ability to proliferate and damage organs. Thanks to these treatments, HIV/AIDS has become a chronic disease, not a death sentence (Komaroff 2005). Clinical trials are currently under way to evaluate the effectiveness and safety of inhaled and oral administration of insulin for patients with Type II diabetes. A substitute for injectable insulin will greatly enhance the quality of life for diabetic patients, particularly the elderly who require assistance with insulin injections.

Impact on Health Care Costs

Technological innovations have been the single most important factor in medical cost inflation over the second half of the 20th century. It has accounted for about half of the total rise in real (after eliminating the effects of general inflation) health care spending during the period 1950–2000 (Institute of Medicine. 2002). Technology in the health care field demonstrates a unique characteristic. In virtually all other industries, new technology has the effect of reducing labor force and production costs, and price considerations often play an important role in the adoption of new technologies. In health care, however, new technology has usually increased both labor and capital costs (Iglehart 1982). There is the cost of acquiring the new technology and equipment. Specially trained physicians and technicians are often needed to operate the equipment and to analyze the results, which often leads to increases in labor costs. New technology may also require special housing and setting requirements, resulting in facility costs (McGregor 1989).

Littell and Strongin (1996) argued that technology's purchase price itself has a minimal effect on systemwide health care costs. The total purchase price of medical products represents only a small fraction, estimated to be a little over 5 percent, of total annual US health care expenditures. Costs associated with utilization of technology, once it becomes available, may be more important because a technology's clinical performance is often evaluated on the basis of its effectiveness—no matter how small—and ease of operation, rather than cost reduction (Gelijns and Rosenberg 1994).

Among medical expenditures related directly to patient care (personal health expenditures—see Chapter 6), the cost of prescription drugs has risen the fastest in recent years. Three factors account for spending increases associated with drugs, as well as other technology: price inflation, increase in utilization, and product shift. In the case of prescription drugs, price increases for existing drugs have been very similar to the rates of inflation for all goods and services as measured by the Consumer Price Index (CPI); increased use of existing drugs has been the main cost driver. Surprisingly, product shift, which occurs when new drugs replace older ones, has had the least impact (Institute of Medicine 2002). This is because there is increased utilization among an aging population, and new uses have been found for existing drugs. Nevertheless, when new drugs enter the market, they not only bear higher price tags than existing drugs, but over time their utilization can expand, particularly if the newer drugs promise greater benefits.

While it is true that many new technologies increase costs, some have reduced costs most indirectly. For example, antiretroviral therapies have been largely credited with the dramatic reduction in hospitalization of AIDS patients (Centers for Disease Control and Prevention 1999). Thanks to technology, the initially estimated cost burden of the AIDS epidemic has not materialized. Technology should also be credited for an overall reduction in the average length of inpatient hospital stays. Many services that previously could be provided only in hospitals can now be delivered in less costly home and outpatient settings without adversely affecting health outcomes. Whereas many new technologies may increase labor costs, some actually produce labor cost savings. For example, when Northwestern University Medical Center in Chicago automated its lab, it dropped the human handling steps from 14 to 1.5, and the turnaround time from eight hours to 90 minutes. Largely because of a significant drop in labor costs, a savings of 30 percent have been realized. Not only that, the error rate dropped to zero since the system was installed (Flower 2006).

Instead of focusing solely on the excessive costs that new technologies may produce, increasing attention is being given to the value or worth of the advances in medical care. In a groundbreaking study, Cutler and colleagues (2006) addressed this issue by examining how medical spending has translated into additional years of life saved based on the assumption that 50 percent of the improvements in life expectancy have resulted from medical care. These authors concluded that the increases in medical spending in the 1960–2000 period in terms of increased life expectancy have rendered reasonable value for the money spent. For example, a 45-year-old American who has a remaining life expectancy of 30 years, the value of remaining life is more than $200,000 per year (Murphy and Topel 2003). For this 45-year-old person, the average annual spending in health care for each year of life gained was $53,700 (Cutler et al. 2006).

Impact on Access

Geography is an important factor in access to technology. If a technology is not physically available to a patient population, access is limited. Geographic access can be improved for many technologies by providing mobile equipment or by employing new communications technologies to allow remote access to centralized equipment and specialized personnel. Mobile equipment can be transported to rural and remote sites, making it accessible to those populations. Mobile cardiac catheterization laboratories, for example, can provide high technology in rural settings. Such services not only provide needed health care to the community, but they also protect a patient base from migrating to tertiary referral centers (Lewis 1989). Access to specialized medical care for rural and other hard-to-reach populations has been transformed through the innovations of telemedicine.

Although technology has had a positive effect on access in rural and geographically remote areas, access in general may be reduced for those who lack insurance, regardless of where they live, because medical care involving high technology becomes less affordable.

Impact on the Structure and Processes of Health Care Delivery

Modern technology has turned hospitals into capital-intensive institutions (Iglehart 1982). Large urban hospitals have been transformed into medical centers where the latest diagnostic and therapeutic remedies are offered. Recent growth in alternative settings (home health and outpatient) has also been made possible primarily by technology. Financial pressures may have prompted the use of outpatient and home settings for health care delivery, but without technological innovations, extensive adaptations of modern treatments to these alternative sites may not have been possible. Lithotripsy (a noninvasive procedure for crushing kidney and bile stones by using shockwaves) and MRI have become increasingly available in outpatient settings. More patients, who only a few years ago would have required lengthy hospital stays, are now undergoing outpatient surgery. Extensive home health services have brought many hospital and nursing home services to the patient's home. Monitoring devices can permit cardiac implants to transmit vital information over telephone lines; respirators maintain breathing in the home; and kidney dialyzers are commonly used at home, as is parenteral feeding—an intravenous technology used to provide full nutritional supplements to help feed patients who cannot swallow or digest food (Luce 1993).

Certain technologies adopted from other industries have improved health care delivery. For example, the bar-coding system has found several new applications in hospitals, including automation of drug dispensing that drastically reduces medication errors. Scanning of information on nurses' badges, patients' wristbands, and drugs to be administered ensures that the right drug is given in the right dose to the right patient (Nicol and

Huminski 2006). In some applications, radio frequency identification (RFID) has started to replace bar-coding technology in the areas of patient identification, equipment management, inventory control, and automatic supply and equipment billing (Replacing bar coding 2006).

Telecommunications technology used in telemedicine is also being used for administrative teleconferencing and continuing medical education. For example, interactive compressed videoconferencing allows for an almost face-to-face meeting in which vendors can demonstrate new products or services and discuss their utilization, costs, and delivery schedules. Significant savings can be achieved by eliminating airfares, hotel expenses, and other travel-related costs. Interactive videoconferencing is also being used for continuing education in the United States and abroad, with a high degree of satisfaction from participants. This technology is particularly helpful to rural health practitioners in overcoming barriers of distance to keep their knowledge and skills up to date (Klein et al. 2005). Recently, videoconferencing applications have been tried to provide language interpretation to translate physician orders and medication regimens for patients who have limited English proficiency (Hamblen 2006).

Managed care has been instrumental in transforming the way in which health services are delivered in the United States. Simpson (1994) observed that without technology, managed care would not be possible because it is based on managing information, and managing information requires technology. For example, information management is the backbone needed for monitoring cost-effectiveness and quality and for tracking referrals to specialized services. Consequently, between 1999 and 2002, managed care organizations (MCOs) doubled their spending on information technology (IT spending doubles 2003).

Impact on Global Medical Practice

Technology development in the United States has significantly impacted the practice of medicine worldwide. Many nations wait for the United States to develop new technologies that can then be introduced into their systems in a more controlled and manageable fashion. This process gives them access to high-technology medical care with less national investment. If technology development were to be slowed by a modest amount in the United States, it would likely have serious health consequences globally (Massaro 1990). Telehealth has made clinical care, distance education, and medical research possible in parts of the world traditionally unexposed to such advances (Umar 2003).

Impact on Bioethics

Increasingly, technological change is raising serious ethical and moral issues. For example, when in vitro fertilization is applied in medical practice and leads to the production of spare embryos, the moral question is what to do with these embryos. Gene mapping of humans, genetic cloning, stem cell research, and other areas of growing interest to scientists may hold potential benefits, but they also present serious ethical dilemmas. Life-support technology raises serious ethical issues, especially in medical decisions regarding continuation or cessation of mechanical support, particularly when a patient exists in a permanent vegetative state.

The Assessment of Medical Technology

Technology assessment, or more specifically, ***health technology assessment*** (HTA) refers to "any process of examining and reporting properties of a medical technology used in health care, such as safety, effectiveness, feasibility, and indications for use, cost, and cost-effectiveness, as well as social, economic, and ethical consequences, whether intended or unintended" (Institute of Medicine 1985, 2). HTA is concerned with the appropriateness of medical technology and can help decide which technology is best suited for a given clinical situation. Questions related to the adoption of new technology and decisions to control its diffusion should also be governed by HTA (Garber 1994). Hence, the results of HTA are meant to provide a rational basis to manage the development and dissemination of technology within a health care delivery system. Considering that one-fourth to one-third of US health care dollars are spent on services that provide only minimal benefit (Brook and Lohr 1986), technology assessment can play a critical role in distinguishing between services that are appropriate and those that are not. Efficacy and safety are the basic starting points in evaluating the overall utility of medical technology. Cost-effectiveness and cost benefit go a step further in evaluating the safety and efficacy in relation to the cost of using technology.

Efficacy and safety are evaluated through clinical trials. A ***clinical trial*** is a carefully designed research study in which human subjects participate under controlled observations. Clinical trials are carried out over three or four phases, starting with a small number of subjects to evaluate the safety, dosage range, and side effects of new treatments. Subsequent studies using larger groups of people are undertaken to confirm the effectiveness and to further evaluate safety. Compliance with rigid standards is required under HIPAA to protect the rights of study participants and to ensure that the experimentation protocols are ethical. Every institution that conducts or supports biomedical or behavioral research involving human subjects must establish an Institutional Review Board (IRB) that initially approves and periodically reviews the research.

Efficacy

Determination of efficacy is based on the premise that if a technology is not efficacious, it should not be used. Without the information on efficacy, it is almost impossible to know a technology's usefulness.

In a broad sense, ***efficacy*** may be defined simply as the health benefit derived from the use of technology. Some authors see a technical distinction between efficacy and ***effectiveness*** (see Wan 1995, 145). Although such a distinction may be important in the actual process of assessment, in a general sense efficacy is synonymous with effectiveness. If a product or service actually produces some health benefits, it can be considered efficacious or effective. Decisions about efficacy require that one ask the right questions. For example, is the current diagnosis satisfactory? What is the likelihood that a different procedure would result in a better diagnosis? If the problem is more accurately diagnosed, what is the likelihood of a better cure? The question of benefits is not as simple as it seems at first because health outcomes have traditionally been measured in terms of mortality and morbidity. Psychosocial and functional factors are also now recognized as important outcomes, but they are difficult to measure. Moreover, the same technology employed by different caregivers can sometimes yield different results, although such variations can be minimized by education and training.

Safety

Safety considerations are designed to protect patients against unnecessary harm from technology. In other words, benefits should outweigh any negative side effects from its use. The negative consequences cannot always be foreseen, however. Hence, clinical trials involving patients who may stand to gain the most from a technology are employed to get a reasonable consensus on safety. Also, the outcomes from the wider use of a certain procedure are closely monitored to identify any problems related to safety.

Cost-Effectiveness

An evaluation of efficacy and safety alone is not sufficient. Cost-effectiveness (or ***cost-efficiency***) is a step beyond the determination of efficacy. Whereas efficacy is concerned only with the benefit to be derived from the technology, cost-effectiveness evaluates the additional (marginal) benefits to be derived in relation to the additional (marginal) costs to be incurred. It thus weighs benefits against costs. A new technology may be clinically effective, that is, it may provide some benefit, but it is not cost-effective if the benefit is small and the cost is high.

As shown in Figure 5–2, at the start of medical treatment, each unit of technology utilization is likely to provide benefits in excess of its costs. At some point (Point A in Figure 5–2), an additional unit of technology utilization would result in parity between benefits and costs. This is where the slopes of the benefit and cost lines are equal, as illustrated by the parallel lines. From an economic standpoint, this is the optimum point of health resource inputs. From this point on, it is highly unlikely that additional technological interventions would result in benefits equal to, or in excess of, the additional costs. As costs continue to increase, the health benefit curve becomes flatter. At Point B (Figure 5–2), the marginal benefits from additional care approach zero, which is referred to as the ***flat of the curve***. In general, much of the medical care delivered in America is at the flat of the curve, where additional care adds little or no health benefits. Hence, high-intensity care is often wasteful. In general, differences in intensity of care play, at most, a minor role in explaining

Figure 5–2 Cost-Effectiveness and Flat of the Curve.

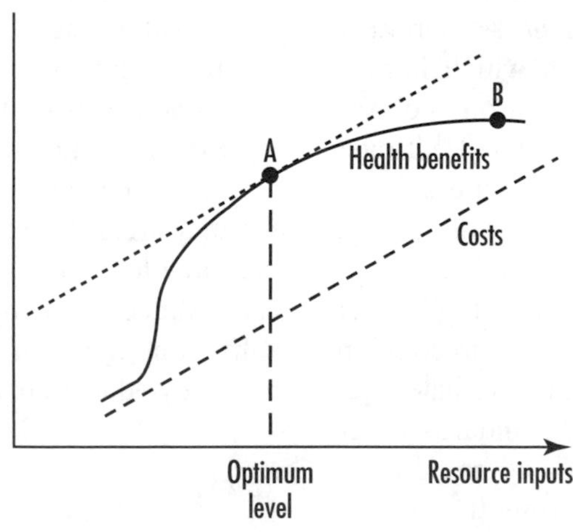

Source: Adapted from T.A. Massaro, Impact of New Technologies on Health Care Costs and on the Nation's Health, *Clinical Chemistry,* Vol. 36, no. 8B, p. 1612, © 1990, The American Association for Clinical Chemistry, Inc.

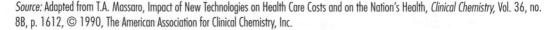

cross-section differences in health outcomes, which are primarily determined by nonmedical factors: the physical and psychosocial environments, socioeconomic factors, personal behavior, and genetics (see Blum's model in Chapter 2) (Fuchs 2004).

A more expensive procedure may actually be more cost-efficient when used appropriately. For instance, computerized axial tomography (CAT) scans are more expensive than traditional X-ray images, but the use of CAT scans has markedly reduced the need for exploratory surgery (Nitzkin 1996). When their use is warranted, the benefits of CAT scans can outweigh their cost. Their use also bypasses the risks associated with exploratory surgery that may otherwise be necessary.

A ***cost-effectiveness analysis*** incorporates the elements of both costs and benefits, especially when the costs and benefits are not expressed in terms of dollars (Wan 1995, 152). In this case, costs may or may not be calculated in monetary terms. If costs cannot be monetarily measured, they may be evaluated in terms of resource inputs, such as staff time, number of service units, space requirements, and degree of specialization needed (specialist versus generalist, physician versus allied health professional). Benefits, evaluated in terms of health outcomes, include elements such as efficacy of treatment, prognosis or expected outcomes, number of cases of a certain disease averted, years of life saved, increase in life expectancy, hospitalization and sick days avoided, early return to work, patient satisfaction, and quality of life. Benefits are then evaluated in relation to dollar costs or resource inputs.

Risk is another type of nonmonetary cost. Most medical procedures are not totally safe. They may have the potential for significant benefits, but they are also accompanied by certain risks. Sometimes, these risks are small; at other times, they can be significant. The process of medical care can result in undesired side effects, iatrogenic illnesses, medical complications, injuries, or death, all of which carry a cost that is often difficult to measure. Hence, the effectiveness of medical interventions should be evaluated not only in terms of costs but also in terms of risks. Thus, Figure 5–2 can also be used to determine the optimum point at which the benefits equal the risks. Beyond that point, the risks from additional technological interventions are likely to exceed the benefits.

Cost (and risk) and benefit evaluations are not precise or objective determinations. Such assessments are generally based on professional judgments and expert opinions. However, standardization of clinical guidelines based on clinical evidence or expert medical consensus is expected to be one step toward making this process more objective.

Cost Benefit

In contrast to cost-effectiveness analysis, ***cost benefit analysis*** is used to evaluate benefits in relation to costs when both are expressed in dollar terms (Seidel et al. 1995, 136; Wan 1995, 152). Hence, cost benefit analysis is subject to a more rigorous quantitative analysis compared to cost-effectiveness analysis. Cost benefit analysis is based on four main assumptions: (1) The problem or health condition can be identified or diagnosed. (2) The problem can be controlled or eradicated using an appropriate intervention. (3) The benefit or outcome can be assigned a dollar value. (4) The cost of intervention can be determined in dollars.

The same principles that apply to cost-effectiveness are also used for assessing cost benefit. If the estimated benefits exceed costs, the additional spending on medical care is worth the extra costs. The ***quality-adjusted life year*** (QALY) is commonly used as a measure of health benefit. QALY is defined as the value of one year of high-quality life, which in recent years has been assigned a value of $100,000. Using this approach, Cutler and McClellan (2001) demonstrated that at least in the case of four selected conditions, namely, heart attacks, low birth-weight infants, depression, and cataracts, the estimated benefit of technological change was much greater than the cost. For breast cancer treatment, the costs and benefits were found to be equal in magnitude.

Current and Future Directions in Health Technology Assessment

Private Sector Initiatives

In the United States, HTA is conducted predominantly in the private sector, unlike nations such as Sweden, the Netherlands, and Canada, which have centralized technology assessment agencies (Neumann and Sandberg 1998). In the public sector, it is mainly the Department of Veterans Affairs and the Department of Defense that conduct clinical trials and other evaluations of technology. Hence, much of the talent needed to assess medical technology is also located, organized, and financed in the private sector. Pharmaceutical firms, for example, have developed pharmacoeconomics departments concerned with internal analysis of the cost-effectiveness of new products (Rettig 1994). Before new drugs are introduced, their economic evaluation has become almost as important as the clinical trials used to determine their safety and efficacy. Private agencies, among them the Blue Cross and Blue Shield Association, Kaiser Permanente, the American Medical Association (AMA), and other professional societies, have undertaken technology assessment for several years now.

Need for Coordinated Effort

At present, efforts in HTA remain fragmented and poorly funded, with little or no coordination between public or private sector groups to deliberately address the assessment and diffusion of technologies. Also, information garnered from HTA studies is not efficiently shared among medical organizations, health care systems, and policymakers. The response has been a demand for broad regional and national HTA programs that would study the effects of health care technology more systematically and involve providers, policymakers, patient advocacy groups, and government representatives (Bozic et al. 2004). Provisions under the Medicare Prescription Drug Improvement and Modernization Act of 2003 provides for increased funding for the Agency for Healthcare Research and Quality (AHRQ) to support clinical effectiveness and cost-effectiveness research on new medical technology (Wechsler 2004).

Need for Standardization

Future efforts in HTA will require greater transparency of methods employed and standardization that would allow comparison of efficacy and cost-effectiveness results across studies. In 1993, the US Public Health Service commissioned the Panel on Cost-Effectiveness in Health and Medicine. The Panel recommended that investigators should also make every effort to include information about both direct medical costs and nonmedical costs (e.g., time and lost productivity) as well as consider costs and benefits that accrue both now and in the future (Gold et al. 1996).

Balance Between Clinical Efficacy and Economic Worth

American consumers often want all available medical resources to be utilized regardless of how little health benefit is received in relation to costs. Physicians often find themselves in a precarious situation when they are required to withhold treatment because of its cost-inefficiency. Payers generally are blamed as uncaring profit-mongers when they intervene in the delivery of medical care based on costs. Even US policymakers are generally not at ease with bringing cost-effectiveness into the equation of health care delivery. Consequently, cost-effectiveness has not taken central stage in the United States, and its application is not openly discussed in health care decision-making. In contrast, European countries, Canada, and Australia use cost-effectiveness openly and explicitly in their centralized health planning decisions (Neumann and Sullivan 2006).

Current research has highlighted the value or worth of medical care spending in terms of gains in life expectancy in the United States (see Cutler and colleagues 2006, discussed earlier). Although such findings may suggest that current levels of expenditures for health care are acceptable, rising health care costs in the United States and excessive spending according to international comparisons are of growing concern to most Americans. Policymakers are likely to respond to any public outcry over health care expenditures. Hence, pressures to grant cost-effectiveness analysis a larger role in the approval process for drugs and devices and new regulatory initiatives to contain future costs are likely to demand greater emphasis on the economic worth of individual technologies.

Clinical Practice Guidelines

Clinical practice guidelines (or medical practice guidelines) are systematically developed protocols to assist practitioners in delivering appropriate health care for specific clinical circumstances (Field and Lohr 1990). The goal is to assist practitioners in adopting a "best practice" approach in delivering care to a given patient population with a given condition (Ramsey 2002). Practice guidelines result from an evaluation of medical procedures regarding their effectiveness, appropriateness, and safety, and the integration of these assessments into clinical practice. Such evidence-based guidelines provide a mechanism for standardizing the practice of medicine and improving the quality of care. The benchmark practice patterns become norms governing what is and is not appropriate in clinical practice. However, cost-effectiveness information is not commonly incorporated in the development of clinical practice guidelines (Wallace et al. 2002). Ramsey (2002) suggested that this disconnect between practice guidelines and economic analyses emanates mainly from clinicians' inclination to treat patients until there is no more health benefit to be gained (flat of the curve, discussed earlier). Conversely, economic analyses weigh treatments based on their incremental health value at a given cost, and they provide a reference point at which additional medical interventions must be discontinued to achieve maximum value in the delivery of medical care. In view of the escalating health care expenditures and the ongoing development and diffusion of expensive new technology, in the future, the concept of value—improved benefits at lower costs—will become increasingly important to both public and private payers of health care.

Ethical Issues

With the rapid pace of innovation, concerns in HTA transcend the traditional questions about safety, effectiveness, and economic value. New technologies also raise social, ethical, and legal concerns. These issues raise complex questions, but provide few answers. Yet, in an era of resource constraints, HTA will have to take into account social, ethical, economic, and legal concerns.

Health care budgets are under constraint not only in the United States, but in other developed countries as well. How to provide the latest and best in health care within limited resource parameters has become a major concern for all developed countries. Insurers, pharmaceutical companies, medical device manufacturers, MCOs, and physician advocacy institutions often act and advocate out of their own self interests. For example, physicians' representatives, such as medical associations, and the medical device and pharmaceutical industries almost always argue in favor of increasing resource inputs in delivering health care (Wild 2005). They often claim that quality would deteriorate and/or harm would ensue unless new innovations are funded. Since these same groups have also assumed major roles in HTA, the probability of circulating biased results is high. Biases might also arise in studies funded by sources that have a financial stake in the results. Such concerns have stimulated interest in developing standards for assessments, perhaps under the aegis of a governmental body.

Within social, ethical, and legal constraints, public and private insurers face the problem of deciding whether or not to cover novel treatments. Recent challenges include, for example, decisions about new reproductive techniques such as intracytoplasmic sperm injection in vitro fertilization (ICSI IVF), new molecular genetic predictive tests for hereditary breast cancer, and new drugs such as sildenafil (Viagra) for sexual dysfunction (Giacomini 2005). The question arises as to whether society should even bear the cost of infertility treatments, genetic tests, and lifestyle remedies that do not affect people's health and longevity.

Therapies classified as experimental are generally not covered by insurance. When new treatments promise previously unattainable health benefits, decisions about assessment of such treatments are often surrounded by controversy. Often critical to the debate, but defying easy answers, are questions regarding the adequacy of studies used to determine whether a certain treatment should be considered experimental, ethical questions about the needs of patients who could possibly benefit from the treatment, and financial questions concerning the responsibility of payers (Reiser 1994). Concerns about withholding treatment from patients are not easily juxtaposed against equally valid concerns about exposing these patients to unjustified risk.

Ethical issues also surround the conduct of clinical research. Emanuel and colleagues (2000) contended that ethical clinical research must fulfill seven requirements: (1) The research must have social or scientific value for improving health or enhancing knowledge. (2) The study must be scientifically valid and methodologically rigorous. (3) The selection of subjects in clinical trials must be fair. (4) The potential benefits to patients and the knowledge gained for further scientific work must outweigh the risks. (5) Independent review of the research methods and findings must be conducted by unaffiliated individuals. (6) Informed, voluntary consent must be obtained from subjects. (7) The privacy of enrolled subjects must be protected, they must be offered the opportunity to withdraw, and their well-being must be maintained throughout the trial.

Summary

Medical technology is the practical application of scientific knowledge produced by biomedical research and the adaptation of scientific advances from other fields to the delivery of health care. The application of information technology and informatics is becoming indispensable in efficient delivery of care and in the effective management of modern health care organizations. With the growth of Internet applications, e-health is becoming a growing field in health care delivery. Telemedicine and telehealth are being used in both synchronous and asynchronous applications to deliver medical care when the provider and client are separated by distance.

Medical technology has greatly enhanced the capabilities of the delivery system to provide more effective and less invasive treatments. The problem is that the development and diffusion of technology are closely intertwined with its use. The United States is foremost in the world in developing new technology, but the uncontrolled use of technology has prompted deep concerns about rising costs.

The growth of technology has been influenced by several factors: beliefs and values in the American culture, medical specialization, financing, competition, and expenditures in research and development. Most other developed countries apply supply-side controls to limit technology diffusion and its use. It curtails cost, but also restricts access to care. Such direct controls over the innovation, diffusion, and utilization of technology through government policy have not been possible in the United States. However, health policy does play a role through the FDA's drug and device approval process and government funding for biomedical research.

Technology has had a tremendous impact on the delivery of health care. It has positively influenced the quality of care, enhanced the quality of life, and improved access in remote areas. Many large institutional providers and MCOs cannot function efficiently without computer-based information systems. Because much of the technology developed in the United States is either purchased or reproduced by other countries, technology development in the United States also has a profound effect on the practice of medicine globally. Advances in genetics and many other areas have the potential to provide unprecedented benefits, but they also raise critical ethical issues.

Given the costs and risks associated with the use of technology, its assessment has become an area of growing interest. Current thought in technology assessment calls for a balance between benefits (efficacy) and costs/risks. Additional interventions beyond the point where costs and/or risks begin to exceed the benefits are considered inappropriate, but the assessment of cost-effectiveness is not an exact science. Evidence-based clinical practice guidelines are paving the way toward standardizing medical practice. However, currently, there is a disconnect between practice guidelines and economic analysis. As escalating health care expenditures reach a critical point, appropriateness of medical treatments may have to be based on their incremental health value at a given cost.

Use of technology is not without controversy. Critical moral dilemmas arise from the use of experimental therapies, delays in the assessment and approval process, life-sustaining treatments, and waste of resources when interventions are not cost-effective.

Test Your Understanding

Terminology

administrative information systems
clinical information systems
clinical practice guidelines
clinical trial
cost benefit analysis
cost-effectiveness analysis
cost-efficiency
decision support systems
effectiveness
efficacy
e-health
electronic health records
flat of the curve
health informatics
health technology assessment
information technology
orphan drugs
quality-adjusted life year (QALY)
self-referral
smart card
technological imperative
technology diffusion
telehealth
telemedicine
value
xenografting

Review Questions

1. Medical technology encompasses more than just sophisticated equipment. Discuss.
2. What role does an information systems (IS) department play in a modern health care organization?
3. Provide brief descriptions of clinical information systems, administrative information systems, and decision support systems in health care delivery.
4. Distinguish between information technology (IT) and health informatics.
5. According to the Institute of Medicine, what are the four main components of a fully developed electronic health records (EHR) system?
6. Why have EHR systems not been widely adopted in the United States?
7. What are the main provisions of HIPAA with regard to the protection of personal medical information?
8. What is telemedicine? How do the synchronous and asynchronous forms of telemedicine differ in their applications?
9. Which factors have been responsible for the low diffusion and low use of telemedicine?
10. Generally speaking, why is medical technology more readily available in the United States than it is in other countries?
11. How does competition lead to greater levels of technology diffusion? How does technological diffusion, in turn, lead to greater competition?
12. Summarize the government's role in technology diffusion.
13. What was the effect of the Kefauver-Harris Drug Amendments of 1962? Why was the law criticized?

14. Provide a brief overview of how technology influences the quality of medical care and quality of life.
15. Discuss the relationship between technological innovation and health care expenditures.
16. What impact has technology had on access to medical care?
17. Discuss the roles of efficacy, safety, and cost-effectiveness in the context of technology assessment.
18. Why is it important to achieve a balance between clinical efficacy and economic worth (cost-effectiveness) of medical treatments?
19. What purpose do clinical practice guidelines serve in health care delivery? What main shortcoming exists in the practice guidelines currently in use?
20. What are some of the ethical issues surrounding the development and use of medical technology?

REFERENCES

Anderson, G., and P.S. Hussey. 2001. Comparing health system performance in OECD countries. *Health Affairs* 20, no. 3: 219–232.

Austin, C.J. 1992. *Information systems for health services administration*, 4th ed. Ann Arbor, MI: AUPHA Press/Health Administration Press.

Baker, L. 2002. Managed care, medical technology, and the well-being of society. *Topics in Magnetic Resonance Imaging* 13, no. 2: 107–113.

Baker, L.C., and C.S. Phibbs. 2002. Managed care, technology adoption, and health care: The adoption of neonatal intensive care. *RAND Journal of Economics* 33, no. 3: 524–548.

Baker, L.C., and S.K. Wheeler. 1998. Managed care and technology diffusion: The case of MRI. *Health Affairs* 17, no. 5: 195–207.

Blumenthal, D. 2002. Doctors in a wired world: Can professionalism survive connectivity? *The Milbank Quarterly* 80, no. 3: 525–546.

Bozic et al. 2004. Health care technology assessment: Basic principles and clinical applications. *The Journal of Bone and Joint Surgery* 86A, no. 6: 1305–1314.

Brailer, D.J. 2005. Interoperability: The key to the future health care system. *Health Affairs*: *Web Exclusive* 24, Supplement 1: w5–19 to w5–21.

Bronzino, J.D. et al. 1990. *Medical technology and society: An interdisciplinary perspective*. Cambridge, MA: MIT Press.

Brook, R.H. 1989. Practice guidelines and practicing medicine: Are they compatible? *Journal of the American Medical Association* 262: 3027–3030.

Brook, R.H., and K.N. Lohr. 1986. Will we need to ration effective health care? *Issues in Science and Technology* (Fall): 68–77.

Centers for Disease Control and Prevention. 1999. New data show AIDS patients less likely to be hospitalized. Available at: *http://www.cdc.gov/od/oc/media/pressrel/r990608.htm*. Accessed June 8, 1999.

Clayton, P.D. 2001. Confidentiality and medical information. *Annals of Emergency Medicine* 38, no. 3: 312–316.

Cohen, A.B. 2004a. The adoption and use of medical technology in health care organizations. In *Technology in American healthcare: Policy directions for effective evaluation and management*, eds. A.B. Cohen and R.S. Hanft, 105–147. Ann Arbor: The University of Michigan Press.

Cohen, A.B. 2004b. Critical questions regarding medical technology and its effects. In *Technology in American healthcare: Policy directions for effective evaluation and management*, eds. A.B. Cohen and R.S. Hanft, 15–42. Ann Arbor: The University of Michigan Press.

Cohen, A.B. 2004c. The diffusion of new medical technology. In *Technology in American healthcare: Policy directions for effective evaluation and management*, eds. A.B. Cohen and R.S. Hanft, 79–104. Ann Arbor: The University of Michigan Press.

Culter, D.M., and M. McClellan. 2001. Is technological change in medicine worth it? *Health Affairs* 20, no. 5: 11–29.

Cutler, D.M. et al. 2006. The value of medical spending in the United States, 1960–2000. *The New England Journal of Medicine* 355, no. 9: 920–927.

Danzon, P.M., and M.V. Pauly. 2001. Insurance and new technology: From hospital to drugstore. *Health Affairs* 20, no. 5: 86–100.

Davis, M.P. 2006. Management of cancer pain: Focus on new opioid analgesic formulations. *American Journal of Cancer* 5, no. 3: 171–182.

Devaraj, A. et al. 2007. PET/CT in non-small cell lung cancer staging—promises and problems. *Clinical Radiology* 62, no. 2: 97–108.

Drake, D. et al. 1993. *Hard choices: Health care at what cost?* Kansas City, MO: Andrews and McMeel.

Ellis, D. 2000. *Technology and the future of health care: Preparing for the next 30 years*. San Francisco: Jossey-Bass Publishers and Chicago: Health Forum, Inc.

Emanuel, E.J. et al. (2000). What makes clinical research ethical? *Journal of the American Medical Association* 283, no. 20: 2701–2711.

Esmail, N., and G. Walker. 2006. *Waiting your turn: Hospital waiting lists in Canada,* 16th ed. Vancouver, British Columbia: The Fraser Institute.

Field, M.J., and J. Grigsby. 2002. Telemedicine and remote patient monitoring. *Journal of the American Medical Association* 288: 423–425.

Field, M.J., and K.N. Lohr, eds. 1990. *Clinical practice guidelines: Directions for a new agency.* Washington, DC: National Academy Press.

Flannery, E.J. 1986. Should it be easier or harder to use unapproved drugs and devices? *Hastings Center Report* 16, no. 1: 17–23.

Flower, J. 2006. Imagining the future of health care. *The Physician Executive* 32, no. 1: 64–66.

Fonkych, K. and R. Taylor. 2005. *The state and pattern of health information technology adoption.* Santa Monica, CA: RAND Corporation.

Fuchs, V.R. 2004. More variation in use of care, more flat-of-the curve medicine. *Health Affairs* 23 (Variations Supplement): 104–107.

Garber, A.M. 1994. Can technology assessment control health spending? *Health Affairs* 13, no. 3: 115–126.

Gelijns, A., and N. Rosenberg. 1994. The dynamics of technological change in medicine. *Health Affairs* 13, no. 3: 28–46.

Giacomini, M. 2005. One of these things is not like the others: The idea of precedence in health technology assessment and coverage decisions. *The Milbank Quarterly* 83, no. 2: 193–223.

Gold, M.R. et al. 1996. *Cost effectiveness in health and medicine*. New York: Oxford University Press.

Goldsmith, J. 2000. How will the Internet change our health system? *Health Affairs* 19, no. 1: 148–156.

Haglund, C.L., and W.L. Dowling. 1993. The hospital. In *Introduction to health services*, 4th ed., eds. S.J. Williams and P.R. Torrens, 135–176. Albany, NY: Delmar Publishers.

Halamka, J. et al. 2005. Exchanging health information: Local distribution, national coordination. *Health Affairs* 24, no. 5: 1170–1179.

Hamblen, M. 2006. Hospitals expand videoconferencing. *Computerworld* 40, no. 23: 21.

Hillestad, R. et al. 2005. Can electronic medical record systems transform health care? Potential health benefits, savings, and costs. *Health Affairs* 24, no. 5: 1103–1117.

Hudson, T. 1993. "Stark II" limits physician referrals, but may help hospital. *Trustee* 46, no. 12: 20.

Iglehart, J.K. 1982. The cost and regulation of medical technology: Future policy directions. In *Technology and the future of health care*, ed. J.B. McKinlay, 69–103. Cambridge, MA: MIT Press.

Institute of Medicine. 1985. *Assessing medical technologies*. Washington, DC: National Academy Press.

Institute of Medicine. 2002. *Medical innovation in the changing healthcare marketplace*. Washington, DC: National Academy Press.

Institute of Medicine. 2003. *Key capabilities of an electronic health records system*. Washington, DC: National Academy Press.

IT spending doubles. 2003. IT spending doubles at MCOs. *Health Management Technology* 24, no. 7: 6.

Jha, A.K. et al. 2006. How common are electronic health records in the United States? A summary of the evidence. *Health Affairs* 25, no. 6: w496–507.

Johnston, B. et al. 2000. Outcomes of the Kaiser Permanente telehome health research project. *Archives of Family Medicine* 9: 40–45.

Kher, U. 2006. The hospital wars. *Time* 168, no. 24 (December 11, 2006): 64–68.

Kim, M. et al. 2001. How interested are Americans in new medical technologies? A multicountry comparison. *Health Affairs* 20, no. 5: 194–201.

Klein, D. et al. 2005. Videoconferencing for rural physicians' continuing health education. *Journal of Telemedicine and Telecare* 11, Suppl. 1: 97–99.

Kleinke, J.D. 2001. The price of progress: Prescription drugs in the health care market. *Health Affairs* 20, no. 5: 43–60.

Komaroff, A.L. 2005. Beyond the horizon. *Newsweek* 146, no. 24 (December 12, 2005): 82–84.

Lewis, S. 1989. Mobile cardiac catheterization services: Invasive diagnostic for small hospitals in the 1990s. *Hospital Technology Series Special Report* 8, no. 29.

Littell, C.L., and R.J. Strongin. 1996. The truth about technology and health care costs. *IEEE Technology and Society Magazine* 15, no. 3: 10–14.

Luce, B.R. 1993. Medical technology and its assessment. In *Introduction to health services*, 4th ed., eds. S.J. Williams and P.R. Torrens, 245–268. Albany, NY: Delmar Publishers.

Maheu, M.M. et al. 2001. *E-health, telehealth, and telemedicine: A guide to start-up and success*. San Francisco: Jossey-Bass.

Massaro, T.A. 1990. Impact of new technologies on health care costs and on the nation's health. *Clinical Chemistry* 36, no. 8B: 1612–1616.

McClellan, M., and D. Kessler. 1999. A global analysis of technological change in health care: The case of heart attacks. *Health Affairs* 18, no. 3: 250–257.

McGregor, M. 1989. Technology and the allocation of resources. *New England Journal of Medicine* 320, no. 2: 118–120.

Merrill, R.A. 1994. Regulation of drugs and devices: An evolution. *Health Affairs* 13, no. 3: 47–69.

Milewa, T. 2006. Health technology adoption and the politics of governance in the UK. *Social Science and Medicine* 63, no. 12: 3102–3112.

Miller, R.H. et al. 2005. The value of electronic health records in solo or small group practices. *Health Affairs* 24, no. 5: 1127–1137.

Morrissey, J. 2002. Hospitals offer remote control. *Modern Healthcare* 32, no. 51: 32–35.

Moses, H. et al. 2005. Financial anatomy of biomedical research. *Journal of the American Medical Association* 294, no. 11: 1333–1342.

Muilner, R.M., and K. Chung. 2006. Current issues in health care informatics. *Journal of Medical Systems* 30, no. 1: 1–2.

Mullan, F., and G. Lundberg. 2000. Looking back, looking forward: Straight talk about US medicine. *Health Affairs* 19, no. 1: 117–123.

Murphy, K.M., and R.H. Topel. 2003. The economic value of medical research. In *Measuring the gains from medical research: An economic approach*, eds. K.M. Murphy and R.H. Topel, 41–73. Chicago: University of Chicago Press.

Neumann, P.J., and E.A. Sandberg. 1998. Trends in health care R&D and technology innovation. *Health Affairs* 17, no. 6: 111–119.

Neumann, P.J., and S.D. Sullivan. 2006. Economic evaluation in the US: What is the missing link? *Pharmacoeconomics* 24, no. 11: 1163–1168.

New leadership for the FDA. 2002. *Lancet* 360, no. 9341: 1183.

Nicol, N., and L. Huminski. 2006. How we cut drug errors. *Modern Healthcare* 36, no. 34: 38.

Nitzkin, J.L. 1996. Technology and health care—Driving costs up, not down. *IEEE Technology and Society Magazine* 15, no. 3: 40–45.

The Oklahoma Medical Research Foundation. 2000. Breakthrough Discovery in Alzheimer's Disease. Available at *http://www.omrf.net*. Accessed February 15, 2000.

Rakich, J.S. et al. 1992. *Managing health services organizations*. Baltimore, MD: Health Professions Press.

Ramsey, S.D. 2002. Economic analyses and clinical practice guidelines: Why not a match made in heaven? *Journal of General Internal Medicine* 17, no. 3: 235–237.

Reed, M.C., and J.M. Grossman. 2004. *Limited information technology for patient care in physician offices*. Issue Brief 89 (September 2004). Washington, DC: Center for Studying Health System Change.

Reiser, S.J. 1994. Criteria for standard versus experimental therapy. *Health Affairs* 13, no. 3: 127–136.

Replacing bar coding. 2006. Replacing bar coding: Radio frequency identification. *Nursing* 36, no. 12: 30.

Research America. 2006. National survey, 2006. Available at: *http://www.researchamerica.org/polldata/2006/NationalPoll2006.pdf.*

Rettig, R.A. 1994. Medical innovation duels cost containment. *Health Affairs* 13, no. 3: 7–27.

Riley, J.G., and H.P. Brehm. 1989. Technological innovations and their impact on care delivery. In *Health care, technology, and the competitive environment*, eds. H.P. Brehm and R.M. Mullner, 21–39. New York: Praeger Publishers.

Seidel, L.F. et al. 1995. *Applied quantitative methods for health services management*. Baltimore, MD: Health Professions Press.

Shaw, L.J. et al. 2000. Clinical and economic outcomes assessment in nuclear cardiology. *Quarterly Journal of Nuclear Medicine* 44, no. 2: 138–152.

Short, A.C. et al. 2003. *Disease management: A leap of faith to lower-cost, higher-quality health care*. Issue Brief No. 69 (October 2003). Washington, DC: Center for Studying Health System Change.

Simpson, R.L. 1994. The role of technology in a managed care environment. *Nursing Management* 25, no. 2: 26–28.

Skinner, A.E.G., and G. Latchford. 2006. Attitudes to counseling via the Internet: A comparison between in-person counseling client and Internet support group users. *Counseling and Psychotherapy Research* 6, no. 3: 92–97.

Spann, S.J. 2001. The future of family medicine: Clinical practice. *Journal of Family Practice* 50, no. 7: 584–585.

Statistics Canada. 2004. *Access to health care services in Canada, 2003*. Ottawa, Ontario: Statistics Canada.

Steinbrook, R. 2006. Private health care in Canada. *The New England Journal of Medicine* 354, no. 16: 1661–1664.

Tan, J.K.H. 1995. *Health management information systems: Theories, methods, and applications*. Gaithersburg, MD: Aspen Publishers, Inc.

Tuffnell, S., and J. Kirby. 1994. *Price controls and global budgets: Lessons from Canada*. Brief Analysis No. 104. Washington, DC: National Center for Policy Analysis.

Umar, K. 2003. *Telemedicine works: Quality, access, and cost impacts cited*. Closing the Gap (January/February), Office of Minority Health Resource Center, Department of Health and Human Services.

US Census Bureau. 1999. Statistical Abstract of the United States. Washington, DC: US Census Bureau.

Wan, T.T.H. 1995. *Analysis and evaluation of health care systems: An integrated approach to managerial decision making*. Baltimore, MD: Health Professions Press.

Warner, K.E. 1982. Effects of hospital cost containment on the development and use of medical technology. In *Technology and the future of health care*, ed. J.B. McKinlay, 41–65. Cambridge, MA: MIT Press.

Wennberg, J.E. 1988. Improving the medical decision-making process. *Health Affairs* 7, no. 1: 99–106.

Wild, C. 2005. Ethics of resource allocation: Instruments for rational decision making in support of a sustainable health care. *Poiesis & Praxis* 3, no. 4: 296–309.

Ybarra, M.L., and W.W. Eaton. 2005. Internet-based mental health interventions. *Mental Health Services Research* 7, no. 2: 75–87.

Wallace, J.F. et al. 2002. The limited incorporation of economic analyses in clinical practice guidelines. *Journal of General Internal Medicine* 17, no. 3: 210–220.

Wechsler, J. 2004. Streamlining clinical research oversight. *Applied Clinical Trials* 13, no. 6: 24–26.

Wright, E. 2006. Here comes the future. *Health Affairs* 25, no. 2: 570.

Zimmerman, E. 2006. The implications of reimbursement changes for specialty hospitals. *Healthcare Financial Management* 60, no. 7: 42–45.

Chapter 6

Health Services Financing

Learning Objectives

- To study the role of health care financing and its impact on the delivery of health care
- To understand the basic concept of insurance and how general insurance terminology applies to health insurance
- To differentiate between the concepts of group insurance, self-insurance, individual health insurance, and managed care
- To examine the distinctive features of public programs, such as Medicare, Medicaid, Department of Defense, Veterans Administration, SCHIP, and PACE
- To understand the various methods of reimbursement
- To discuss national health care and personal health care expenditures
- To get acquainted with the key trends, problems, and issues in health care financing

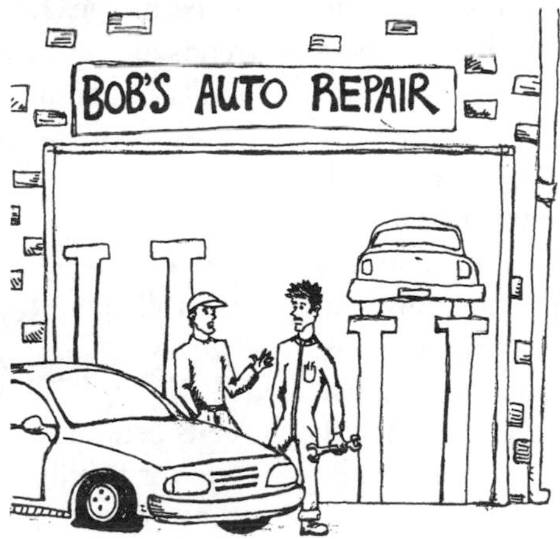

"I have comprehensive insurance."

Introduction

Complexity of financing is one of the primary characteristics of medical care delivery in the United States. Both private and public resources are used to purchase health care services through a multitude of programs and health plans. The actual payment to providers of care is also handled in numerous ways. Some services are paid for directly by patients themselves, but most of the services are paid for indirectly through a variety of insurance plans, managed care organizations (MCOs), and government programs. The government and some large employers use the services of third-party administrators (TPAs) to process payment claims from providers.

The financing mechanisms are commonly referred to as health insurance. People who are not covered by either private or government-sponsored health insurance programs are referred to as ***uninsured***. The voluntary system of health insurance in America is the primary reason that a segment of the US population is uninsured. Many Americans are uninsured because employers in the private sector are not mandated to provide health insurance to their employees, employees are not required to sign up even when health insurance is offered as an employment benefit, and the public programs cover only certain defined categories of people who meet the criteria established for eligibility. This situation is unlike national health care programs that provide universal coverage to all citizens. Since the mid-1960s, when the Medicare and Medicaid programs were established, public outlays for health care financing have steadily increased while private financing has decreased.

Chapter 1 characterized the structure of health services delivery in terms of its four main functions: financing, insurance, delivery, and payment. Because the dollars to fund health insurance come primarily from employers and the government, they are referred to as the financiers of health services delivery. Unless the basic financing function is assumed by these financiers, the burden for health care expenses falls on the individual consumers of health care, the patients. However, when financing is discussed in broad terms, as in this chapter, the concepts of financing, insurance, and payment are generally included. But this does not mean that the three functions are structurally integrated. For example, the government-financed programs, Medicare and Medicaid, integrate the functions of financing and insurance, but contracted TPAs make the actual payments to the providers after services have been delivered. Commercial insurance companies integrate the functions of insurance and payment, whereas employers largely constitute the source of financing. Managed care has gone one step further in integrating all four functions.

This chapter focuses on the financing mechanisms in both private and public programs and discusses national health care spending, which continues to be a matter of concern. The chapter concludes with current trends and directions in financing, and also points out some of the main problems and issues in financing health care services.

The Role and Scope of Health Services Financing

As its central role, health services financing pays for health insurance premiums to cover individuals and families. Health insurance is the primary mechanism that enables people to obtain health care services. Hence, the insurance function is often regarded as a key component of health care financing in its broad sense. Providers often rely on the patients' insurance status to be assured that they will receive payment for the services they provide. The various methods used to determine how much the providers should be paid (i.e., reimbursement) for their services are also closely intertwined with the broad financing function.

Financing determines who has access to health care and who does not. Thus, the demand for health care is directly related to its financing. Health insurance increases the demand for covered services; the demand would be less if the same services were not covered. Increased demand means greater utilization of health services, given adequate supply. According to economic theory, insurance lowers the out of pocket cost of medical care to the consumers. Hence, they will consume more health services than if they had to pay the entire price out of their own pockets. Consumer behavior that leads to a higher utilization of health care services when the services are covered by insurance is referred to as ***moral hazard*** (Feldstein 1993, 125).

Financing also exerts powerful influences on the supply-side factors, such as how much health care is produced. New services proliferate when private insurance plans or Medicare start paying for them. Indeed, financing has given rise to new subindustries within the health care delivery system. Subacute care and home health care are two such examples. Similarly, when new technologies are covered by health plans, their diffusion and utilization increase, as discussed in Chapter 5. When reimbursement is constrained, supply of services is curtailed accordingly.

Issues pertaining to reimbursement for services are critical in health services management decision-making. Health services managers are typically guided by demand-side factors, including reimbursement, in evaluating the type and extent of services to offer. Management decisions, such as acquisition of new equipment, renovation or expansion of facilities, and launching of new programs, are also heavily influenced by the amount of reimbursement needed to recoup capital costs over time.

Financing can also influence the supply and distribution of health care delivery professionals. Employer financing for dental insurance has spawned the growth of dentists and dental hygienists. Mechanisms for reimbursing physicians, such as the resource-based relative value scales (RBRVS) used by Medicare, directly affect physicians' incomes. One main intent of RBRVS, implemented in 1992, was to entice more medical residents into general practice by increasing the reimbursement for services provided by generalists. Due to other factors, however, the imbalance between generalists and specialists continues (see Chapter 4).

Financing eventually affects, directly as well as indirectly, the total health care expenditures (also referred to as health care costs or health care spending) incurred by a health care delivery system. The level of health care spending and the rise of these expenditures in the United States has been a matter of ongoing concern. The next section discusses the relationship between financing and health care expenditures and provides a general framework for controlling health care costs.

Financing and Cost Control

Health care financing and cost control are closely intertwined. As Figure 6–1 illustrates, in the US health care delivery system, insurance is the main factor that determines

Figure 6–1 Influence of Financing on the Delivery of Health Services.

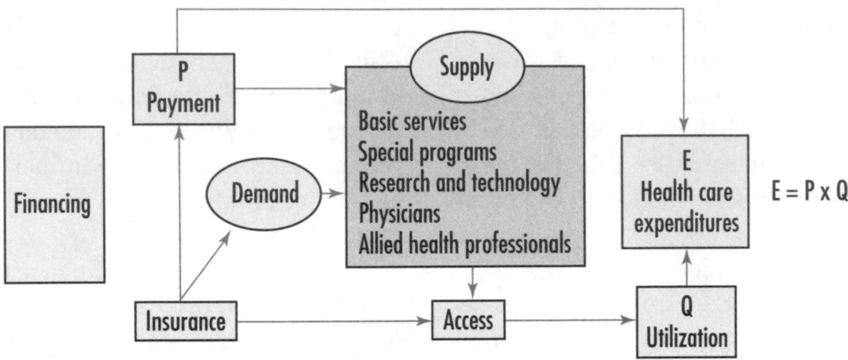

the level of demand for health services. Total health care expenditures are eventually controlled by restricting financing for health insurance. This is referred to as demand-side rationing (see Chapter 2). Conversely, extension of health insurance to the uninsured, without other restrictions, will increase total health care expenditures (E). Such increases for 1994, when a national health care program was last proposed by President Clinton, have been estimated to range between $16.3 and $24.8 billion (Short et al. 1997). Even though these estimates represent only about 2 to 3 percent of total health care spending, moral hazard and provider-induced demand could substantially raise the actual costs. Various types of supply-side approaches to ration health care would have to be employed to restrain cost escalations, as shown by the experiences of other nations that have national health care programs. Apart from the extent of insurance coverage, systemwide health care expenditures are also affected by how much health insurance premiums cost.

Insurance, along with payment (i.e., price = P), influences the supply or availability of health services. Restricting payment to providers by cutting reimbursement has a direct influence on E, as well as an indirect influence through shrinkage in supply. Cuts in reimbursement have been used in the United States, as well as in other countries, to contain the growth of health care expenditures.

As discussed in Chapter 5, diffusion of technology and other types of services can be directly restricted through health planning to limit supply (supply-side rationing—see Chapter 2). When supply of technology is rationed, people may be insured, but do not have free access to those services. Reduced utilization of expensive technology results in direct savings. This approach to cost containment is common in national health care programs. In addition to the direct savings realized by rationing technology, nations that have national health care achieve indirect savings by having fewer specialist physicians and specialized technicians, and by spending less money on research and development.

Insurance and supply of health care services together determine access, and eventually the utilization of services (i.e., quantity of services consumed = Q). Utilization can also be directly controlled. For example, private health plans, as well as Medicare and

Medicaid, contain utilization by specifying which services are not covered. Managed care uses various mechanisms to directly control utilization (discussed in Chapter 9).

Because E = P × Q, rising health care costs can be controlled by managing the numerous factors that influence P and Q. Many of these factors are external to the health care delivery system. P, for example, includes general economy-wide inflation as well as medical inflation that exceeds general inflation. In addition to the intrinsic factors discussed in this section, Q is also a function of changes in the size and demographic composition (age, sex, and racial mix) of the population (Levit et al. 1994). These factors are discussed more extensively in Chapter 12.

The Insurance Function

Insurance is a mechanism for protection against risk; that is its primary purpose. The notion of risk is central to the concept of insurance. In this context, ***risk*** refers to the possibility of a substantial financial loss from an event whose probability of occurrence is relatively small (at least in a given individual's case). For example, even though auto accidents are common in the United States, the likelihood is quite small that a specific individual will have an auto accident in a given year. Even though the risk is small, people buy insurance to protect their assets against catastrophic loss.

An individual who is protected by insurance against risk is called the ***insured***. The insuring agency that assumes risk is called the ***insurer*** or underwriter. ***Underwriting*** is a systematic technique for evaluating, selecting (or rejecting), classifying, and rating risks. Four fundamental principles underlie the concept of insurance (Health Insurance Institute 1969, 9; Vaughn and Elliott 1987, 17): (1) Risk is unpredictable for the individual insured. (2) Risk can be predicted with a reasonable degree of accuracy for a group or a population. (3) Insurance provides a mechanism for transferring or shifting risk from the individual to the group through the pooling of resources. (4) Actual losses are shared on some equitable basis by all members of the insured group.

Technically, health services for all Americans 65 and over are provided through Medicare. For those below the age of 65, private insurance is the predominant avenue for receiving health care. Medicaid covers many of the poor. A small number of people are covered under other public programs, such as VA and SCHIP. The remainder, without any coverage, are the uninsured. Sources for health insurance for all Americans appear in Figure 6–2.

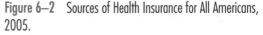

Figure 6–2 Sources of Health Insurance for All Americans, 2005.

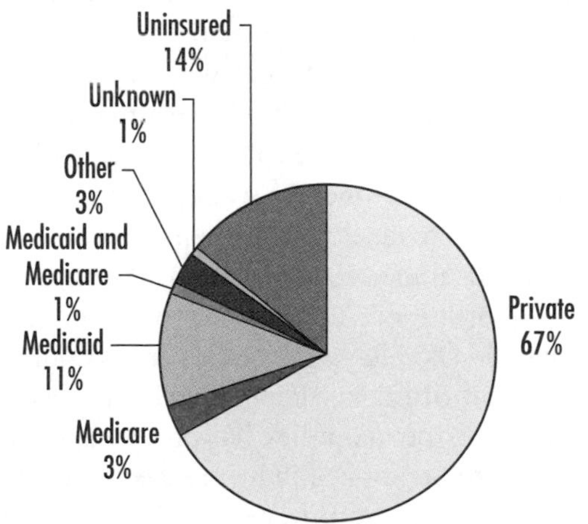

Source: Data from *Summary health statistics for the US population: National health interview survey, 2005*, National Center for Health Statistics, p. 46.

Private Financing

Private health insurance is also referred to as "voluntary health insurance" because it is not mandatory. The modern health insurance industry is pluralistic. Private insurance includes many different types of health plan providers, such as commercial insurance companies (e.g., Aetna, Cigna, Metropolitan Life, and Prudential), Blue Cross/Blue Shield, self-insured employers, and managed care organizations (MCOs). The nonprofit Blue Cross and Blue Shield Associations are similar to private health insurance companies.

Types of Private Insurance

Group Insurance

Group insurance can be obtained through an employer, a union, or a professional organization. A ***group insurance*** program anticipates that a substantial number of people in the group will purchase insurance through its sponsor. Risk, and often the cost of insurance, is spread out among the insured individuals. As discussed in Chapter 3, health insurance became an attractive fringe benefit to workers when wages were frozen during World War II. Around that time, fringe benefits also received favorable tax treatment. Unlike monetary wages, benefits are not subject to taxes. Consequently, a dollar of health insurance received from the employer is worth more than the same amount received in taxable wages or an after-tax dollar spent out of pocket for medical care. For a long time, the tax policy has provided an incentive to obtain health insurance as a benefit paid by the employer.

Early health insurance policies were often inadequate to cover extended illnesses or long hospital stays. With the rapid growth of health insurance as a fringe benefit, which expanded competition among insurance companies, major medical insurance became common starting in the 1950s. ***Major medical*** was designed to cover catastrophic situations that could subject families to substantial financial hardships, such as hospitalization, extended illness, and expensive surgery. Blue Cross/Blue Shield followed the lead of insurance companies and offered similar plans. The most common type of health insurance coverage available in the 1950s and 1960s included hospital care, surgical fees, and related physicians' expenses. Since the 1970s, health insurance plans have commonly combined major medical coverage with all-inclusive comprehensive coverage, which includes basic and routine physician office visits and diagnostic services (Health Insurance Association of America [HIAA] 1991, 2–5). Today, the term "major medical" is no longer limited to a single type of expense but applies broadly to almost all types of medical care (Somers and Somers 1977, 113).

Self-Insurance

Some big employers realized that their work force was large enough and sufficiently well diversified in terms of risk that they could safely predict their medical expenditures from year to year. Rather than pay insurers a dividend to bear the risk, large employers could simply assume the risk by budgeting a certain amount to pay medical claims incurred by their employees. Being self-insured also gives such employers a greater degree of control, and costs are contained through a slower rise in premiums during periods of rapid inflation (Gabel et al. 2003). Self-insured employers can protect themselves against any potential risk of high losses by purchasing ***reinsurance*** from a private insurance company.

Self-insurance was spurred by government policies. Self-insured employers were exempt from a premium tax that insurance companies had to pay, the cost of which was passed on to customers through higher premiums. Further, the Employee Retirement Income Security Act (ERISA) of 1974 exempts self-insured plans from certain mandatory benefits that regular health insurance plans are required to provide in many states. Self-insured plans also avoid other types of state insurance regulations, such as reserve requirements and consumer protection requirements. Premium taxes and other regulatory requirements would increase the cost of health insurance. Thus, employers that are large enough to make it feasible for themselves have viewed self-insurance as a better economic alternative. In 2006, 55 percent of all covered workers in private firms were in self-insured plans (The Kaiser Family Foundation and Health Research and Educational Trust 2006).

Individual Private Health Insurance

Although most Americans obtain health insurance coverage through employer-sponsored group plans or government programs, individually purchased private health insurance (non-group plans) is an important source of coverage for many Americans. The family farmer, the early retiree, the self-employed, and the employee of a business that does not offer health insurance make up most of those relying on private health insurance. Unlike group insurance in which risk is spread over the entire group, individual private insurance determines premium price and eligibility based on the risk indicated by each individual's health status and demographics (General Accounting Office [GAO] 1996). Consequently, high-risk individuals are often unable to obtain privately purchased health insurance. For those who can obtain coverage, premiums are much higher than they are in group plans, and the covered individuals also incur high deductibles and co-payments. In 2002, approximately 6 million Americans under the age of 65 were covered under private non-group plans. The average annual premium in 2002 for a non-group plan was estimated at $2,531 for single coverage (ranging from $1,661 for those younger than 40 to $3,703 for those between the ages of 55 and 64) and $4,442 for family coverage (Agency for Healthcare Research and Quality 2005). In comparison, in 2002, the total premium costs for employer-sponsored group plans averaged $3,060 for a single plan and $7,956 for a family plan (The Henry J. Kaiser Family Foundation 2002). One would expect the group plans to cost less. However, the differences between individually purchased plans and employer-sponsored group plans most likely reflect the fact that tax-advantaged treatment of employer-provided benefits gives both employers and employees strong incentives to replace taxable wages with non-taxable benefits. Such benefits lead to the purchase of excessive health insurance coverage—more than what people may actually need. These same people would likely purchase less generous health insurance plans if they had to pay all the premiums out of pocket.

Managed Care Plans

MCOs, such as health maintenance organizations (HMOs) and preferred provider organizations (PPOs), emerged in response to the rapid escalation of health care costs. Managed care plans can be regarded as a type of health insurance because they assume risk in exchange for an insurance premium. The full range of functions of MCOs, however, extends beyond the simple insurance function. In a nutshell, MCOs provide a broad range of services, generally emphasizing primary and preventive care. Services are provided through the MCOs' own internally employed professionals, through contractual arrangements with external providers, or through a combination of the two. MCOs also use a variety of mechanisms to monitor utilization and a variety of methods to reimburse providers for the services rendered. Whereas internal providers are salaried, external providers are commonly paid capitated or discounted fees. A detailed discussion on managed care is presented in Chapter 9.

Some Health Insurance Concepts

The Insured

The insured, also called a ***beneficiary***, is anyone covered under a particular health insurance plan. Two types of employer-sponsored plans are single coverage plans and family coverage plans. The latter cover the spouse and dependent children of the working employee. The number of dependents covered under employer plans far exceeds the number of primary insured. In all, approximately 160 million Americans are covered under employer-sponsored health insurance plans.

Medicare and Medicaid plans recognize only individual beneficiaries. In the case of married couples, for instance, each spouse is recognized as an independent beneficiary.

Premiums

A ***premium*** is the amount charged by the insurer to insure against specified risks. The premium is usually paid every month. For most job-based health insurance, the employee is asked to share in the cost of premiums. The employee's contribution is generally paid through payroll deductions. In most cases both individual and family coverage are subject to premium cost sharing. The average monthly cost, including the shares paid by employers and employees, in 2006 was $354 for a single plan and $957 for a family plan (Claxton et al. 2006). In 2000, these costs were $202 and $529 respectively (The Kaiser Family Foundation and Health Research and Educational Trust 2000). The average annual increase in premiums between 2000 and 2006 was 9.8 percent for a single plan and 10.4 percent for a family plan. Workers on average paid 16 percent of the premium cost for a single plan and 27 percent for a family plan in 2006 (Claxton et al. 2006).

Premiums are determined by the actuarial assessment of risk. Two methods have been commonly used to determine premiums: The first, called ***experience rating***, is based on a group's own medical claims experience. Under this method, premiums differ from group to group because different groups have different risks. For example, people working in various industries are exposed to various levels and types of hazards, people in certain occupations are more susceptible to certain illnesses or injuries, and older groups represent higher risks than younger groups. High-risk groups are expected to incur high utilization of medical care services so they are charged higher premiums compared to preferred or favorable risk groups. Experience rating was the common method adopted by insurance companies (HIAA 1991, 3), but several states have passed legislation that requires insurers to price their premiums according to community rating or modified community rating. ***Community rating*** spreads the risk among members of a larger community and establishes premiums based on the utilization experience of the whole community. Under pure community rating, the same rate applies to everyone regardless of age, gender, occupation, or any other indicator of health risk (Goodman and Musgrave 1992, 125). For example, a person who has AIDS would pay the same premium as someone who does not. Under "modified" community rating, price differences could be based on age and sex while ignoring other risk factors. When premiums are based on community rating, the good risks actually help pay for the poor risks (Somers and Somers 1977, 113). In other words, cost is shifted from people in poor health to the healthy. It makes health insurance less affordable for those who are healthy.

Cost Sharing

In addition to paying a share of the cost of premiums through payroll deductions, insured individuals also generally pay a portion of the actual cost of medical services out of their own pockets. These out of pocket expenses are in the form of deductibles and co-payments, and are incurred only if and when medical services are used. ***First-dollar coverage plans***, plans without deductibles and co-payments, are now practically nonexistent. A ***deductible*** is the amount the insured must first pay before any benefits are payable by the plan. A deductible commonly must be paid on an annual basis. For example, suppose a plan requires the insured to pay a $250 deductible. When medical care is received, the plan starts paying only after the cost of medical services received by the insured has exceeded $250 in a given year. The insured must pay the first $250 out of pocket each year. The second type of out of pocket cost is ***co-payment***. It is the amount the insured must pay each time health services are received. A co-payment is set either as a dollar amount or as a proportion of the medical costs incurred. In the latter case, co-payment is established in the form of what is referred to as ***coinsurance***. As an example, for an office visit the co-payment amount could be $20. On the other hand, a plan may require 80–20 coinsurance. In this case, once the deductible requirement has been met, the plan starts paying 80 percent of all covered medical expenditures; the insured pays the remaining 20 percent as co-payment. The 80–20 ratio of cost sharing between the insurance plan and the insured is called coinsurance. Most plans include a ***stop-loss*** provision, which is the maximum out of pocket liability an insured would incur in a given year. In case of a catastrophic illness or injury, the co-payment amount can add up to a substantial sum. The purpose of the stop-loss provision is to limit the total out of pocket costs to a certain amount, for example, $2,000. This means that once the deductible and co-payments have totaled $2,000 in a given year, no further co-payments are required and the plan pays 100 percent of any additional expenses. Some plans have set lifetime benefits limits of $1 to $2 million; others have no limits.

The rationale for cost sharing is to control utilization of health care services. Since insurance creates moral hazard by insulating the insured against the cost of health care, making the insured pay part of the cost promotes more responsible behavior in health care consumption. A comprehensive study employing a controlled experimental design conducted in the 1970s, commonly referred to as the Rand Health Insurance Experiment, demonstrated that cost sharing had a material impact on lowering utilization without any significant negative health consequences.

Indemnity and Service Plans

Technically, health insurance plans can be classified as either "indemnity" or "service." Today, most health insurance plans are service plans. An ***indemnity plan*** provides reimbursement to the insured, without regard to the expenses actually incurred (Health Insurance Institute 1969, 21). For example, a predetermined cash amount is paid to the beneficiary per procedure or per day in the hospital. The insured is responsible for paying the provider. There is no relationship between the insurer and the provider of services. If the actual expense is more than the indemnity amount, the balance becomes an out of pocket expense. A ***service plan*** provides specified services to the insured. The plan pays the hospital or physician directly, except for the deductible and co-payments for which the insured is responsible. The insured does not get a bill from the providers except for the out of pocket portion of the charges. Traditionally, private insurance companies offered indemnity plans, whereas Blue Cross/Blue Shield offered service plans (HIAA 1991, 1–2). Plans offered by MCOs are also regarded as service plans. Charges are prenegotiated with the providers in the form of capitated payments or discounted fees. Co-payments in managed care plans are generally smaller than those in traditional plans to provide an inducement for enrollment. Even though, technically, the term "indemnity plan" carries a specific meaning, all traditional health insurance plans, other than managed care plans, are now loosely referred to as indemnity plans.

Covered Services

Services covered by an insurance plan are referred to as ***benefits***. Each health insurance plan spells out the type of medical services it covers. It also specifically lists services that are not covered. Covered and noncovered services are outlined in a contract, a copy of which is provided to the insured. A typical disclaimer included in most contracts states that only "medically necessary" health services are covered, regardless of whether or not such services are provided by a physician. Most plans include medical and surgical services, hospitalizations, emergency services, prescriptions, maternity care, and delivery of a baby. Most plans also provide, within specified limits, mental health services, substance abuse services, home health care, skilled nursing care, rehabilitation, supplies, and equipment. Services such as eyeglasses and dental care may or may not be covered. Services most commonly excluded are those not ordered by a physician, such as self-care and over-the-counter products. Other services commonly excluded from health insurance coverage are cosmetic and reconstructive surgery, work-related illness and injury (covered under workers' compensation), rest cures, genetic counseling, and the like. Many plans had excluded coverage of preexisting medical conditions for new enrollees until a certain time had elapsed. The Health Insurance Portability and Accountability Act (HIPAA) of 1996 has made this practice illegal in cases of employees who had health insurance coverage in their previous job. Some managed care plans, especially HMOs, exclude certain services unless the insured's primary care physician prescribes them or refers the insured to them. Other plans may require preauthorization (also called precertification) or second opinions for certain surgical procedures or hospitalizations.

Dental insurance is often a separate plan, independent of major medical plans. Dental insurance generally covers oral examinations, routine cleanings, X-rays, fillings, extractions, inlays, bridgework, dentures, root canal therapy, and orthodontia (Health Insurance Institute 1969, 33).

Public Financing

Historically, delivery of health care in the United States has been privately financed. However, since 1965, government financing has played a significant role in expanding services, particularly to those who otherwise would not be able to afford them. Today, a significant proportion of health services in the United States is supported through public programs. In 2005, approximately 18 percent of the US population was covered under various public insurance programs (see Figure 6–2). The inception of Medicare and Medicaid programs was discussed in Chapter 3. This section discusses the financing, eligibility requirements, and services covered under the major public health insurance programs.

Public financing supports ***categorical programs***, each designed to benefit a certain category of people. Examples are Medicare for the elderly and certain disabled individuals, Medicaid for the indigent, Defense Department programs for active service people, and Veterans Affairs (VA) programs for former armed forces personnel. The government finances Medicare and Medicaid, but services are purchased from providers in the private sector. Similarly, in two other government programs, TriCare (formerly called CHAMPUS—Civilian Health and Medical Program of the Uniformed Services) and CHAMPVA (Civilian Health and Medical Program of the Department of Veterans Affairs), the government provides the financing, but insurance and health care services are obtained through the private sector. In contrast, the government finances health care services for the uniformed armed forces and veterans, and delivery of services, with few exceptions, is also through the public sector.

Medicare

The Medicare program, also referred to as Title XVIII of the Social Security Act, finances medical care for (1) persons 65 years and older, (2) disabled individuals who are entitled to Social Security benefits, and (3) people who have end-stage renal disease (permanent kidney failure requiring dialysis or a kidney transplant). People in these three categories can enroll regardless of income status. Among Medicare enrollees, 88 percent are 65 years and older, 56 percent are female, and 41 percent have income levels below 200 percent of the federal poverty level. Roughly, one-third of the beneficiaries are in fair to poor health (The Henry J. Kaiser Family Foundation 2006).

The Medicare program was first implemented in 1966. It is a federal program operated under the administrative oversight of the Centers for Medicare and Medicaid Services (CMS, which was formerly named Health Care Financing Administration [HCFA]), a branch of the US Department of Health and Human Services (DHHS). Being a federal program, eligibility criteria and benefits are consistent throughout the United States.

Shortly after the program was created, it had 19.5 million enrollees in 1967. In July 2005, Medicare enrollees totaled 42.4 million in all US states, the District of Columbia, and US territories (Centers for Medicare and Medicaid Services 2006a). With the aging of the population, as the baby-boomers begin reaching the age of 65 in 2011, the program is expected to grow to 61 million enrollees by the year 2020.

The Balanced Budget Act of 1997 established an independent federal agency, the Medicare Payment Advisory Commission (MedPAC), to advise the US Congress on various issues affecting the Medicare program. MedPAC's statutory mandate extends beyond payments to private health care providers participating in Medicare. The Commission is also tasked with analyzing access to care, quality of care, and other issues affecting Medicare.

For almost 30 years after its inception, Medicare had a dual structure comprising two separate insurance programs referred to as Part A and Part B. Now Medicare has a four-part structure.

Part A (Hospital Insurance)

Part A, the Hospital Insurance (HI) portion of Medicare, is financed primarily by special payroll taxes. The employer and employee share equally in financing the Hospital Insurance Trust Fund. Tax deductions for Medicare are distinctly identified on employee pay stubs. All working individuals, including those who are self-employed, pay these mandatory taxes. Prior to 1994, a maximum taxable ceiling was set each year. The Omnibus Budget Reconciliation Act of 1993 (OBRA-93) eliminated the maximum taxable earnings base, so all earnings are now subject to Medicare tax (Davis and Burner 1995).

Part A covers hospital inpatient services, care in a skilled nursing facility (SNF), home health visits, and hospice care. Following is an overview of the type of benefits:

1. A maximum of 90 days of inpatient hospital care is allowed per benefit period. Once the 90 days are exhausted, a lifetime reserve of 60 additional hospital inpatient days remains. A ***benefit period*** is a spell of illness beginning with hospitalization and ending when a beneficiary has not been an inpatient in a hospital or an SNF for 60 consecutive days. The number of benefit periods is not limited.
2. Medicare pays for up to 100 days of care in a Medicare-certified SNF subsequent to inpatient hospitalization for at least three consecutive days, not including the day of discharge. Admission to the SNF must occur within 30 days of hospital discharge.
3. Medicare pays for home health care when a person is homebound and requires intermittent or part-time skilled nursing care or rehabilitation care. Part A covers the first 100 visits following a three-day stay in a hospital or an SNF. Additional visits may be covered under Part B.
4. For terminally ill patients, Medicare pays for care provided by a Medicare-certified hospice.

The Part A program requires the beneficiaries to pay a deductible (except for home health and hospice) for each benefit period and to make co-payments based on the duration of services (except for home health). Most people 65 years of age or older do not have to pay a premium if they paid Medicare taxes while working. Some who do not meet the Social Security Administration's qualifications for premium-free coverage can get Part A by paying a monthly premium. Details of the Part A program are given in Exhibit 6–1.

Part B (Supplementary Medical Insurance)

Part B, the supplementary medical insurance (SMI) portion of Medicare, is a voluntary program financed partly by general tax rev-

Exhibit 6–1 Medicare Part A Financing, Benefits, Deductible, and Copayments for 2007

Financing

The Hospital Insurance Trust Fund is financed by a payroll tax of 1.45 percent from the employee and 1.45 percent from the employer. All income is taxed.

Premiums	None (Those who do not qualify for premium-free coverage can buy coverage at a monthly premium of $410)
Deductible	$992 per benefit period

Benefits	Copayments
Inpatient hospital (Room, meals, nursing care, operating room services, blood transfusions, special care units, drugs and medical supplies, laboratory test, rehabilitation therapies, and medical social services)	None for the first 60 days [benefit period] $248 per day for days 61–90 [benefit period] $496 per day for days 91–150 [nonrenewable lifetime reserve days]
Skilled nursing facility (after a 3-day hospital stay)	None for the first 20 days [benefit period] $124 per day for days 21–100 [benefit period]
Home health services (Part-time skilled nursing care, home health aide, rehabilitation therapies, medical equipment, social services, and medical supplies)	None for home health visits 20% of approved amount for durable medical
Hospice care	A small copayment for drugs
Inpatient psychiatric care (190 days lifetime limit)	Same as for inpatient hospital

Noncovered Services

Long-term care

Custodial services

Personal convenience services (televisions, telephones, private-duty nurses, private rooms when not medically necessary)

Source: Data from Centers for Medicare and Medicaid Services.

enues and partly by required premium contributions. Effective 2007, CMS implemented income-based Part B premiums as mandated by the Medicare Prescription Drug, Improvement, and Modernization Act of 2003 (MMA 2003). Single beneficiaries earning less than $80,000 per year ($160,000 per couple) will pay the standard premium. Those whose incomes exceed the threshold amount will pay a higher income-based premium (see Exhibit 6–2).

Almost all persons entitled to HI also choose to enroll in SMI because they cannot get similar coverage at that price from private

Exhibit 6–2 Medicare Part B Financing, Benefits, Deductible, and Coinsurance for 2007

Financing

The general tax revenues of the federal government support approximately 75 percent of the program costs. The remaining 25 percent is financed through monthly premiums paid by persons enrolled in Part B.

Standard premium	$93.50 per month
Income-adjusted premium*	$105.80 to $161.40 annually
Deductible	$131 annually
Coinsurance	80–20 (50–50 for outpatient mental health)

Main Benefits

Physician services
Emergency department services
Outpatient surgery
Diagnostic tests and laboratory services
Outpatient physical therapy, occupational therapy, and speech therapy
Outpatient mental health services
Part-time home health care
Ambulance
Renal dialysis
Artificial limbs and braces
Blood transfusions and blood components
Organ transplants
Medical equipment and supplies
Rural health clinic services
Some limited preventative services (Pap smears, mammography, colorectal and prostate cancer screening, glaucoma screening, and flu shots)

Noncovered Services

Routine physical examinations
Most preventive care
Outpatient prescription drugs
Dental services
Hearing aids or eyeglasses
Services not related to treatment or injury

Source: Data from Centers for Medicare and Medicaid Services.

*For single beneficiaries whose annual incomes exceed $80,000.

insurers. In 2004, 93 percent of all Medicare enrollees had SMI coverage (CMS 2004). The main services covered by SMI are physician services; hospital outpatient services, such as outpatient surgery, diagnostic tests, and radiology and pathology services; emergency department visits; ambulance services; outpatient rehabilitation services; renal dialysis; radiation treatment; tissue transplants; prostheses; medical equipment and supplies; and limited preventive services (see Exhibit 6–2 for additional details). Part B also covers limited home health services that are not associated with a hospital or SNF stay.

Part C (Medicare Advantage)

Part C is, in reality, not a new program because it does not add specifically-defined new services. It merely provides some additional choices of health plans with the objective of channeling a greater number of beneficiaries into managed care plans. The Balanced Budget Act (BBA) of 1997 (Public Law 105–33) authorized the Medicare+Choice program which took effect on January 1, 1998. The law expanded the role of private health plans such as health maintenance organizations (HMOs), preferred provider organizations (PPOs), provider-sponsored organizations (PSOs), and private fee-for-service (PFFS) plans to serve Medicare beneficiaries who could either choose to enroll in Medicare+Choice or remain in the original Medicare fee-for-service program. Medicare+Choice was renamed Medicare Advantage through the passage of the MMA of 2003. In 2005, 247 private plans (mostly HMOs) participated in the Medicare Advantage program, and approximately 12 percent of the Medicare beneficiaries were enrolled in these plans, down from a high of 16 percent in 2000 (The Henry J. Kaiser Family Foundation 2005a).

Medicare Advantage plans may offer additional benefits that are not offered by the Original Medicare Plan, and/or may have lower out of pocket costs. In many cases, enrollees may not need private Medigap policies (discussed later). Hence, it is a good option particularly for lower income Medicare beneficiaries.

The MMA of 2003 required that Medicare Advantage include special needs plans. These plans were first offered in 2005 to meet the special needs of people who were institutionalized, enrolled in both Medicare and Medicaid, or had chronic or disabling conditions. Medicare Advantage Special Needs Plans (MA-SNP) are available in limited areas. The program is designed to benefit people who have special needs and to coordinate services between Medicare and Medicaid for those enrolled in both programs.

Part D (Prescription Drug Coverage)

Like Part B, the prescription drug program is voluntary because it requires payment of a monthly premium by those who want the coverage. The program is available to anyone, regardless of income, who has coverage under Part A or Part B. Part D was added to the existing Medicare program under the MMA of 2003, and was fully implemented in January 2006. Coverage is offered through two types of private plans approved by Medicare: (a) Stand-alone Prescription Drug Plans that offer only drug coverage are available to those who want to stay in the original Medicare fee-for-service program. (b) Medicare Advantage Prescription Drug Plans are available to those who want to obtain all health care services through managed care organizations participating in Part C. Exhibit 6–3 summarizes the standard benefit, which is the minimum required by law regardless of the choice of plan. Some plans may offer additional benefits or have lower out of pocket costs for the enrollees than what the standard benefit mandates.

The program is likely to be well received by those beneficiaries who previously had no drug coverage. Also, special provisions in the program are designed to help low-income enrollees by keeping their out of pocket costs to a minimum. However, it remains to be seen whether the large majority of beneficiaries will be satisfied with the program, how much the program will eventually cost the taxpayers, and any mid-course corrections that Congress may have to make. According to the Congressional Budget Office's 2004 estimates, the program would cost $409 billion over an eight-year period. The cost estimates were based on a projected rise in monthly premiums from $35 to $58, an increase in annual deductibles from $250 to $445, and an increase in the catastrophic coverage threshold (out of pocket spending before qualifying for the catastrophic level—see Exhibit 6–3) from $3,600 to $6,400 (Holtz-Eakin 2004). Benefits and cost estimates for 2007 are summarized in Exhibit 6–4.

Medicare Financing and Spending

The sources of financing for Parts A, B, and D are given in Exhibits 6–1, 6–2, and 6–3 respectively. For the Medicare program as a whole, in 2001, 56 percent of the total financing was attributed to payroll taxes, 27 percent to general tax revenues, 8 percent to premiums from participants, and 9 percent to other sources (The Henry J. Kaiser Family Foundation 2003). The addition of Part D in 2006 has substantially altered the proportion of financing dollars derived from payroll taxes, general tax revenues, premiums paid by beneficiaries, and miscellaneous sources. Fig-

Exhibit 6–3 Medicare Part D Financing and Standard Benefit for 2006

The general tax revenues of the federal government support approximately 78 percent of the program costs. Roughly 10 percent is financed through monthly premiums paid by the beneficiaries, 11 percent through payments by states, and 1 percent from other sources.

Premiums $32.20 per month (estimated national average)*
Deductible $250 annually

Three levels of benefits and out-of pocket costs beyond the $250 deductible:

	Drug costs	Medicare pays	Beneficiary pays
Basic level	$251 – 2,250	75% up to $1,500	25% up to $500
Gap or "Doughnut hole"	$2,251 – 5,100	no coverage	100% up to $2,850
Catastrophic level	Over $5,100	95%	5%

Note: Catastrophic coverage (95—5 coinsurance) begins after a beneficiary has spent $3,600 annually out of pocket [$750 at the basic level ($2,250–$1500) and $2,850 ($5,100–$2,250) in the doughnut hole].

The Extra Help program

A special part of the Medicare drug coverage program called Extra Help is designed to serve people who have low incomes and savings. This group of beneficiaries includes those who receive Medicaid or Supplemental Security Income. For those who qualify, the out-of-pocket costs are minimal.

*Actual premium varies according to the plan selected by the beneficiary.

Exhibit 6–4 Part D Standard Benefits and Individual Out-of-Pocket Costs for 2007

Premiums $37 per month (estimated)*
Deductible $265 annually

Three levels of benefits and out-of pocket costs beyond the $265 deductible:

	Drug costs	Medicare pays	Beneficiary pays
Basic level	$266 – 2,400	75% up to $1,601.25	25% up to $533.75
Gap or 'Doughnut hole'	$2,401 – 5,451.25	no coverage	100% up to $3,051.25
Catastrophic level	Over $5,100	95%	5%

Note: Catastrophic coverage threshold: $3,850

*Holtz-Eakin, D. 2004. *CBO testimony: Estimating the cost of the Medicare Modernization Act.* Washington, DC: Congressional Budget Office.

Figure 6–3 Sources of Financing Medicare, 2006 (projected).

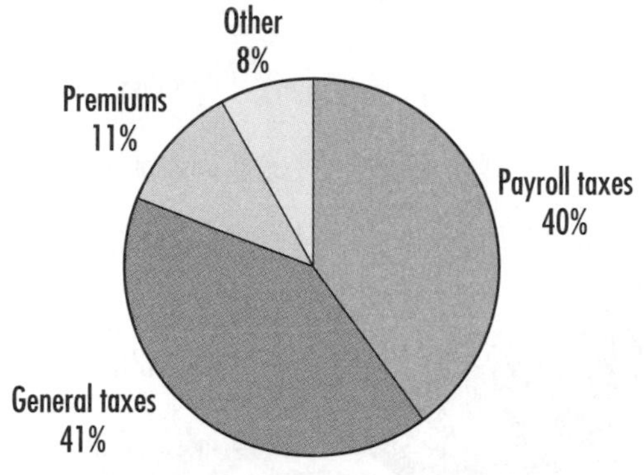

Source: Data from The Henry J. Kaiser Foundation, *Medicare Spending and Financing,* April 2005.

Table 6–1 Status of HI and SMI Trust Funds, 2005 (billions of dollars)

	HI	SMI
Assets at the end of 2004	$269.3	$ 19.4
Income	199.4	158.1
Disbursements	182.9	153.5
Net increase in assets	16.4	4.6
Assets at the end of 2005	285.8	24.0

Source: Social Security Administration. 2006. *A summary of the 2006 Annual Reports: Social Security and Medicare Board of Trustees.* Available at: *http://www.ssa.gov/OACT/TRSUM/trsummary.html.*

ure 6–3 provides the 2006 estimated sources of financing for the Medicare program.

Medicare has established two main trust funds: The HI trust fund provides the money pool for Part A services, and the SMI trust fund provides the money pool for Parts B and D. Each trust fund accounts for incomes and disbursements. Taxes, premiums, and other incomes are credited to the respective trust funds, and benefit payments and administrative costs are the only purposes for which disbursements from the funds can be made. The excess of revenues over expenditures generates interest income that stays in each fund (Social Security Administration 2006). The trust fund results for 2005 are shown in Table 6–1.

Projected depletion of the trust funds has been a matter of concern for quite some time. A combination of three main factors raises such concerns: (1) The cost of delivering health care continues to grow at a rate faster than the rate of inflation in the general economy. (2) An aging population will consume a greater quantity of health care services. (3) The workforce is shrinking, and wage increases to support tax revenues are smaller than the rise in medical inflation.

Even though the trust funds currently show surpluses (i.e., revenues exceed expenses), starting in 2006, expenditures are projected to exceed revenues in the HI trust fund. Deficits are expected to grow rapidly starting in 2010 as baby boomers begin to retire. According to current forecasts, the HI trust fund would be depleted in 2018 unless current financing arrangements are overhauled. The SMI trust fund is projected to remain adequately financed into the indefinite future under current law (Social Security Administration 2006). However, rapid cost increases will place a substantial burden on the taxpaying workforce, and will require hefty increases in Part B and Part D premiums. It is highly unlikely that working Americans would be willing to pay significantly higher taxes.

The distribution of Medicare expenditures for the various covered services provided under HI and SMI funding is shown in Figure 6–4. Data on enrolled population and expenditures are given in Exhibit 6–5.

Figure 6–4 Percentage Distribution of Medicare Expenditures, 2005.

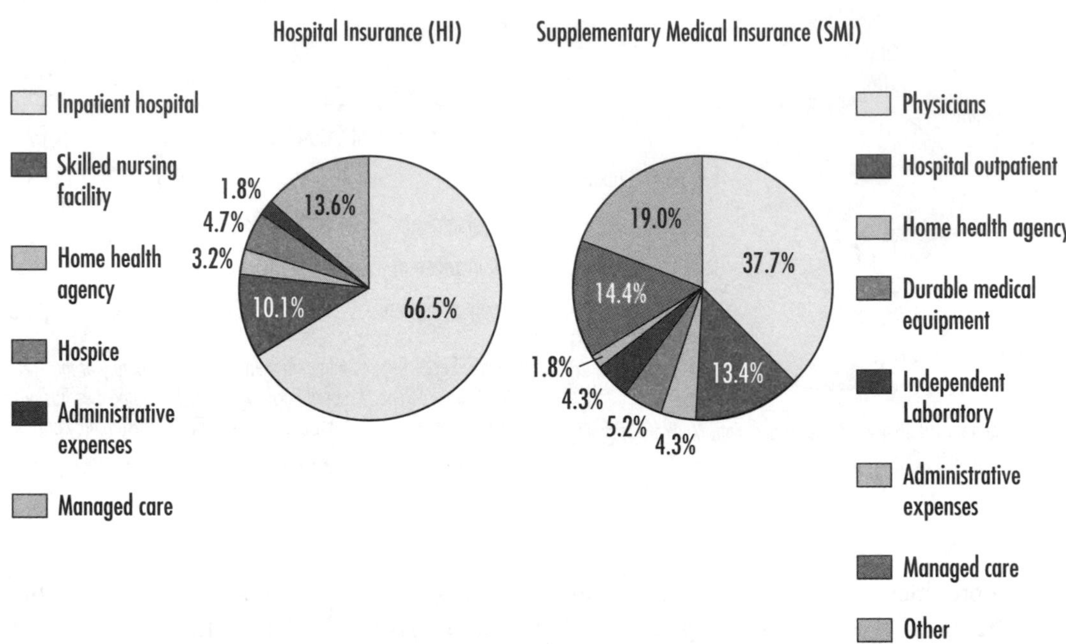

Source: Data from *Health, United States, 2006*, p. 404, US Department of Health and Human Services, National Center for Health Statistics.

Note: The "other" category under SMI includes free-standing surgery centers, free-standing dialysis centers, ambulance services, outpatient rehabilitation facilities, psychiatric facilities, rural health clinics, and community health centers.

Exhibit 6–5 Medicare: Enrolled Population and Expenditures in Selected Years

	1970	1985	1990	1995	2000	2005
Population Covered (in millions)	20.4	31.1	34.3	37.6	39.7	42.5
Expenditures (in billions)	$7.5	$72.3	$111.00	$184.2	$221.7	$336.4
Proportion of Total US Health Care Expenditures	10.0%	16.9%	15.5%	18.1%	16.3%	16.9%

Source: Data from *Health, United States, 2000*, pp. 325, 348; *Health, United States, 2006*, pp. 377, 404. National Center for Health Statistics.

Noncovered Services under Medicare

Neither Part A nor Part B offers comprehensive coverage. Services such as vision care, eyeglasses, dental care and dentures, hearing exams and hearing aids, routine foot care, and routine physical exams are not covered by either plan. Exceptions are bone mass measurement, cardiovascular screening, screening for colorectal and prostate cancer, diabetes screening, glaucoma screening, Pap smears, screening mammography, flu shots, and vaccinations against pneumonia. These preventive services are covered for Part B enrollees.

Many elderly think that when they need nursing home care, they will be covered under Medicare. Long-term care benefit, however, is very limited. Under Part A, the patient must first meet the criteria for skilled nursing care. Even after this condition is met, services are fully paid for just 20 days. In other words, Medicare is not a program for long-term care.

Deductibles, co-payments, and premiums (see Exhibits 6–1, 6–2, and 6–3) leave the elderly with high out of pocket expenses. For example, in 2002, Medicare covered about 45 percent of the beneficiaries' total health care expenses. In 2003, the average (mean) income of an elderly individual in the United States was estimated to be $23,200, of which an estimated 22 percent was consumed by Medicare out of pocket costs (The Henry J. Kaiser Family Foundation 2005b).

Medicaid

Medicaid, also referred to as Title XIX of the Social Security Act, finances health care services for the indigent; however, Medicaid does not provide medical assistance for all poor persons. Certain categories of people are automatically eligible under federal guidelines: (1) Families with children receiving support under the Temporary Assistance for Needy Families (TANF) program. (2) People receiving Supplemental Security Income (SSI), which includes many of the elderly, the blind, and the disabled with low incomes. (3) Children and pregnant women whose family income is at or below 133 percent of the Federal Poverty Level, which was $20,650 for a family of four in 2007. The amount was $25,820 for Alaska and $23,750 for Hawaii (Federal Register 2007). (4) Other categories defined by federal law. In addition, most states, at their discretion, have defined other "medically needy" categories based on people's income and assets. Most important of these are individuals who are institutionalized in nursing or psychiatric facilities, and individuals who are receiving community-based services but would otherwise be eligible for Medicaid if institutionalized. All these people have to qualify based on assets and income, which must be below the threshold levels established by each state. Hence, Medicaid is a ***means-tested program***.

All US states, the District of Columbia, and US territories, such as Guam, Puerto Rico, American Samoa, and the Virgin Islands, operate Medicaid plans. Each state administers its own Medicaid program. Hence, eligibility criteria, covered services, and payments to providers vary considerably from state to state. However, for a state to receive federal matching funds, federal law mandates that every state provide some specific basic health services (see Exhibit 6–6). In addition, states may also receive federal matching funds for providing certain optional services, such as prescription drugs and prostheses, optometrist services and eyeglasses, transportation services, rehabilitation, home and community-based care for people with chronic impairments, and services in intermediate

Exhibit 6–6 Federally Mandated Services for State Medicaid Programs

Hospital inpatient care
Hospital outpatient services
Physician services
Laboratory and X-ray services
Nursing faciltiy services
Home health services for those eligible for skilled nursing (SNF) services
Prenatal care
Family planning services and supplies
Rural health clinic services
Preventive, diagnostic, and treatment services (including vaccinations) for dependent children under the age of 21
Nurse-midwife services
Certain federally qualified ambulatory and health center services
Pediatric and family nurse practioner services

Source: Data from *Health Care Financing Review, Statistical Supplement, 2001*: 14.

care facilities for the mentally retarded (ICF/MR). States may impose nominal deductibles and co-payments on some Medicaid recipients for certain services, but some exclusions exist. Emergency services, family planning services and supplies, and hospice care are exempt from co-payments.

Changes to Medicaid benefits have been legislated under the Deficit Reduction Act of 2005. The law requires states to institute premium and cost sharing based on income.

Medicaid Financing and Spending

The federal and state governments jointly finance the Medicaid program. The federal government provides matching funds to the states based on the per capita income in each state. By law, federal matching—known as the Federal Medical Assistance Percentage (FMAP)—cannot be less than 50 percent nor greater than 83 percent of total state Medicaid program costs. Wealthier states have a smaller share of their costs reimbursed by the federal government. For the federal fiscal year 2007, the FMAPs varied from 50 percent (for 12 states) to 75.9 percent (for Mississippi). The actual cost sharing between the federal and state governments in 2005 was 57:43 (Catlin et al. 2007).

The Medicaid program serves approximately 45 million low-income Americans. Figure 6–5 presents the main characteristics of people covered by Medicaid. The pie chart on the left gives the proportion of recipients in each classification; the one on the right gives the proportion of payments made to health care providers on behalf of each category of recipient. Notice that children under 21 years of age, who constitute a little less than half of all Medicaid recipients, incur 17 percent of total expenditures. The blind and disabled, on the other hand, constitute approximately 15 percent of the recipients but incur almost 44 percent of all expenditures. Also, the elderly, who constitute 8 percent of all recipients, incur 24 percent of the expenses.

Medicaid enrollment and spending vary according to the state of the US economy. For example, the level of spending rose at an annual rate of 12 percent between 2000 and 2002, and moderated down to 7.6 percent from 2002 to 2004 as the economy improved following the 2001 recession (The Kaiser Commission on Medicaid and the Uninsured 2006). Managed care enrollment has been increasingly used to control costs. In 2005, at least 10 states (Nevada, Tennessee, South Dakota, Georgia, Colorado, Iowa, Kentucky, Utah, Oregon, and Pennsylvania) had 90 per-

Figure 6–5 Medicaid Recipients and Medical Vendor Payments According to Basis of Eligibility, 2003 Data.

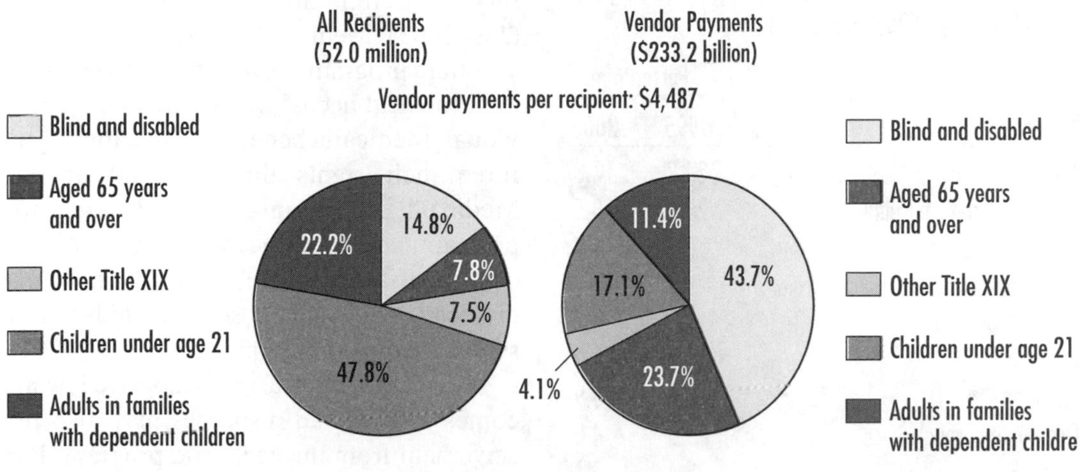

Source: Data from *Health, United States, 2006*, p. 409, Department of Health and Human Services.

cent or more of their Medicaid recipients enrolled in managed care plans.

Data on enrolled population, including children under the age of 21, and expenditures are given in Exhibit 6–7. Proportional payments to the various types of vendors providing services to Medicaid recipients are shown in Table 6–2.

Exhibit 6–7 Medicaid: Population Covered and Expenditures in Selected Years

Population Covered (in millions)					
1970	1985	1990	1995	2000	2003
17.6	21.8	25.3	36.3	42.8	52.0
Number of Under Age 21 Children Covered (in billions)					
	9.8	11.2	17.2	20.2	24.9
Expenditures (in billions)					
$5.4	$41.7	$76.6	$144.3	$205.0	$275.8
Proportion of Total US Health Care Expenditures					
7.2%	9.7%	10.7%	14.1%	15.1%	15.8%

Source: Data from *Health, United States, 1998*, pp. 348, 369; *Health, United States, 2006*, pp. 388, 409. National Center for Health Statistics.

Table 6–2 Medicaid Vendor Payments According to Type of Service, 1995 and 2003

	Percentage	
Type of Service	1995	2003
Nursing facilities	24.2	17.3
Inpatient general hospital	21.9	13.5
Prescribed drugs	8.1	14.5
Mentally retarded intermediate care facilities	8.6	4.7
Home health	7.8	1.9
Physician	6.1	3.9
Outpatient hospital	5.5	4.0
Clinic	3.6	3.1
Mental health facility	2.1	0.9
Laboratory and radiological	1.0	1.0
Dental	0.8	1.1
Managed care and other prepaid care	None	16.0
Miscellaneous	10.3	18.1

Total payments: 1995 $120.1 billion
2003 233.2 billion

Source: Data from *Health, United States, 2006*, p. 410, and National Center for Health Statistics.

Main Distinctions and Relationships Between Medicare and Medicaid

Although Medicare and Medicaid may both be loosely referred to as entitlement programs, technically there is an important distinction between the two. Similar to Social Security, Medicare is an ***entitlement*** program. Because people have contributed to Medicare through taxes, they are "entitled" to the benefits regardless of the amount of income and assets they may have. Medicare beneficiaries are specifically given the legal right to enforce in federal courts, if necessary, their eligibility and access to services (Jost 2003). Medicaid, on the other hand, is a welfare program to assist the indigent with their medical needs. Unlike Medicare, individual Medicaid beneficiaries cannot enforce their rights through legal action. Medicaid is a comprehensive health care program, unlike Medicare. However, dental care benefits are severely limited; only children can receive dental services under most states' Medicaid programs.

Medicare beneficiaries who have low incomes and limited resources may also receive help from the Medicaid program. For the elderly and disabled who qualify for Medicaid, the program pays their Medicare premiums, deductibles, and co-payments. For such dually covered persons, Medicaid is the payer of last resort, that is, the Medicare program pays for any services covered under Medicare before Medicaid kicks in. Dually covered persons are estimated to comprise roughly 18 percent of all Medicare beneficiaries.

Dually eligible beneficiaries are covered under two separate programs. Under the Qualified Medicare Beneficiary (QMB) program, Medicaid picks up Medicare Part A and Part B premiums, as well as all deductibles and co-payments. Depending on the state's Medicaid guidelines, beneficiaries may also qualify for full Medicaid benefits (about half actually do). The QMB program covers individuals whose incomes are at, or below, the federal poverty level. The second program, Specified Low-income Medicare Beneficiary (SLMB) program, pays only the Part B premiums for people whose incomes are higher than the Medicaid threshold but still less than 120 percent of the federal poverty level. Two additional, but less important, programs are also available to low-income or disabled people. The qualified individual (QI) program provides states with block grants to pay Medicare premiums for individuals with incomes between 120 and 135 percent of the federal poverty level. Under this program, qualified people are served on a first-come first-served basis until the available funds are exhausted. These block grants were originally set to expire in 2002, but have been reauthorized through September 2007 (Ebeler et al. 2006). Under the Qualified Disabled and Working Individual (QDWI) program, states are required to pay Part A premiums for certain low-income people who qualified for Medicare because of disability but then returned to work and hence lost the entitlement.

Public Programs Initiated under the Balanced Budget Act of 1997

PACE

A program that spans both Medicare and Medicaid is the Program of All-inclusive Care for the Elderly (PACE), but it is not available in all states. PACE provides community-based care for persons aged 55 years or older who otherwise qualify for placement in a nursing facility. The care is provided in day-care centers, homes, hospitals, and nursing homes. All medical care and social services are coordinated by a PACE team. Providers of PACE services receive payment only through the PACE agreement and not separately from Medicare or Medicaid, but they must make available all services covered under both Medicare and Medicaid. PACE has no deductibles and co-payments, which is an incentive for qualified individuals to join the program. The main aim of the program is to provide long-term care services in community settings to people who otherwise risk being in nursing homes.

SCHIP

The State Children's Health Insurance Program (SCHIP), codified as Title XXI of the Social Security Act, is another program enacted under the BBA of 1997. The program was initiated in response to the plight of uninsured children, who were estimated to number 10.1 million (nearly one-quarter of all uninsured) in 1996. The program offers additional funds to states to expand Medicaid eligibility to enroll children under 19 years of age who otherwise would not qualify for coverage because their families' incomes exceed the Medicaid threshold levels. SCHIP is available to families with incomes up to 200 percent of the federal poverty level, which was $41,300 for a family of four in 2007 (the thresholds are higher in Alaska and Hawaii), and if they are not covered under another private or public health insurance plan. SCHIP offers participating states two basic options: (1) expansion of Medicaid, or (2) establishment of a special child health assistance program. A state also has the option to combine the two approaches. States are required to screen applicants for Medicaid eligibility and to enroll eligible children in Medicaid rather than in the new SCHIP program. The law was authorized for 10 years and allocated $40 billion in federal funding to the states during the period 1998–2007. As enrollment has grown over time, SCHIP has been serving roughly 3.9 million children since 2003. Research has shown that SCHIP has had a significant impact in reducing uninsurance among children (Hudson et al. 2005). SCHIP has also been credited with improved access, continuity of care, and quality of care for all racial/ethnic groups, and a reduction in preexisting racial/ethnic disparities in access, unmet need, and continuity of care (Shone et al. 2005). Unless reauthorized by Congress, SCHIP will expire on September 30, 2007.

The Military Health Services System

The United States Department of Defense operates a substantial program to provide medical services to the active duty and retired members of the armed forces, their dependents, and survivors through the Military Health Services System (MHSS). In 2005, the MHSS operated 75 hospitals and 461 clinics to serve an eligible population of 8.9 million. These hospitals and clinics are mainly for active-duty service members, but dependents of service members, retirees and their dependents, and survivors of deceased members can also obtain services at military facilities if space is available. Otherwise, they can receive medical care under a program known as TriCare (previously called CHAMPUS).

The TriCare program was developed in response to the growing health care needs of military personnel, an increasing number of whom are retirees. Closing of military bases and other downsizing efforts during the Clinton administration resulted in the closure of 35 percent of the military hospitals that existed in the United States in 1987. Yet the total number of people seeking health care through the MHSS dropped by only 9 percent. Consequently, military facilities no longer had the capacity to meet the demand for health care (Department of Defense 1996).

TriCare has three main features: (1) It is regionally managed to facilitate administration of the program; (2) it is structured after managed care; and (3) it brings together the medical resources of the Army, Navy, and Air Force, and supplements them with networks of civilian health care professionals and facilities. There are 11 TriCare regions in the United States, plus TriCare Europe, TriCare Latin America, and TriCare Pacific.

TriCare offers three health plan options. (1) TriCare Prime functions like an HMO. Enrollees must choose a primary care manager (PCM) from a list of providers. The PCM coordinates the beneficiary's total health care needs. The PCM can be located in a military hospital or clinic or in a civilian network, but most of the care is delivered through the military's own medical treatment facilities (MTFs). The TriCare Prime option offers additional wellness and preventive care services. Enrollees choosing this option must agree to a one-year enrollment. Of the three options, this plan is the most cost-efficient for the enrollees. (2) TriCare Extra is a preferred provider option. Enrollees receive medical care from participating civilian network providers at a discount. Compared to TriCare Prime, TriCare Extra offers an expanded network of providers. This program has no enrollment requirement. (3) TriCare Standard is a traditional fee-for-service plan similar to the former CHAMPUS program. Civilian providers provide the services. Beneficiaries using this option have the greatest choice of physicians, but at a higher cost. None of the options requires premiums from active-duty personnel, but deductibles and co-payments generally apply (Best 2005; Department of Defense 1999).

For elderly beneficiaries who are enrolled in Medicare Part B, TriCare for Life (TFL) serves as a second payer to Medicare, paying out of pocket costs for services covered under Medicare. The program also provides benefits not covered by Medicare but covered by TriCare (Best 2005).

Veterans Health Administration

Formerly called Veterans Administration, the Department of Veterans Affairs (VA) is an executive department of the US government. Veterans Health Administration (VHA), the health services branch of the VA, operates the largest integrated health services system in the United States, with approximately 163 hospitals, 913 outpatient clinics, and 137 nursing homes and various other facilities (Department of Veterans Affairs 2004). VHA employs approximately 180,000 health care professionals (Department of Veterans Affairs 2003). The VA health care system was originally established to treat veterans with war-related injuries and to help rehabilitate past service members with war-related disabilities. This original mission was expanded, and nonservice-related conditions actually account for the bulk of the care provided because the system has been increasingly used by poor veterans with medical conditions unrelated to military combat services. A little over 60 percent of the veterans served by VHA have no service-connected disabilities (National Center for Health Statistics 2005, 402). However, Congress requires VHA to provide services on a priority basis to veterans with service-connected illnesses and disabilities, low incomes, or special health care needs. Eligible veterans are classified into one of eight priority groups upon enrollment. Priority Group 1 receives the highest priority. These veterans have service-connected disabilities rated as 50 percent or more disabling. Apart from delivering health care services, the VHA system also actively participates in medical education and research.

In 2004, the veteran population was estimated to be 24.6 million. Almost 5 million people received services through the VA system. Total medical expenditures were $28.1 million (Department of Veterans Affairs 2004). Each year, a growing number of veterans use VA medical services.

The VA is a tax-financed agency that, for the most part, delivers care directly through salaried physicians and government-owned facilities. Funding for the VHA program is appropriated in the annual presidential budget approved by Congress. The structure of VA funding is patterned after the global budget model, in which budget appropriations are determined in advance for the entire system. The VHA then distributes the funds to its organizational units having oversight for the delivery of health care.

In 1996, the VHA restructured its delivery system by creating 22 geographically distributed Veterans Integrated Service Networks (VISNs). Each VISN is responsible for coordinating the activities of the hospitals, outpatient clinics, nursing homes, and other facilities located within its jurisdiction. The VHA also implemented the Veterans Equitable Resource Allocation (VERA) system to allocate funds to the 22 VISNs. Each VISN is then responsible for allocating those resources among the facilities in its prescribed geographic area to ensure care and equitable access within the network. Before the organizational restructuring, problems existed with equitable distribution of resources and access to services in certain regions of the country. Another role of the VISNs is to improve efficiency by reducing duplicate services by consolidating medical facilities and programs, by emphasizing preventive services, and by shifting services from costly inpatient care to less costly outpatient care (GAO 1998). As a result of these efforts, between 1996 and 2001, expenditures for acute hospital care actually decreased by 4 percent even as total VA expenditures increased by 30 percent (Department of Veterans Affairs 2002).

The VA also operates a health care benefits program for the eligible dependents of veterans. The program is called CHAMPVA, which covers (1) dependents of permanently disabled veterans and (2) survivors of veterans who died in the line of duty, died from service-related conditions, or were permanently disabled at the time of death.

The VHA system offers some insight into what a tax-financed national health care system with an increased number of participants may look like. The system is under severe capacity and financing constraints. Between 1996 and 2002, the number of veterans seeking care doubled. Enrollment to the lowest priority category, Priority Group 8, has been frozen. Approximately 235,000 veterans waited six months or more for an appointment (Fong 2003). Another major challenge VHA will face in the near future is the growing need for efficient long-term care and geriatric services to an aging veteran population.

Indian Health Service

The federal program administered by the Indian Health Service (IHS), a division of the DHHS, provides comprehensive health care services directly to members of federally recognized American Indian and Alaska Native Tribes and their descendants. Approximately 1.8 million of the estimated 3.3 million Native Americans receive services under the program, which has an annual budget appropriation of roughly $3 billion. The beneficiaries live primarily on reservations and in rural communities, mostly in the western United States and Alaska. Besides medical and dental care, services include health promotion and disease prevention, and programs in substance abuse, maternal and child health, sanitation, and nutrition. The IHS system includes 33 hospitals, 59 health centers, and 50 health stations. Additional services are contracted from tribally operated health programs and private providers (IHS 2006). A more detailed discussion on the IHS is presented in Chapter 11.

Miscellaneous Private and Public Programs

Medigap

As mentioned earlier, Medicare covers less than half of an average beneficiary's total health care costs, and leaves them with substantial out of pocket expenses. To cover these expenses, Medicare beneficiaries can receive supplemental coverage from one of four sources: (1) Medicaid becomes the source of supplemental coverage for dually eligible enrollees. (2) Enrollment in Medicare Advantage (Part C) can provide supplemental coverage. (3) Employer-sponsored retiree insurance is available to some of the elderly. (4) The remaining Medicare participants have the option to purchase supplemental insurance policies from private insurance companies. These policies are referred to as ***Medigap*** policies.

Medigap policies cover all or a portion of Medicare deductibles and co-payments, and they may pay for services not covered by Medicare. To protect consumer interests and to simplify plan selection, the Omnibus Budget Reconciliation Act of 1990 mandated that Medicare designate standardized plan categories containing uniform benefits that consumers could choose from. Insurance companies could sell only these standardized plans. The 10 original plans were labeled A through J. Since Medicare now provides prescription drug coverage, plans H, I, and J can no longer be sold (except for those who already have this coverage). Two new Medigap plans, K and L, have been added. These are high deductible plans designed to cover catastrophic costs. The most common out of pocket costs covered by most plans include hospital co-payments (all Medigap plans), hospital deductible (all but plan A), and skilled nursing facility co-payments (all but plans A and B). Premiums vary according to the plan selected, and they also vary from company to company.

Workers' Compensation

The theory underlying workers' compensation is that all accidents that occur during the course of employment and all illnesses directly attributable to the workplace must be regarded as risks of industry. In other words, the employer is financially liable for such injuries and illnesses, regardless of who is at fault. Since workers' compensation is a state-administered program, financing and benefits vary among states. There are four categories of benefits: (1) cash payment for lost wages, (2) payment for medical treatment, (3) indemnification for loss of occupational capacity and skills, and (4) survivors' death benefits. Employers finance these benefits through one of three mechanisms: private insurance, a state fund to which the employers contribute, or self-insurance.

Federal programs cover only specific categories of workers. Civilian employees of the federal government are covered under the Federal Employees' Compensation Act administered by the Office of Workers' Compensation Programs. The Longshore and Harbor Workers' Compensation Act provides benefits to approximately 500,000 workers when they are injured, disabled, or contract an occupational disease occurring on the navigable waters of the United States. The Black Lung Benefits program covers coal miners who are totally disabled from black lung disease (pneumoconiosis) (US Department of Labor 2006).

Workers' compensation is not considered a regular health insurance program, although it provides a significant amount of medical benefits. The medical component may account for 50 percent or more of workers' compensation costs (Harty 2005). Nearly all standard employer sponsored health insurance programs contain provisions that exclude coverage for medical care for work-related accidents and illnesses to avoid duplicate payments by both the medical plan and workers' compensation (Whitted 1993). Workers' compensation differs significantly from regular health insurance in that employers are required by law to bear the full cost of the benefits. There is no employee cost sharing. Managed care and physician networks specializing in workers' compensation are being increasingly used to contain medical costs for worker's compensation beneficiaries.

Other Public Programs

In addition to Medicaid, Medicare, MHSS, TriCare, VHA, CHAMPVA, and IHS programs, the government acts as financier and provider for other types of services. Such programs are administered mainly by state and local governments and are limited in scope. Notable among these programs are state mental hospitals, general hospitals operated by county and municipal governments (discussed in Chapter 8), and community health centers and public health services (discussed in Chapter 7).

The Payment Function

Insurance companies, MCOs, Blue Cross/Blue Shield, and the government (for Medicare and Medicaid) are referred to as ***third-party payers***, the other two parties being the patient and the provider. The payment function has two main facets: (1) the determination of the methods and amounts of reimbursement for the delivery of services and (2) the actual payment after services have been rendered. The set fee for a service is commonly referred to as a charge or rate. Technically, a ***charge*** is set by the provider and is akin to price in general commerce; a ***rate*** is a price set by a third-party payer. An index of charges listing individual fees for each type of service is referred to as a ***fee schedule***. In general, to receive payment for services rendered, the provider must file a ***claim*** with the third-party payer. For the sake of simplicity, in this section we will refer to the determination of charges as "reimbursement" and to the payment of claims as "disbursement."

Reimbursement Methods

Various methods for determining how much providers should be paid are in use. Traditionally, providers have preferred the fee-for-service method, which has fallen out of favor with payers because of cost escalations. Private payers, as well as the government, have devised various methods aimed at limiting the amount of reimbursement, but the main thrust for devising innovative reimbursement methods has come from Medicare. The reimbursement methods discussed below are all in use depending on the nature of service. Physicians, dentists, optometrists, therapists, hospitals, nursing facilities, etc. may be reimbursed according to different reimbursement mechanisms.

Fee-for-Service

Fee-for-service reimbursement is based on the assumption that health care is provided in a set of identifiable and individually distinct units of services, such as examination, X-ray, urinalysis, and a tetanus shot, in the case of physician services. For surgery, such individual services may include an admission kit, numerous medical supplies each accounted for separately, surgeon's fees, anesthesia, anesthesiologist's fees, recovery room charges, and so forth. Each of these services is separately itemized on one bill, and there can be more than one bill. For example, the hospital, the surgeon, the pathologist, and the anesthesiologist generally bill for their services separately.

Initially, fee-for-service charges were set by providers, and insurers passively paid the claims. Later, insurers started to limit reimbursement to a "usual, customary, and reasonable" (UCR) amount. Each insurer determined on its own what the UCR charge should be, generally through community or statewide surveys of what providers were charging. If the actual charges exceed the UCR amount, then reimbursement from insurers is limited to the UCR amount. Providers then ***balance bill***, that is, ask the patients to pay the difference between the actual charges and the payments received from insurers.

The main problem under fee-for-service arrangements is that providers have an incentive to deliver additional services that are not essential. Providers can increase their incomes by increasing the volume of services (see "Imperfect Market" section in Chapter 1). (For a more detailed study of this phenomenon, see Rice and Labelle 1989.)

Bundled Charges (Package Pricing)

Fee-for-service essentially pays for unbundled services. Bundled-fee or package pricing includes a number of related services in one price. For example, normal vaginal delivery may have one set fee that includes the procedure and pre- and post-delivery care (Williams 1995, 114). Optometrists sometimes advertise package prices that include the charges for eye exams, frames for eyeglasses, and corrective lenses. However, dentists, therapists, and some physicians continue to receive payment according to fee-for-service. The various prospective payment systems of reimbursement, discussed later, are also examples of payments for bundled services.

Resource-Based Relative Value Scale

Under the Omnibus Budget Reconciliation Act of 1989 (OBRA-89), Medicare developed a new initiative to reimburse physicians according to a "relative value" assigned to each physician service. The RBRVS method was implemented in 1992. Prior to this date, physician services under Part B were reimbursed according to fee-for-service. Over the years, third-party payers other than Medicare have also adopted variations of RBRVS.

Relative value units (RVUs) are based on the time, skill, and intensity (physician work) it takes to provide a service. Hence, RVUs reflect resource inputs—time, effort, and expertise—to deliver a service. RVUs are established for different types of services that are identified by their ***Current Procedural Terminology*** (CPT) codes—an accepted standard for coding physician services. For each CPT, in addition to RVUs associated with physician work, separate RVUs are included for the cost of practice (overhead costs) and for malpractice insurance. Because of geographical cost variations, each of the RVU categories is multiplied by its own geographic adjustment factor (Geographic Practice Cost Index). Finally, for each year's Medicare budget for physician payments, a conversion factor (CF) is established. The payment for each CPT equals its RVU multiplied by the CF. Medicare establishes a national ***Medicare Physician Fee Schedule*** (MPFS), a price list for physician services, based on which individual payments are made when its physicians file their claims.

Managed Care Approaches

Various types of MCOs have concentrated on three main approaches, which are discussed in greater detail in Chapter 9. The first is the preferred-provider approach, which may be regarded as a variation of the fee-for-service approach. The main distinction is that an MCO establishes fee schedules based on discounts negotiated with providers. These providers are then referred to as preferred providers. Emphasis is placed on using the preferred providers when enrollees need medical services. The second mechanism for reimbursing providers is called capitation. The provider is paid a set monthly fee per enrollee (sometimes referred to as per member per month or PMPM rate), regardless of whether or not an enrollee sees the provider and regardless of how often an enrollee sees the provider. Capitation removes the incentive for providers to increase the volume of services to generate additional revenues. It also makes them prudent in providing only necessary services. A potential problem with capitation is that providers may limit services. When providers withhold necessary services because of cost constraints, it is referred to as ***underutilization***. Salary is the third method used by some MCOs that employ their own physicians.

Cost-Plus Reimbursement

Cost-plus was the traditional method used by Medicare and Medicaid to establish per diem (daily) rates for inpatient stays in hospitals, nursing homes, and other institutions. Home health was also reimbursed based on cost. Under the cost-plus method, reimbursement rates for institutions are based on the total costs incurred in operating the institution. The institution is required to submit a cost report to the third-party payer. Complex formulas are developed that may designate certain costs as "nonallowable" and place cost ceilings in other areas. The formulas are used to calculate the per diem reimbursement rate, also referred to as a per-patient-day (PPD) rate. The method is called ***cost-plus*** because, in addition to the total operating costs, the reimbursement formula also generally allows a portion of the capital costs in arriving at the PPD rate. Because the reimbursement methodology sets rates after evaluating the costs retrospectively, this mechanism is broadly referred to as ***retrospective reimbursement***.

Under the cost-plus system, the total reimbursement is directly related to length of stay, services rendered, and cost of providing the services. Providers have an incentive to provide services indiscriminately, thus increasing costs. There is little motivation for efficiency and cost containment in the delivery of services. Paradoxically, health care institutions could increase their profits by increasing costs. Because of the perverse financial incentives inherent in retrospective cost-based reimbursement, it has been largely replaced by other methods of reimbursement discussed in the following sections. The federal critical access hospital program continues to allow certain rural hospitals to be paid under the cost-plus reimbursement system.

Prospective Reimbursement

In contrast to retrospective reimbursement, where historical costs are used to determine the amount to be paid, ***prospective reimbursement*** uses certain established criteria to determine the amount of reimbursement in advance, before services are delivered. Prospective reimbursement not only minimizes some of the abuses inherent in cost-plus approaches, it also enables providers, such as Medicare, to better predict future health care spending.

Medicare has been using the prospective payment system (PPS) to reimburse inpatient hospital acute care services under Medicare Part A since 1983. Subsequently, the BBA of 1997 mandated implementation of a PPS for hospital outpatient services, and post-acute care providers, such as skilled nursing facilities (SNFs), home health agencies, and inpatient rehabilitation facilities.

Depending on the type of service setting, the three main prospective reimbursement methods, discussed in the following sections, are based on diagnosis-related groups (DRGs), ambulatory payment classification (APC), case-mix methods, and home health resource groups (HHRGs).

In January 2005, Medicare implemented a prospective payment system, using a modified DRG approach, for inpatient psychiatric facilities that previously had been paid according to the cost-plus methodology. The initiative was authorized under the Balanced Budget Refinement Act of 1999. The change affected all of the nearly 2,000 freestanding psychiatric hospitals and certified psychiatric units located in general hospitals. The program is being phased in over a three-year period, to be fully implemented in 2008.

Diagnosis-Related Groups

The PPS for hospital inpatient reimbursement was enacted under the Social Security Amendments of 1983. The predetermined reimbursement amount is set according to DRGs. Each DRG group represents principal diagnoses that are expected to have similar hospital resource use. The approximately 500 DRGs correspond to the most prevalent diagnoses among patients using acute-care inpatient services. The amount of payment is set per discharge rather than per diem. Hence, reimbursement rates are established for bundled services. The bundle of services consists of whatever medical care the patient requires for a given principal diagnosis at the time of admission to an acute-care hospital. The hospital receives the predetermined fixed rate for the particular DRG classification.

The primary factor governing the amount of reimbursement is the type of case, but additional factors can create differences in reimbursement for the same DRG. Such factors include differences in wage levels in various geographic areas; location of the hospital in urban versus rural areas; whether or not the institution is a teaching hospital, that is, it has residency programs for medical graduates (adjustments in reimbursement are based on the intensity of teaching); and an adjustment related to treating a disproportionately large share of low-income patients (HCFA 1996). The latter provision was authorized by Congress under the Consolidated Omnibus Budget Reconciliation Act of 1985 (COBRA-85) to support "safety net" hospitals (also called disproportionate share hospitals) in inner cities and rural areas, many of which would otherwise have been forced to close, leaving underserved and uninsured persons without access to health care (Davis and Burner 1995). Additional payments are made for cases that involve extremely long hospital stays or are extremely expensive, which are referred to as ***outliers***.

Inpatient psychiatric facilities receive a per diem rate (rather than a case-specific rate) based on psychiatric DRGs. The program also includes a stop-loss provision to protect psychiatric hospitals against significant losses. In other respects, the factors considered in arriving at reimbursement rates are similar to those used for reimbursing acute-care hospitals. In 2003, long-term care hospitals (hospitals serving complex post-acute cases) were brought under PPS reimbursement.

The prospective rate-setting methodology has enabled Medicare to control the growth in Part A hospital expenditures. By keeping the actual costs of services below the fixed reimbursement amount, a hospital gets to keep the difference as profit. A hospital loses money when its costs exceed the prospective reimbursement rate. Initially, concerns were voiced that hospitals may discharge patients too early or underprovide necessary services. However, an interplay of several factors, such as competition among hospitals to attract patients, internal ethics committees, external peer review organizations, and development of post-acute care services, such as home health and subacute care, have been largely successful in mitigating such concerns.

Ambulatory Payment Classification

This prospective payment method, implemented in August 2000, is associated with Medicare's Outpatient Prospective Payment System (OPPS) for services provided by hospital outpatient departments. Main services included in OPPS are outpatient surgeries, radiology and other diagnostic procedures, clinic visits, and emergency services. Ambulatory payment classification (APC) divides all outpatient services into more than 300 procedural groups. The services within each group are clinically similar and require comparable resources. Each APC is assigned a relative payment weight based on the median cost of services within the APC. The reimbursement rates are adjusted for geographic variation in wages. APC reimbursement is a bundled rate that includes services such as anesthesia, certain drugs, supplies, and recovery room charges in a packaged price established by Medicare.

Case-Mix Methods

Case-mix is an aggregate of the intensity of conditions requiring medical intervention. Case-mix categories are mutually exclusive and differentiate patients according to the extent of resource use. On a case-mix index, higher score categories comprise patients who have more severe conditions than those in lower score categories. The case mix for an inpatient facility is determined by a comprehensive assessment of each patient's condition. Patients who require similar levels of services are then categorized into groups that are relatively uniform in their consumption of the amount of resources. Reimbursement may be on a per diem basis (e.g., skilled nursing facilities) depending on an institution's case-mix composite, or it may be based on a case-specific basis depending on the case-mix category in which a given patient is placed (e.g., inpatient rehabilitation facilities).

Resource Utilization Groups

The Medicare program has adopted a case-mix method to reimburse SNFs, replacing the old cost-based reimbursement. Implemented in July 1998, the PPS provides for a per diem prospective rate based on the acuity level (clinical severity) of patients. The case-mix for an SNF is determined through a comprehensive assessment of each patient using an assessment instrument called the Minimum Data Set (MDS). The MDS consists of a core set of screening elements that must be used to assess the clinical, functional, and psychosocial needs of each patient admitted to an SNF. Using MDS data, a classification system, called resource utilization groups, version 3 (RUG-III), has been designed to differentiate patients by their levels of resource use. Among the variables used to differentiate resource utilization are patient characteristics, such as principal diagnosis, functional limitations, negative health conditions, skin problems, and special treatments and procedures needed. RUG-III classifies patients into 44 categories according to their health care needs. Twenty-seven of these categories have been used for per diem rate setting (HCFA 1998, 84–85). The aim of RUG-III–based PPS is to ensure that Medicare payments are related to the care requirements of the patient and are made equitably to SNFs with different patient caseloads. The per diem rate is all-inclusive, which means that it includes payment for all covered SNF services provided in a nursing facility. Adjustments to the PPS rate are made for differences in wages prevailing in various geographic areas and for facility location in urban versus rural areas.

Case-Mix Groups

As of January 2002, inpatient rehabilitation facilities (rehabilitation hospitals and distinctly certified rehabilitation units in general hospitals) are reimbursed according to case-mix groups (CMGs). Each patient must undergo a patient assessment at admission and discharge. Based on information from the assessment, the patient is first placed into one of 21 rehabilitation impairment categories (RICs) such as stroke, brain injury, spinal cord injury, amputation, etc. Next, the patient is placed into a CMG within the RIC, depending primarily on the patient's physical and cognitive functioning. There are 100 CMGs. For each patient Medicare pays a predetermined fixed amount. Reimbursement is adjusted for early transfers, patients who expire, and outliers (Grimaldi 2002).

Home Health Resource Groups

Implemented in October 2000, the PPS for home health pays a fixed, predetermined rate for each 60-day episode of care, regardless of the specific services delivered. Thus, all services provided by a home health agency are bundled under one payment made on a per-patient basis. The episode reimbursement amount depends on each patient's home health resource group (HHRG). It means that the rate is adjusted to reflect the home health recipient's classification according to a case-mix system for home health. The HHRG classification uses 80 distinct groups to indicate severity of a patient's condition. Since PPS also requires consolidated billing of all home health services while a beneficiary is under a home health plan of care authorized by a physician, payment for all such items and services is made to a single home health agency overseeing that plan. Costs of any durable medical equipment (DME) and osteoporosis drugs are not included in the bundled rate.

Disbursement of Funds

After services have been delivered, some agency has to perform the administrative task of verifying and paying the claims received from the providers or, in some cases, indemnifying the patients. Disbursement of funds (or claims processing) is carried out in accordance with the reimbursement policy adopted by the particular program. Commercial insurance companies and MCOs generally have their own claims departments to process payments to providers. Self-insured employers typically contract the services of a ***third-party administrator*** (TPA) to process and pay claims. The TPA may also monitor utilization and perform other oversight functions. The government contracts with contractors in the private sector to process Medicare and Medicaid claims. These contractors generally include Blue Cross/Blue Shield and commercial insurance companies. While ***fiscal intermediaries*** process Part A Claims, Medicare refers to claims processors for Part B services as ***carriers***. These are also Blue Cross/Blue Shield and commercial insurance companies. Even though Medicare makes a technical distinction between the two, fundamentally, fiscal intermediaries and carriers are the same.

National Health Care Expenditures

In 2005, national health expenditures (or health care spending) in the United States amounted to almost $2 trillion, or an average per capita spending of $6,697 for each American. It represented 16 percent of the gross domestic product (GDP) (Catlin et al. 2007). The ***GDP*** is the total value of goods and services produced in the United States and is an indicator of total economic production (or total consumption). Hence, 16 percent of GDP refers to the share of the total economic output consumed by health care products and services. National health expenditures from 1960 to 2005 are presented in Table 6–3. Total spending grew at an average annual rate of 6.6 percent from 1990 to 2000, and at 7.9 percent from 2000 to 2005. National health care expenditures are projected to grow at a higher rate than GDP and are expected to account for 20 percent of GDP and $4 trillion by 2015 (Centers for Medicare and Medicaid Services 2006b). The reasons for the growth in health care spending, international comparisons, and cost-containment measures are discussed in Chapter 12.

Table 6–3 National Health Expenditures, Selected Years

Year	Amount (in billions)	Percentage of Gross Domestic Product	Amount per Capita
1960	$26.9	5.1	$141
1965	41.1	5.7	202
1970	73.2	7.1	341
1975	130.7	8.0	582
1980	247.3	8.9	1.052
1985	428.7	10.3	1,735
1990	717.3	12.4	2,821
1995	1020.4	13.8	3,762
2000	1,358.5	13.8	4,729
2005	1,987.7	16.0	6,697

Source: Data from US Department of Health and Human Services, National Center for Health Statistics, *Health, United States, 1999*, p. 284; *Health, United States, 2006*, pp. 374, 377; Catlin, A. et al. 2007. National health spending in 2005: The slowdown continues. *Health Affairs* 26, no. 1: 142–153.

Difference between National and Personal Health Expenditures

National health expenditures are an aggregate of the amount the nation spends for all health services and supplies, public health services, health-related research, administrative costs, and investment in structures and equipment during a calendar year. The proportional distribution of national health expenditures into the various categories of health services (a comparison between 2000 and 2005) appears in Table 6–4.

National health expenditures are distinct from ***personal health expenditures***. The latter expenditures are for services and goods related directly to patient care. More specifically, personal health expenditures constitute the amount remaining after subtracting from national health expenditures, spending for research, structures (construction, additions, alterations, etc.), and equipment; administrative expenses incurred in health insurance programs, and costs of government public health activities. In 2005, 83.6 percent of total national health expenditures were spent on personal health services and products, which include hospital care, physician services, dental care, other professional services, nursing home care, home health care, prescription drugs, nondurable products, durable medical equipment, vision care, and other personal health care (see Table 6–4). The remaining 16.4 percent of national expenditures is accounted for by public health services, noncommercial medical re-

Table 6–4 Percentage Distribution of National Health Expenditures, 2000 and 2005

Type of Expenditure	Percentage Distribution 2000	2005
National health expenditures	**100.0**	**100.0**
Personal health care	**87.0**	**83.6**
Hospital care	31.7	30.8
Physician and clinical services	22.0	21.2
Dentist services	4.6	4.4
Nursing home care	7.1	6.1
Other professional services	3.0	2.9
Home health care	2.5	2.4
Prescription drugs	9.4	10.1
Other personal health care	2.8	2.9
Other medical products	3.8	2.9
Government administration and net cost of private health insurance	**6.2**	**7.2**
Government public health activities	**3.4**	**2.8**
Investment	**3.4**	**6.4**
Noncommercial research	2.0	2.0
Structures & equipment	1.4	4.4

Total amount: 2000 $1,299.5 billion
2005 $1,987.7 billion

Source: Data from *Health, United States, 2002*, pp. 291–292, National Center for Health Statistics; Catlin, A. et al. 2007. National health spending in 2005: The slowdown continues. *Health Affairs* 26, no. 1: 142–153.

search, expenditures by health care establishments on structures and equipment, costs related to administration of government programs, and net cost of private health insurance. The latter costs represent the difference between the premiums collected and benefits paid by private insurers. The ratio of benefits paid by insurance to revenue from premiums is referred to as the ***medical loss ratio***. For example, a medical loss ratio of 75 percent means that 25 percent of the premiums are retained for administrative costs and profits, and 75 percent is spent on health care services. When the loss ratio is low, it indicates that a substantial portion of premiums is retained for administration, overhead, and profits. Between 2000 and 2005, a greater proportion of health care spending went into prescription drugs, but structures and equipment is where the biggest jump occurred.

Public and Private Share of Health Care Expenditures

The shift from private financing to public financing since 1960 is illustrated in Figure 6–6. In recent years, the ratio of private to public financing has been stable at around 55 to 45. In 1960, private funds—including out of pocket payments, private health insurance premiums, and other private funds—paid for three-quarters of all health care. The introduction of Medicare and Medicaid in 1966 transferred a large portion of the private expenditures to the public sector while increasing access for many who previously could not afford the growing costs of health care. A few years later, in 1972, when Medicare began coverage of the disabled population, the proportion of health care expenditures from private sources declined to 62 percent. The share of private funds reached its lowest point in 1997 when 53.6 percent of the nation's health dollars came from private sources, and 46.4 percent came from public sources. Although the shift from private to public seems to have stabilized, creation of new public programs such as Medicare Part D are likely to increase the public share of expenditures on health care unless the government employs measures to control escalating costs.

Figure 6–7 summarizes the sources of financing and the proportionate consumption of health care dollars by various services.

Figure 6–6 Proportional Distribution of Private and Public Shares of National Health Expenditures.

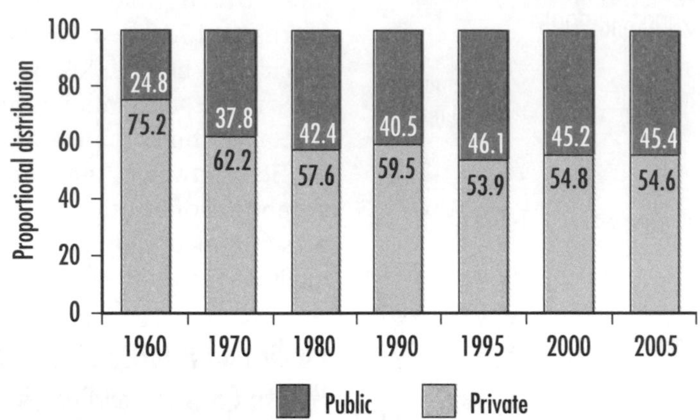

Source: Data from *Health, United States, 2002*, p. 288, Department of Health and Human Services; Catlin, A. et al. 2007. National health spending in 2005: The slowdown continues. *Health Affairs* 26, no. 1: 142–153.

Figure 6–7 The Nation's Health Dollar: 2005.

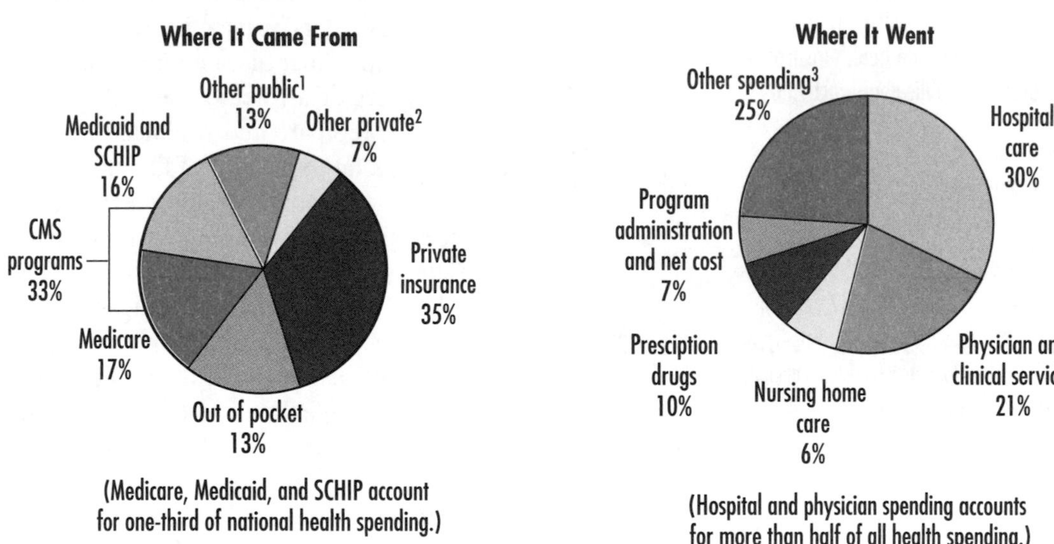

Source: CMS, Office of the Actuary, National Health Statistics Group.

[1]Other public includes programs such as workers' compensation, public health activity, Department of Defense, Department of Veterans Affairs, Indian Health Service, state and local hospital subsidies, and school health.

[2]Other private includes industrial in-plant, privately funded construction, and non-patient revenues, including philanthropy.

[3]Other spending includes dentist services, other professional services, home health, durable medical products, over-the-counter medicines and sundries, public health care, other personal health care, research, and structures and equipment.

Of the combined private health insurance and out of pocket expenses, 26.4 percent were paid by the insured, and 73.6 percent were paid by insurers. Of the total public share of national health spending, 71.3 percent was borne by the federal government, the remainder was paid by state and local governments (data from Catlin et al. 2007).

Trends, Problems, and Issues in Insurance and Financing

Pay-for-Performance

The objective of ***pay-for-performance*** (P4P) initiatives is to link reimbursement to quality and efficiency as an incentive to improve the quality of health care as well as reduce systemwide costs. Government agencies and private health plans are establishing programs that encourage hospitals, physicians, and other providers to meet quality standards. Providers who can demonstrate improvement in care and more efficient performance stand to reap financial rewards (Wechsler 2006). With approximately 30 percent of all health care spending going to hospitals, payers have particularly targeted hospitals to reduce costs. Petersen and colleagues (2006) concluded that the cost-effectiveness of pay-for-performance incentives was unknown. Hence, despite the enthusiasm about the potential for aligning financial incentives with high-quality health care, many fundamental questions about their optimal design and implementation remain unanswered, and much work needs to be done to make pay-for-performance schemes effective in accomplishing their primary objective. Even though P4P programs are in their infancy, due to their intuitive appeal, such programs are likely to increase in popularity.

Insurance Portability and Continuity

The ability to have continuous health insurance coverage has long been an issue when changing jobs or waiting out periods of unemployment. For fear of losing health insurance, people were often reluctant to change jobs, a phenomenon referred to as ***job lock***. In response, Congress passed the Consolidated Omnibus Budget Reconciliation Act of 1985 (COBRA), which allows employees to pay for continued group coverage for 18 months after leaving a job. The individuals are required to pay 102 percent of the group rate to continue health benefits, but without employer subsidy, the high cost of premiums prevents many from keeping their health insurance. This is the main reason why many people lose insurance for part of the year when they are between jobs.

HIPAA provides for continued coverage beyond the COBRA provisions. Higher tax deductions for the cost of premiums than what was allowed under previous rules help reduce the cost burden for the individual, although the problem of affordability persists for some. HIPAA was also instrumental in removing certain barriers that had previously prevented some people from obtaining health insurance or continuing coverage under their existing plans. The law places severe limitations on a plan's ability to deny health insurance coverage to people who have a ***preexisting condition***, that is, a health problem that a person has prior to obtaining health insurance coverage. Before HIPAA, many people were unable to obtain health insurance, especially if they had an expensive-to-treat health problem. For example, the GAO estimated that 33 percent of all applicants were denied coverage by insurance companies because of preexisting health conditions (GAO 1996). As a result of HIPAA, use of preexisting condition clauses in health plans declined dramatically (Gabel et al. 2003). HIPAA also prohibits health plans from dropping an employee or a dependent from coverage or charging higher premiums because the insured's health status has deteriorated. Similarly, an insurance company cannot drop an employer's plan because of adverse experience in utilization of health services. The main health insurance provisions of the law are summarized in Exhibit 6–8.

Erosion of Private Insurance Coverage

According to the US Census Bureau, the number of uninsured in America increased from approximately 40 million in 2000 to nearly 46 million in 2004. In percentage terms, the proportion of the uninsured population increased from 14.2 percent to 15.7 percent in the four-year period (DeNavas-Walt et al. 2005). It should be pointed out that part-year coverage for a segment of the population introduces some errors in tracking the data. Hence, any figures dealing with the uninsured are broad estimates. Since almost all of the elderly are insured under Medicare, uninsurance is primarily experienced by the younger age groups. An examination of the 1998–2000 National Expenditure Panel Survey data by Klein and colleagues (2005) revealed that 69 percent of the nonelderly population is always insured, 9 percent is always uninsured, and the remaining 22 percent experience health insurance ***churning***, a phenomenon in which people gain and lose coverage multiple times. In addition to the uninsured, it is estimated that 16 million adults were ***underinsured*** in 2003, meaning their insurance did not adequately protect them against catastrophic health care expenses (Schoen et al. 2005).

Lack of health insurance is slowly rising among families earning moderate and middle incomes. For example, according to one nationally representative survey, the per-

Exhibit 6–8 Main Provisions of the Health Insurance Portability and Accountability Act, 1996

- Employer-sponsored group health insurance can be denied only for the first 12 months if a preexisting condition is diagnosed within the previous 6 months. If the employee changes jobs, the right to full coverage is portable to another place of employment without another 12 months of waiting.
- Employers or insurance companies (including MCOs) cannot drop coverage when a covered person becomes seriously ill.
- As long as the premiums are paid, an employer's plan cannot be dropped because of high utilization experience.
- An insured who has had coverage for at least 18 months, and has exhausted the 18 months of coverage under COBRA after leaving a job, can continue coverage on payment of premiums if coverage is not available under any other employment-based plan.
- Small employers that have between 2 and 50 employees cannot be refused insurance.
- Self-employed people are allowed an increased tax deduction for health-insurance premiums. The deduction increases from 30% to 80% by 2006.
- On an experimental basis, tax-deductible medical savings accounts can be set up by small businesses, the self-employed, and the uninsured.

centage of adults in the 19–64 age category who were found to be uninsured rose from 17 percent to 28 percent of those with incomes between $20,000 and $35,000, and from 6 percent to 9 percent for those with incomes between $35,000 and $60,000. One in five of all nonelderly adults is in debt from past medical bills (Collins et al. 2006), and medical bills are a factor in nearly half of all personal bankruptcy filings (Institute of Medicine 2003). The main reason behind this trend is the gradual erosion of private employer-based health insurance. First, between 2000 and 2005, the percentage of private firms offering health benefits to their employees fell from 69 percent to 60 percent. The cutback has been particularly sharp among small businesses. For example, only 59 percent of small firms (3–199 workers) in 2005 offered health benefits, compared to 98 percent of firms with 200 or more workers (Claxton 2005).

When employers offer health insurance, 80 percent of the employees are eligible for coverage. Waiting periods or minimum work-hour rules make the rest ineligible. However, of those eligible, 83 percent elect to enroll (Claxton et al. 2005). One reason for nonenrollment is the share of premium costs that the employee must pay. Secondly, globalization has put increasing pressure on US corporations to keep their costs down. Consequently, employers have increased the use of nontraditional workers, i.e., temporary or part-time workers, and use of contracted labor. It is estimated that almost 10 percent of the American workforce, or 13 million people, fit the nontraditional workforce category (Dessler 2005, 12). They are twice as likely as regular, full-time workers to be uninsured unless they can rely on insurance through a working spouse or be eligible for a public insurance program (Ditsler 2005).

Community Rating and Adverse Selection

Community rating has been advocated as a way to promote widespread and affordable health insurance coverage, particularly for those purchasing individual private policies. Several states require underwriting of such policies using community rating. Under community rating, healthy people subsidize the insurance cost for the less healthy, particularly those with high-cost chronic conditions. High-risk people find community rating to be more advantageous, and they enroll in greater numbers. This ***adverse selection*** leads to a larger pool of high-risk individuals participating in the plan than would be the case if everyone were paying according to true risk. This arrangement leads to premiums rising in a continuous upward spiral (Goodman and Musgrave 1992, 125). Adverse selection occurs because people who anticipate being high users of medical services are likely to buy extensive coverage, whereas those who expect to have low use either do not buy insurance or buy less comprehensive policies (Pauly et al. 1992, 31).

Favorable Risk Selection

Favorable risk selection or, simply, ***risk selection***, occurs when healthy people are disproportionately enrolled into a health plan. It amounts to "cream skimming." For example, health plans may selectively enroll healthier people and avoid sicker ones, or they may induce risk selection through selective advertising. Since patients with chronic health problems are likely to consume more services, risk selection can help insurers to increase their profitability. It has been estimated that the most expensive 1 percent of the population, the very sick, accounts for 30 percent of all health spending, and the least expensive 50 percent of the population, the healthy, accounts for only 3 percent of health spending. These estimates have been shown to stay stable over time (Berk and Monheit 2001). This disparity is the reason why insurers may go to extra lengths to identify and select below-average risks and to avoid high-risk populations (Blumberg and Nichols 1996). Provisions of the Medicare Prescription Drug, Improvement, and Modernization Act of 2003 are designed to deter risk selection, but there is concern that these provisions will be insufficient. Private plan choices in Medicare Part D are likely to provide new opportunities to risk select through advertising (Mehrotra et al. 2006). There is also some evidence that favorable risk selection may occur with pay-for-performance contracting in some settings (Shen 2003).

Although adverse selection and risk selection are regarded as unfair, practices that are more likely to reflect actual risk have also been criticized. Adjusting premiums to reflect health status, and making potential high-cost enrollees pay more, a practice called ***risk rating***, is also criticized on equity grounds. It has also been politically unacceptable to have the sick pay higher costs for coverage, particularly because ill health may also have reduced their ability to work. Also, very high-risk individuals may be unable to obtain coverage at affordable rates (Pauly et al. 1992, 32).

Cost Shifting

When the amount of reimbursement from some payer source becomes inadequate, or when uncompensated services are rendered, providers resort to ***cost shifting*** by charging extra to payers who do not exercise strict cost controls. The uninsured, for instance, can obtain needed catastrophic services at times of acute illness, although they generally go without routine preventive and primary care (Altman and Reinhardt 1996). Uninsured families are able to pay less than half of their outpatient care costs, but only 7 percent of hospital costs (Institute of Medicine 2003). Cross-subsidization by those who bear the burden of cost shifting has been the traditional way to provide needed health care services to the uninsured. However, over the years, most payers have implemented some form of cost-containment mechanisms. Capitation and prospective reimbursement methods, in particular, have eroded the margins for cost shifting. Consequently, providers have less ability to provide uncompensated care through cost shifting than was previously possible.

Financing for the Uninsured

Despite lacking coverage, many of the approximately 41 million uninsured Americans do get health care. In dollar terms, they receive about half as much care as those who are fully insured. The work of Hadley and Holahan (2003) indicates that for 2001, the value of uncompensated care may amount to $35 billion, of which approximately 66 percent came from hospitals, 20 percent from clinics and community health care providers, and 14 percent from physicians. Total government spending may be covering as much as 80 to 84 percent of uncompensated care, mainly in the form of indirect payment arrangements that are built into Medicare and Medicaid reimbursement to providers. Based on these findings, Hadley and Holahan (2003) argued that since the government is already the main source of this health care financing, these funds could be used to establish a new insurance program for the uninsured.

Fraud and Abuse

Health care fraud and program abuse is one of the most troubling aspects of health care financing. The GAO estimated in 1992 that 10 percent of all health spending might be lost to fraud and abuse (Anders and McGinley 1997). Since 1994, Medicare and Medicaid programs have been able to recoup billions of dollars in fines, settlements, restitutions, and other recoveries. Even though fraud is a significant problem, it is difficult to detect. In most cases, fraudulent schemes have been exposed by whistleblowers. The system lacks routine monitoring and control procedures. Although fiscal intermediaries have been delegated the responsibility of reviewing claims for appropriateness, their audits focus mainly on making sure that claims are submitted in a standard fashion rather than checking whether Medicare is paying for appropriate care (Anders 1997, A2).

The False Claims Act is the longstanding legislation dealing with cheating and false claims. In 1986, Congress enacted the False Claims Act Amendments, which clarified that the Act applied to Medicare and Medicaid. It also made it easier for private parties, called relators, to bring cases on behalf of the government under the *qui tam* provisions. HIPAA of 1996 also contains strong provisions against fraud and abuse. First, it provides for budget appropriations to prosecute fraud and abuse cases. Second, it provides for tough sanctions and penalties. In fighting fraud, the CMS has strengthened its own efforts by working with the Office of the Inspector General, the Department of Justice, and the Federal Bureau of Investigation. Investigative activities will only grow as federal agencies are recovering $13 for every dollar spent on investigating health care fraud (Judge 2005).

Summary

Financing is the lifeblood of any health care delivery system. At a basic level, it determines who will pay for health care services for whom. Access to continuous and comprehensive services hinges on coverage through a health insurance program. Thus, demand for health care services is directly linked to financing. Financing also determines indirectly how much and what type of health care services are produced.

Health care financing in the United States is a patchwork of mechanisms that are largely uncoordinated, adding to the complexity of the health care delivery system. Most health care in the United States is provided through employment-based group health insurance. As a general rule, employees are required to share the costs. Many large employers are self-insured. Managed care has become the predominant avenue for providing insurance and delivery of services in an integrated fashion. Medicare and Medicaid are the major health programs for most of the civilian population not covered under private health insurance plans. The Department of Defense and the Department of Veterans Affairs also operate large health care delivery systems to care for armed forces personnel, their dependents, military retirees, and veterans. Over the years, the share of public financing relative to private financing has gradually increased, but it seems to have leveled off. However, there are forces at work, such as creation of Medicare Part D to offer a prescription drug benefit to seniors, that may shift the balance.

Insurers, TPAs, and fiscal intermediaries handle most payment functions. Fee for service has been the traditional method for reimbursing providers. However, cost pressures have led to the development of innovative approaches designed to realign incentives to provide services more efficiently and at lower cost. Bundling of charges, RBRVS, and prospective payment mechanisms are some examples. The most dramatic shift in reimbursement was initiated in the 1980s to pay for hospital inpatient care under a PPS based on DRGs. Reimbursement based on case-mix is another prospective payment method adopted for paying nursing homes and inpatient rehabilitation facilities.

In the past several years, the United States has experienced a dramatic growth in national health care expenditures. These expenditures have surpassed growth rates in the GDP, as well as the rise in general inflation. After a brief respite during the 1990s, health care spending has resumed its inflationary track, and controlling health care costs will be a major challenge in the years ahead, particularly as national health care expenditures are projected to double between 2005 and 2015.

Test Your Understanding

Terminology

adverse selection
balance bill
beneficiary
benefit period
benefits
carriers
case mix
categorical programs
charge
churning
claim
coinsurance
community rating
copayment
cost-plus
cost shifting
Current Procedural Terminology (CPT)
deductible
entitlement
experience rating
fee schedule
first-dollar coverage plans
fiscal intermediaries
GDP
group insurance
indemnity plan
insurance
insured
insurer
job lock
major medical
means-tested program
medical loss ratio
Medicare Physician Fee Schedule (MPFS)
Medigap
moral hazard
national health expenditures
outliers
pay-for-performance
personal health expenditures
preexisting condition
premium
prospective reimbursement
rate
reinsurance
relative value units (RVUs)
retrospective reimbursement
risk
risk rating
risk selection
service plan
stop-loss
third-party administrator
third-party payers
underinsured
underutilization
underwriting
uninsured

Review Questions

1. What is meant by health care financing in its broad sense? What impact does financing have on the health care delivery system?

2. Discuss the general concepts of insurance. Describe the various types of private health insurance options, pointing out the differences among them.
3. Discuss how the concepts of premium, covered services, and cost sharing apply to health insurance.
4. What is the difference between experience rating and community rating?
5. What is Medicare Part A? Discuss the financing and cost-sharing features of Medicare Part A. What benefits does Part A cover? What benefits are not covered?
6. What is Medicare Part B? Discuss the financing and cost-sharing features of Medicare Part B. What benefits are covered under Part B? What benefits are not covered?
7. Briefly describe the Medicare Advantage program.
8. Briefly explain the prescription drug program under Medicare Part D.
9. Discuss the financing, eligibility, and covered benefits for the Medicaid program.
10. What provisions has the federal government made for providing health care to military personnel and to veterans of the US armed forces?
11. What are the major methods of reimbursement for outpatient services?
12. What are the differences between the retrospective and prospective methods of reimbursement?
13. Discuss the prospective payment system under DRGs.
14. Distinguish between national health expenditures and personal health expenditures.
15. What is pay-for-performance? What is its main objective?
16. Discuss the main provisions of HIPAA in health insurance portability and continuity.
17. How has globalization affected the number of uninsured Americans?
18. How does community rating lead to adverse selection?
19. What incentive do insurers have to engage in risk selection? Why is risk rating criticized?
20. Pertaining to fraud and abuse, what are the main provisions of the 1986 False Claims Act Amendments?

REFERENCES

Agency for Healthcare Research and Quality. 2005. *Trend data on individual health insurance policies*. AHQR News and Numbers, May 10, 2005. Agency for Healthcare Research and Quality, Rockville, MD. Available at: *http://www.ahrq.gov/news/nn/nn051005.htm.*

Altman, S.H., and U.E. Reinhardt. 1996. Where does health care reform go from here? An uncharted odyssey. In *Strategic choices for a changing health care system*, eds. S.H. Altman and U.E. Reinhardt, xxi–xxxii. Chicago: Health Administration Press.

Anders, G. 1997. Improper Medicare spending is frequent. *The Wall Street Journal*, 11 June, A2.

Anders, G., and L. McGinley. 1997. A new brand of crime now stirs the Feds: Health care fraud. *The Wall Street Journal*, 6 May, A1.

Berk, M.L., and A.C. Monheit. 2001. The concentration of health expenditures, revisited. *Health Affairs* 20, no. 2: 9–18.

Best, R.A. 2005. *Military medical care services: Questions and answers*. Congressional Research Service. Available at: *http://www.fas.org/sgp/crs/misc/IB93103.pdf.*

Blumberg, L.J., and L.M. Nichols. 1996. First, do no harm: Developing health insurance market reform packages. *Health Affairs* 15, no. 3: 35–54.

Catlin, A. 2007. National health spending in 2005: The slowdown continues. *Health Affairs* 26, no. 1: 142–153.

Centers for Medicare and Medicaid Services (CMS). 2004. *News release: HHS announces Medicare premium, deductibles for 2005*. CMS Public Affairs Office, September 3, 2004.

Centers for Medicare and Medicaid Services (CMS). 2006a. *Medicare enrollment: National trends 1966–2005*. Available at: *http://www.cms.hhs.gov/MedicareEnRpts/Downloads/HISMI05.pdf.*

Centers for Medicare and Medicaid Services (CMS). 2006b. *National health care expenditures projections: 2005–2015*. Available at: *http://www.cms.hhs.gov/NationalHealthExpendData/downloads/proj2005.pdf.*

Claxton, G. et al. 2006. *Employer health benefits: 2006 annual survey*. Washington, DC: The Kaiser Family Foundation and Health Research and Educational Trust.

Collins, S.R. et al. 2006. *Gaps in health insurance: An all-American problem*. New York, NY: The Commonwealth Fund.

Davis, M.H., and S.T. Burner. 1995. Three decades of Medicare: What the numbers tell us. *Health Affairs* 14, no. 4: 231–243.

DeNavas-Walt et al. 2005. *Income, poverty, and health insurance coverage in the United States: 2004*. Washington, DC: US Census Bureau.

Department of Defense. 1996. *Your military health plan: TriCare*. Falls Church, VA.

Department of Defense. 1999. *Frequently asked questions*. Available at: *http://www.tricare.osd.mil/tricare/news/market.html*.

Department of Veterans Affairs. 2002. *Veteran data and information*. Available at: *http://www.va.gov/vetdata/*.

Department of Veterans Affairs. 2003. *2001 national survey of veterans*. Available at: *http://www.va.gov/vetdata/SurveyResults/final.htm*.

Department of Veterans Affairs. 2004. *Veteran data and information*. Available at: *http://www.va.gov/vetdata/ProgramStatics/index.htm*.

Dessler, G. 2005. *Human resource management*, 10th ed. Upper Saddle River, NJ: Pearson/Prentice Hall.

Ditsler, E. et al. 2005. *On the fringe: The substandard benefits of workers in part-time, temporary, and contract jobs*. New York, NY: The Commonwealth Fund.

Ebeler, J. et al. 2006. *Improving the Medicare savings program*. Washington, DC: National Academy of Social Insurance.

Federal Register. 2007. Vol. 72, No. 15, January 24, 2007, pp. 3147–3148. Available at: *http://www.aspe.hhs.gov/poverty/07fedreg.htm*.

Feldstein, P.J. 1993. *Health care economics,* 4th ed. New York: Delmar Publishers.

Fong, T. 2003. An army of patients: The VA struggles with a growing population of veterans using its healthcare system as it works to boost quality and capacity. *Modern Healthcare* 33, no. 2: 48–50.

Gabel, J.R. et al. 2003. Self-insurance in times of growing and retreating managed care. *Health Affairs* 22, no. 2: 202–210.

General Accounting Office. 1996. *Private health insurance: Millions relying on individual market coverage face cost and coverage trade-offs*. Washington, DC.

General Accounting Office. 1998. *VA health care: More veterans are being served, but better oversight is needed. Chapter Report*, 08/28/98, GAO/HEHS-98–226. Washington, DC.

Goodman, J.C., and G.L. Musgrave. 1992. *Patient power: Solving America's health care crisis*. Washington, DC: CATO Institute.

Grimaldi, P.L. 2002. Inpatient rehabilitation facilities are now paid prospective rates. *Journal of Health Care Finance* 28, no. 3: 32–48.

Hadley, J., and J. Holahan. 2003. How much medical care do the uninsured use, and who pays for it? *Health Affairs* 22, no. 2: 13.

Harty, S. 2005. Health insurers try to bring managed care to workers comp. *Business Insurance* 39, no. 31: 11–13.

Health Care Financing Administration. 1996. *Medicare and Medicaid statistical supplement, 1996*. Pub. No. 03386. Baltimore, MD: Department of Health and Human Services.

Health Care Financing Administration. 1998. *Medicare and Medicaid statistical supplement, 1998*. Pub. No. 03409. Baltimore, MD: Department of Health and Human Services.

Health Care Financing Administration. 2001. *Medicare and Medicaid statistical supplement, 2000*. Pub. No. 03424. Baltimore, MD: Department of Health and Human Services.

Health Insurance Association of America. 1991. *Source book of health insurance data*. Washington, DC.

Health Insurance Institute. 1969. *Modern health insurance*. New York.

The Henry J. Kaiser Family Foundation. 2002. *Employer health benefits: 2002 annual survey*. Menlo Park, CA: Kaiser Family Foundation.

The Henry J. Kaiser Family Foundation. 2003. *Medicare fact sheet: Medicare at a glance*, February 2003. Available at: *http://www.kff.org*.

The Henry J. Kaiser Family Foundation. 2005a. *Medicare fact sheet: Medicare Advantage*, September 2005. Available at: *http://www.kff.org*.

The Henry J. Kaiser Family Foundation. 2005b. *Medicare fact sheet. Medicare at a glance*, September 2005. Available at: *http://www.kff.org*.

The Henry J. Kaiser Family Foundation. 2006. *Medicare fact sheet: Medicare at a glance*, July 2006. Available at: *http://www.kff.org*.

Holtz-Eakin, D. 2004. *CBO testimony: Estimating the cost of the Medicare Modernization Act*. Washington, DC: Congressional Budget Office.

Hudson, J.L. 2005. The impact of SCHIP on insurance coverage of children. *Inquiry* 42, no. 3: 232–254.

Indian Health Service. 2006. *Fact sheet*. Available at: *http://www.ihs.gov/PublicInfo/PublicAffairs/Welcome_Info/ThisFacts.asp*.

Institute of Medicine. 2003. *A shared destiny: Effects of uninsurance on individuals, families, and communities*. Washington, DC: National Academies Press.

Jost, T.S. 2003. The tenuous nature of the Medicaid entitlement. *Health Affairs* 22, no. 1: 145–153.

Judge, J.M. 2005. Key compliance areas for healthcare financial executives. *Healthcare Financial Management* 59, no. 6: 95–96.

The Kaiser Commission on Medicaid and the Uninsured. 2006. Medicaid Facts. The Henry J. Kaiser Family Foundation. Available at: *http://www.kff.org*.

The Kaiser Family Foundation and Health Research and Educational Trust. 2006. *Employer health benefits: 2006 annual survey*. Menlo Park, CA: Kaiser Family Foundation.

The Kaiser Family Foundation and Health Research and Educational Trust. 2000. *Employer health benefits: 2000 annual survey*. Menlo Park, CA: Kaiser Family Foundation.

Klein, K. et al. 2005. *Entrances and exits: Health insurance churning, 1998–2000*. New York, NY: The Commonwealth Fund.

Levit, K.R. et al. 1994. National health spending trends, 1960–1993. *Health Affairs* 13, no. 5: 14–31.

Mehrotra A. et al. 2006. The relationship between health plan advertising and market incentives: Evidence of risk-selective behavior. *Health Affairs* 25, no. 3: 759–765.

National Center for Health Statistics. 1997. *Health, United States, 1996–97*. Hyattsville, MD: US Department of Health and Human Services.

National Center for Health Statistics. 2005. *Health, United States, 2005*. Hyattsville, MD: US Department of Health and Human Services.

Pauly, M.V. et al. 1992. *Responsible national health insurance*. Washington, DC: AEI Press.

Petersen, L.A. et al. 2006. Does pay-for-performance improve the quality of health care? *Annals of Internal Medicine* 145, no. 4: 265–278.

Rice, T.H., and R.J. Labelle. 1989. Do physicians induce demand for medical services? *Journal of Health Policies*, Policy and Law 14, no. 3: 587–600.

Schoen, C. et al. 2005. Insured but not protected: How many adults are underinsured? *Health Affairs, January–June 2005 Supplement Web Exclusives* 24: 289–302.

Shen Y. 2003. Selection incentives in a performance-based contracting system. *Health Services Research* 38, no. 2:535–52.

Shone, L.P.et al. 2005. Reduction in racial and ethnic disparities after enrollment in the State Children's Health Insurance Program. *Pediatrics* 115, no. 6: e697–705.

Short, P.F. et al. 1997. The effect of universal coverage on health expenditures for the uninsured. *Medical Care* 35, no. 2: 95–113.

Social Security Administration. 2006. *A summary of the 2006 Annual Reports: Social Security and Medicare Board of Trustees*. Available at: *http://www.ssa.gov/OACT/TRSUM/trsummary.html.*

Somers, A.R. and H.M. Somers. 1977. *Health and health care: Policies in perspective*. Germantown, MD: Aspen Systems.

US Department of Labor. 2006. Workers' compensation programs: Fact sheets. Available at: *http://www.dol.gov/esa/regs/compliance/owcp/owcpfact.htm.*

Vaughn, E.J., and C.M. Elliott. 1987. *Fundamentals of risk and insurance*. New York: John Wiley & Sons.

Wechsler, J. 2006. Pay for performance. *Managed Healthcare Executive* 16, no. 8: 30–32.

Whitted, G. 1993. Private health insurance and employee benefits. In *Introduction to health services*, 4th ed., eds. S.J. Williams and P.R. Torrens, 332–360. Albany, NY: Delmar Publishers.

Williams, S.J. 1995. *Essentials of health services*. Albany, NY: Delmar Publishers.

PART III

System Processes

Chapter 7

Outpatient and Primary Care Services

Learning Objectives

- To understand the meanings of outpatient, ambulatory, and primary care
- To identify the reasons why there has been a dramatic growth in outpatient services
- To develop an understanding of the various types of outpatient settings and services

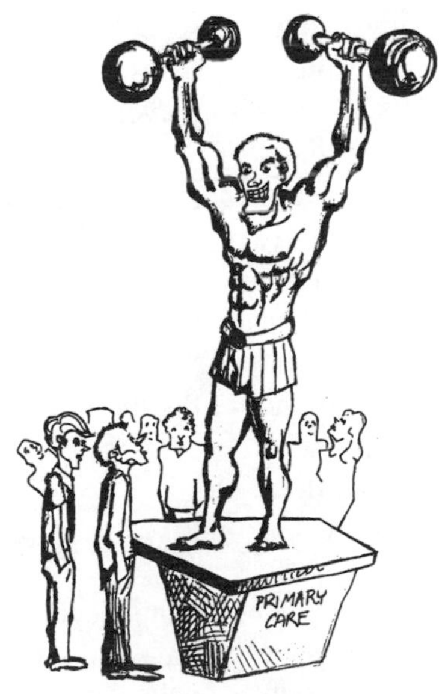

"I suppose a system based on primary care is more robust."

Introduction

Outpatient health care services originated with the healing arts themselves (Williams 1993) and have been in existence for a long time. Historically, outpatient care has been independent from services provided in health care institutions. In earlier days, physicians saw patients in their clinics, and most physicians also made home visits to treat patients. Given the limitations of medical science in those days, physicians generally provided the full spectrum of medical services, including diagnosis, treatment, surgery, and dispensing of medications. Institutions for inpatient care, such as hospitals and nursing homes, developed later. With advances in medical science, the locus of health care delivery concentrated around the institutional core of community hospitals. As the range of services that could be provided on an outpatient basis continued to expand, hospitals gradually became the dominant players in providing the vast majority of outpatient care as well, with the exception of cognitive and basic diagnostic care provided in physicians' offices (Barr and Breindel 1995). Hospitals were better equipped to provide such services because they increasingly capitalized on technological innovation. Hospital laboratories and diagnostic units, for example, were better equipped to perform most tests and diagnostic procedures. Independent providers, on the other hand, faced capital constraints and competitive pressures in the health care marketplace. To better cope with the changing realities of the new marketplace, most solo practitioners consolidated into group practices.

Various changes in the health care delivery system, both financial and social, have led to new alignments in the delivery of outpatient services. In recent years, the process of health care delivery, in a broad sense, has increasingly shifted outside of expensive acute care hospitals, and the trend is likely to continue. Although basic primary care has traditionally been the foundation of outpatient ambulatory services, certain intensive procedures are increasingly being performed on an outpatient basis.

State and local government agencies have also actively sponsored limited outpatient services to meet the needs of underserved populations, mainly indigent patients who lack personal resources to obtain health care in the private sector. Examples include public clinics and dispensaries. Delivery of outpatient care by public agencies has been limited in scope and detached from the dominant private system of health services delivery. Community health centers, which primarily depend on federal and state funds, serve a number of rural and inner city areas, providing a wider array of outpatient services. As discussed in Chapter 3, public health functions, in most cases, have been limited to child immunizations, care of mothers and infants, health screening in public schools, monitoring for certain contagious diseases like tuberculosis, family planning, and prevention of sexually transmitted diseases.

The terms "outpatient" and "ambulatory" have been used interchangeably, as they are in this book, but the term "outpatient" is more comprehensive. It better describes the range of services now being referred to as "ambulatory." Apart from that, there is little distinction between the two terms.

What Is Outpatient Care?

Outpatient services do not require an overnight inpatient stay in an institution of health care delivery, such as a hospital or long-term care facility, although certain outpatient services may be offered by a hospital or nursing home.

Many hospitals, for instance, have emergency departments (EDs) and other outpatient service centers, such as outpatient surgery, rehabilitation, and specialized clinics.

Outpatient services are also referred to as ***ambulatory care.*** Strictly speaking, ambulatory care constitutes diagnostic and therapeutic services and treatments provided to the "walking" (ambulatory) patient. Hence, in a restricted sense, the term "ambulatory care" refers to care rendered to patients who come to physicians' offices, hospital outpatient departments, and health centers to receive care. The term is also sometimes used synonymously with "community medicine" (Wilson and Neuhauser 1985, 43) because the geographic location of ambulatory services is intended to serve the surrounding community, providing convenience and easy accessibility.

Patients do not always walk to the service centers to receive ambulatory care, however. For example, in a hospital ED, patients may arrive by land or air ambulance. EDs, in most cases, are equipped mainly to provide secondary and tertiary care services rather than primary care. In other instances, such as mobile diagnostic units and home health care, services are transported to the patient instead of the patient coming to receive the services. Hence, the terms "outpatient" and "inpatient" are more precise, and the term ***outpatient services*** refers to any health care services that are not provided on the basis of an overnight stay in which room and board costs are incurred.

The Scope of Outpatient Services

In recent years, extraordinary growth has occurred in the volume of outpatient services and the emergence of new types of settings in which outpatient services are delivered. The most basic outpatient services, such as physical exams and minor treatments, are still delivered in a physician's office, which is now more likely to be part of a group practice or a medical complex rather than an independent solo practice. Advanced outpatient care has traditionally been provided in hospital-based facilities, generally in various building complexes surrounding the main hospital. In addition, explosive growth has occurred in the type and ownership of nonhospital-based facilities offering ambulatory care (see examples in Table 7–1).

The shift to ambulatory care is expected to endure. Hospital occupancy rates have continued to decline during the past decade. Consequently, hospital executives have been forced to view ambulatory care as an essential portion of their overall health care business rather than a supplemental product line of an inpatient facility (Barr and Breindel 1995). Seeing their inpatient business erode, hospital administrators have realized that establishing a firm position in the ambulatory care market is critical to the continued survival of their organizations. To meet the growing demand for outpatient services, hospitals have expanded into services that previously were not considered a part of their core business.

The growth of nonhospital-based ambulatory services has intensified competition for outpatient medical services between hospitals and community-based providers. Examples of such competition include home health care, ambulatory clinics for routine and urgent care, and outpatient surgery. On the other hand, several other services, such as dental care and optometric services, continue to be office based. Financing is the main reason why dental and optometric services have not been integrated with other outpatient medical services. Traditionally, medical insurance plans have been separate from dental and vision care plans.

Table 7–1 Owners, Providers, and Settings for Ambulatory Care Services

Past	Present
Owners/Providers	
• Independent physician practitioners	• Independent physician practitioners
• Hospitals	• Hospitals
• Community health agencies	• Community health agencies
• Home health agencies	• Managed care organizations
	• Insurance companies
	• Corporate employers
	• Group practices
	• National physician chains
	• Home health companies
	• National diversified health care companies
Service Settings	
• Hospital outpatient departments	• Physicians' offices
• Physicians' offices	• Walk-in clinics/Urgent care centers
• Outpatient surgery centers	• Outpatient surgery centers
• Hospital emergency departments	• Chemotherapy and radiation therapy centers
• Home health agencies	• Dialysis centers
• Neighborhood health centers	• Community health centers
	• Diagnostic imaging centers
	• Mobile imaging centers
	• Fitness/wellness centers
	• Occupational health centers
	• Psychiatric outpatient centers
	• Rehabilitation centers
	• Sports medicine clinics
	• Hand injury rehab clinics
	• Women's health clinics
	• Wound care centers

Source: Data from K.W. Barr and C.L. Breindel, "Ambulatory Care," *Health Care Administration: Principles, Practices, Structure, and Delivery*, © 1995, Aspen Publishers, Inc.

Philosophical and technical differences account for other variations. Chiropractic care, for instance, is generally covered by most health plans but remains isolated from the mainstream practice of medicine. Other services, such as alternative therapies and self-care, are not covered by insurance; yet continue to experience remarkable growth.

Primary care is the conceptual foundation for ambulatory health services, but not all ambulatory care is primary care. For example, hospital ED services are not intended to be primary in nature. On the other hand, services other than primary health care have now become an integral part of outpatient services. Thanks to the technological advances in medicine, many secondary and tertiary treatments are now provided in ambulatory care settings. Examples include conditions requiring urgent treatment, outpatient surgery, rehabilitative therapies, and tertiary treatments, such as renal dialysis and chemotherapy.

Primary Care

Primary care plays a central role in a health care delivery system. Other essential levels of care include secondary and tertiary care (distinct from primary, secondary, and tertiary prevention discussed in Chapter 2). Compared to primary care, secondary and tertiary care services are more complex and specialized. Primary care is distinguished from secondary and tertiary care according to its duration, frequency, and level of intensity. ***Secondary care*** is usually short-term, involving sporadic consultation from a specialist to provide expert opinion and/or surgical or other advanced interventions that primary care physicians are not equipped to perform. Secondary care thus includes hospitalization, routine surgery, specialty consultation, and rehabilitation. ***Tertiary care*** is the most complex level of care, needed for conditions that are relatively uncommon. Typically, tertiary care is institution-based, highly specialized, and technology-driven. Much of tertiary care is rendered in large teaching hospitals, especially university hospitals. Examples include trauma care, burn treatment, neonatal intensive care, tissue transplants, and open heart surgery. In some instances, tertiary treatment may be extended, and the tertiary care physician may assume long-term responsibility for the bulk of the patient's care. It has been estimated that 75–85 percent of people in a general population require only primary care services in a given year; 10–12 percent require referrals to short-term secondary care services; and 5–10 percent use tertiary care specialists (Starfield 1994). These proportions vary in populations with special health care needs.

Definitions of primary care often focus on the type or level of services, such as prevention, diagnostic and therapeutic services, health education and counseling, and minor surgery. Although primary care specifically emphasizes these services, many specialists also provide the same spectrum of services. For example, the practice of most ophthalmologists has a large element of prevention, as well as diagnosis, treatment, follow-up, and minor surgery. Similarly, most cardiologists are engaged in health education and counseling. Hence, primary care should be more appropriately viewed as an approach to providing health care rather than as a set of specific services (Starfield 1994).

World Health Organization Definition

Traditionally, primary care has been the cornerstone of ambulatory care services. The World Health Organization (WHO) describes ***primary health care*** as:

> Essential health care based on practical, scientifically sound, and socially acceptable methods and technology made universally accessible to individuals and families in the community by means acceptable to

> them and at a cost that the community and the country can afford to maintain at every stage of their development in a spirit of self-reliance and self-determination. It forms an integral part of both the country's health system of which it is the central function and the main focus of the overall social and economic development of the community. It is the first level of contact of individuals, the family, and the community with the national health system, bringing health care as close as possible to where people live and work and constitutes the first element of a continuing health care process (World Health Organization 1978, 25).

Three elements in this definition are particularly noteworthy for an understanding of primary care: point of entry, coordination of care, and essential care.

Point of Entry

Primary care is the point of entry into the health services system in which health care delivery is organized around primary care (Starfield 1992, vii). Primary care is the first contact a patient makes with the health care delivery system. This first contact feature is closely associated with the "gatekeeper" role of the primary care practitioner. ***Gatekeeping*** implies that patients do not visit specialists and are not admitted to a hospital without being referred by their primary care physicians. On the surface, gatekeeping may appear to be a controlling mechanism for denying needed care. In most cases, however, the interposition of primary care protects patients from unnecessary procedures and overtreatment (Franks et al. 1992) because specialists use medical tests and procedures to a much greater extent than primary care providers, and such interventions carry a definite risk of ***iatrogenic*** (caused by the process of health care) complications (Starfield 1994).

One of the goals of primary care is to bring health care as close as possible to where people live and work. In other words, true primary care is community based. It represents convenience and easy accessibility. To make such services widely available to communities in urban, suburban, and rural areas, the nature of primary care services must remain basic, routine, and inexpensive. Yet, appropriate technology must be incorporated into the delivery of primary care so that costly referrals to other components of the health delivery system are made only when necessary.

The British National Health Service (NHS) is an example of a health care delivery system founded on the principles of gatekeeping. In the NHS, primary care is the single portal of entry to secondary care and acts as a filter so that 90 percent of care is provided outside hospitals in ambulatory care settings (Orton 1994). General practitioners (GPs) are primary care gatekeepers in the British system. In the United States, under the managed care gatekeeping arrangement, patients initiate the care with their primary care physicians and obtain authorization when specialized services are needed.

Coordination of Care

One of the main functions of primary care is to coordinate the delivery of health services between the patient and the myriad delivery components of the system. Hence, in addition to providing basic services, primary care professionals serve as patient advisors, advocates, and system gatekeepers. In this coordinating role, the provider refers patients to sources of specialized care, gives advice regarding various diagnoses and therapies, discusses treatment options, and provides continuing care for chronic conditions (Williams 1993). Coordination of an individual's total health care needs is meant to ensure continuity and comprehensiveness. These desirable goals of primary care are best achieved when the patient and provider have formed a close mutual relationship over time. Primary care can be regarded as the hub of the health care delivery system wheel. The various components of the health care delivery system are located around the rim, and the spokes signify the coordination of continuous and comprehensive care (see Figure 7–1).

Countries whose health systems are oriented more toward primary care achieve better health levels, higher satisfaction with health services among their populations, and lower expenditures in the overall delivery of health care (Starfield 1994). Countries with weak primary care infrastructures incur poorer health outcomes and higher health care costs. Even in the United States, better health outcomes are achieved in states with higher ratios of primary care physicians and better availability of primary care (Shi 1994; Shi and Starfield 2000, 2001; Shi et al. 2002). Higher ratios of family and general physicians in the population are also associated with lower hospitalization rates for conditions treatable with good primary care (Parchman and Culler 1994). Adults who have primary care physicians as their regular source of care experience lower mortality and incur lower health care costs (Franks et al. 1998). Research has also shown that primary care may play an important role in mitigating the adverse health effects of income inequality (Shi et al. 1999).

Figure 7–1 The Coordination Role of Primary Care in Health Delivery.

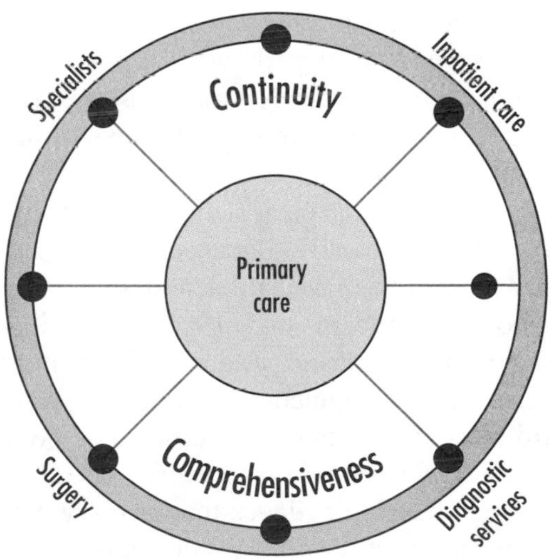

An ideal system of health care delivery is based on primary care but is closely interlinked to adequate and timely specialized services. Continuous and coordinated care requires secondary and tertiary services to be integrated with primary care through appropriate interaction and consultation among physicians. Coordination of health care has certain definite advantages. Studies have shown that both the appropriateness and the outcomes of health care interventions are better when patients are referred to specialists by primary care physicians, as opposed to being self-referred (Bakwin 1945; Roos 1979).

Essential Care

Primary health care is regarded as essential health care. The goal of the health care delivery system is to optimize population health, not just the health of individuals who have the means to access health services. Achievement of this goal requires that disparities across population subgroups be minimized to ensure equal access. Because financing of health care is a key element in determining access, the goal of universal access is better achieved under a national health care program. For this reason, lack of access to primary care for countless millions remains a nagging concern in the United States.

Most Western nations have adopted programs based on universal coverage financed through general tax revenues. As a result, primary care has been an integral part of the national health policy of these nations and is fundamental to the structure of their national health care systems. In the United States, the amalgam of public and private financing has created a fragmented system in which primary care does not form the organizing hub for continuous and coordinated health services. Although the primary care model has gained increased popularity under the managed care system, its current role appears to be limited to low-cost general medicine and gatekeeping to the rest of the health care system. In reality, primary care is much more than that.

Institute of Medicine Definition

The Institute of Medicine (IOM) Committee on the Future of Primary Care recommended that primary care be the usual and preferred, but not the only, route of entry into the health care system. As part of this emphasis, the IOM defined ***primary care*** as: (Vanselow et al. 1995, 192) "The provision of integrated, accessible health care services by clinicians who are accountable for addressing a large majority of personal health care needs, developing a sustained partnership with patients, and practicing in the context of family and community."

The term "integrated" embodies the concepts of comprehensive, coordinated, and continuous services that provide a seamless process of care. Primary care is *comprehensive* because it addresses any health problem at any given stage of a patient's life cycle. The *coordinating* function ensures the provision of a combination of health services to best meet the patient's needs. *Continuity* refers to care over time by a single provider or a team of health care professionals. The IOM definition goes further to emphasize accessibility and accountability as key characteristics of primary care. *Accessibility* refers to the ease with which a patient can initiate an interaction with a clinician for any health problem. It includes efforts to eliminate barriers, such as those posed by geography, financing, culture, race, and language. The IOM Committee recognizes that both clinicians and patients have ***accountability***. The clinical system is accountable for providing quality care, producing patient satisfaction, using resources efficiently, and behaving in an ethical manner. On the other hand, patients are responsible for their own health to the extent that they can influence it. Patients also are responsible for judicious use of resources when they need health care. Partnership between a patient and a clinician does not necessarily imply equal roles. The role played by each party will vary over time and from case to case. Mutual trust, respect, and responsibility are the hallmarks of this partnership. The IOM Committee has proposed that primary care clinicians possess the knowledge and skills necessary to manage most of the physical, mental, social, and emotional concerns that affect the functioning of patients. Primary care clinicians must use their best judgment to involve other practitioners in diagnosis, treatment, or both, when it is appropriate to do so. The IOM Committee also believes that primary care clinicians should be able to address most personal health needs, including health promotion and disease prevention. The definition recognizes that primary care clinicians must consider the influence of the family on a patient's health status and be aware of the patient's living conditions, family dynamics, and cultural background. Finally, exemplary primary care requires an understanding of, and a responsibility for, the community's health (Vanselow et al. 1995).

Community-Oriented Primary Care

The 1978 International Conference on Primary Health Care (held at Alma-Ata in the former Soviet Union, under the auspices of WHO) concluded that people throughout the world had very little control over their own health care and that emphasis should be placed on attaining health through a response from the community to their health problems (WHO 1978). More positive outcomes occur when people have a greater sense of ownership of health programs that address their needs. It requires a partnership between health care providers and the communities in which they serve. It has been suggested that collective action by communities may enhance their competence in mitigating risk factors and thereby reduce their vulnerability to social problems and disease (Minkler 1992).

Community-oriented primary care (COPC) incorporates the elements of good primary care delivery and adds a population-based approach to identifying and addressing community health problems. Current thoughts about primary care delivery have extended beyond the traditional biomedical paradigm, which focuses on medical care for the individual in an encounter-based system. The broader biopsychosocial paradigm emphasizes the health of the population, as well as that of the individual (Lee 1994). A system of health care delivery based on COPC would require developments on at least four fronts.

1. Primary care must take a central place in the delivery of health services.
2. The biomedical model that has dominated both research and health professions' education must be broadened to include a stronger element of the social and behavioral sciences (Engle 1977).
3. Primary and secondary prevention (see Chapter 2) must be appropriately linked in a clinical setting with population-based health programs. Indeed, primary and secondary prevention, as well as certain aspects of tertiary prevention, are essential elements of primary care.
4. Public health functions must be strengthened as an adjunct to clinical interventions because clinicians alone cannot deal with most population-based health problems. Community organizations, such as schools, social service agencies, churches, and employers, must become partners in strengthening public health programs (Lee 1994).

Primary Care Providers

Specialization is oriented toward treating disease. Hence, delivery of health care with a central focus on specialization cannot maximize health because preventing illness and promoting optimal health require a broader perspective than can be achieved by the disease specialist. Specialization focuses on a specific disease or organ system, and specialists may provide the most appropriate care for particular illnesses within their area of competence. A generalist is needed, however, to integrate care for the variety of health problems that individuals experience over time (Starfield 1992, 3).

Physicians in general practice are most commonly the providers of primary care in Europe. In the United States, primary care practitioners are not restricted to physicians trained in general and family practice. Providers of primary care include physicians trained in internal medicine, pediatrics, and obstetrics and gynecology. One cannot assume, however, that these various types of practitioners are equally skilled in rendering primary care services (Starfield 1994). Unless a medical training program is dedicated to providing instruction in primary care, significant differences are likely to exist (Noble et al. 1992). In fact, some controversy and competition have arisen among practitioners as to which specialists should be providing primary care. The specialty of family practice, in particular, represents a challenge to internal medicine in providing adult primary care and to pediatrics in providing child primary care. On the other hand, the role of family practice is now firmly established in some managed care organizations (MCOs) (Petersdorf 1975). As discussed in Chapter 4, it is also important to note the expanded role that nonphysician practitioners (NPPs) are playing in the delivery of primary care. In view of the increasing emphasis on health care cost containment, physician extenders, such as nurse practitioners, physician assistants, and certified nurse midwives, are in great demand in primary care delivery settings, particularly in medically underserved areas. In addition to more effective health care, evidence suggests that a high proportion of primary care professionals in a population results in lower health care expenditures (Welch et al. 1993). Data from Medicaid managed care organizations demonstrate that patients receiving care from nurse practitioners at Nurse-Managed Health Centers experience significantly fewer emergency room visits, hospital inpatient days, and specialist visits, and are at a significantly lower risk of giving birth to low birth weight infants compared to patients in conventional health care (National Nursing Centers Consortium 2003).

Two key factors determine the proportion of primary care personnel to specialists needed for the adequate provision of primary care. The first is how rigidly a health care delivery system employs the concept of gatekeeping. The British National Health Service, for instance, employs this concept more rigidly than the Canadian health system. Consequently, the proportion of primary care physicians is approximately 50 percent in Canada compared to 70–72 percent in Britain (Hodge 1994). In the United States, gatekeeping has gained prominence in the managed care system, and the proliferation of health care delivery through managed care has created an increased demand for primary care physicians. For instance, a growth of 54 percent in family practice residency programs between 1993 and 2000 (Colwill and Cultice 2003) coincided with the rapid expansion of managed care. The second factor driving the need for primary care providers is the propensity of people in a given population to use primary care services. Utilization of primary care is greater in a system offering universal access, hence the need for more primary care professionals in national health care systems.

After a healthy trend in the growth of medical school graduates who chose careers in primary care, a reversal is occurring.

The trend has leveled off, and may even be declining. Block and colleagues (1996) concluded that the culture, values, and educational practices prevailing in the academic medical community are poorly aligned with the goals of enhancing the education and environment for primary care practice. One reason cited is the numerical dominance of specialists and subspecialists on the clinical faculties of medical schools, which is reflected in a negative cultural bias toward primary care. The situation is perhaps difficult to rectify without substantial changes in the composition of medical school faculties, including an infusion of community-based generalists who can serve as teachers, role models, and advocates for primary care (Petersdorf 1993; Roos and Roos 1980). Moreover, current reimbursement systems must be realigned to create financial incentives for people to enter primary care (Reuben 2007). At a time when the United States needs a robust system built on the foundation of primary care, it is unfortunate that the values of traditional biomedicine and medical education continue to emphasize specialization as opposed to breadth of knowledge and training, biological factors as opposed to social and emotional factors in health, and inpatient as opposed to outpatient care and training (Block et al. 1996).

Growth in Outpatient Services

As mentioned earlier, outpatient care now includes much more than primary care services. Duffy and Farley (1995) studied the 150 most frequently performed procedures in hospitals in 1980. By 1987, 37 of the 150 procedures had declined in use by more than 40 percent (Table 7–2). Some of these

Table 7–2 Hospital Weighted Mean Procedure Rates per 1,000 Inpatients, Rates of Decline, and Reason for Decline, 1980–1987

ICD-9-CM Code	Procedure	1980 Mean Rate per 1,000	Mean % Decline 1980–87	Mean % Reasons for Decline: Outpatient	Other
04.07	Peripheral nerve excision[1]		1.84	55	X
04.43	Carpal tunnel release		3.93	76	X ...
06.39	Other partial thyroidectomy[1]	1.09	39	X	...
13.19	Intracapsular lens extraction[1]	20.14	97	X	...
20.01	Myringotomy with intubation	13.60	70	X	...
23.19	Surgical tooth extraction[1]	18.56	80	X	...
28.3	Tonsillectomy, adenoidectomy	13.07	48	X	Practice change
44.00	Vagotomy[2]	1.15	49	...	Replaced
44.15	Open gastric biopsy	7,025.00	74	...	Replaced
48.23	Rigid proctosigmoidoscopy	22.40	67	X	Replaced
48.25	Open rectal biopsy	1.64	66	X	...
49.12	Anal fistulectomy	1.62	48	X	...

(continues)

Table 7–2 Hospital Weighted Mean Procedure Rates per 1,000 Inpatients, Rates of Decline, and Reason for Decline, 1980–1987 (*continued*)

ICD-9-CM Code	Procedure	1980 Mean Rate per 1,000	Mean % Decline 1980–87	Mean % Reasons for Decline	
				Outpatient	Other
49.3	Local destruction of anal lesion[1]	4.59	52	X	. . .
58.6	Urethral dilation	13.49	49	X	. . .
62.5	Orchiopexy	1.18	46	X	. . .
63.1	Excision of spermatic varicocele	2.10	61	X	. . .
67.12	Cervical biopsy[1]	13.25	86	X	. . .
67.2	Conization of cervix	3.25	76	X	. . .
67.39	Destruction of cervical lesion[1]	1.64	70	X	. . .
69.09	D&C[1]	35.06	79	X	. . .
72.1	Low forceps operation with episiotomy	26.87	52	. . .	Practice change
77.59	Bunionectomy[1]	5.28	50	X	. . .
80.16	Other arthrotomy—knee	3.85	66	X	. . .
80.6	Excision of semilunar cartilage of knee	8.61	68	X	. . .
82.21	Excision of lesion of tendon sheath of hand	2.32	90	X	. . .
85.12	Open breast biopsy	4.70	49	X	. . .
85.21	Local excision of breast lesion	6.01	67	X	. . .
86.21	Excision of pilonidal cyst or sinus	1.94	57	X	. . .
86.23	Nail removal	1.42	49	X	. . .
86.3	Other local skin destruction or excision	11.14	49	X	. . .
86.51	Replantation of scalp	1.99	72	. . .	Other
87.59	Biliary tract X-ray[1]	42.02	92	X	Replaced
87.62	Upper gastrointestinal series	73.58	68	X	Replaced
87.73	Intravenous pyelogram	57.97	71		Replaced
92.02	Liver scan, radioisotope function study	25.78	75	X	. . .
92.11	Radioisotope cerebral scan	30.77	97	X	Replaced
97.71	Intrauterine device removal	2.14	84	X	Reduced need

[1]Not elsewhere classified.

[2]Not otherwise specified.

Each hospital's rate of decline is the percentage change from 1980 to 1987 in the number of procedures per 1,000 admissions. Each mean is weighted by the number of times the procedure was performed in 1980. Weighting prevents hospitals with low volumes in 1980 from unduly affecting the analysis. That is, a decline from 200 to 100 procedures is more important than a decline from 4 to 2, even though both are 50 percent reductions.

Source: Reprinted from Public Health Reports, Vol. 110, no. 6, p. 677, 1995, *Journal of the US Public Health Service.*

procedures have been replaced by more advanced procedures, and a few have been largely abandoned as ineffective. The most prominent reason (for 33 of the 37 procedures) for the decline, however, was that most of these procedures were shifted to outpatient settings, especially for patients who did not need to be hospitalized for other health reasons. Patients who did receive one of the 37 procedures in 1987 on an inpatient basis tended to be more severely ill compared to those in 1980. By 1990, more than one-half of all surgeries performed by hospitals took place in an outpatient setting. The proportion of total surgeries performed in outpatient departments of community hospitals increased from 16.3 percent in 1980 to 63.3 percent in 2004 (Figure 7–2). The fact that it is not a simple tradeoff is of some concern. The decline in inpatient procedures has actually been outweighed by the growth of ambulatory procedures. Also, for patients older than 65 years of age, the rate of inpatient surgeries has not decreased (Kozak et al. 1999).

Reasons for the Growth in Outpatient Services

Over the years, several noteworthy changes have occurred in the health care delivery system and in the social environment in which health services are delivered. As a result of these changes, many hospital admissions are regarded as unwarranted. A Rand Corporation study based on a sample of hospital records from 1974 to 1982 concluded that 17 percent of the admissions could have been avoided through the use of outpatient surgery (Siu et al. 1986). Several key changes have been instrumental in shifting the balance between inpatient and outpatient services. These factors can be broadly classified as

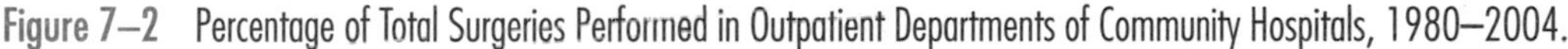
Figure 7–2 Percentage of Total Surgeries Performed in Outpatient Departments of Community Hospitals, 1980–2004.

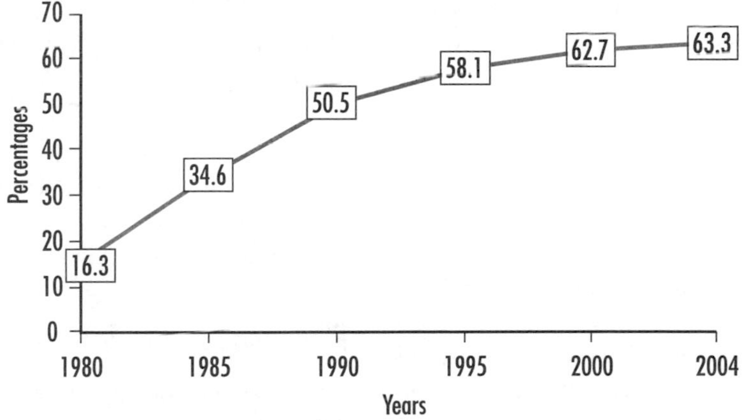

Source: Data from *Health, United States, 2006*, p. 350, National Center for Health Statistics, US Department of Health and Human Services.

reimbursement, technological factors, utilization control factors, physician practice factors, and social factors.

Reimbursement

Until the 1980s, health insurance coverage was usually more generous for inpatient services than for outpatient services. For years, many interventions that could have been performed safely and effectively on an outpatient basis remained inpatient procedures because third-party reimbursement for outpatient care was limited. These payment policies began to change during the 1980s. Today, private and public payers clearly prefer outpatient treatments. In response to the changes in financial incentives, hospitals aggressively developed outpatient services to offset declining inpatient income. The financial factors, for instance, have provided a major impetus for the unprecedented growth of home health care.

In the mid-1980s, Medicare substituted a prospective payment system (PPS) for the cost-plus system to reimburse inpatient hospital services (see Chapter 6). PPS reimbursement based on diagnosis-related groups provides fixed case-based payment to hospitals. The outpatient sector, on the other hand, had no payment restrictions. Hospitals, therefore, had a strong incentive to minimize inpatient lengths of stay and to provide continued treatment in outpatient settings. To contain costs in the mushrooming outpatient sector, in 2000, Medicare implemented prospective reimbursement mechanisms, such as the Medicare Outpatient Prospective Payment System (OPPS) for services provided in hospital outpatient departments and Home Health Resource Groups (HHRGs) for home health care (see Chapter 6).

Cost-containment strategies adopted by managed care also stress lower inpatient use, with a corresponding emphasis on outpatient services. Capitation methods used by many MCOs discourage hospital stays in favor of outpatient services because inpatient care is more expensive.

Technological Factors

Development of new diagnostic and treatment procedures and less invasive surgical methods has made it possible to provide services in outpatient settings that previously had required hospital stays. Shorter-acting anesthetics are now available. The diffusion of arthroscopes, laparoscopes, lasers, and other minimally invasive technologies have made many surgical procedures less traumatic. These modern procedures have dramatically curtailed recuperation time, which has made same-day surgical procedures very common. As pointed out in Chapter 5, many office-based physicians have expanded their capacity to perform outpatient diagnostic, treatment, and surgical services, because acquisition of technology has become more feasible and cost-effective.

Utilization Control Factors

Hospital stays have been strongly discouraged by various payers. Prior authorization for inpatient admission and close monitoring during hospitalization have been actively pursued with the objective of minimizing the length of stay. Utilization control methods are discussed in Chapter 9.

Physician Practice Factors

The growth of managed care and consolidation by large hospital-centered institutions weakened physician autonomy and professional control over the delivery of medical care. Physicians also lost income. To counter these forces, an increasing number of physicians have broken their ties with hospitals and have started their own specialized care centers, such as ambulatory surgery centers and cardiac care centers. In specialized ambulatory care centers, physicians find that they can perform more procedures in less time and earn higher incomes (Jackson 2002). As one would expect to find in the industrial mass-production model, in a study of hospital outpatient procedures, a higher case volume for the same procedures resulted in significant reduction in average cost per procedure (Center for Healthcare Industry Performance Studies 1997). Higher volumes may also be associated with better quality. Such factors may be behind the growth in specialized centers of excellence for cataract and hernia surgeries and cardiac procedures.

Social Factors

In addition to the financial, technological, and utilization control factors just mentioned, social factors have contributed to the growth of outpatient services. Patients generally have a strong preference for receiving health care in home and community-based settings. Unless absolutely necessary, most patients do not want to be institutionalized. Staying in their own homes gives people a strong sense of independence and control over their lives, elements considered important for quality of life.

Large hospitals have traditionally been located in congested urban centers. These locations have been perceived as inconvenient by increasing numbers of suburbanites. During the past two decades, many freestanding outpatient centers as well as satellites operated by inner city hospitals, have emerged in the expanding suburbs.

Types of Outpatient Care Settings and Methods of Delivery

The myriad of outpatient care and community-based services now operating sometimes makes it difficult to adequately differentiate between the structural settings in which these services are provided. For example, agencies providing home health services can be freestanding, hospital based, or nursing home based. Many physician group practices are merging with hospitals; hospitals and freestanding surgical clinics often compete for various types of surgical procedures. Therefore, the classifications used in this section are only illustrative, because many exceptions exist. Also, in this constantly evolving system, new settings and methods are likely to emerge. The various settings for outpatient service delivery found in the US health care delivery system can be grouped as:

- private practice
- hospital-based services
- freestanding facilities
- mobile medical, diagnostic, and screening services
- home health care
- hospice services
- ambulatory long-term care services
- public health services
- public and voluntary clinics
- telephone access
- alternative medicine

Private Practice

Physicians, as office-based practitioners, are the backbone of ambulatory care and constitute the vast majority of primary care services. Most visits entail relatively limited examination and testing, and encounters with the physician are generally brief. The waiting time in the office is typically longer than the actual time spent with the physician.

In the past, the solo practice of medicine and small partnerships attracted the most practitioners. Self-employment offered a degree of independence not generally available in large organizational settings. During the past few years, group practice and institutional affiliations, such as employment by an MCO, have expanded dramatically. Few graduates of residency programs are entering solo practice. Several factors account for this shift, including uncertainties created by rapid changes in the health care delivery system, contracting by MCOs with consolidated rather than solo entities, competition from large health care delivery organizations, high cost of establishing a new practice, complexity of billings and collections in a multiple-payer system, and increased external controls over the private practice of medicine. Group practice and other organizational arrangements offer the benefits of a patient referral network: negotiating leverage with MCOs; sharing overhead expenses; ease of obtaining coverage from colleagues for personal time off; and, in a growing number of instances, attractive starting salaries, with benefits and profit-sharing plans. Most young physicians find that these advantages far outweigh the allure of being an independent solo practitioner.

For these reasons, group practice of medicine in the United States has experienced a sharp increase (Figure 7–3). An estimated one-fourth of all US physicians now practice in a group clinic (SMG Solutions 2000). Most of these groups are small, with about 69 percent having no more than six physicians. Twenty-seven percent have 7 to

Figure 7–3 Growth in the Number of Medical Group Practices.

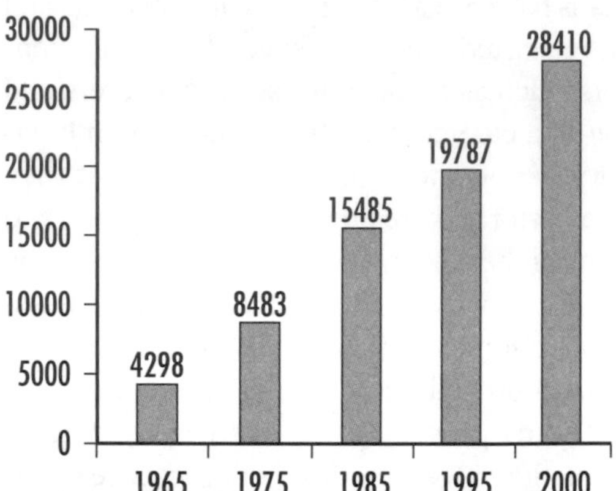

Sources: Data from VHA Inc. and Deloitte & Touche, *1997 Environmental assessment: Redesigning health care for the millennium,* Irving, TX: VHA Inc.; SMG Solutions, *2000 Report and directory: Medical group practices,* Chicago, IL: SMG Solutions.

25 physicians. Only 4 percent have 26 or more physicians; however, nearly one-half of all physicians working in group practices have 26 or more partners (VHA Inc. and Deloitte & Touche 1997). In other words, roughly 4 percent of group practices employ nearly one-half of all physicians.

Group practice clinics also offer important advantages to patients. In many instances, patients can receive up-to-date diagnostic, treatment, pharmaceutical, and certain surgical services. All but the most advanced secondary and tertiary procedures can generally be performed within these large clinics. Patients also often see cross-referrals among partner physicians located near each other as an added convenience.

Apart from physicians, other private practitioners often work in solo or group practice settings, for example: dentists; optometrists; podiatrists; psychologists; and physical, occupational, and speech therapists. Group practice among these health care providers is becoming increasingly common, generally for the same reasons as physicians.

Figure 7–4 shows the distribution of total ambulatory visits among physician offices, hospital-based outpatient departments, and hospital EDs. In 2004, approximately 82.4 percent of all ambulatory care visits occurred in physicians' offices. It is interesting to note that hospitals have made substantial strides in gaining market share for outpatient services.

Hospital-Based Outpatient Services

Not too long ago, hospital professionals regarded outpatient departments of urban hospitals with certain contempt. The outpatient department was often viewed as the stepchild of the institution and the least popular area of the hospital in which to work (Knowles 1965). Hospital outpatient clinics, which were mainly operated by city and county government hospitals and located in urban centers, served primarily indigent populations because these people lacked access to private medical care (Sultz and Young 1997, 99). Even today, many hospital outpatient clinics, particularly those in inner city areas, function as the community's safety net, providing primary care to medically indigent and uninsured populations. Some of the early voluntary hospitals, that is, nonprofit community hospitals, also had outpatient departments. For example, in the mid-1770s, the Pennsylvania Hospital in Philadelphia treated almost 200 patients a year in its outpatient department (Raffel and Raffel 1994, 113). However, these voluntary hospitals preferred to serve paying patients.

Outpatient services are now a key source of profit for hospitals. Consequently, hospitals have expanded their outpatient departments, and utilization has grown (see Figure 7–4). This trend is the result of fierce competition in the health care industry, in which MCOs emphasizing preventive and outpatient care have waged a relentless drive to cut costs. As hospitals have seen inpatient revenues steadily erode, they have begun sprucing up and expanding outpatient services. In doing so, they are competing for privately insured patients who favor private physicians'

Figure 7–4 Ambulatory Care Visits.

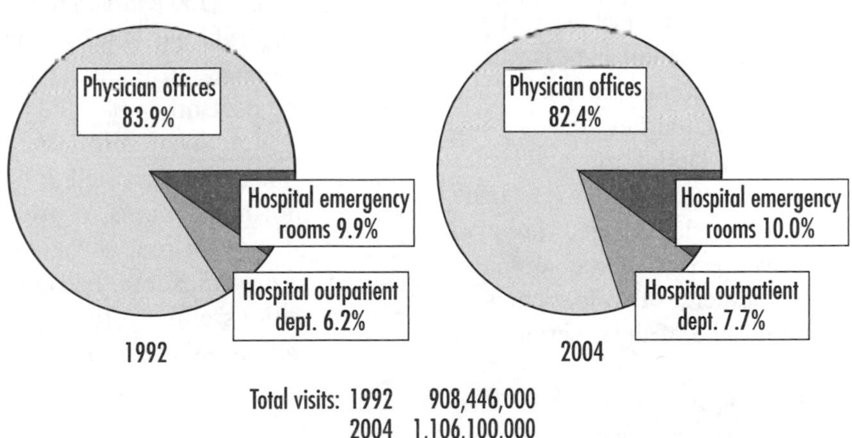

Source: Data from National Center for Health Statistics, US Department of Health and Human Services. *Statistical Abstracts of US*, 2001, p. 108; and *Statistical Abstracts of US*, 2007, p. 112.

offices. Beth Israel Hospital of New York City has struggled over the years to compete for patients with the city's more prestigious academic medical centers. In 1996, the hospital opened the Phillips Ambulatory Care Center in a gleaming building that looks like a medical mall. Inside are cozy offices, plush glass-walled waiting rooms looking out on an atrium with a waterfall, and state-of-the-art examining rooms (Fein 1996). The center provides a full range of outpatient services from primary care to over 50 different on-site diagnostic services, a cancer center, ambulatory surgery, a spine institute, and a wellness library (Phillips Ambulatory Care Center 2000).

A continuum of inpatient and outpatient services developed by a hospital offers opportunities for cross-referral among services to keep patients within the same delivery system. A hospital providing both inpatient and outpatient services can enhance its revenues by referring postsurgical cases to its affiliated units for rehabilitation and home care follow-up. Patients receiving various types of outpatient services constitute an important source of referrals back to hospitals for inpatient care. A hospital can thus expand its patient base. Quicker discharge of patients from hospital beds under prospective and capitated reimbursement methods has created a substantial market for ongoing outpatient services. Under managed care arrangements, better cost-efficiencies can be achieved when all needed services are provided within a well-established continuum, regardless of whether both inpatient and outpatient, or only one of these services, is capitated.

Prior to 1985, outpatient care had less than 15 percent of the total gross patient revenue for all US hospitals. This ratio has now grown to nearly 40 percent (AHA 2006). Between 1996 and 2000, hospital outpatient revenues grew by approximately 54.4 percent, whereas the growth of inpatient revenues was merely 32 percent (data from Health Forum 2002). Given the growing competition in the delivery of outpatient services, hospitals and hospital systems are increasingly operating freestanding ambulatory care facilities (see Freestanding Facilities). Sports medicine, women's health, and renal dialysis are some of the specialized services being provided in both hospital- and nonhospital-based facilities. Many hospitals have also developed health promotion/disease prevention and health fitness programs as outreaches to the communities they serve.

Most hospital-based outpatient services can be broadly classified into five main types: clinical, surgical, emergency, home health, and women's health.

Clinical Services

Many clinical services in hospital outpatient departments correspond to the services provided by private physicians in their offices. Acquisition of group practices has enabled hospitals to increase their market share for outpatient care. Downstream referrals for inpatient, surgical, and other specialized services have generated additional revenues for these hospitals. Both public and private nonprofit hospitals located in inner city locations provide uncompensated care to patients who do not have access to private practitioners' offices for routine care, mainly because they are uninsured. Teaching hospitals operate various clinics offering highly specialized, research-based services.

Surgical Services

Hospital-based ambulatory surgery centers originated in Washington, DC, Los Angeles, and other large cities. They provide same-day surgical care; patients are sent home after a few hours of recovery time following surgery. Follow-up care generally continues in the physician's office. Although most procedures are still performed on an inpatient basis, hospitals also have the upper hand over freestanding centers in the provision of outpatient medical procedures (see Figure 7–5).

Emergency Services

The ED has been a vital outpatient component of many community hospitals. The main purpose of this department is to have services available around the clock for patients who are acutely ill or injured, particularly those with serious or life-threatening conditions requiring immediate attention. When deemed medically appropriate, prompt hospitalization can occur directly from the ED. Emergency departments are generally staffed by full-time physicians 24 hours a day. These physicians commonly have specialized training in emergency medicine. In small hospitals, the staff may be members of the regular medical staff in rotation (Wilson and Neuhauser 1985, 32). Another option is to contract ED staffing to physician groups specializing in that type of work.

Figure 7–5 Medical Procedures by Location.

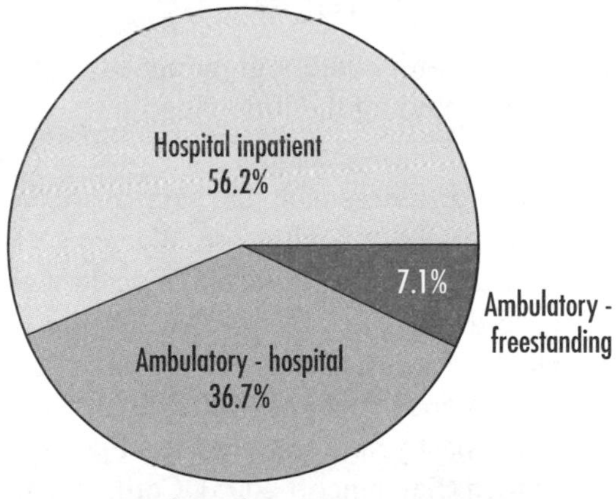

Source: Data from *Vital and Health Statistics: Ambulatory and Inpatient Procedures in the United States, 1996,* p. 25, November 1998, National Center for Health Statistics, US Department of Health and Human Services.

Weinerman and colleagues (1966) defined three categories of conditions for which patients present themselves to the ED: ***emergent conditions*** are critical and require immediate medical attention; time delay is harmful to patient; and the disorder is acute and potentially threatening to life or function. ***Urgent conditions*** require medical attention within a few hours; a longer delay presents possible danger to the patient; and the disorder is acute but not severe enough to be life threatening. ***Nonurgent conditions*** do not require the resources of an emergency service, and the disorder is nonacute or minor in severity.

It has been well documented that, in the United States, EDs are overused for nonurgent or routine care that could be more appropriately addressed in a primary care setting (Glick and Thompson 1997). Actually, fewer than half of the visits are for emergency conditions (McCaig 2002). For many of the uninsured lacking access to routine primary care, the ED has become the family physician, especially at night and on weekends (Raffel and Raffel 1994, 142). Reasons for ED use for nonurgent care include erroneous self-assessment of severity of ailment or injury, the 24-hour open-door policy, convenience, and unavailability of primary care providers (Liggins 1993). The uninsured and people on Medicaid and Medicare use disproportionately more ED services than those who have private insurance coverage (McCaig and Burt 2002). Many private physicians do not provide services to Medicaid enrollees because of low Medicaid reimbursement. Thus, people on Medicaid often have no primary care provider (McNamara et al. 1993). On the other hand, people who have a source of ongoing primary care are less likely to use EDs (Rosenblatt et al. 2000). The Emergency Medical Treatment and Labor Act of 1986 (EMTALA) requires screening and evaluation of every patient, necessary stabilizing treatment, and admitting when necessary, regardless of ability to pay. Hence, Medicaid patients and the uninsured often use EDs for primary care treatments. Thus, EDs often function as a public "safety net."

Crowding in EDs has also been exacerbated by hospital and emergency department closings nationwide. In 1992, approximately 6,000 hospitals had EDs. Less than 4,000 remain today. On the other hand, the demand for ED visits has increased considerably, as reflected by the growth in the annual number of ED visits from 93.4 million to 110.2 million between 1994 and 2004 (McCaig and Newar 2006). Causes of ED overcrowding include hospital bed shortages in some areas, high medical acuity of patients, increasing patient volume, too few examination spaces, and a shortage of registered nurses (Derlet and Richards 2002).

Overcrowded hospital EDs reflect a lack of well-structured ambulatory services in the community. Because EDs require sophisticated facilities and highly trained personnel and must be accessible 24 hours a day, costs are high and services are not designed for nonurgent care (Williams 1993, 127). Inappropriate use of emergency services wastes precious resources. Hence, alternatives to the ED for nonurgent and routine care are critically needed, especially for Medicaid and uninsured patients. Freestanding walk-in clinics and urgent care centers provide extended hours, but their services are mainly available to insured patients. Because of competition from such freestanding clinics, some hospitals now offer extended evening and weekend hours at their own outpatient centers. After-hours telephone access to trained professionals, which is discussed later, is another alternative that is both economical and convenient. EDs are also using triage mechanisms to screen patients for the level of severity and for the referral of nonemergency cases to primary care physicians.

Home Health Care

Many hospitals have opened separate home health departments, which provide mainly postacute care and rehabilitation therapies. Hospitals have entered the home health business to keep discharged patients within the hospital system. Hospitals operate about 24 percent of all Medicare-certified home health agencies in the United States (National Association of Home Care and Hospice 2004). Home health care is discussed in detail later in this chapter.

Women's Health Centers

Women's health centers grew out of social changes, including the following:

- A market assessment that women are the major users of health care. Women seek health care more often than men do. According to the 2004 Kaiser Women's Health Survey, 87 percent of women had at least one visit to a health care provider in the past year, compared to 74 percent of men (Salganicoff 2005). Compared to men, women have only a slightly higher mean number of specialty care visits and emergency department visits. However, women have higher annual charges than men do for all types of care, including primary, specialty, emergency, and diagnostic services, indicating that women receive more intensive services (Bertakis et al. 2000). Morbidity is greater among women than among men, even after childbearing-related conditions are factored out. For instance, nearly 38 percent of women report having chronic conditions that require ongoing medical treatment compared to 30 percent of men (Salganicoff 2005).

- A change in philosophy in American culture toward women, including gender equality. Advocacy groups voiced growing concern that research in women's health was not being appropriately funded. Concern was also expressed that what was known about health and disease was based on conditions in men, because males primarily constituted the research populations.
- A recognition that the female majority in the United States will continue to grow as the aging population includes more females. Table 7–3 shows current population trends.
- Response to the call to make women's health a national priority. In the 1980s, the US Public Health Service established a coordinating committee and special task force on women's health, leading to the creation of the Office of Women's Health in July 1991 (Looker 1993). Women's issues are covered in greater detail in Chapter 11.

Since the 1980s, the emerging recognition of the prominence of women as a major health market has led medical institutions to develop specialized women's health centers in hospital-based and/or hospital-affiliated settings. These new programs have focused on outpatient services, as indicated by industry trends. Hospital-sponsored women's health centers have a variety of service provision models on a continuum that includes telephone information and referral, educational programs, health screening and diagnostics, comprehensive primary care for women, and mental health services. In addition to services in obstetrics, gynecology, and primary care, women's health centers offer mammography, ultrasound, osteoporosis screening, and other health screenings. Specialized inpatient programs for women, such as special units, pavilions, and women's hospitals, are also in operation (Looker 1993).

Table 7–3 Growth in Female US Resident Population by Age Groups between 1980 and 2004 (in thousands)

	Age Groups						
	<15	15 to 44	45 to 64	65 to 74	75 to 84	85+	total
1980	25,073	52,833	23,342	8,824	4,862	1,559	116,493
2004	29,698	62,034	36,245	10,036	7,753	3,352	149,118
growth	4,625	9,201	12,903	1,212	2,891	1,793	32,625

Source: Data from *Health, United States, 2006*, p. 127, National Center for Health Statistics.

Freestanding Facilities

During the past several years, various types of proprietary, community-based freestanding medical facilities have opened across the country. They are known as walk-in clinics, urgent care centers, and surgi-centers. Other types of outpatient facilities include outpatient rehabilitation centers, optometric centers, and dental clinics. Such facilities have given patients a wider range of health care choices and have attempted to meet consumer needs of convenience and cost reduction (Lowell-Smith 1994). These clinics, which are often owned or controlled by corporations, commonly employ practitioners on salary. The growing number of ambulatory centers might be expected to reduce the use of hospital EDs for nonurgent care. However, because these centers cater mainly to insured patients, the use of hospital EDs by the uninsured is likely to continue unless other alternatives are developed to meet the routine medical needs of the uninsured population.

Walk-in clinics provide ambulatory services ranging from basic primary care to urgent care, but they are generally used on a nonroutine, episodic basis. The main advantages of these clinics are convenience of location, evening and weekend hours, and availability of services on a "walk-in" (no appointment) basis. Many ***urgent care centers*** are open 24 hours a day, 7 days a week, and accept patients with no appointments. These centers generally offer a wide range of routine services for basic and acute conditions on a first-come first-served basis, but they are not comparable to hospital EDs. Often, the distinctions between these two types of outpatient facilities are rather blurred. They all compete with hospital EDs and office-based physicians. ***Surgi-centers*** are freestanding ambulatory surgery centers independent of hospitals. They usually provide a full range of services for the types of surgery that can be performed on an outpatient basis and do not require overnight hospitalization. On the other hand, office-based specialists still use their own offices for routine procedures, such as oral surgery, plastic surgery, and ophthalmology (Williams 1993).

Outpatient rehabilitation centers provide physical therapy, occupational therapy, and speech pathology services. In the past, generous Medicare reimbursement attracted various operators to open outpatient rehabilitation centers, but caps ($1,500 annually for speech and physical therapies, and another $1,500 annually for occupational therapy) instituted under the Balanced Budget Act of 1997 will have a lasting impact on such clinics. Due to protests from therapists and their patients, the caps have been suspended, but similar efforts to curtail reimbursement are likely to reemerge.

Neighborhood optical centers providing vision services have become quite popular in recent years, replacing many office-based opticians. Other freestanding facilities include audiology clinics, dental centers, hemodialysis centers, pharmacies, and suppliers of durable medical equipment (DME). A growing number of the various types of freestanding facilities are part of large regional and nationwide chains, which are opening new facilities at an unprecedented rate in new geographic locations.

Mobile Medical, Diagnostic, and Screening Services

Mobile health care services are transported to patients. Ambulance service and first aid treatment provided to the victims of severe illness, accidents, and disasters by trained emergency medical technicians (EMTs) are the most commonly encountered mobile medical services. Such services are also referred to as prehospital medicine. Early attention following traumatic injury is often lifesaving. EMTs are specially trained to provide such attention at the site and in transit to the hospital. Most ambulance personnel have a Basic-EMT rating. Advanced training can lead to EMT-Paramedic certification. Paramedics are trained to administer emergency drugs and provide advanced life support emergency medical services. Examples include intravenous administration of fluids and drugs, treatment for shock, electrocardiograms, electrical interventions to support cardiac function, and endotracheal intubation (insertion of a tube as an air passage through the trachea).

To provide a speedy response to emergencies, most urban centers have developed formal emergency medical systems that incorporate all area hospital EDs along with transportation and communication systems. Most such communities have established 911 emergency phone lines to provide immediate access to those needing emergency care. An ambulance is dispatched by a central communications center that also identifies and alerts the hospital most appropriately equipped to deal with the type of emergency and located closest to the site where the emergency has occurred. Specialized ambulance services or advanced life support ambulances include mobile coronary care units, shock-trauma vans, and disaster relief vans. They are staffed by paramedics and EMTs with advanced training.

Mobile medical services also constitute an efficient and convenient way to provide certain types of routine health services. Mobile eye care, podiatric care, and dental care units, for example, can be brought to a nursing home site where they can efficiently serve many patients residing in the facility. They are a convenient service for the patients, many of whom are frail elderly who can then avoid an often difficult and tiring trip to a regular clinic.

Mobile diagnostic services include mammography and magnetic resonance imaging (MRI). Such mobile units take advanced diagnostic services to small towns and rural communities. They offer the advantages of convenience to patients and cost-efficiency in the delivery of diagnostic care. Other screening services are more basic in nature. Screening vans, staffed by volunteers who are trained professionals and generally operated by various nonprofit organizations, are often seen at malls and fair sites. Various types of health education and health promotion services and screening checks, such as blood pressure and cholesterol screening, are commonly performed for anyone who walks in.

Home Health Care

For most ambulatory care, patients must voluntarily leave their homes to go to the settings where such care is delivered. In ***home health care***, services are brought to patients in their own homes. Without home services, the only alternative for most such patients would be institutionalization in a hospital or nursing home. Home health is consistent with the philosophy of maintaining people in the least restrictive environment possible. Most people express a strong preference for receiving health services at home rather than in an institution.

Before the home health boom, the Visiting Nurse Associations (VNAs) provided nursing and other services in patients' homes. The first VNAs were established in Buffalo, Boston, and Philadelphia in 1885 and 1886 (Wilson and Neuhauser 1985, 52). VNAs now account for only 6 percent of all Medicare-certified agencies (National Association for Home Care and Hospice 2004).

Following a lawsuit in 1989, Medicare rules for home health care were clarified, making it easier for Medicare beneficiaries to receive home health services. Patients are eligible to receive these services under Medicare if they are homebound, have a plan of treatment and a periodical review by a physician, and require intermittent or part-time skilled nursing and/or rehabilitation therapies (Waid 1998).

Home health services typically include nursing care, such as changing dressings, monitoring medications, and providing help with bathing; short-term rehabilitation, such as physical therapy, occupational therapy, and speech therapy. Other services include homemaker services, such as meal preparation, shopping, transportation, and some specific household chores; and certain medical supplies and equipment, such as ostomy supplies, hospital beds, oxygen tanks, walkers, and wheelchairs—all called ***durable medical equipment*** (DME). Not every home health agency provides all of these services, however. For example, home health agencies often assume responsibility for arranging for DME, but private DME companies actually furnish the equipment.

Under Medicare, home health benefits do not include full-time nursing care, food, blood, and drugs. Since the early 1980s, specialized high-technology home therapies have also proliferated. Before that, those services could only be delivered in hospitals. Such specialized services include intravenous antibiotics, oncology therapy, hemodialysis, parenteral and enteral nutrition, and ventilator care (Evashwick 1993). For specialized services, home health care is cost-effective and enhances the patient's quality of life. For example, home hemodialysis costs about one-third of what in-center dialysis costs. Especially for younger patients, the option of dialyzing at home is providing greater independence and flexibility, such as the ability to dialyze at night. It has enabled people to maintain employment and, in many cases, saved hours of time spent traveling to and from dialysis centers (Stahl 1997). Overall costs were reduced on average by more than $13,000 per patient when a pulmonary specialty team managed the in-home health care of patients suffering from advanced chronic obstructive pulmonary disease (COPD) because of decreased use of hospital, emergency department, and skilled nursing facility resources (Steinel and Madigan 2003).

Figure 7–6 shows the demographic characteristics of home health care patients in 2000. Because of variations in data sources,

Figure 7–6 Demographic Characteristics of Home Health Patients, 2000.

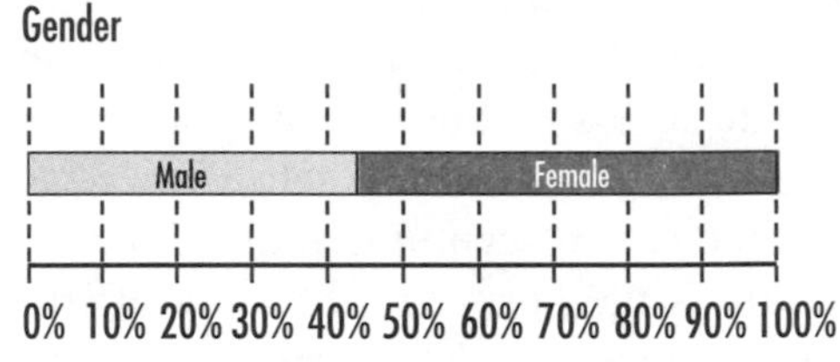

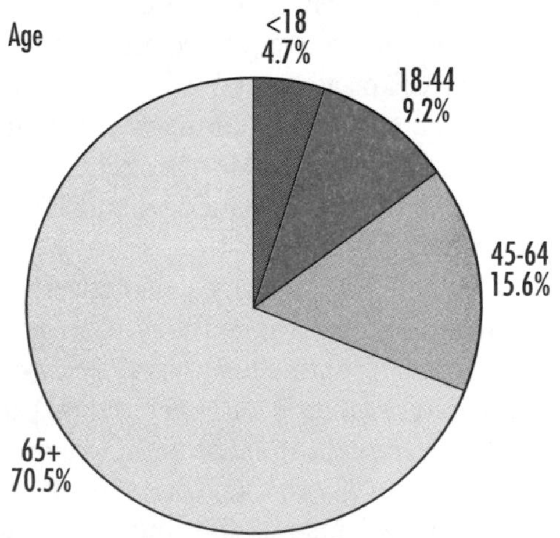

Source: Data from National Center for Health Statistics, *2000 National Home and Hospice Care Survey.*

national expenditures for home health care are difficult to calculate. However, estimates from the Centers for Medicare & Medicaid Services (2006) indicate that total expenditures for home health were $43.2 billion in 2004 (CMS 2006). Medicare is the largest single payer for home care services. It financed approximately $16.4 billion of home health care expenditures in 2004, compared to $13.7 billion for Medicaid, $5.2 billion for private insurance, and $4.9 billion for out-of-pocket payments (CMS 2006). Payments to home health agencies were sharply cut under the Balanced Budget Act of 1997. As a result, home health expenditures accounted for 4 percent of total Medicare spending in 2004, compared to 9 percent in 1997 (National Association of Home Care and Hospice 2004). An estimated 3.5 million Medicare enrollees received fee-for-service home health care in 1997, twice the number in 1990. However, since 1997, use of the home health benefit has decreased significantly (National Association of Home Care and Hospice 2004).

Medicaid payments for home care are divided into three main categories: the traditional home health benefit that is a federally mandated service provided by all states, and two optional programs—the personal care option, and home and community-based waivers. Together, these three home health services represent a relatively small but growing portion of total Medicaid payments. In 2000, approximately 14.4 percent of the total Medicaid benefit payments to vendors were for home care services, compared to 9.8 percent in 1997 (National Association of Home Care and Hospice 2004).

Various private payers also prefer to minimize the high costs associated with hospital inpatient care and opt for home health services wherever possible. Private home health care is increasingly being financed through managed care organizations. Hence, home health care is no longer synonymous with long-term home-based care for the elderly, although the elderly are the largest users of home health care.

Reimbursement cuts implemented under the Balanced Budget Act had a marked impact on the home health industry. Between 1997 and 2000, the number of home health agencies in the United States declined from 15,069 to 13,067 (Hoechst Marion Roussel 1999; Aventis Pharmaceuticals 2001). Thirty percent of Medicare-certified agencies are hospital-based, 40 percent are proprietary, and the remaining 24 percent have other types of ownership. Figure 7–7 shows sources of revenue and average distribution of revenues from these sources for home health care. Tables 7–4 and 7–5 provide additional statistics.

Figure 7–7 Estimated Payments for Home Care by Payment Source, 2010.

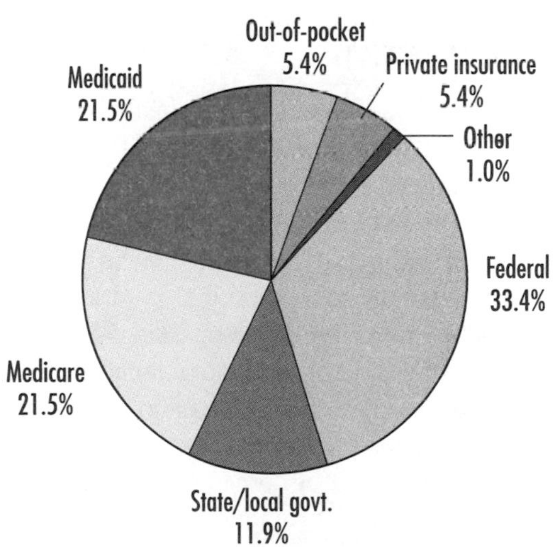

Source: Data from Centers for Medicare and Medicaid Service, Office of the Actuary, *National Health Expenditures Projections: 2005–2015.*

Table 7–4 Home Health and Hospice Care Agencies, by Selected Characteristics, 1998

Agency Characteristic	Agencies, Total	Current Patients			Discharges		
		Total	Home Health Care	Hospice Care	Total	Home Health Care	Hospice Care
Total (1,000)	13.3	1,961.6	1,881.8	79.8	8,117.7	7,621.8	496.0
Percentage distribution							
Ownership							
Proprietary	53.9	46.1	47.1	23.0	38.4	39.1	26.7
Voluntary nonprofit	36.2	45.4	44.2	73.0	54.3	53.2	69.9
Government and other	9.9	8.5	8.7	4.1	7.4	7.6	3.9
Certification							
Medicare	84.3	84.0	83.5	96.6	42.9	92.8	93.9
Medicaid	85.1	85.1	84.8	92.3	89.3	89.3	90.0
Region							
Northeast	16.7	34.4	35.4	10.7	34.8	34.8	18.7
Midwest	25.8	21.5	21.4	23.9	25.7	25.7	22.9
South	42.0	33.9	33.4	44.6	25.9	25.9	33.3
West	15.5	10.2	9.7	20.8	13.5	13.5	25.1

Source: Reprinted from US National Center for Health Statistics, *Statistical Abstracts of the United States,* p. 115, 2001.

Hospice Services

The term ***hospice*** refers to a cluster of comprehensive services for the terminally ill with a life expectancy of six months or less. Over half of the patients are diagnosed with cancer upon admission. Hospice, whose programs provide services that address the special needs of dying persons and their families, is a method of care, not a location, and services are taken to patients and their families wherever they are located. Thus, hospice can be a part of home health care when the services are provided in the patient's home. In other instances, hospice services are taken to patients in nursing homes, retirement centers, or hospitals. Services can be organized out of a hospital, nursing home, freestanding hospice facility, or home health agency. The dollar outlays in these four types of hospice operations gives a fair indication of the volume of services provided through each setting (see Figure 7–8).

Hospice regards the patient and family as the unit of care. This special kind of care includes (Miller 1996):

- meeting the patient's physical needs
- meeting the patient's and family's emotional and spiritual needs
- delivery of care in the patient's home or in a home-like setting

Table 7–5 Home Health Care and Hospice Patients, 2000

Type of Patient and Characteristic	Home Health Care	Hospice Patients
Number of current patients	1,355,300	105,500
Percentage distribution of primary admission diagnosis		
Malignant neoplasm of	5.0	52.0
Large intestine and rectum	—	4.9
Trachea, bronchus, and lung	—	12.3
Breast	—	4.8
Prostate	—	7.7
Diabetes	7.9	—
Diseases of the nervous system and sense organs	6.1	—
Diseases of the circulatory system	23.6	15.6
Heart disease	10.9	12.8
Cerebrovascular diseases	7.3	—
Diseases of the respiratory system	6.8	6.5
Decubitus ulcers	1.9	—
Diseases of the musculoskeletal system and connective tissue	9.8	—
Osteoarthritis	3.5	—
Fractures, all sites	4.1	—
Fracture of neck of femur (hip)	1.5	—
Other	31.3	25.9

Source: Data from National Home and Hospice Care Survey 2000, Centers for Disease Control and Prevention, National Center for Health Statistics, Division of Health Care Statistics.

- emphasis on making the patient free of pain and as comfortable as possible so the patient can make the most of the time that remains
- support for the family members before and after the patient's death
- focus on maintaining the quality of life rather than prolonging life

Hospice services include medical, psychological, and social services provided in a holistic context. The two primary areas of emphasis in hospice care are (1) pain and symptom management, which is referred to as ***palliation***, and (2) psychosocial and spiritual support. The pharmacologic technology of pain management is particularly essential to hospice care. Psychological services focus on relieving mental anguish. Counseling and spiritual help are made available to help the patient deal with his or her death. After the patient's death, bereavement counseling is offered to the family. Social services include help with arranging final affairs (Dychtwald et al. 1990, 150–151). Apart from medical, nursing, and social

Figure 7–8 Medicare Dollar Outlays by Type of Hospice, 2003.

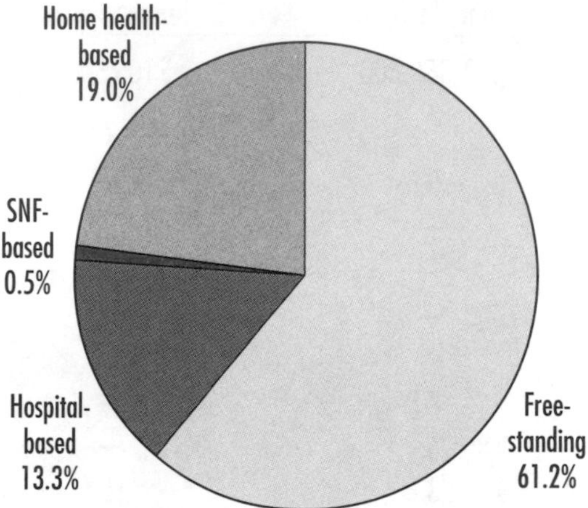

Source: Data from Centers for Medicare and Medicaid Services 2005.

services staff, hospice organizations rely heavily on volunteers.

The idea of providing comprehensive care to terminally ill patients was first promoted by Dame Cicely Saunders in the 1960s in England. In the United States, the first hospice was established in 1974 by Sylvia Lack in New Haven, Connecticut (Beresford 1989). Hospice organizations expanded after Medicare extended hospice benefits in 1983. Hospice is a cost-effective option for both private and public payers. It is estimated that for every dollar spent on hospice, Medicare saves $1.52 in Part A and Part B expenditures (National Hospice and Palliative Care Organization 2003). The difference in costs is mainly due to the intensity of services. Many states now provide hospice benefits under Medicaid.

To receive Medicare certification, a hospice must meet these basic conditions:

- Physician certification that the patient's prognosis is for a life expectancy of six months or less
- Make nursing services, physician services, and drugs and biologicals available on a 24-hour basis
- Provide nursing services under the supervision of a registered nurse
- Make arrangements for inpatient care when necessary
- Provide social services by a qualified social worker, under the direction of a physician
- Make counseling services available to both the patient and the family, including bereavement support after the patient's death
- Provide needed medications, medical supplies, and equipment for pain management and palliation
- Provide physical, occupational, and speech therapy services when necessary
- Provide home health aide and homemaker services when needed

There were approximately 2,444 Medicare-certified hospices in the United States in 2003 (National Association of Home Care and Hospice 2004). Medicare is the largest source of financing for hospice services. Under the provisions of the Balanced Budget Act of 1997, Medicare provides for two 90-day benefit periods. Subsequently, an unlimited number of 60-day periods are available, based on recertification by a physician that a patient has six months or less to live. Figure 7–9 shows the sources of coverage for hospice services. Tables 7–4 and 7–5 provide additional statistics.

Ambulatory Long-Term Care Services

Long-term care has typically been associated with care provided in nursing homes, but during the past several years, a number of al-

Figure 7–9 Coverage of Patients for Hospice Care at the Time of Admission.

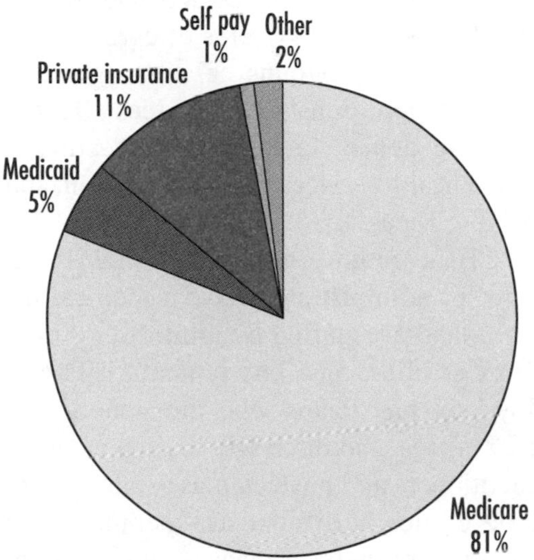

Source: Data from the National Hospice and Palliative Care Organization, NHPCO Facts and Figures, January 2003. *http://www.nhpco.org.*

ternative settings that form a continuum have emerged. Two types of ambulatory long-term care services are case management and adult day care. ***Case management*** provides coordination and referral among a variety of health care services. The objective is to find the most appropriate setting to meet a patient's health care needs. ***Adult day care*** complements informal care provided at home by family members with professional services available in adult day care centers during the normal workday. Both services are discussed in more detail in Chapter 10.

Public Health Services

Public health services in the United States are typically provided by local health departments, and the range of services offered varies greatly by locality. Generally, public health programs are limited in scope. They include well-baby care, venereal disease clinics, family planning services, screening and treatment for tuberculosis, and ambulatory mental health. For reasons pointed out in Chapter 3, public health programs generally offer services that do not directly compete with those provided by private practitioners. Typically, such services are restricted to those areas in which private practitioners have little interest, or they are targeted to serve inner city, poor, uninsured populations. All are ***categorical programs*** specifically designed to address certain categories of disease or to serve specific categories of persons. School health programs in public schools fall under the public health domain, but they are limited to vision and hearing screening and assistance with dysfunctions that prevent learning. Ambulatory clinics in prisons also fall in the public health domain.

The public school setting is a growing area of practice for physical therapists, occupational therapists, and speech/language pathologists. They help children with special physical and emotional dysfunctions. The Individuals with Disabilities Education Act (IDEA) of 1975 (subject to reauthorization every three years) has been instrumental in allowing children with special needs to receive services in public schools so that they can obtain optimum access to education.

Public and Voluntary Clinics

Examples of public and voluntary clinics include community health centers, free clinics, and others. Most of them serve mainly underprivileged populations.

Community Health Centers

Creation of community health centers (CHCs) was authorized during the 1960s, mainly to provide for the medically underserved regions of the United States. CHCs operate under the auspices of the Bureau of Primary Health Care (BPHC), US Public Health Service, and US Department of Health and Human Services. CHCs are required by law to locate in medically underserved areas and provide services to anyone seeking care, regardless of insurance status or ability to pay (McAlearney 2002). The federal government determines the ***medically underserved*** designation. It indicates a dearth of primary care providers and delivery settings, as well as poor health indicators for the populace.

CHCs provide family-oriented preventive care, primary care, and dental care at over 3,650 clinic sites across America (Shi 2007). CHCs work to improve the health of underserved populations and provide access to critical health care services for the uninsured. Hence, CHCs are a primary care safety net for the nation's poor and underserved in both inner city and rural areas. Such areas are often characterized by economic, geographic, or cultural barriers that limit access to primary health care for a substantial portion of the population. CHCs tailor their services to family-oriented primary and preventive health care.

Section 330 of the Public Health Service Act provides federal grant funding for CHCs. Formerly called neighborhood health centers (NHCs), CHCs are private, nonprofit organizations that nonetheless depend heavily on funding through the Medicaid program and federal grants. Private-pay patients are charged on sliding-fee scales determined by the patient's income. According to 2004 national data, more than 40 percent of the patients served by CHCs are uninsured, 73 percent have incomes below 200 percent of the federal poverty level, and about 60 percent are racial/ethnic minorities (Shi 2007).

During their long tenure as the primary source of care for the medically underserved, CHCs have developed considerable expertise in managing the health care needs of these populations. Many centers have developed long-standing systems of care that include outreach programs, case management, transportation, translation services, alcohol and drug abuse screening and treatment, mental health services, health education, and social services.

CHCs are governed by an executive director or administrator, have a medical director, and are staffed by multidisciplinary teams of clinicians. The typical CHC employs six physicians who are generalists, eight nurses, and three NPPs, such as nurse practitioners and physician assistants. Also, some clinics have dentists, mental health practitioners, and pharmacists on site. Other members of the team may include case managers and education specialists (BPHC 1996; Shi 2007).

Approximately 13 million people were served by CHCs in 2004 (Shi 2007). Expanding the services of CHCs is a central element of President Bush's plan for expanding health care access to the uninsured and underserved. In 2002, the Bush Administration proposed a $1.5 billion budget to continue a long-term strategy that would add 1,200 new and expanded CHC sites over five years and serve an additional 6.1 million patients. Between 2001 and 2004, the President's Health Center Initiative created 600 new or expanded CHC sites (Shi 2007).

Free Clinics

Modeled after the 19th century dispensary (see Chapter 3), a related category of provider, the ***free clinic*** is a general ambulatory care center serving primarily the poor, the homeless, and the uninsured. Free clinics have three main characteristics: (1) services are provided at no charge or at a very nominal charge, (2) they are not directly supported or operated by a government agency or health department, and (3) services are delivered mainly by trained volunteer staff. The number of such clinics throughout the United States is estimated at 500. A survey of five major US cities disclosed that these clinics are open for limited hours and typically provide services to about 30 to 200 patients per month. They are funded by churches, hospitals, or private donations (Felt-Lisk et al. 2002). Some of these clinics receive government grants to partially support their operations. Free clinics focus on the delivery of primary care. Other services vary, depending on the number and training of their volunteer staff. The number of free clinics appears to be growing. Although mainly a voluntary effort, it is increasingly taking the form of an organized movement. In 1992, the Free Clinic Foundation of America was founded. It has published a manual on how to start a free clinic and maintains a national free clinic directory. Several states, such as Pennsylvania, Virginia, and North Carolina, have formed professional associations of free clinics in their states.

Other Clinics

Other CHCs that have been developed through federal funding are migrant health centers serving transient farm workers in agricultural communities and rural health centers in isolated underserved rural areas. The Community Mental Health Center program was established to provide ambulatory mental health services in underserved areas. The combination of free clinics, CHCs, public health services, and some hospitals now forms a significant safety net of providers for individuals who lack private or public health insurance. The various types of clinics discussed in this section generally face serious problems because of inadequate funding and a shortage of primary care providers. Other challenges include the difficulty of recruiting and retaining physicians and other qualified health professionals and the inability to diversify patient mix, particularly regarding patients with private insurance or those who have the ability to pay for services (Williams 1993).

Telephone Access

Telephone access is a means of bringing expert opinion and advice to the patient, especially during the hours when physicians' offices are generally closed. Referred to as ***telephone triage***, this type of access has expanded under managed care. The example of the Park Nicollet Clinic of the Minneapolis-based HealthSystem Minnesota illustrates how such a system functions. The telephone call-in system operates 7 days a week, 24 hours a day. The system is staffed by specially trained nurses who receive patients' calls. Using a computer system, they can access a patient's medical history and view the most recent radiology and laboratory test results. The nurses use standardized protocols to guide them in dealing with the patient's problem and consult with primary care physicians when necessary (Appleby 1995). If necessary, the staff can direct patients to appropriate medical services, such as an ED or a physician's office. The URAC organization now accredits Telephone Triage and Health Information programs.

Alternative Medicine

Because of their tremendous growth, the roles of alternative medicine (also referred to as "complementary medicine," "nonconventional therapies," or "natural medicine") and self-care cannot be ignored by the health care establishment. In the United States, the dominant health care practice is the biomedicine-based allopathic medicine. ***Alternative medicine***, or complementary and alternative medicine (CAM), refers to the broad domain of all health care resources other than those intrinsic to biomedicine to which people have recourse (CAM Research Methodology Conference 1997). Alternative therapies are regarded as nontraditional and include a wide range of treatments, such as homeopathy, herbal formulas, use of other natural products as preventive and treatment agents, acupuncture, meditation, yoga exercises, biofeedback, and spiritual guidance or prayer. Chiropractic is also largely regarded as a complementary treatment. Alternative medicine is not yet a system of healing endorsed by conventional Western medicine, although the traditional medical establishment has shown growing interest in the efficacy of these therapies.

No particular settings of health care delivery are involved in alternative treatments. With few exceptions, most therapies are self-administered or at least require active patient participation. The types of trained and licensed health care professionals discussed in Chapter 4 are generally not involved in the delivery of unconventional care. The efficacy of most of the alternative treatments has not been scientifically established, yet their use has exploded. Alternative medicine's growth has happened mainly for these reasons:

- Most people who seek alternative therapies believe that they have already explored conventional Western treatments but have not been helped. Most have chronic disorders, such as persistent pain, for which Western medicine can usually offer only symptomatic relief, not definitive treatment. According to recent investigations, individuals reporting serious health problems are more likely to use alternative treatments than healthier individuals are.
- People generally are persuaded that at least there is no harm in trying alternative treatments.
- Many fear the harms of iatrogenic effects of modern western medicine more than any potential dangers inherent in nonconventional therapies.
- The holistic concepts of health and medicine discussed in Chapter 2 are finding a growing appeal in the American belief and value system.
- Most people feel empowered by access to a vast amount of medical and health-related information available through the Internet, and they feel in control to pursue what they think is best for their own health.
- Many patients report that they seek alternative therapies and individuals who practice them because they want practitioners to take the time to listen to them, understand them, and deal with their personal life as well as their pathology. They believe that alternative practitioners will meet those needs (Gordon 1996).

A landmark study by Eisenberg and colleagues (1998) estimated that between 1990 and 1997, the proportion of the US adult population over 18 years of age using alternative therapies increased from 33.8 percent (60 million people) to 42.1 percent (83 million people). While the estimated number of visits to primary care physicians remained stable, visits to alternative medical practitioners increased by 47 percent (39 million people in 1997 versus 22 million in 1990).

The most common reasons given for seeking alternative therapies were back problems, allergies, fatigue, arthritis, and headaches. In both the 1990 and 1997 surveys, 96 percent of the respondents who saw a practitioner of alternative therapy for a principal condition also saw a medical doctor, but only a minority discussed these therapies with the conventional physician. Based on conservative estimates, Americans spent $14.6 billion in 1990 and $21.2 billion in 1997 on visits to alternative medicine practitioners. Among people who saw alternative therapy practitioners, 58.3 percent paid for the services out of pocket in 1997. The prevalence of CAM use in the United States remained fairly steady in a follow-up study conducted by Eisenberg and others in 2002 (Tindle 2005). Complementary medicine also appears to be popular in Europe, Canada, and other industrialized countries. Even though most of these countries provide universal access to medical care, a significant number of people try alternative treatments.

Although health insurance coverage for chiropractic has been widely available for some time, only some plans include coverage for other alternative therapies. Chiropractic, and even osteopathy, was once a pariah in medical practice. Doctors of osteopathy now work alongside MDs in medical institutions. Chiropractic, even though largely alienated from mainstream modern medicine, has been increasingly recognized for its healing values. Given the growing public demand for complementary medicine and its claims for health promotion, disease prevention, and promise for certain chronic conditions, mainstream medicine is showing a genuine interest in better understanding the value of alternative treatments. On the other hand, skepticism is justifiable because alternative medicine is predominantly unregulated. Also, the efficacy of most treatments, and the safety of some, have not been scientifically evaluated. Only rigorous scientific inquiry and research-based evidence will bring about a genuine integration of alternative therapies into the conventional practice of medicine.

Nevertheless, some recent developments are noteworthy. In 1993, Congress established the Office of Alternative Medicine (OAM), which became the National Center for Complementary and Alternative Medicine (NCCAM) in 1998. Budget allocations for the center have increased from $2 million in 1993 to $122.7 million in 2006 (NCCAM 2007). The center has three main objectives: (1) explore complementary and alternative healing practices in the context of rigorous science, (2) train complementary and alternative medicine researchers, and (3) disseminate authoritative information to the public and professionals. A growing number of US medical schools now offer some instruction in alternative medicine.

As cost containment in health care continues to occupy center stage, insurance companies, MCOs, and the government are eager to learn about the cost-effectiveness, as well as safety, of alternative therapies. Meanwhile, they are slowly and cautiously proceeding toward accepting the integration of certain unorthodox treatments with traditional medical interventions. At the same time, natural medicine-based private clinics are emerging across the United States.

Utilization of Outpatient Services

In 2004, Americans made approximately 910.9 million visits, or three visits per person, to office-based physicians (Table 7–6).

Table 7–6 Annual Number, Percentage Distribution, and Rate of National Ambulatory Office Visits by Selected Physician Practice Characteristics and Patient Age, Sex, and Race, 2004

Table 1. Number, percent distribution, and annual rate of office visits with corresponding standard errors, by selected physician practice characteristics: United States 2004

Physician practice characteristic	Number of visits in thousands	Percent distribution	Number of visits per 100 persons per year[1, 2]
All visits	910,857	100.0	315.9
Physician specialty			
General and family practice	207,879	22.8	72.1
Internal medicine	146,324	18.1	50.7
Pediatrics	116,659	12.8	192.0
Obstetrics and gynecology	65,291	7.2	55.5
Ophthalmology	47,333	5.2	16.4
Orthopaedic surgery	43,899	4.8	15.2
Dermatology	33,852	3.7	11.7
Psychiatry	30,657	3.4	10.6
Cardiovascular diseases	22,973	2.5	8.0
Otolaryngology	19,807	2.2	6.9
General surgery	19,320	2.1	6.7
Urology	18,295	2.0	6.3
Neurology	14,780	1.6	5.1
All other specialties	123,787	13.6	42.9
Professional identity			
Doctor of medicine	844,828	92.8	293.0
Doctor of osteopathy	66,029	7.2	22.9
Specialty type[3]			
Primary care	532,420	58.5	184.6
Surgical specialty	176,431	19.4	61.2
Medical specialty	202,006	22.2	70.0
Geographic region			
Northeast	169,899	18.7	316.1
Midwest	197,507	21.7	305.2
South	353,852	38.8	341.5
West	189,600	20.8	286.0
Metropolitan status[4]			
MSA	790,630	86.8	325.1
Non-MSA	120,227	13.2	266.1

— Category not applicable.

[1]Visit rates for age, sex, race, and region are based on the July 1, 2004, set of estimates of the civilian noninstitutional population of the United States as developed by the Population Division, US Census Bureau.

[2]Population estimates of metropolitan statistical area status are based on data from the 2004 National Health Interview Survey, National Center for Health Statistics, adjusted to the US Census Bureau definition of core-based statistical areas as of December 2004. See http://www.census.gov/population/www/estimates.metrodef.html for more about metropolitan statistical definitions.

[3]Physician specialty and specialty type defined in "Physician specialty groups" section of "Methods."

[4]MSA is metropolitan statistical area.

Note: Numbers may not add to totals because of rounding.

(*continues*)

Table 7–6 Annual Number, Percentage Distribution, and Rate of National Ambulatory Office Visits by Selected Physician Practice Characteristics and Patient Age, Sex, and Race, 2004 *(continued)*

Table 2. Number and percent distribution of office visits with corresponding standard errors, by selected physician practice characteristics: United States 2004

Physician practice characteristic	Number of visits in thousands	Percent distribution
All visits	910,857	100.0
Employments status		
Owner	684,074	75.1
Employee	201,339	22.1
Contractor	25,444	2.8
Ownership		
Physician or group	791,456	86.9
Other health care corporation	36,656	4.0
Other hospital	25,824	2.8
HMO[1]	*21,006	*2.3
Medical or academic health center	18,957	2.1
Other[2]	*16,957	*1.9
Practice size		
Solo	320,042	35.1
2–4	286,980	31.5
5–9	194,200	21.3
10–39	92,870	10.2
40 or more	*16,785	*1.8
Blank	*	*
Type of practice		
Single-specialty group	374,988	41.2
Multispecialty group	215,826	23.7
Solo	320,042	35.1
Office type		
Private practice	833,597	91.5
Clinic or urgicenter	39,488	4.3
Other[3]	37,773	4.1

— Category not applicable.

* Figure does not meet standards of reliability or precision.

[1]HMO is health maintenance organization.

[2]"Other" includes owners such as local government (state, county, or city) and charitable organizations.

[3]"Other" includes the following office types: HMO, nonfederal government clinic, mental health center, federally qualified health center, and facility practice plan.

Note: Numbers may not add to totals because of rounding.

(*continues*)

Table 7–6 Annual Number, Percentage Distribution, and Rate of National Ambulatory Office Visits by Selected Physician Practice Characteristics and Patient Age, Sex, and Race, 2004 *(continued)*

Table 3. Number, percent distribution, and annual rate of office visits with corresponding standard errors, by patient characteristics: United States 2004

Physician practice characteristic	Number of visits in thousands	Percent distribution	Number of visits per 100 persons per year[1, 2]
All visits	910,857	100.0	315.9
Under 15 years	147,910	16.2	243.4
Under 1 year	27,107	3.0	665.4
1–4 years	44,659	4.9	279.3
5–14 years	76,144	8.4	187.1
15–24 years	70,593	7.8	173.8
25–44 years	194,261	21.3	236.5
45–64 years	264,103	290.	376.2
65 years and over	233,991	25.7	675.2
65–74 years	113,426	12.5	622.6
75 years and over	120,565	13.2	733.6
Sex and age			
Female	535,541	58.8	363.3
Under 15 years	70,184	7.7	236.5
15–24 years	45,232	5.0	224.8
25–44 years	133,318	14.6	321.0
45–64 years	152,319	16.7	421.5
65–74 years	63,202	6.9	638.1
75 years and over	71,286	7.8	710.1
Male	375,316	41.2	266.3
Under 15 years	77,726	8.5	250.0
15–24 years	25,361	2.8	123.7
25–44 years	60,943	6.7	150.1
45–64 years	111,784	12.3	328.16
65–74 years	50,224	5.5	604.0
75 years and over	49,279	5.4	770.6
Race and age[2]			
White	775,019	85.1	333.6
Under 15 years	123,842	13.6	266.8
15–24 years	59,121	6.5	186.8
25–44 years	160,173	17.6	244.9
45–64 years	226,319	24.8	386.4
65–74 years	96,996	10.6	618.5
75 years and over	108,568	11.9	742.6
Black or African American	98,001	10.8	271.3
Under 15 years	16,626	1.8	176.9
15–24 years	7,799	0.9	132.0

(continues)

Table 7–6 Annual Number, Percentage Distribution, and Rate of National Ambulatory Office Visits by Selected Physician Practice Characteristics and Patient Age, Sex, and Race, 2000 *(continued)*

25–44 years	24,767	2.7	239.2
45–64 years	28,903	3.2	381.6
65–74 years	11,763	1.3	703.1
75 years and over	8,143	0.9	666.2
All other races[2]			
Asian only	29,131	3.2	237.7
Native Hawaiian or other Pacific Islander	2,869	0.3	577.7
American Indian or Alaska Native	2,615	0.3	94.4
Multiple races	3,223	0.4	73.5
Ethnicity[2]			
Hispanic or Latino	92,370	10.1	226.4
Not Hispanic or Latino	818,487	89.9	330.6

—Category not applicable.

[1]Visit rates for age, sex, race, and region are based on the July 1, 2004, set of estimates of the civilian noninstitutional population of the United States as developed by the Population Division, US Census Bureau.

[2]The race groups, white, Black or African American, Asian, Native Hawaiian or other Pacific Islander, American Indian or Alaska Native, and multiple races, include persons of Hispanic and non-Hispanic origin. Persons of Hispanic origin may be of any race. Starting with data year 1999, race-specific estimates have been tabulated according to 1997 Standards for Federal Data on Race and Ethnicity and are not strictly comparable with estimates for earlier years. However, the percentage of visit records with multiple races indicated is small and lower than what is typically found for self-reported race in household surveys.

Note: Numbers may not add to totals because of rounding.

Source: Data from *Advance Data*, No. 374, pp. 11–13, US Department of Health and Human Services, Public Health Service, Centers for Disease Control and Prevention, National Center for Health Statistics, June 23, 2006.

Physicians in general and family practice accounted for the largest share of these visits (22.8 percent), followed by physicians in internal medicine (16.1 percent), pediatrics (12.8 percent), and obstetrics and gynecology (7.2 percent). Doctors of osteopathy accounted for 7.2 percent of the visits. The South led the nation in the proportion of physician visits (38.8 percent), followed by the Midwest (21.7 percent), the Northeast (18.7 percent), and the West (20.8 percent). Ambulatory visits per person were the highest in the South (3.4 visits) and lowest in the West (2.9 visits). Most physician office visits (86.8 percent) took place in metropolitan areas. Visits per person were also higher in metropolitan areas (3.2) compared to rural areas (2.7), reflecting poorer access to primary care in rural areas of the United States. Some of the other general conclusions regarding the utilization of primary care services that can be drawn from data in Table 7–6 include the following: older individuals use more services than younger people; females see doctors more frequently (3.6 visits per person per year) than males (2.7 visits per person per year); and whites incur more visits per person (3.3) than blacks (2.7). The latter reflects access barriers for the US African American population.

Table 7–7 presents the most frequently mentioned principal reasons for visiting a

Table 7–7 Ambulatory Visits by the 20 Principal Reasons for Visit Most Frequently Mentioned by Patients, 2004

Principal Reason for Visit	Number of Visits (in thousands)
All visits	910,857
General medical examination	56,703
Progress visit, not otherwise specified	48,302
Postoperative visit	26,299
Cough	25,951
Prenatal examination, routine	24,816
Medication, other and unspecified kinds	16,483
Gynecological examination	14,716
Hypertension	14,510
Symptoms referable to throat	14,470
Knee symptoms	14,241
For other and unspecified test results	13,159
Stomach pain, cramps, and spasms	13,080
Diabetes mellitus	13,053
Depression	12,110
Back symptoms	11,892
Skin rash	11,548
Vision dysfunctions	11,364
Well-baby examination	11,023
Headache, pain in head	10,780
Earache or ear infection	10,125
All other reasons	536,232

Source: Data from *Advance Data*, No. 374, p. 17, US Department of Health and Human Services, Public Health Service, Centers for Disease Control and Prevention, National Center for Health Statistics, June 23, 2006.

physician in 2004. The top 10 reasons were general medical examination, follow-up progress visit, postoperative visit, cough, routine prenatal examination, medication, gynecological exam, hypertension, symptoms referable to throat, and knee symptoms. Table 7–8 shows the most frequent principal diagnoses cared for by office-based physicians.

In a comparative survey, physicians and nurses in the United States spent more time with patients (average 25 minutes) than their counterparts in Canada and Germany (average 19 minutes). The differences were found to be statistically significant. Despite receiving more time in face-to-face provider contact, the Americans were more inclined to think that the amount of time was inadequate. In the same survey, the waiting time in physicians' offices averaged approximately 30 minutes in the United States and Canada, but 36 minutes (statistically significant) in Germany (Donelan et al. 1996).

Table 7–8 Ambulatory Visits by the 20 Principal Diagnoses for Visit Most Frequently Rendered by Physicians, 2004

Principal Diagnosis	Number of Visits (in thousands)	Percentage Distribution
All visits	910,857	100.0
Essential hypertension	37,843	4.2
Routine infant or child health check	31,349	3.4
Malignant neoplasms	27,776	3.0
Acute upper respiratory infections, excluding pharyngitis	27,687	3.0
Diabetes mellitus	27,167	3.0
Arthropathies and related disorders	24,711	2.7
Spinal disorders	23,988	2.6
Normal pregnancy	23,222	2.5
Rheumatism, excluding back	18,562	2.0
Specific procedures and aftercare	15,392	1.7
Gynecological examination	15,173	1.7
Allergic rhinitis	14,058	1.5
General medical examination	14,041	1.5
Asthma	13,607	1.5
Chronic sinusitis	12,545	1.4
Follow-up examination	12,199	1.3
Heart disease, excluding ischemic	11,944	1.3
Otitis media and eustachian tube disorders	11,733	1.3
Disorders of lipoid metabolism	10,763	1.2
Potential health hazards related to personal and family history	10,353	1.1
All other diagnoses	526,742	57.8

Source: Data from *Advance Data*, No. 374, p. 22, US Department of Health and Human Services, Public Health Service, Centers for Disease Control and Prevention, National Center for Health Statistics, June 23, 2006.

Summary

In the history of health care delivery, the main settings for ambulatory services have come full circle. First came a shift from outpatient settings to hospitals. Now, ambulatory services outside the hospital have mushroomed. The reasons for this shift are mainly economic, social, and technological. Thanks to new technology, many physicians have broken their ties with hospitals and have started their own specialized care centers, such as ambulatory surgery centers and cardiac care centers. A variety of general medical and surgical interventions is provided in ambulatory care settings. Thus, ambulatory services now transcend the basic and routine primary care services. On the other hand, primary care itself has become "specialized." Primary care is no longer concerned simply with the treatment of colds, sprains, and other simple ailments, and with determining who is ill enough to require the attention of a specialist (Cassell 1996). Primary care physicians must coordinate a plethora of services to maintain the long-term viability of a patient's health. Continuity of care over a period of time is essential not just for individuals but also for an entire community. A health services delivery system that lacks universal access is ill-equipped to meet such an objective. Apart from coordination and continuity, other essential functions served by primary care include point of entry and comprehensiveness. In the United States, the gatekeeping aspect of primary care is sometimes regarded as a threat to free choice, but when a person's comprehensive health care needs are coordinated by a trained primary care professional, it leads to better health outcomes and cost efficiency.

In response to the changing economic incentives within the health care delivery system, numerous types of outpatient services have emerged and a variety of settings for the delivery of services has developed. In most settings, patients go to the delivery sites to receive services. In other cases, services are brought to the patients. The growing interest in alternative medicine is largely consumer driven. Compared to our corporate-dominated health care megalithic system, alternative medicine, with its emphasis on self-care and individual holism, is one area where many patients feel more in control of their own destiny. Indications are that alternative medicine is likely to have a growing influence on the delivery of health care.

Americans, on average, make three visits a year to physician offices. The most common reason is for a general medical examination; however, use of primary care is not consistent across geographic regions and races. There is evidence of barriers to care in rural areas and for racial/ethnic minorities.

Test Your Understanding

Terminology

accountability
adult day care
alternative medicine
ambulatory care
case management
categorical programs
community-oriented primary care
durable medical equipment
emergent condition
free clinic
gatekeeping
home health care
hospice
iatrogenic
medically underserved
nonurgent conditions
outpatient services
palliation
primary health care
secondary care
surgi-center
telephone triage
tertiary care
urgent care center
urgent conditions
walk-in clinic

Review Questions

1. Describe how some of the changes in the health services delivery system have led to a decline in hospital inpatient days and a growth in ambulatory services.
2. What implications has the decline in hospital occupancy rates had for hospital management?
3. All primary care is ambulatory, but not all ambulatory services represent primary care. Discuss.
4. What are the main characteristics of primary care?
5. Discuss the gatekeeping role of primary care.
6. What is community-oriented primary care? Explain.
7. Discuss the two main factors that determine what should be an adequate mix between generalists and specialists.
8. What are some of the reasons solo practitioners are joining group practices?
9. Why is it important for hospital administrators to regard outpatient care as a key component of their overall business strategy?
10. Discuss the main hospital-based outpatient services.
11. What are some of the social changes that led to the creation of specialized health centers for women?
12. Why is the hospital emergency department sometimes used for nonurgent conditions? What are the consequences?
13. What are mobile health care services? Discuss the various types of mobile services.
14. What is the basic philosophy of home health care? Describe the services it provides.
15. What are the conditions of eligibility for receiving home health services under Medicare ?
16. Explain the concept of hospice care and describe the types of services a hospice provides.
17. What are some of the main requirements for Medicare certification of a hospice program?
18. Describe the scope of public health ambulatory services in the United States.
19. Describe the main public and voluntary outpatient clinics, and the main problems they face.
20. What is alternative medicine? What role does it play in the delivery of health care?
21. Briefly explain how a telephone triage system functions.

REFERENCES

Appleby, C. 1995. Boxed in? *Hospitals and Health Networks* 69, no. 18: 28–34.

American Hospital Association. 2006. *TrendWatch Chartbook, 2006*. Washington, DC: AHA.

Aventis Pharmaceuticals. 2001. *Managed care digest series, 2001: Institutional highlights digest*. Bridgewater, NJ: Aventis Pharmaceuticals.

Bakwin, H. 1945. Pseudodoxia pediatrica. *New England Journal of Medicine* 232: 691–697.

Barr, K.W., and C.L. Breindel. 1995. Ambulatory care. In *Health care administration: Principles, practices, structure, and delivery*. 2nd ed., ed. L.F. Wolper, 547–573. Gaithersburg, MD: Aspen Publishers, Inc.

Beresford, L. 1989. *History of the National Hospice Organization*. Arlington, VA: The National Hospice Organization.

Bertakis, K.D. et al. 2000. Gender differences in the utilization of health services. *Journal of Family Practice* 49: 147–152.

Block, S.D. et al. 1996. Academia's chilly climate for primary care. *Journal of the American Medical Association* 276, no. 9: 677–682.

Bureau of Primary Health Care (BPHC). 1996. *Community Health Center Program* fact sheet. Bethesda, MD: Bureau of Primary Health Care, US Department of Health and Human Services.

CAM Research Methodology Conference. 1997. Defining and describing complementary and alternative medicine. *Alternative Therapies* 3, no. 2: 49–56.

Cassell, E.J. 1996. The two faces of primary care. *The Wilson Quarterly* 20, no. 2: 28–30.

Center for Healthcare Industry Performance Studies. 1997. Economies of scale in outpatient surgery. *Healthcare Financial Management* 51, no. 9: 105–107.

Centers for Medicare & Medicaid Services. 2006. National Health Expenditures Projections: 2005–2015. Table 10: Home Health Care Expenditures. http://www.cms.hhs.gov/NationalHealthExpendData/downloads/proj2005.pdf.

Colwill, J.M., and J.M. Cultice. 2003. The future supply of family physicians: Implications for rural America. *Health Affairs* 22, no. 1: 190–198.

Derlet, R.W., and J.R. Richards. 2002. Emergency department crowding in Florida, New York, and Texas. *Southern Medical Journal* 95, no. 8: 846–849.

Donelan, K. et al. 1996. All payer, single payer, managed care, no payer: Patients' perspectives in three nations. *Health Affairs* 15, no. 2: 255–265.

Duffy, S.Q., and D.E. Farley. 1995. Patterns of decline among inpatient procedures. *Public Health Reports* 110, no. 6: 674–681.

Dychtwald, K. et al. 1990. *Implementing eldercare services: Strategies that work*. New York: McGraw-Hill.

Eisenberg, D.M. et al. 1998. Trends in alternative medicine use in the United States, 1990–1997. *Journal of the American Medical Association* 280, no. 18: 1569–1575.

Engle, G.L. 1977. The need for a new medical model: A challenge for biomedicine. *Science* 196, no. 1: 127–136.

Evashwick, C.J. 1993. *The continuum of long-term care*. In *Introduction to health services*. 4th ed., eds. S.J. Williams and P.R. Torrens, 177–218. Albany, NY: Delmar Publishers.

Fein, E.B. 1996. Region's hospitals have seen the future, and it's an outpatient clinic. *The New York Times*, 19 February, B1.

Felt-Lisk, S. et al. 2002. Monitoring local safety-net providers: Do they have adequate capacity? *Health Affairs* 21, no. 5: 277–283.

Franks, P. et al. 1992. Gatekeeping revisited: Protecting patients from overtreatment. *New England Journal of Medicine* 327, no. 4: 424–429.

Franks, P. et al. 1998. Primary care physicians and specialists as personal physicians: Health care expenditures and mortality experience. *Journal of Family Practice* 47: 105–109.

Glick, D.F., and K.M. Thompson. 1997. Analysis of emergency room use for primary care needs. *Nursing Economics* 15, no. 1: 42–49.

Gordon, J.S. 1996. Alternative medicine and the family practitioner. *American Family Physician* 54, no. 7: 2205–2212.

HCIA Inc. and Deloitte & Touche. 1997. *The comparative performance of US hospitals: The sourcebook*. Baltimore, MD: HCIA Inc.

Health Forum. 2002. *Hospital Statistics*. Chicago: Health Forum.

Hodge, R. 1994. The evolving role of the primary care physician. *Physician Executive* 20, no. 10: 15–18.

Hoechst Marion Roussel. 1999. *Managed care digest series 1999: Institutional digest*. Kansas City, MO: Hoechst Marion Roussel, Inc.

Jackson, C. 2002. Cutting into the market: Rise of ambulatory surgery centers. *American Medical News* (April 15). www.amednews.com/2002/bisa0415.

Knowles, J.H. 1965. The role of the hospital: The ambulatory clinic. *Bulletin of the New York Academy of Medicine* 41, no. 1: 68–70.

Kozak, L.J. et al. 1999. Changing patterns of surgical care in the United States, 1980–1995. *Health Care Financing Review* 21, no. 1: 31–49.

Lee, P.R. 1994. Models of excellence. *The Lancet* 344, no. 8935: 1484–1486.

Liggins, K. 1993. Inappropriate attendance at accident and emergency departments: A literature review. *Journal of Advanced Nursing* 18, no. 7: 1141–1145.

Looker, P. 1993. Women's health centers: History and evolution. *Women's Health Issues* 3, no. 2: 95–100.

Lowell-Smith, E.G. 1994. Alternative forms of ambulatory care: Implications for patients and physicians. *Social Science and Medicine* 38, no. 2: 275–283.

McAlearney, J.S. 2002. The financial performance of community health centers, 1996–1999. *Health Affairs* 21, no. 2: 219–225.

McCaig, L.F., and E.W. Newar. 2006. *National hospital ambulatory medical care survey: 2004 emergency department summary*. Atlanta, GA: Centers for Disease Control and Prevention, National Center for Health Statistics.

McCaig, L.F., and C.W. Burt. 2002. *National hospital ambulatory medical care survey: 1999 emergency department summary*. Atlanta, GA: Centers for Disease Control and Prevention/National Center for Health Statistics.

McNamara, P. et al. 1993. Pathwork access: Primary care in EDs on the rise. *Hospitals* 67, no. 10: 44–46.

Miller, G. 1996. Hospice. In *The continuum of long-term care: An integrated systems approach*, ed. C.J. Evashwick, 98–108. Albany, NY: Delmar Publishers.

Minkler, M. 1992. Community organizing among the elderly poor in the United States. *International Journal of Health Services* 22, no. 2: 303–316.

Misra, D. ed. 2001. *Women's health data book: A profile of women's health in the United States*, 3rd ed. Washington, DC: Jacobs Institute of Women's Health and The Henry J. Kaiser Family Foundation.

National Association of Home Care and Hospice. 2004. *Basic statistics about home care. http://www.nahc.org/04HC_Stats.pdf*

National Hospice and Palliative Care Organization. 2003. *NHPCO Facts and Figures, January 2003*. http://www.nhpco.org.

National Center for Complementary and Alternative Medicine (NCCAM). 2007. http://nccam.nih.gov/about/appropriations/index.htm

National Nursing Centers Consortium. 2003. *Nurse-managed health centers briefing*. May 2003: 1–4.

Noble, J. et al. 1992. Career differences between primary care and traditional trainees in internal medicine and pediatrics. *Annals of Internal Medicine* 116, no. 7: 482–487.

Orton, P. 1994. Shared care. *The Lancet* 344, no. 8934: 1413–1415.

Parchman, M., and S. Culler. 1994. Primary care physicians and avoidable hospitalization. *Journal of Family Practice* 39: 123–128.

Petersdorf, R. 1975. Internal medicine and family practice: Controversies, conflict and compromise. *New England Journal of Medicine* 293, no. 3: 326–332.

Petersdorf, R. 1993. The doctor is in. *Academic Medicine* 68, no. 2: 113–117.

Phillips Ambulatory Care Center. 2000. *http://wehealny.org/patients/pace_description.html.*

Raffel, M.W., and N.K. Raffel. 1994. *The US health system: Origins and functions*. 4th ed. Albany, NY: Delmar Publishers.

Reuben, D.B. 2007. Saving primary care. *The American Journal of Medicine* 120, no. 1: 99–102.

Roos, N. 1979. Who should do the surgery? Tonsillectomy and adenoidectomy in one Canadian province. *Inquiry* 16, no. 1: 73–83.

Roos, N.P., and L.L. Roos. 1980. Medical school impact on student career choice: A longitudinal study. *Evaluation and the Health Professions* 3, no. 1: 3–19.

Rosenblatt, R.A. et al. 2000. The effect of the doctor-patient relationship on emergency department use among the elderly. *American Journal of Public Health* 90: 97–102.

Salganicoff, A., U.R. Ranji, and R. Wyn. 2005. *Women and health care: A national profile*. Menlo Park, CA: The Henry J. Kaiser Family Foundation.

Shi, L., P.B. Collins, K.F. Aaron, et al. 2007. Health center financial performance: National trends and state variation, 1998–2004. *Journal of Public Health Management and Practice* 13, no.2: 133–50.

Shi, L. 1994. Primary care, specialty care, and life chances. *International Journal of Health Services* 24, no. 3: 431–458.

Shi, L. et al. 1999. Income inequality, primary care, and health indicators. *The Journal of Family Practice* 48: 275–284.

Shi, L., and B. Starfield. 2000. Primary care, income inequality, and self-related health in the US: Mixed-level analysis. *International Journal of Health Services* 30: 541–555.

Shi, L., and B. Starfield. 2001. Primary care physician supply, income inequality, and racial mortality in US metropolitan areas. *American Journal of Public Health* 91: 1246–1250.

Shi, L. et al. 2002. Primary care, self-rated health care, and reduction in social disparities in Health. *Health Services Research* 37, no. 3: 529–550.

Siu, A.L. et al. 1986. Inappropriate use of hospitals in a randomized trial of health insurance plans. *New England Journal of Medicine* 315, no. 2: 1259–1266.

SMG Solutions. 2000. *2000 report and directory: Medical group practices*, Chicago, IL: SMG Solutions.

Stahl, C. 1997. Home hemodialysis enjoying a comeback. *ADVANCE for Occupational Therapists* 13, no. 25 (June 23): 4.

Starfield, B. 1992. *Primary care: Concept, evaluation, and policy*. New York: Oxford University Press.

Starfield, B. 1994. Is primary care essential? *The Lancet* 344, no. 8930: 1129–1133.

Steinel, J.A., and E.A. Madigan. 2003. Resource utilization in home health chronic obstructive pulmonary disease management. *Outcomes Management* 7, no. 1: 23–27.

Sultz, H.A., and K.M. Young. 1997. *Health care USA: Understanding its organization and delivery*. Gaithersburg, MD: Aspen Publishers, Inc.

Tindle, H.A., R.B. Davis, R.S. Phillips, and D.M. Eisenberg. 2005. Trends in use of complementary and alternative medicine by U.S. adults, 1997–2002. *Altern Ther Health Med* 11, no.1: 42–9.

Vanselow, N.A. et al. 1995. From the Institute of Medicine. *Journal of the American Medical Association* 273, no. 3: 192.

VHA Inc. and Deloitte & Touche. 1997. *1997 Environmental assessment: Redesigning health care for the millennium*. Irving, TX: VHA Inc.

Waid, M.O. 1998. Overview of the Medicare and Medicaid programs. *Health Care Financing Review: Medicare and Medicaid Statistical Supplement, 1998*.

Welch, W.P. et al. 1993. Geographic variation in expenditure for physicians' service in the United States. *New England Journal of Medicine* 328, no. 9: 621–627.

Weinerman, E.R. et al. 1966. Yale studies in ambulatory medical care. V. Determinants of use of hospital emergency services. *American Journal of Public Health* 56, no. 7: 1037–1056.

Williams, S.J. 1993. *Ambulatory health care services*. In *Introduction to Health Services*. 4th ed., eds. S.J. Williams and P.R. Torrens. Albany, NY: Delmar Publishers.

Williams, S.J. 1995. *Essentials of health services*. Albany, NY: Delmar Publishers.

Wilson, F.A., and D. Neuhauser. 1985. *Health services in the United States*. 2nd ed. Cambridge, MA: Ballinger Publishing Co.

World Health Organization (WHO). 1978. *Primary health care*. Geneva.

Chapter 8

Inpatient Facilities and Services

Learning Objectives

- To get a functional perspective on the evolution of hospitals
- To survey the factors that contributed to the growth of hospitals prior to the 1980s
- To understand the reasons for the subsequent decline of hospitals and their utilization
- To learn some key measures pertaining to hospital operations and inpatient utilization
- To differentiate between various types of hospitals
- To differentiate between nonprofit and for-profit hospitals and understand some of the issues surrounding the nonprofit status of voluntary hospitals
- To comprehend some basic concepts in hospital governance
- To get a perspective on some key ethical issues and the erosion of public trust

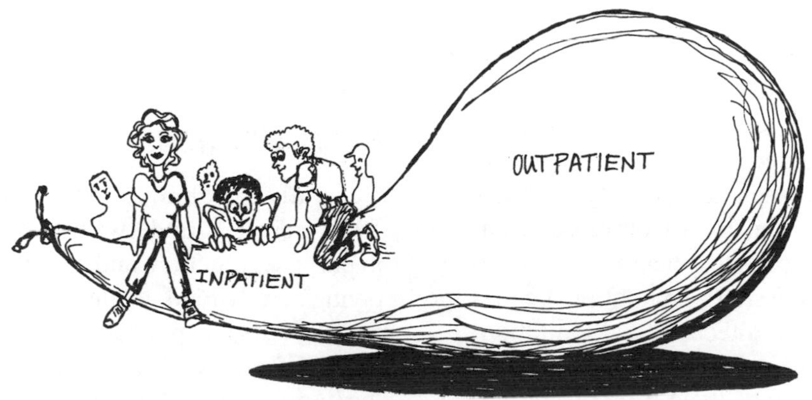

"We have the inpatient sector under control."

Introduction

The term ***inpatient*** is used in conjunction with an overnight stay in a health care facility, such as a hospital. On the other hand, outpatient refers to services provided while the patient is not lodged in a health care facility. Although the primary function of hospitals is to deliver inpatient acute care services, many hospitals have expanded their scope of services to include non-acute and outpatient care.

According to the American Hospital Association (AHA), a ***hospital*** is an institution with at least six beds whose primary function is "to deliver patient services, diagnostic and therapeutic, for particular or general medical conditions" (AHA 1994). In addition, a hospital must be licensed, it must have an organized physician staff, and it must provide continuous nursing services under the supervision of registered nurses. Other characteristics of a hospital include an identifiable governing body that is legally responsible for the conduct of the hospital, a chief executive with continuous responsibility for the operation of the hospital, maintenance of medical records on each patient, pharmacy services maintained in the institution and supervised by a registered pharmacist, and food service operations to meet the nutritional and therapeutic requirements of the patients (Health Forum 2001). The construction and operation of the modern hospital is governed by federal laws; state health department regulations; city ordinances; standards of the Joint Commission on Accreditation of Healthcare Organizations (Joint Commission); and national codes for building, fire protection, and sanitation.

In the past 200 years or so, hospitals have gradually evolved from ordinary institutions of refuge for the homeless and poor to ultramodern facilities providing the latest medical services to the critically ill and injured. The term "medical center" is used by some hospitals, reflecting their high level of specialization and wide scope of services, which may include teaching and research. Growth of multihospital chains, especially those providing a variety of health care services, has led to the nomenclature "hospital system" or "health system."

Hospital care consumes the biggest share of national health care spending (see Figure 6–7). Hence, the hospital inpatient sector was the first to be targeted by prospective reimbursement methods during the 1980s. Subsequently, as new technologies emerged to treat patients outside the hospital setting, outpatient services for various types of medical procedures and treatments mushroomed. Managed care also played a significant role in curtailing inpatient utilization.

This chapter describes institutional care delivery with specific reference to acute care—mostly characterized by secondary and tertiary levels of care—in community hospitals. It also discusses various ways to classify hospitals and points out important trends and critical issues that will continue to shape the delivery of inpatient services.

Transformation of the Hospital in the United States

Generally speaking, from about 1840 to 1900, hospitals underwent a drastic change in purpose, function, and number. From supplying merely food, shelter, and meager medical care to the pauper sick, to armies, to those infected with contagious diseases, to the insane, and to those requiring emergency treatment, they began to provide skilled medical and surgical attention and nursing care to all people (Raffel 1980, 241). Subsequently, hospitals became centers of medical training and research. More recent transformations are mainly organizational in nature, as hospitals have consolidated into medical systems delivering a broad range of health care services. Medical technology also continues to transform the delivery of health care; in recent years, it has been a significant factor in shaping the organizational structures within the health care industry. These transformations can be neatly categorized according to five dominant functions in the evolution of hospitals:

1. Primitive institutions of social welfare
2. Distinct institutions of care for the sick
3. Organized institutions of medical practice
4. Advanced institutions of medical training and research
5. Consolidated systems of health services delivery

Primitive Institutions of Social Welfare

As discussed in Chapter 3, except for a few hospitals that were located in some of the major US cities, municipal almshouses (or poorhouses) and pesthouses existed during the 1800s to provide food and shelter to the destitute. Financed through charitable gifts and local government funds, these institutions essentially served a social welfare function. Medical care, or more properly, nursing care, was only secondary and was quite primitive. Some almshouses had adjoining infirmaries where the sick were isolated. People generally stayed in these institutions for months rather than days.

Pesthouses were used to quarantine people who were sick with contagious diseases so the rest of the community would be protected. Later hospitals evolved from these almshouses and pesthouses, but even after hospitals developed, people generally did not want to be admitted to these establishments for treatment because a hospital could do little for them. Most illnesses were treated at home, using folk medicine or the services of physicians who made home visits.

Distinct Institutions of Care for the Sick

Not until the late 1800s did the infirmaries or hospital departments of city poorhouses break away to become independent medical care institutions. These were the first public hospitals (Haglund and Dowling 1993), in this case operated by local governments. For example, the Kings County Almshouse and Infirmary, organized in Brooklyn in 1830, later became the Kings County Hospital (Raffel 1980, 221), but such hospitals still served mainly the poor. A few hospitals serving all classes of society and built specifically to care for the sick also emerged during the 19th century. These hospitals were voluntary or nongovernment.

The founding of ***voluntary hospitals***—community hospitals financed through local philanthropy as opposed to taxes—was often inspired by influential physicians with the financial backing of local donors and philanthropists. These hospitals accepted both indigent and paying patients, but to cover their operating expenses they required charitable contributions from private citizens.

In the United States, most voluntary hospitals had private rather than religious or government sponsorship. In Europe, by contrast, the first hospitals were established predominantly by religious orders. Nurses, who were primarily monks and nuns, attended to the physical as well as the spiritual needs of the patients. Later, many of these hospitals became tax-financed public institutions as less church money became available for hospitals and monasteries. In England, the "royal hospitals" were supported by private donations and taxes. Later hospitals in Britain were voluntary hospitals, which served as a model for such hospitals in the United States (Raffel and Raffel 1994, 108, 110).

The first voluntary hospital in the United States established specifically to care for the sick was the Pennsylvania Hospital in Philadelphia, opened in 1752. It was patterned after the British voluntary hospitals. The city already had an almshouse. Similar to other seaports, Philadelphia also had pesthouses to isolate people with contagious diseases, such as smallpox and yellow fever. However, Dr. Thomas Bond, a London-trained physician, brought to prominence the need for a hospital to care for the sick poor of the city. Benjamin Franklin, who was a friend and advisor of Dr. Bond, was instrumental in promoting the idea and in raising voluntary subscriptions. According to the charter, the contributors had the right to make all laws and regulations relating to the hospital's operation. The contributors also elected members to form the governing board or the ***board of trustees***. Thus, the control of voluntary hospitals was in the hands of influential community laypeople rather than physicians (Raffel and Raffel 1994, 110–111). The tradition of the voluntary hospital following this early model has continued to this day, as the majority of hospitals in the United States have private nonprofit status.

Other prominent voluntary hospitals included the New York Hospital in New York, which was completed in 1775, but, due to the Revolutionary War, was not opened to civilian patients until 1791. The Massachusetts General Hospital in Boston was incorporated in 1812 and opened in 1821. During this period, the almshouses continued to serve an important function by receiving overflow patients who could not be admitted to the hospitals because of the unavailability of beds or who had to be discharged from hospitals because they were declared incurable (Raffel and Raffel 1994, 115–116). Later hospitals in the United States were modeled after Pennsylvania, New York, and Massachusetts General.

Organized Institutions of Medical Practice

Social and demographic change, but above all, the advance of medical science, transformed hospitals into institutions of medical practice. From the latter half of the 19th century, technological progress led to the development of advanced equipment, facilities, and personnel training, which became centered in the hospital. Medicine was revolutionized as investigators discovered the causes of disease and developed technological devices for diagnosis and treatment (Raffel 1980, 235). Most notable in terms of their impact on hospitals were (1) the discovery of anesthesia, which aided significantly in advancing new surgical techniques, (2) development of the germ theory of disease, which led to the subsequent discovery of antiseptic and sterilization techniques, and (3) X-ray for diagnostic imaging. Use of antiseptic procedures, and later, introduction of sulfa drugs and penicillin in the mid-20th century produced significant reductions in mortality from infections (Snook 1981). The application of medical science and technology in hospitals also made it necessary for physicians to receive their training and to practice medicine in hospitals.

Drastic improvements in the environmental conditions and the practice of medicine in hospitals made them more acceptable to the middle and upper classes. Hospitals actually began to attract affluent patients who could afford to pay privately. Hospitals also came to be regarded as a necessity because the superior medical services and surgical procedures could not be obtained at home. Thus, the hospital was transformed from a charitable institution into one that could generate a profit. In many instances, physicians started opening small hospitals, financed by wealthy and powerful sponsors. These facilities were the first proprietary hospitals.

In the early 20th century, the field of hospital administration became a discipline in its own right. Administrators with expertise in financial management and organizational skills were needed to manage hospitals. The administrative structure of the hospital was organized into departments, such as food service, pharmacy, X-ray, and laboratory. It became necessary to employ professional staff to manage the delivery of services. Efficiency began to emerge as an important element in the management of hospitals. The term was defined broadly, encompassing not only economy but also quality and breadth of services, as well as access to care. This early emphasis on efficiency foreshadowed two main issues that affect health policy and hospital management to this day: the pressure on hospitals to introduce new technology while containing cost, and the assumption that hospitals should act like businesses (Arndt and Bigelow 2006). With greater pressure for cost containment, hospitals began to limit care to the more acute periods of illness, rather than the full course of a disease.

Advanced Institutions of Medical Training and Research

The hospital had a profound influence on medical education in the United States. With the advance of medical science, hospitals became important centers for the dissemination of biomedical knowledge. Hospitals provided the desirable venue for clinical studies. The vast number of clinical records and a large array of medical conditions among patients seeking care in major hospitals provide a wealth of data to conduct investigative studies to advance medical knowledge.

Recognition of the critical role hospitals played in medical education led to collaborations between hospitals and universities. The Pennsylvania Hospital, for example, taught courses required by the College of Philadelphia's medical school, which later became the University of Pennsylvania School of Medicine. Similarly, New York Hospital served as a teaching hospital for medical students of Columbia Medical School, and Massachusetts General Hospital provided practical clinical instruction for Harvard Medical School (Raffel and Raffel 1994, 113–116). In affiliation with university based medical schools, many hospitals became centers of medical research where new discoveries were made, and the findings were disseminated through publications in medical journals.

The Johns Hopkins Hospital (opened in 1889), with its adjoining medical school (opened in 1893), inaugurated a new era in combining clinical practice with teaching and the promotion of scientific inquiry in medicine. Patterned after the great European hospitals connected with medical schools, the hospital was to teach students the best methods then known of caring for the sick, and to serve as a great laboratory to advance the knowledge of the causes, processes, and treatment of disease (Raffel 1980, 245). From the 1920s, the hospital's teaching role became even more prominent as specialization in medicine led to a proliferation of internships and residencies (Haglund and Dowling 1993).

More recently, the increasing use of noninstitutional settings has shifted some aspects of medical education from inpatient to outpatient sectors and to other delivery settings such as nursing homes, hospices, and community health centers. Nevertheless, the hospital continues to play a central role in the training of physicians. Nursing education has also evolved largely around hospitals as the role of nursing has become more technically complex. The same is true of many other health care professions (Williams 1995, 56, 57). For both the training and the subsequent employment of virtually the whole spectrum of health professionals, hospitals play a significant role.

Consolidated Systems of Health Services Delivery

In the late 20th century, the major impact of radical changes in the health care delivery system has been experienced by hospitals because they constitute the institutional nucleus of health care delivery. The most profound changes are seen in the drastic reductions in the length of inpatient stays brought about by prospective and capitated payment methods and aggressive utilization review practices. The declining utilization of acute care beds had left most hospitals with excess capacity in the form of empty beds. Hence, consolidation of hospitals was particularly intense during the mid-1990s mainly because of economic necessity. As the acute inpatient care sector of health care delivery has become less profitable, hospitals have diversified into nonacute services, such as outpatient centers, home health care, long-term care, subacute care, assisted living, and inpatient and outpatient rehabilitation. Local market pressures have also prompted many hospitals to merge or enter into formal affiliations with other hospitals. The three main types of consolidations, discussed more fully in Chapter 9, have occurred through mergers and acquisitions, vertical integration, and participation in networks through contractual arrangements. These strategies have offered patients increased access to care across a continuum of services. However, intense consolidation in certain hospital markets has also diluted competition. Research suggests that hospital consolidation in the 1990s raised prices by at least 5 percent as competition eroded. Evidence also suggests that increasing hospital concentration may also lower quality, but the findings are not robust (Vogt and Town 2006).

The Expansion Phase: Late 1800s to Mid-1980s

Hospitals grew in numbers when they became a necessary local adjunct of medical practice. Growth in the volume of surgical work especially provided the basis for expansion of hospital beds. The expansion in surgical practice coincided with biomedical discoveries and growth of medical technology.

Profits from surgery enabled physicians to build small hospitals without upper-class sponsorship. The number of hospitals grew from 178 (35,604 beds) in 1872 to 4,359

(421,065 beds) in 1909. By 1929, 6,665 hospitals provided 907,133 beds (Haglund and Dowling 1993). As new beds were built, their availability almost ensured that they would be used. This phenomenon led Milton Roemer (1916–2001) to proclaim, "a built bed is a filled bed," known popularly as Roemer's Law (Roemer 1961).

Haglund and Dowling (1993) pointed to six significant factors in the growth of hospitals: advances in medical science, development of specialized technology, advances in medical education, development of professional nursing, growth of health insurance, and the role of government. The first three factors were discussed in the previous section; this section covers the last three.

Development of Professional Nursing

During the latter half of the 19th century, Florence Nightingale was instrumental in transforming nursing into a recognized profession in Britain. Following the founding of the Nightingale School of Nursing in England, nursing schools in the United States were established at Bellevue Hospital (New York City), New Haven Hospital (New Haven, Connecticut), and Massachusetts General Hospital (Boston). The benefits of having trained nurses in hospitals became apparent as increased efficacy of treatment and hygiene improved patient recovery (Haglund and Dowling 1993). As a result of these advances, hospitals increasingly came to be regarded as places of healing and found acceptance with the middle and upper classes.

Growth of Private Health Insurance

During and after the Great Depression of the 1930s, many hospitals were forced to close, and the financial solvency of many more was threatened. Thus, the number of hospitals in the United States dropped from 6,852 in 1928 to 6,189 in 1937. Subsequently, the growth of private health insurance became a vehicle for enabling people to pay for hospital services, and the flow of insurance funds helped revive the financial stability of hospitals. Insurance also contributed to the increased demand for health services. Historically, insurance plans provided generous coverage for inpatient care. Consequently, there were few restrictions on patients and physicians opting for more expensive hospital services (Feldstein 1971). Note that private health insurance in the United States first began as a hospital insurance plan (see Chapter 3).

Role of Government

Government funding for hospital construction perhaps played the most important role in the expansion of hospitals. Subsequently, Medicare and Medicaid provided indirect funding to the hospital industry by vastly expanding public-sector health insurance.

The Hill-Burton Act

Relatively little hospital construction took place during the Great Depression and World War II, so by the end of the war, the nation was severely short of hospitals. The Hospital Survey and Construction Act of 1946, commonly referred to as the Hill-Burton Act, provided federal grants to states for the construction of new community hospital beds; however, the hospitals would not be under federal control. This legislation required that each state develop and upgrade annually a plan for health facility construction—based on bed-to-population ratios—that would serve as a basis for allocation of federal construction grants (Raffel 1980, 588).

In 1946, after the war, 3.2 community hospital beds were available per 1,000 civilian population. The objective of Hill-Burton was to reach 4.5 beds per 1,000 population (Teisberg et al. 1991). The Hill-Burton program assisted in the construction of nearly 40 percent of the beds in the nation's short-stay general hospitals and was the greatest single factor in the increase in the nation's bed supply during the 1950s and 1960s (Haglund and Dowling 1993). Hill-Burton made it possible for even small, remote communities to have their own hospitals (Wolfson and Hopes 1994). By 1980, the United States had reached its goal of 4.5 community hospital beds per 1,000 civilian population (DHHS 2002) even though the Hill-Burton program terminated in 1974.

Hill-Burton was also instrumental in promoting the growth of non-profit community hospitals because it had required that hospitals constructed with federal funds must provide a certain amount of uncompensated care. Competition from these new hospitals led to the closure of many smaller proprietary for-profit hospitals. Most of the remaining proprietary hospitals began delivering free or discounted services to those who could not afford to pay (Muller 2003). Thanks to Hill-Burton, nonprofit community hospitals in the United States far outnumber all other types of hospitals.

Public Health Insurance

The creation of Medicare and Medicaid programs in the mid-1960s also had a significant, although indirect, impact on the increase in the number of hospital beds and their utilization (Feldstein 1993, 215) as government-funded health insurance became available to a large number of elderly and poor Americans. Between 1965 and 1980, the number of community hospitals in the United States increased from 5,736 (741,000 beds) to 5,830 (988,000 beds); total admissions per 1,000 population increased from 130 to 154; and total inpatient days per 1,000 population increased from 1,007 to 1,159. The percentage occupancy also remained relatively stable at around 76 percent (AHA 1990). Figure 8–1 shows trends from 1940 to 2004 in the number of beds per 1,000 resident population.

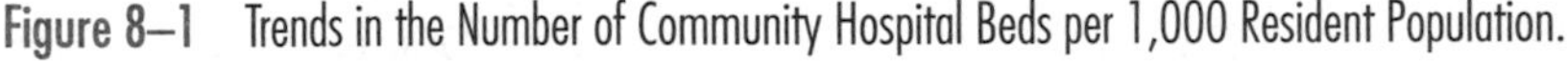

Figure 8–1 Trends in the Number of Community Hospital Beds per 1,000 Resident Population.

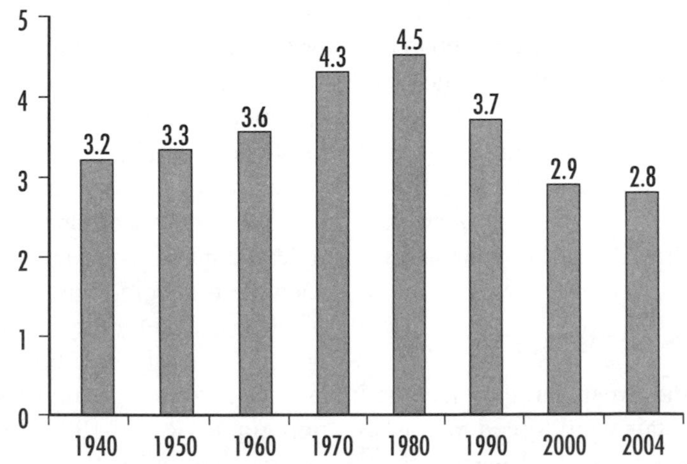

Source: Data from *Health United States, 2002*, p. 281; *Health United States, 2006*, p. 366; National Center for Health Statistics.

The Downsizing Phase: Mid-1980s Onward

The mid-1980s marked a turning point in the growth and use of hospital beds. After a sharp decline in 1985, the number of community hospitals and the total number of beds have declined fairly consistently (Figure 8–2). A sharper decline in the number of hospitals compared to hospital beds illustrates the closure of smaller hospitals, particularly in rural areas. At the same time, the average bed capacity per hospital declined from 196 beds in 1980 to 166 beds in 2004 (DHHS 2006, 364).

Even as the number of hospitals and capacity have contracted, further declines have occurred in the actual utilization of the shrunken capacity. Occupancy rates (percentage of beds occupied) in community hospitals declined from 75.6 percent in 1980 to around 64 percent in 2000. Since then, occupancy rates have increased slightly (67 percent in 2004) mainly because capacity (number of available beds) has steadily declined, from 823,560 total community hospital beds in 2000 to 808,127 in 2004. Similarly, the average length of stay (ALOS) in community hospitals has declined from 7.5 days in 1980 to 4.8 days in 2004 (DHHS 2006, 339, 364).

Within hospitals, a tremendous shift from inpatient to outpatient utilization occurred, as illustrated in Figure 8–3 in the form of increasing ratios between hospital outpatient visits and inpatient days. Along with this shift in the use of hospital services, the share of national expenditures on hospital care has also consistently declined (Table 8–1). It does not appear that hospitals were able to recoup the loss of inpatient revenues

Figure 8–2 The Decline in the Number of Community Hospitals and Beds.

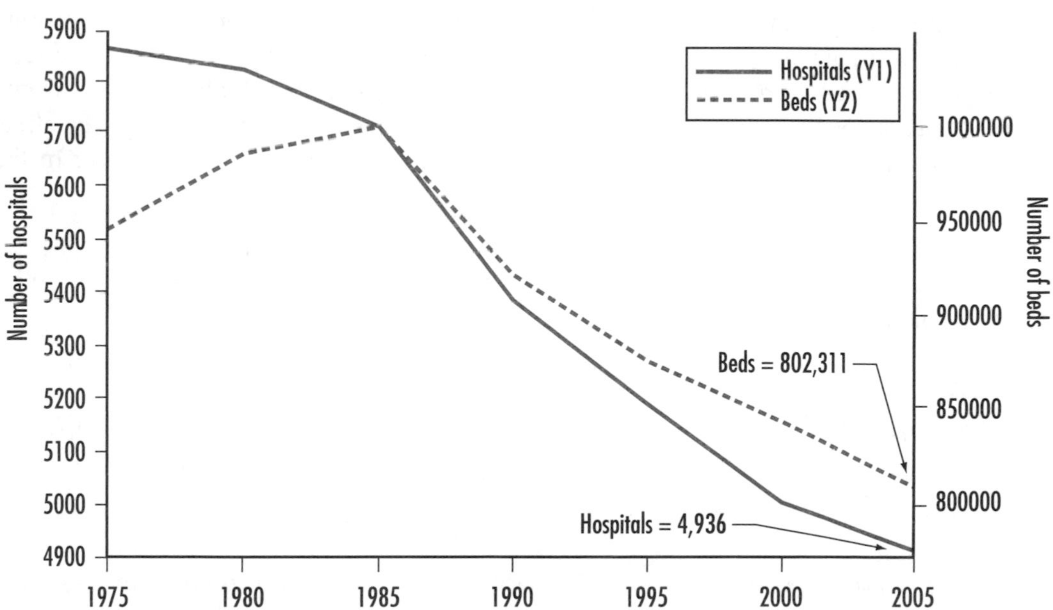

Source: Data from *Health United States, 2002*, p. 279; AHA Hospital Statistics, 2007, Health Forum LLC.

Figure 8–3 Ratio of Hospital Outpatient Visits to Inpatient Days (all hospitals), 1980–2004.

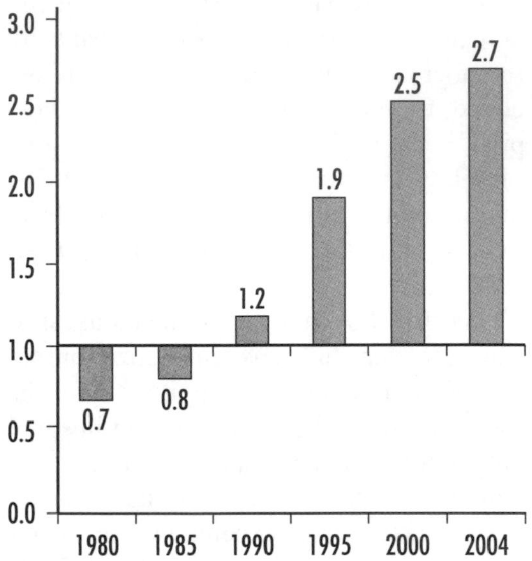

Source: Data from *Statistical Abstract of the United States, 2002*, p. 110; *Statistical Abstract of the United States, 2007*, p. 114; US Census Bureau.

by developing outpatient services. This is mainly due to the development of, and increased competition from, new outpatient services that are not affiliated with hospitals. In the future, however, we can expect to see a pick-up in hospital inpatient use as the US population continues to age. Aging is a key driver of hospital inpatient utilization.

The downward pressures on hospital utilization have been exerted by three main forces: changes in hospital reimbursement, closure of small rural hospitals, and the impact of managed care. Of these three, hospital reimbursement had the most dramatic effect on hospitals.

Changes in Reimbursement

The Tax Equity and Fiscal Responsibility Act (TEFRA) of 1982 was implemented in 1983. This legislation authorized the conversion of hospital Medicare reimbursement from cost-plus to a prospective payment system (PPS) based on DRGs (see Chapter 6). PPS marked a major change in the way hospitals were paid for inpatient services. Following Medicare's lead, several states adopted prospective methods to reimburse hospitals for services provided to their Medicaid enrollees. Private payers also resorted to competitive pricing and discounted fees, and closely monitored when patients would be hospitalized and for how long. The effect of PPS on hospitals was dramatic. In the

Table 8–1 Share of National Expenditures for Hospital Care

	1980	1990	1995	2000	2005
National health expenditures (NHE)	$245.8	$696.0	$990.3	$1299.5	1,987.7
Expenditures—hospital care	$101.5	$253.9	$343.6	$412.1	611.6
Hospital expenditures as a percent of NHE	41.3%	36.5%	34.7%	31.7%	30.8%

Source: Data from *Health United States, 2002*, p. 291, National Center for Health Statistics; Catlin, A. et al. 2007. National Health Spending in 2005: The Slowdown Continues. *Health Affairs* 26, no. 1: 142–153.

1980s, 550 hospitals closed and 159 mergers and acquisitions occurred (Balotsky 2005).

Rural Hospital Closures

During the 1990s, many small rural hospitals had to close because of economic constraints. Hospitals of all sizes throughout the country had to close entire wings or convert those beds for alternative uses, such as psychiatric care or long-term care. To rescue many of the remaining small hospitals from closure, in 1983, the then Health Care Financing Administration (HCFA) initiated a swing bed program for rural hospitals. ***Swing beds*** were authorized under the Omnibus Reconciliation Act of 1980 (Public Law 96499). The program created additional revenues for small rural hospitals by allowing them to switch the use of hospitals beds between acute-care and long-term care skilled nursing facility (SNF) as needed. However, in July 2002, the Centers for Medicare and Medicaid Services (formerly called HCFA) brought hospital swing beds under the existing SNF PPS reimbursement (discussed in Chapter 6), which created further financial pressures for these hospitals.

Impact of Managed Care

In the 1990s, managed care became a growing force transforming the delivery of health services. Managed care has emphasized cost containment and the efficient delivery of services. Because inpatient care, especially in acute care hospitals, is costly, managed care has emphasized alternative delivery settings, such as outpatient treatments, home health care, and the use of nursing homes whenever appropriate. Such measures have had a tremendous impact on curtailing the utilization of inpatient services and on the downsizing of individual hospitals. It has been demonstrated that Health Maintenance Organizations' (HMO) penetration in health care markets has played a significant role in lowering hospital profitability (Clement and Grazier 2001). Hospitals, on the other hand, have employed consolidation strategies in an effort to cope with such external pressures.

Some Key Utilization Measures and Operational Concepts

Discharges

The total number of patient discharges per 1,000 population is one indicator of access to hospital inpatient services and of the extent of utilization. Because babies born in the hospital are not included in admissions, discharges provide a more accurate count of the inpatients served by a hospital. ***Discharge*** refers to the total number of patients discharged from a hospital's acute care beds in a given period. Deaths in hospitals are counted as discharges. Discharge rates per 1,000 population (Table 8–2) are important because all other inpatient use patterns depend on them. Discharges per 1,000 population from community hospitals declined from 122.3 in 1990 to 119.2 in 2004 (DHHS 2006, 339), reflecting a lower rate of inpatient hospital utilization.

Inpatient Days

An ***inpatient day*** (also called a patient day or a hospital day) is a night spent in the hospital by a person admitted as an inpatient. The cumulative number of patient days over a certain period is known as ***days of care***. Days of care per 1,000 population over one year generally reflect access to inpatient services and their utilization. When days of care are compared according to demographic characteristics, some interesting facts about access and utilization emerge (Table 8–2). There is a direct relationship between age and days of care in hospitals (with the exception of children between birth and 4 years of age—not shown in Table 8–2). Older people spend more time in hospitals than younger people. In general, females incur higher use of hospital services than men do. However, roughly 27 percent of all dis-

Table 8–2 Discharges, Days of Care, and Average Length of Stay per 1,000 Population in Nonfederal Short-Stay Hospitals, 2004

Characteristics	Discharges	Days of Care	Average Length of Stay
Total	119.2	574.1	4.8
Age			
Under 18 years	43.0	193.2	4.5
18–44 years	91.1	334.9	3.7
45–54 years	99.7	491.1	4.9
55–64 years	143.6	735.2	5.1
65–74 years	259.2	1,405.2	5.4
75+ years	470.2	2,714.9	5.8
Gender[1]			
Male	102.6	541.1	5.3
Male (18+ years)[2]	123.2	659.5	5.4
Female	134.9	599.6	4.4
Female (18+ years after factoring out child-birth-related utilization)[2]	129.0	639.3	5.0
Race[1]			
White	89.0	431.0	4.8
Black	110.0	597.0	5.4
Geographic Region[1]			
Northeast	128.8	687.6	5.3
Midwest	114.4	498.7	4.4
South	125.6	614.2	4.9
West	101.2	457.5	4.5

[1]Age adjusted.

[2]Author's estimate based on 2004 data from the National Center for Health Statistics and US Census Bureau.

Source: Data from *Health, United States, 2006,* pp. 339, 340, US Department of Health and Human Services, National Center for Health Statistics; Statistical Abstract of the United States, 2007, p. 117. US Census Bureau.

charges and 12.5 percent of all days of care among women 18 years of age and older are childbirth-related. After factoring out childbirth-related use, in the 18+ age category, women still incur a higher discharge rate than men, but have 3 percent fewer population-adjusted days of care, and have a shorter average length of stay (see Table 8–2). Hospitalization is higher among blacks than whites. Generally, hospital use is higher among people of lower socioeconomic status than the more affluent because poorer population groups generally have less access to routine primary care, and there are other factors involved. Consequently, poorer population groups in the United States are more likely to suffer from acute conditions, incurring more frequent hospitalization and also longer stays once admitted. In the western United States, hospital utilization is much lower than in other parts of the country. A high rate of managed care penetration is believed to be primarily responsible for the lower utilization. The utilization patterns also suggest that overall hospital use is higher among Medicare and Medicaid recipients than among the rest of the population.

Average Length of Stay

Average length of stay (ALOS) is calculated by dividing the total days of care by the total number of discharges. It provides a measure of how many days a patient, on average, spends in the hospital. Hence, this measure, when applied to individuals or specific groups of patients, is an indicator of severity of illness. It also indicates the average inpatient resources used for specific categories of patients, under the assumption that medical resources are used in conjunction with each day a patient spends in a hospital bed. In 2003, the ALOS for community hospitals in the United States dropped to 4.8 days, the lowest ever recorded (it remained the same in 2004). Table 8–2 shows ALOS based on several patient characteristics (discussed in the previous section). Figure 8–4 shows trends in ALOS by type of hospital ownership. Federal hospitals mainly include those in the Veterans Health Administration system, which serve a population that is getting older. State and local government hospitals disproportionately serve the poor and uninsured. For 2004, the ALOS in voluntary and proprietary hospitals are similar. Figure 8–5 illustrates the downward trend in ALOS from 1970 to 2004. First, the PPS had a marked influence on the decline in the ALOS during the mid-1980s. This was followed by the influence of managed care during the 1990s. The sharp decline in average length of hospital stay during the 1990s became possible with the growth of alternative services, such as home health and subacute long-term care, which enabled people to be discharged earlier. Thanks to the development of these substitute sites of care and better technology, no evidence has emerged that quicker discharges of patients from hospitals under PPS or managed care payment systems resulted in medical harm to patients.

Capacity

The number of beds set up and staffed for inpatient use determines the size or capacity of a hospital. Eighty-four percent of all community hospitals in the United States have fewer than 300 beds (Figure 8–6). The average size of a community hospital is approximately 165 beds, which has remained relatively constant since 1995. Nationally, a typical rural hospital has 65 beds, and an

Figure 8–4 Average Lengths of Stay by Hospital Ownership: 1990–2004.

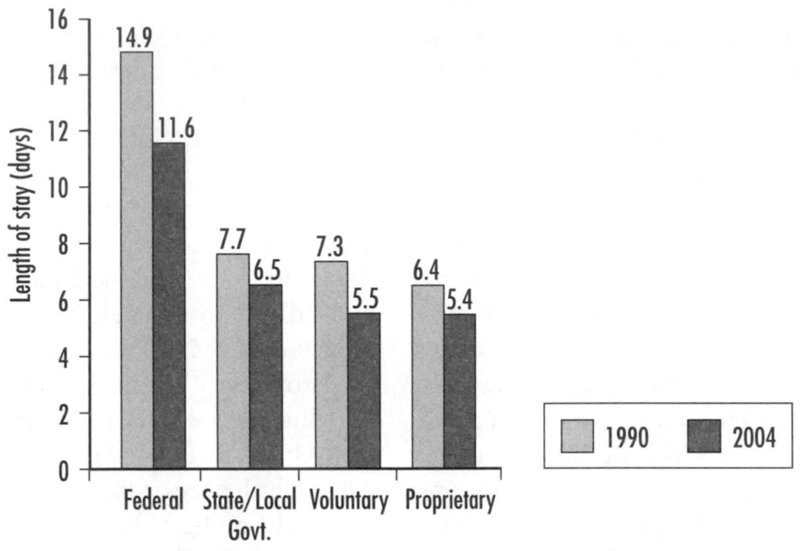

Source: Data from *Health United States, 2006*, p. 350, US Department of Health and Human Services.

Figure 8–5 Change in Average Length of Stay in All US Community Hospitals, 1970–2004.

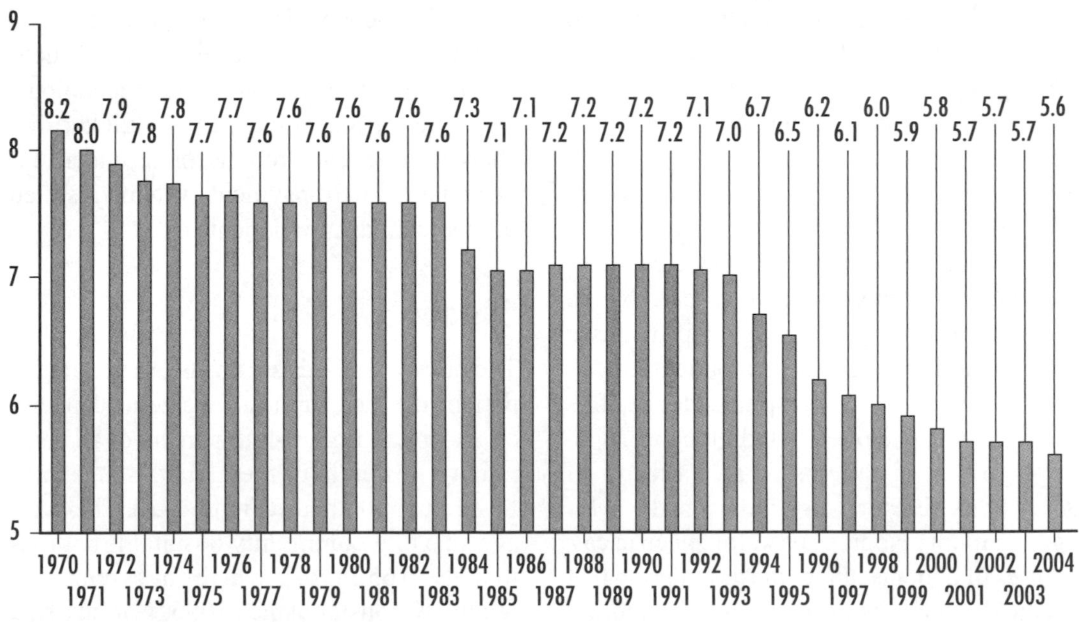

Source: Data from *Hospital Statistics, 1999*, p. 2, © American Hospital Association; *Hospital Statistics 2002*, p. 4, Health Forum; *Health United States, 2003*, p. 285; *Health United States, 2006*, p. 350, National Center for Health Statistics.

Figure 8–6 Breakdown of Community Hospitals by Size, 2004.

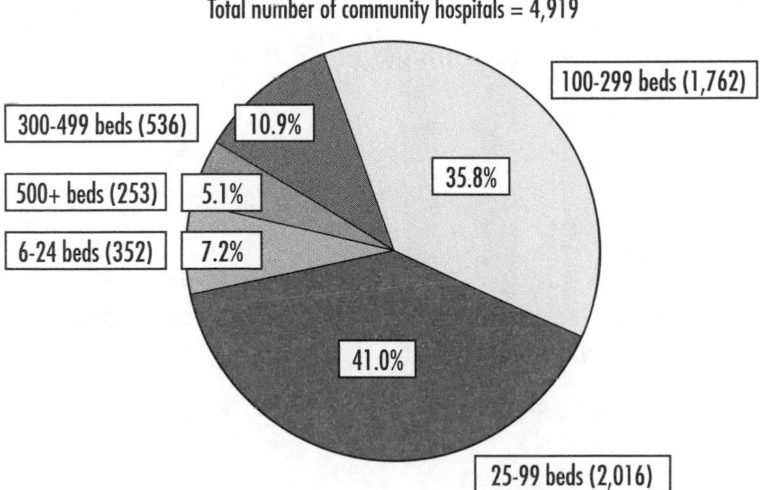

Source: Data from *Health United States, 2006*, p. 364, National Center for Health Statistics, US Department of Health and Human Services.

urban hospital has 231 beds (Anonymous 2002).

Average Daily Census

The average number of beds occupied each day in a hospital is referred to as ***average daily census***. Hence, it is one of the common measures used to define occupancy of inpatient beds in a hospital. The total inpatient days during a given period (days of care) are divided by the number of days in that period to arrive at the average daily census. For example, if the number of total inpatient days for July is 3,131, then the average daily census for July is 101 (3,131/31).

Occupancy Rate

The ***occupancy rate*** for a given period is derived by dividing the average daily census for that period by the number of available beds (capacity). The fraction is expressed as a percentage (percent of beds occupied). It indicates the proportion of a hospital's total inpatient capacity that is actually utilized. Occupancy rate is also commonly used for other types of inpatient facilities, such as nursing homes, and is often used as a measure of performance. Figure 8–7 shows the change in aggregate occupancy rates for US community hospitals from 1960 to 2004. Since hospitals are able to increase or decrease capacity (number of beds that are set up and staffed), trends in occupancy over time may not indicate much. However, individual hospitals can compare their own occupancy rates against the industry. In a competitive environment, facilities with higher occupancy rates are considered more successful than those with lower occupancy rates.

Figure 8–7 Change in Occupancy Rates (percent of beds occupied) in Community Hospitals, 1960–2004 (selected years).

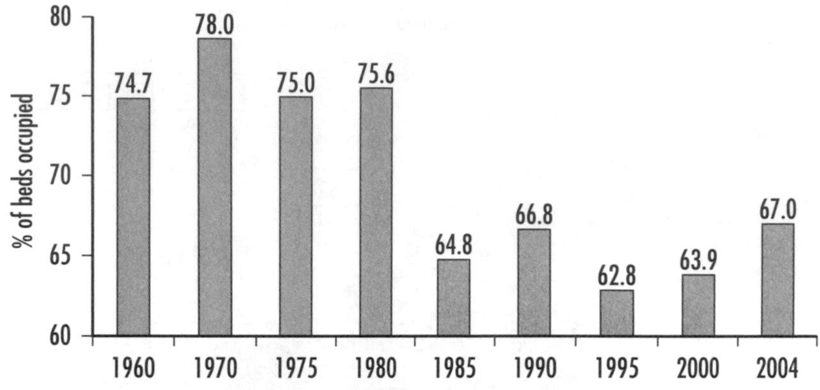

Source: Data from *Health United States, 1995*, p. 231; *Health United States, 1996–7*, p. 243, *Health United States, 2006*, p. 364, National Center for Health Statistics.

Hospital Employment

Employment in hospitals declined by 2.3 percent, to about 4 million workers over the 1983 to 1986 period. Staff cuts, hiring freezes, and the increased use of contract services were part of a belt-tightening effort in response to declining inpatient admissions (Kahl and Clark 1986). But, as hospitals chased more liberal reimbursement in outpatient markets, employment in hospitals in 1989 rose to 4.3 million workers, an increase of 6.9 percent from 1986 (Anderson and Wootton 1991). This trend has continued as hospitals have been employing an increasing number of personnel. In 2003, America's hospitals employed the full-time equivalent of 4.7 million people (Iglehart 2006). Hospital employment constitutes roughly 4 percent of all service-providing jobs in the United States.

Staffing ratios per occupied bed increased substantially between 1995 and 2000, but have moderated since then. Table 8–3 pre-

Table 8–3 Full-Time Equivalent (FTE) Staffing Per Occupied Bed

	Multihospital Systems			Independent Hospitals		
	1995	2000	2005	1995	2000	2005
Staff and resident physicians	0.48	0.63	0.54	0.75	0.92	0.65
RNs and LPNs	2.19	2.54	2.45	2.30	3.07	3.16
Ratio of RN to LPN	4.6	4.5	4.6	3.0	2.9	3.1
Other personnel	5.09	5.89	5.75	5.54	8.00	8.04
Total staff	7.76	9.06	8.74	8.59	11.99	11.85

Sources: Data from *Managed Care Digest Series: Institutional Digest,* 1998, Hoechst Marion Roussel; SMG Marketing-Verispan LLC, 2002, available at www.managedcaredigest.com; Hospitals/Systems Digest, © 2007, Sanofi-Aventis.

sents full-time equivalent staffing data per occupied bed by selected staff categories for facilities affiliated with multihospital systems (a chain of two or more hospitals) and for independent facilities. Compared to other developed nations, American hospitals are much more heavily staffed. Paradoxically, despite more resource-intensive treatments given to patients in US hospitals, quality outcomes are not appreciably greater (Reinhardt 2002).

Types of Hospitals

Instead of a centralized system of hospitals under state ownership, the United States has a variety of institutional forms, with both private and government-owned institutions under independent management. Most hospitals are voluntary, nonprofit, short-stay, general hospitals. State and local government-owned hospitals are next in predominance. Then come the for-profit (investor-owned) hospitals and, finally, federal hospitals. Figure 8–8 shows the distribution of hospitals, and Figure 8–9 shows the distribution of beds among various hospital types.

The endless variations in hospital characteristics defy any simple classification. The following classification arrangements have been commonly used to differentiate between the various types of hospitals. It is important to keep in mind, however, that these classifications are not mutually exclusive.

Figure 8–8 Proportion of Total US Hospitals by Type of Hospital, 2004.

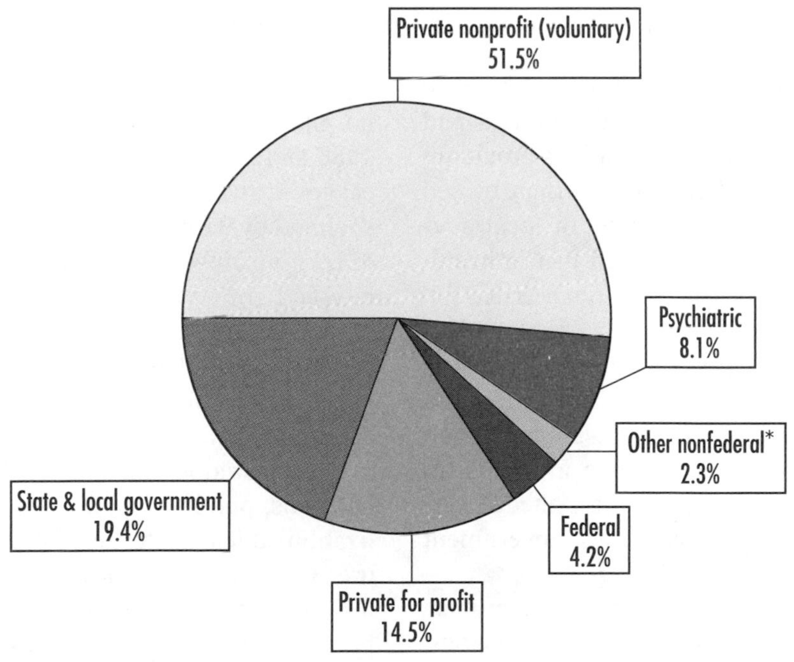

* Mainly nonfederal long-term hospitals.

Source: Data from *Statistical Abstract of the United States, 2007*, p.114, US Census Bureau.

Figure 8–9 Proportion of Total US Hospital Beds by Type of Hospital, 2004.

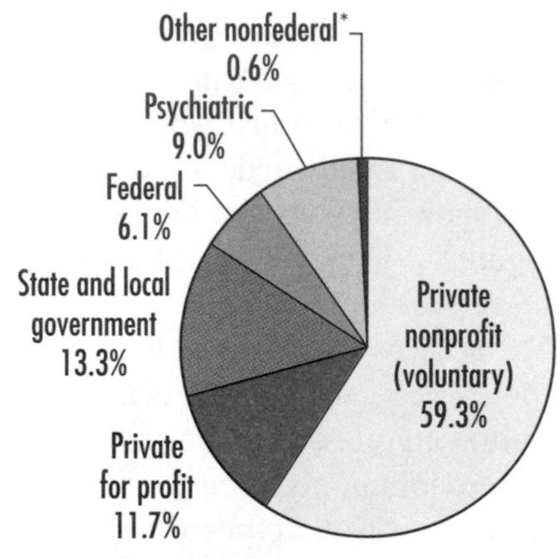

Source: Data from *Statistical Abstract of the United States, 2007*, p. 114. US Census Bureau.

Classification by Ownership

Public Hospitals

Generally speaking, public hospitals were the first to appear when almshouses and pesthouses evolved into hospitals providing medical services. ***Public hospitals*** are owned by agencies of federal, state, or local governments. It should be noted that in health care the word "public" does not carry its ordinary meaning. A public hospital, for instance, is not necessarily a hospital that is open to the general public. In business, a public corporation is one whose stock is publicly traded to attract private investors. In health care, particularly in the United States, the word "public" connotes government ownership.

Federal hospitals are maintained primarily for special groups of federal beneficiaries, such as Native Americans, military personnel, and veterans. As a general rule, federal hospitals do not serve the common public. Veterans Affairs (VA) hospitals constitute the largest group among federal hospitals.

State governments have generally limited themselves to the operation of mental and tuberculosis hospitals, reflecting government's early role in protecting communities by isolating the mentally ill and persons with contagious diseases. During the past several years, the number of state psychiatric hospitals has decreased considerably because of policies favoring deinstitutionalization of mentally ill patients, not only in the United States but also in Europe, Canada, and Australia.

Local governments, such as counties and cities, operate hospitals that are open to the general public. Many of these hospitals are located in large urban areas where they serve mainly the inner city indigent and disadvantaged populations. Medicare, Medicaid, and state and local tax dollars pay for almost 80 percent of the services these hospitals provide (Safety net in shreds 2002). Because of increasing financial pressures, many public hospitals had to privatize or close. Between 1980 and 2004, the number of state and local government-owned community hospitals declined by 37 percent, from 1,778 in 1980 to 1,117 in 2004. Most hospitals operated by city and county governments are small to moderate size. Some large public hospitals are affiliated with medical schools; they play a significant role in training physicians and other health care professionals.

Compared to voluntary and proprietary hospitals, public hospitals incur higher utilization, at least in terms of ALOS (see Figure 8–4). ALOS is the highest in federal hospitals (11.6 days), and veterans are the biggest users of these hospitals. At present, about 43 percent of the veteran population is over 65 (compared to 13 percent of the general US population) and it is aging rapidly. The proportion of veterans over the age of 65 is expected to rise to 51 percent by 2010 (Zeber et al. 2004).

Voluntary Hospitals

Voluntary hospitals are nongovernmental, and therefore, privately-owned hospitals that are operated on a nonprofit basis. They are owned and operated by community associations or other nongovernment organizations. These hospitals are called voluntary because the development and financial backing of the institutions is done voluntarily by citizens without government involvement (Raffel and Raffel 1994, 130). Their primary mission is to benefit the community in which they are located. Their operating expenses are covered from patient fees, third-party reimbursement, donations, and endowments. The private nonprofit sector constitutes the largest group of hospitals (Figure 8–8). In 2004, the private nonprofit sector accounted for over 51 percent of all hospitals and almost 60 percent of all beds with an average capacity of 191 beds per hospital (DHHS 2006, 364).

Proprietary Hospitals

For-profit ***proprietary hospitals***—also referred to as ***investor-owned hospitals***—are owned by individuals, partnerships, or corporations. They are operated for the financial benefit of the entity that owns the institution, that is, the stockholders. At the beginning of the 20th century, more than half of the nation's hospitals were proprietary. Most of these hospitals were small and were established by physicians who wanted a place to hospitalize their own patients (Stewart 1973). Later, most of these institutions were closed or acquired by community organizations or hospital corporations because of population shifts, increased costs, and the necessities of modern clinical practice (Raffel and Raffel 1994, 133). Even though the nonprofit hospital sector has maintained its market dominance, during the past decade, the for-profit sector has gained market share (Table 8–4). However, compared to other types of ownership, proprietary hospitals continue to have the lowest occupancy rates (60.5 percent in 2004 compared to 67 percent for all community hospitals) [DHHS 2006, 364].

Classification by Multiunit Affiliation

Hospitals are part of a multihospital chain (sometimes referred to as a multihospital system—MHS) when two or more hospitals are owned, leased, sponsored, or contractually managed by a central organization (AHA 1994). In recent years, MHSs have gained a

Table 8–4 Changes in Number of Community Hospitals, Beds, Average Size, and Occupancy Rates

	1995	2004	Change
Nonprofit Sector			
Number of hospitals	3,092	2,967	–4.0%
Number of beds	609,729	567,863	–6.9%
Average size	197	191	–2.9%
Occupancy rate	64.5%	68.3%	5.9%
For-Profit Sector			
Number of hospitals	752	835	11.0%
Number of beds	105,737	112,693	6.6%
Average size	141	135	–4.0%
Occupancy rate	51.8%	60.5%	16.8%

Source: Data from *Health, United States, 2006,* p. 364, National Center for Health Statistics.

larger share of all hospitals by acquiring facilities confronting financial problems. Acquired hospitals are more likely to be located in markets with higher numbers of health maintenance organizations (HMOs). They also tend to have lower occupancy rates and older facilities (Harrison et al. 2003). Table 8–5 lists the largest of the multihospital chains according to size. MHSs accounted for 49 percent of all hospitals nationwide in 2005, up from 46 percent five years earlier (Sanofi-Aventis 2007). Despite inroads made by investor-owned groups into MHSs, most such systems are operated by nonprofit corporations (Table 8–6). Some of the advantages of multihospital chain affiliation include economies of scale with administrative overhead, the ability to provide a wide spectrum of care, ability to reach a variety of markets, increased access to capital markets, and access to management resources and expertise.

Table 8–5 The Largest US Multihospital Chains, 2004 (ranked by Staffed Beds)

Name of Hospital System (Location)	Number of Owned Hospitals	Number of Staffed Beds	Average Occupancy %	ALOS
Nonprofit Chains				
Ascension Health (St. Louis, MO)	44	9,966	57.8%	4.8
Catholic Health Initiatives (Denver, CO)	60	9,964	50.2%	4.8
Catholic Healthcare West (San Francisco, CA)	36	8,953	57.6%	5.1
Kaiser Permanente (Oakland, CA)	31	7,234	64.1%	4.1
Catholic Health East (Newtown, PA)	22	7,036	61.2%	5.3
Trinity Health (Novi, MI)	25	5,690	60.4%	4.4
Adventist Health System (Winter Park, FL)	27	5,463	57.3%	4.6
Christus Health (Irving, TX)	22	4,973	61.7%	5.9
Catholic Healthcare Partners (Cincinnati, OH)	21	3,753	63.5%	5.6
SSM Health Care System (St. Louis, MO)	14	3,192	62.1%	4.7
For-Profit Chains				
HCA (Nashville, TN)	171	35,335	58.5%	4.7
Tenet Health System (Dallas, TX)	71	16,182	60.7%	5.2
Community Health Systems (Brentwood, TN)	69	7,292	46.6%	4.8
Health Mgmt. Associates (Naples, FL)	51	6,972	53.1%	4.5
Universal Health Services (King of Prussia, PA)	22	4,157	65.1%	4.9
State and Local Government-Owned Chains				
New York City Health and Hospitals Corporation (New York, NY)	11	4,746	86.7%	6.6
Los Angeles County Department of Health Services (Los Angeles, CA)	5	3,054	47.3%	7.6
University of California (Oakland, CA)	6	2,493	55.1%	5.6
University of Texas Systems (Austin, TX)	3	1,336	71.5%	6.8
North Broward Hospital District (Fort Lauderdale, FL)	4	1,294	69.8%	5.3

Source: Data from *Managed Care Digest Series: Hospital/Systems Digest,* Sanofi-Aventis, 2006, Bridgewater, NJ: Sanofi-Aventis.

Table 8–6 Multihospital Health Care Systems: Number of Hospitals and Beds, 2005
(Includes owned, leased, sponsored and contract-managed hospitals)

Type of Control	Number of Systems	Hospitals	Beds	% Beds*
Catholic church related	42	555	108,538	18.6
Other church related	13	108	21,699	3.7
Total church related	**55**	**663**	**130,237**	**22.3**
Other nonprofit	244	1,210	262,051	44.8
Total nonprofit	**299**	**1,873**	**392,288**	**67.1**
Investor owned	65	1,241	146,541	25.1
Federal government owned	5	223	46,095	7.9
Total	**369**	**3,337**	**584,924**	**100.0**

*As a percentnge of all systems

Source: Data from *AHA Hospital Statistics, 2007*, p. 197, © Health Forum.

The VA operates the single largest hospital system in the country, with 163 medical centers, owned by the federal government. In fiscal year 2000, the Veterans' Health System treated 3.3 million veterans and had over 600,000 hospital discharges. The overall ALOS for a veteran admitted to the hospital was 12.5 days (Pfizer Inc. 2003).

Classification by Length of Stay

A ***short-stay hospital*** is one in which the average length of stay is less than 25 days; that is, most hospitals. Patients admitted to these hospitals suffer from acute conditions. Hospitals with average stays of more than 25 days are long-stay hospitals. These include state-run as well as private psychiatric hospitals, long-term care hospitals (LTCHs) providing subacute care, tuberculosis hospitals, and chronic disease hospitals.

A ***long-term care hospital*** (LTCH) is a special type of long-stay hospital described in section 1886(d)(1)(B)(iv) of the Social Security Act. LTCHs must meet Medicare's conditions of participation for acute (short-stay) hospitals, and must have an ALOS greater than 25 days. LTCHs serve patients who have complex medical needs and may suffer from multiple chronic problems requiring long-term hospitalization. Many LTCH patients are admitted directly from short-stay hospital intensive care units with respiratory/ventilator-dependent or other complex medical conditions. The number of LTCHs has grown rapidly from 105 facilities in 1993 to 318 in 2003 (MedPAC 2004). The demand for other types of long-stay hospitals has generally declined over the years. The number of tuberculosis hospitals, for example, has declined from 103 in 1970 to 4 (US Census Bureau 2007, 114), mainly because the disease has been largely eradicated or controlled with modern drugs.

Classification by Type of Service

General Hospitals

A ***general hospital*** provides a variety of services, including general and specialized medicine, general and specialized surgery, and obstetrics, to meet the general medical needs of the community it serves. It provides diagnostic, treatment, and surgical services for patients with a variety of medical conditions. Most hospitals in the United States are general hospitals.

It is important to note that the term "general hospital" does not imply that these hospitals are less specialized or that their care is inferior to that of specialty hospitals. The difference lies in the nature of services, not their quality. General hospitals provide a broader range of services for a larger variety of conditions; whereas specialty hospitals provide a narrow range of services for specific medical conditions or patient populations.

Specialty Hospitals

According to the North American Industry Classification System of the US Census Bureau, ***specialty hospitals*** are establishments that primarily engage in providing diagnostic and medical treatment to inpatients with a specific type of disease or medical condition, except services for psychiatric care or substance abuse. Specialty hospitals forge a distinct service niche. Traditionally, the two most common specialty hospitals have been rehabilitation hospitals and children's hospitals. With increasing competition, however, other types of specialty hospitals have emerged to provide treatments that are also available in many general hospitals. Examples include orthopedic hospitals, cardiac hospitals, cancer (oncology) hospitals, and women's hospitals. Physicians find such specialized hospitals more efficient, and in many instances, physicians are full or part owners of these hospitals. Affiliation with such hospitals gives physicians control over hospital operations, flexibility with their time, and opportunity to enhance their incomes. However, physician-owned facilities raise legal and ethical issues with regard to self-referrals without full disclosure. Stark Laws that prohibit self-referrals (see Chapter 5) do not apply when physicians self refer to a "whole hospital." Under this exception, physicians may refer patients to a facility if their ownership interest is in the whole hospital, rather than a smaller entity (Guterman 2006). Also, in 2003, Congress amended the Stark Laws to impose an 18-month moratorium during which physician-investors in new specialty hospitals could not refer Medicare patients to those hospitals (Zimmerman 2006). Although, the moratorium had effectively stifled the development of new specialty hospitals, the development boom has reignited as the moratorium ended in 2006. Currently, the Centers for Medicare and Medicaid Services (CMS) has proposed changes in hospital reimbursement with the intent of making private investments in specialty hospitals less lucrative.

Another issue, emergency care, is at the heart of the controversy between specialty hospitals and community general hospitals. Administrators of general hospitals argue that specialty hospitals are cream-skimming insured patients and leaving costly emergency and uncompensated cases to general hospitals (Snyder 2003). Recent studies also suggest that compared to community hospitals, physician-owned specialty hospitals seem to treat less complex and more profitable cases (Guterman 2006).

Psychiatric Hospitals

The primary function of a psychiatric inpatient facility is to provide diagnostic and treatment services for patients who have psychiatric-related illnesses. Specifically, such an institution must have facilities to provide psychiatric, psychological, and social work services. A psychiatric hospital must also have a written agreement with a general hospital for the transfer of patients who may require medical, obstetrics, or surgical services (Health Forum 2001, A3).

Historically, state governments have taken the primary responsibility for establishing facilities for the care of the mentally ill. Trends during the 1970s and 1980s resulted in significant deinstitutionalization of the inpatient population that resided in state mental hospitals. As a result, the responsibility for much psychiatric care shifted to psychiatric units in general hospitals, private psychiatric hospitals, other types of residential facilities, and community care programs (Mechanic 1998). However, state mental institutions continue to provide long-term treatment to people with severe and persistent mental illness (Patrick et al. 2006). In 2004, the United States had 466 psychiatric hospitals (US Census Bureau 2007, 114).

Rehabilitation Hospitals

Rehabilitation hospitals specialize in therapeutic services to restore the maximum level of functioning in patients who have suffered recent disability due to an episode of illness or an accident. These hospitals serve patients who generally cannot be cured but whose functioning can be improved. According to Medicare rules, to be classified as a rehabilitation hospital, 75 percent of a hospital's inpatients must require intensive rehabilitation services for the treatment of stroke, spinal cord injury, major multiple trauma, brain injury, and other specific conditions (Grimaldi 2002). Rehabilitation hospitals also serve amputees and victims of accident or sports injuries. Patients often transfer to these facilities after orthopedic surgery in a general hospital. Facilities and staff are available to provide physical therapy, occupational therapy, and speech and language pathology. Most rehabilitation hospitals have special arrangements for psychological, social work, and vocational services, and are required to have written arrangements with a general hospital for the transfer of patients who need medical, obstetrical, or surgical care not available at the institution (Health Forum 2001, A3).

Children's Hospitals

Children's hospitals are community hospitals that typically have specialized facilities to deal mainly with complex, severe, or chronic illnesses among children. Nearly all children's hospitals provide neonatal intensive care units, pediatric intensive care units, trauma centers, and transplant services. Thus, these hospitals provide a wide range of high-intensity services for children, such as pediatric surgery, cardiology, orthopedic surgery, cancer treatment, HIV/AIDS treatment, and rehabilitation services (DelliFraine 2006).

There are 45 freestanding children's hospitals in the United States. They have an average capacity of 124 beds. All of these hospitals are nonprofit, and are located in major metropolitan areas. Many are affiliated with medical schools and academic medical centers. However, many large communities do not have specialty children's hospitals. In these communities, general acute-care hospitals serve as de facto children's hospitals by providing the same services and treating the same types of patients (DelliFraine 2006).

Classification by Public Access

Most people are familiar with the community hospital. A ***community hospital*** is a nonfederal short-stay hospital whose facilities and services are available to the general public. Its primary mission is to serve the general community. These hospitals are not restricted to serving a certain category of people. A community hospital may be proprietary, voluntary, or owned by the state or local government (but not by the federal government). It may be a general hospital or a specialty hospital. Generally speaking, the larger the community served, the larger the hospital, range of specialties, and range of supporting equipment and services (Raffel and Raffel 1994, 131). Noncommunity hospitals include hospitals operated by the federal government, such as VA hospitals to serve veterans; hospital units of institutions, such as prisons and infirmaries in colleges and universities; and long-stay hospitals.

In 2004, of the 5,759 US hospitals, 4,919 (over 85 percent) were community hospitals (DHHS 2006, 364). Figure 8–10 shows the breakdown of community hospitals by ownership type.

Figure 8–10 Breakdown of Community Hospitals by Types of Ownership, 2004.

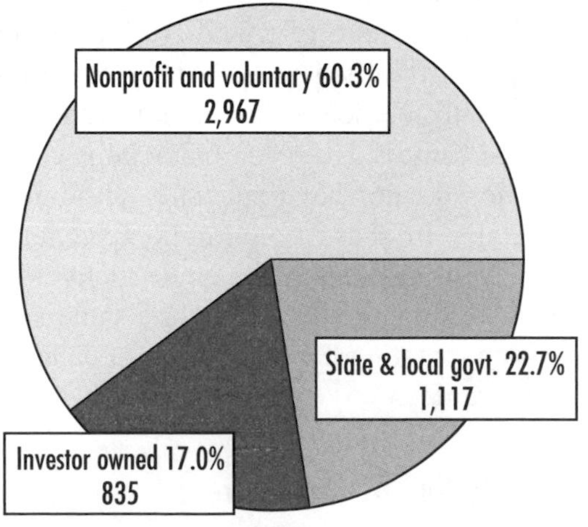

Source: Data from *Health United States, 2006*, p. 364, National Center for Health Statistics.

Classification by Location

Based on location, hospitals can be classified as urban or rural. ***Urban hospitals*** are located in a county that is part of a metropolitan statistical area (MSA). The US Bureau of Census has defined an MSA as a geographical area that includes at least (1) one city with a population of 50,000 or more or (2) an urbanized area of at least 50,000 inhabitants and a total MSA population of at least 100,000. ***Rural hospitals*** are located in a county that is not part of an MSA. It is estimated that rural hospitals deliver health care to 54 million Americans, including 9 million Medicare beneficiaries (Slusky 2006).

From an operational standpoint, compared to rural hospitals, urban hospitals have higher costs because they typically pay higher salaries in more competitive markets, offer a broader scope of more sophisticated services, and generally treat patients requiring more complex care. Urban hospitals are located either in inner cities or in the suburbs. Because suburbs of metropolitan areas are generally more affluent than inner cities or rural areas, both inner city urban hospitals and rural hospitals treat a patient mix that is disproportionately poor and elderly compared to suburban hospital patients (HCIA Inc. and Deloitte & Touche 1997, 64). Because of the disproportionate numbers of the elderly and poor in rural areas, rural community hospitals often find themselves in financial trouble. Conversion to a facility that provides nonacute health care services, such as a primary care clinic, a long-term care facility, or a specialty hospital, is sometimes a viable alternative when these hospitals are threatened with closure.

For example, adoption of long-term care strategies has demonstrated to improve profitability of rural hospitals (Stuart et al. 2006).

The plight of rural hospitals was discussed earlier. To save some of the very small rural hospitals, the Balanced Budget Act of 1997 created the Medicare Rural Hospital Flexibility Program (MRHFP). Under this program, certain rural hospitals can be classified as ***Critical Access Hospitals*** (CAH) if they have no more than 25 acute care beds and if they provide emergency medical services. Although CAH status is not necessarily the best alternative for all small rural hospitals, the number of such hospitals jumped from 850 in 2003 to 1,050 at the end of 2004 (Mantone 2005). If a hospital elects CAH status, and meets the criteria for CAH designation, it can receive cost-plus reimbursement under Medicare Part A. Since cost-plus reimbursement allows inclusion of capital costs, these hospitals have now access to capital for new construction and renovations. The CAH program has provided the financial stability that many small rural hospitals need.

Classification by Size

There is no standard way to classify hospitals by size. According to one classification scheme, hospitals with fewer than 100 beds would be classified as small, those with 100 to 500 beds as medium, and those with 500-plus beds as large. Others may classify by size a little differently. Just a little over half (52 percent) of all hospitals in the United States have 100 beds or more (US Census Bureau 2007, 114).

Figure 8–11 illustrates expenses per inpatient day by hospital size. Experience in the manufacturing and retail sectors of the

Figure 8–11 Expenses per Inpatient Day by Hospital Size, Community Hospitals, 2004.

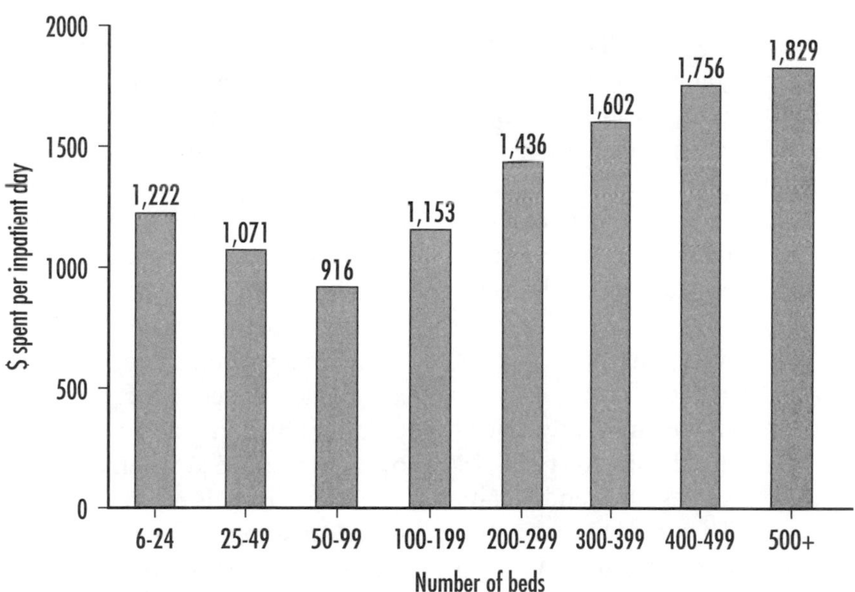

Source: Data from *Health United States, 2006*, p. 392, National Center for Health Statistics.

economy suggests that large enterprises should realize economies of scale. The reason is that certain overhead costs are fixed or semi-fixed—they do not increase proportionally as the size of the enterprise increases. Examples are administrative costs and plant maintenance costs. In the hospital industry, economies of scale seem to evaporate when the size exceeds 100 beds or so. Higher costs in larger hospitals are mainly attributable to a more extensive array of specialized and resource-intensive services that these hospitals must be equipped to provide. Such services require sophisticated technology and personnel with advanced training. Large teaching hospitals incur the additional costs of residency training and medical research.

Other Types of Hospitals

Teaching Hospitals

To be designated as a ***teaching hospital***, a hospital must have one or more graduate residency programs approved by the American Medical Association (AMA). The mere presence of nursing programs or training affiliations for other health professionals, such as therapists and dietitians, does not make an institution a teaching hospital.

The term ***academic medical center*** is commonly used when a hospital or health system is organized around a medical school. Apart from the training of physicians, research activities and clinical investigations become an important undertaking.

Among the largest and most prestigious teaching hospitals are the members of the Council of Teaching Hospitals and Health Systems (COTH). They usually have substantial teaching and research programs and are affiliated with medical schools of large universities. The approximately 400 COTH member institutions train about three-quarters of the physician residents in the United States (AAMC 2003).

Three main traits separate teaching and nonteaching hospitals. First, teaching hospitals provide medical training to physicians, research opportunities to health services researchers, and specialized care to patients. They incur certain costs directly associated with medical education programs, the largest category being the salary and benefits expense for interns and residents. Medicare reimburses the additional costs of graduate medical education in teaching hospitals separately, in addition to the prospective DRG rates (Dalton 1995). Secondly, teaching hospitals have a broader and more complex scope of services than nonteaching hospitals. Teaching hospitals often operate several intensive care units, possess the latest medical technologies, and attract a diverse group of physicians representing most specialties and many subspecialties. Major teaching hospitals also offer many unique tertiary care services not generally found in other institutions, such as burn care, trauma care, and organ transplantation. Because more specialized services are available, teaching hospitals attract patients who frequently have more complicated diagnoses or need more complex procedures. Because of the greater case-mix complexity of teaching hospitals, greater resources are required for treatment. Third, many of the major teaching hospitals are located in economically depressed, older inner city areas, and are generally owned by state or local governments. Consequently, these hospitals often provide disproportional amounts of uncompensated care to uninsured patients (HCIA Inc. and Deloitte & Touche 1997, 66).

Church-Affiliated Hospitals

Various churches established hospitals mainly during the latter half of the 19th and the early 20th centuries. The first church-sponsored hospitals in the United States were established by various Catholic sisterhoods. Later, protestant denominations organized hospitals in accord with their missions of service, and Jewish philanthropic organizations opened hospitals so that Jewish patients could observe their dietary laws more faithfully and Jewish physicians could more easily find sites for training and work opportunities (Raffel 1980, 241).

Church-affiliated hospitals are often community general hospitals. They may be large or small, teaching or nonteaching. Affiliation with a medical school may also vary. They are different only in that they are owned or heavily influenced by the church groups that sponsor them. Church hospitals do not discriminate in rendering care; however, they are generally sensitive to the sponsoring denomination's special spiritual and/or dietary emphasis (Raffel and Raffel 1994, 131–132).

Osteopathic Hospitals

For all practical purposes, osteopathic hospitals are community general hospitals. In 1970, osteopathic hospitals became eligible to apply for registration with the AHA (AHA 1994). Approximately 200 osteopathic hospitals operate in the United States.

Osteopathic medicine represents an approach to medical practice employing all the methods traditionally associated with allopathic medicine, such as pharmaceuticals, laboratory tests, X-ray diagnostics, and surgery. ***Osteopathic medicine***, however, takes a holistic approach and goes a step further in advocating treatment that involves correction of the position of the joints or tissues, and in emphasizing diet and environment as factors that might influence natural resistance. For many years after osteopathy was established as a separate branch of medicine in 1874, osteopaths had to develop their own hospitals because of antagonism from the established allopathic medical practitioners. Both groups have now inspected each other's medical schools and satisfied themselves that each is worth associating with, and that each could serve on the other's faculties and practice side by side in the same hospitals (Raffel and Raffel 1994, 45).

Due to the emphasis on preventive care and less invasive solutions to medical problems, one would expect that osteopathic hospitals would deliver cost-efficient care. However, results of one study show that osteopathic hospitals are more costly and less productive in comparison to their counterparts. Inefficient production of outpatient services and high cost of medical education are two reasons for their poor performance (Sinay 2005).

What Makes a Hospital Nonprofit?

Laypeople make a common assumption that nonprofit (sometimes called not-for-profit) health care corporations are driven by the mission to meet the health care needs of patients regardless of their ability to pay. It is further assumed that these corporations do not make a profit. The fact is that every corporation, regardless of whether it is for profit or nonprofit, has to make a profit (surplus of revenues over expenses) to survive over the long term. No business can survive for long if it continually spends more than it takes in. That is true for both the nonprofit and the for-profit sectors (Nudelman and Andrews 1996).

The Internal Revenue Code, Section 501(c)(3), grants tax-exempt status to nonprofit organizations. As such, these institutions are exempt from federal, state, and local taxes, such as income taxes, sales taxes, and property taxes. In general, these organizations must (1) provide some defined public good, such as service, education, or community welfare, and (2) not distribute any profits to any individuals. A major goal for a for-profit corporation, on the other hand, is to provide its shareholders with a return on their investment, but it achieves this goal primarily by excelling at its basic mission. For any health services provider the basic mission is to deliver the highest quality care at the most reasonable price possible.

Community hospitals owned by various groups, such as local citizens, fraternal orders, churches, and the government, have traditionally been classified as nonprofit. Among all private (non-government) hospitals in the United States, nearly 80 percent (84 percent of beds) are nonprofit. These hospitals receive substantial tax subsidies. Current rules for tax-exempt hospitals require them to provide charity care as well as community benefits. The latter broadly refer to services that the government would otherwise have to undertake (Owens 2005). Also, Section 4958 of the IRS code prohibits executive compensation that may be deemed unreasonable for tax-exempt organizations. Under current scrutiny, nonprofit hospitals have to be prepared to demonstrate not only that they are paying salaries within some reasonable range of industry standards, but also that executives are bringing measurable value in key areas of operations, including community benefits (Appleby 2004). Hence, it is recommended that some portion of hospital chief executive officers' salaries should directly hinge on his or her performance in two critical areas: (1) organizational effectiveness (financial performance, market share, quality, daily operations, and achievement of strategic objectives), and (2) community health (charitable care, health promotion and education, and overall state of the community's health) (Newman et al. 2001).

The problem is that nonprofit hospitals, in many instances, compete head-on with for-profit hospitals. For example, nonprofit hospitals frequently engage in the same kinds of aggressive marketplace behaviors that for-profit hospitals pursue. Institutional theory actually predicts such behavior. When for-profit and nonprofit organizations face similar regulatory, legal, and professional constraints, they will imitate each other, according to institutional theory (O'Connell and Brown 2003). In the hospital industry, competition commonly occurs in the same communities, for the same patients, with revenues coming from the same public and private third-party sources, and often involving the same physician providers who have admitting privileges at more than one hospital.

The empirical evidence indicates that, in general, for-profit and nonprofit hospitals provide similar levels of charity and uncompensated care (Thorpe et al. 2000). Their quality of care and the adoption of new technology are also similar (Sloan 1998). Generally, conversion of nonprofit to for-profit status does not adversely affect the provision of uncompensated care. However, some reduction in uncompensated care may occur particularly when public hospitals are acquired by for-profit owners (Thorpe et al. 2000).

Whether nonprofit hospitals are indeed charitable institutions remains controversial, and there is continued scrutiny of nonprofit hospitals by Congress to determine whether nonprofit hospitals provide sufficient services to warrant their exemption from taxes. The Internal Revenue Service now monitors how well nonprofit hospitals are complying with federal law that requires them to provide social benefits, such as free or low-cost health care for the poor. The viability of nonprofit hospitals will continue to be challenged until they produce decisive evidence of tangible value to their communities beyond that produced by their for-profit counterparts. Nonprofit hospitals could play a unique role if they can refocus on maintaining the delicate balance between market justice and social justice orientations (discussed in Chapter 2). This balance will be jeopardized if nonprofit organizations continue to emulate profit-seeking, investor-owned providers.

Many nonprofit hospitals are in fact engaged in various community outreach programs that directly or indirectly impact the health of their communities. Many hospitals across the nation are engaged in community health assessments, educational activities, support groups, and wellness programs. Some outreach activities even go beyond the hospital's core competencies of delivering health care, extending into improving the social and economic environments or influencing lifestyle behaviors to promote better health and well-being. For example, St. Bernard Hospital and Health Care Center in Chicago has been involved in developing an affordable housing project in its economically depressed neighborhood (Robbins 2002).

The question can arise as to whether nonprofit hospitals merely have a legal obligation to provide community benefits or whether the hospitals could also derive tangible benefits by providing community benefits which cost the hospitals money. A study of a sample of nonprofit hospitals in Massachusetts found a significant positive association between corporate citizenship, such as providing unmet health needs in the community, and financial performance of the hospitals (Longest and Lin 2005).

Some Management Concepts

From a management standpoint, hospitals are complex organizations. Compared to other business enterprises of similar size, both external and internal environments of hospitals are more complex. A hospital is generally responsible to numerous stakeholders in its external environment. These stakeholders include the community, the government, insurers, managed care organizations, and accreditation agencies. Internally, hospital governance involves three major sources of power whose motivations are sometimes at odds. A hospital's organizational structure (Figure 8–12) also differs substantially from that of other large organizations. The CEO receives delegated authority from the board and is responsible for managing the organization with the help of senior managers. In large hospitals, these senior managers often carry the title of senior vice president or vice president for various key service areas, such as nursing services, restorative (rehabilitation) services, human resources, finance, and so forth. The medical staff constitute a separate organizational structure parallel to the administrative structure. Such a dual structure is rarely seen in other businesses and presents numerous opportunities for conflict between the CEO and the medical staff. Matters are further complicated when the lines of authority cross between the two structures. For example, nursing service, pharmacists, diagnostic technicians, and dietitians are

Figure 8–12 Hospitals Governance and Operational Structures.

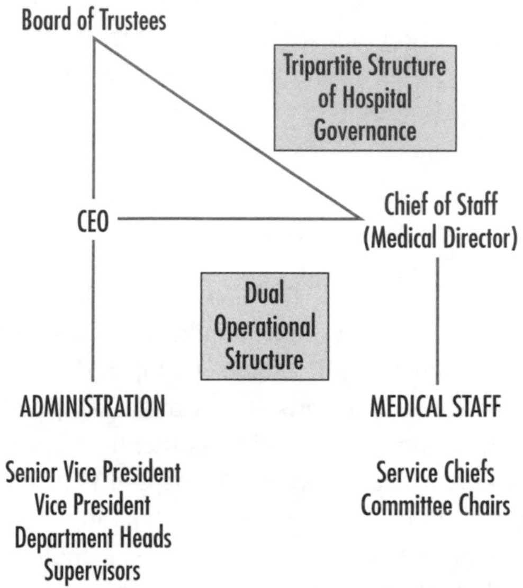

administratively accountable to the CEO (via the vertical chain of command) but professionally accountable to the medical staff (Raffel and Raffel 1994, 139). The medical staff generally are not paid employees of the hospital, yet they play a significant role in its success. It requires special skills on the part of the CEO to manage this dual structure to achieve the organization's overall objectives.

Hospital Governance

Hospital governance has traditionally followed a tripartite structure. The three major sources of authority are the CEO, the board of trustees, and the chief of staff (medical director), as illustrated in Figure 8–12. In earlier periods, when physicians operated their own hospitals, the hospitals were dominated by the trustees. Trustees were often the source of capital investment, and their influence in the community brought prestige to the hospital. Later, as voluntary hospitals increased in number, the balance of power shifted into the hands of physicians because they played a critical role in bringing patients to the hospitals. Changes in the health care environment over the last two decades have made the management of hospitals more complex; administrators now wield considerable power.

Board of Trustees

The ***board of trustees*** (also referred to as the governing body or board of directors) consists of influential business and community leaders. The board is legally responsible for the operations of the hospital. It is also responsible for defining the hospital's mission and long-term direction. It also sets policy guidelines that establish the overall framework for day-to-day operations. It approves long-range plans and annual budgets, and monitors performance against plans and budgets (Griffith 1995). The CEO is generally a member of the board. One or more physicians also sit on the board as voting members. One of the most important responsibilities of the board is to appoint and evaluate the performance of the CEO, who is charged with providing the board timely reports on the institution's progress in achieving its mission and objectives. The board has the power to remove the CEO. In most hospitals, the board also approves the appointment of physicians and other professionals to the hospital's medical staff.

Boards often function through committees. Standing committees usually include executive, medical staff, human resources, finance, planning, quality improvement, and ethics. Special, or ad hoc, committees are established as needed. The two most important committees from a governance standpoint are the executive committee and the medical staff committee. The ***executive committee*** has continuing monitoring responsibility and authority over the hospital. Usually, it receives reports from other committees, monitors policy implementation, and makes recommendations. The ***medical staff committee*** is charged with medical staff relations. For example, it reviews admitting privileges and the performance of the medical staff. There is also increased emphasis on the legal and ethical obligations of the hospital regarding patient safety, quality improvement, and patient satisfaction.

Chief Executive Officer

Formerly, the titles of "superintendent" and later "administrator" were commonly used for a hospital's chief executive. Now, "chief executive officer" and "president" are the common titles used. The CEO's job is to accomplish the organization's mission and objectives through leadership within the organization. He or she has the ultimate responsibility for day-to-day operations.

Medical Staff

The hospital's medical staff is an organized body of physicians who provide medical services to the hospital's patients and perform related clinical duties. The physicians, in most hospitals, are in private practice outside the hospital. The hospital grants them admitting privileges that enable them to admit and care for their patients in the hospital. Other clinicians, such as dentists and podiatrists, may also be granted admitting privileges. Appointment to the medical staff is a formal process outlined in the hospital's medical staff bylaws. The medical staff use a framework of self-governance, which represents the strong tradition of physician independence. The medical staff are formally accountable to the board. Lines of communication to the CEO and the board of trustees are established through various committee representations.

A medical director or ***chief of staff*** heads the medical staff. In all but the smallest hospitals, medical staff are organizationally divided by major specialties into departments, such as anesthesiology, internal medicine, obstetrics and gynecology, orthopedic surgery, pathology, cardiology, and radiology. A ***chief of service***, such as chief of cardiology, heads each specialty.

The medical staff generally have their own executive committee that sets general policies and is the main decision-making body in medical matters. Other medical staff committees, such as the following, are common to most hospitals. The ***credentials committee*** grants and reviews admitting privileges for those already credentialed and for new doctors whose skills are yet untested. The ***medical records committee*** ensures that accurate documentation is maintained on the entire regimen of care given to each patient. This committee also oversees confidentiality issues related to medical records. The ***utilization review committee*** performs routine checks to ensure that inpatient placements, as well as the length of stay, are clinically appropriate. The ***infection control committee*** is responsible for reviewing policies and procedures for minimizing infections in the hospital (Griffith 1995; Rakich et al. 1992). The ***quality improvement committee*** is responsible for overseeing the program for continuous quality improvement.

Licensure, Certification, and Accreditation

A license to operate a certain number of hospital beds is a basic regulatory requirement. State governments oversee the ***licensure*** of health care facilities, and each state sets its own standards for licensure. All facilities must be licensed to operate, but they do not have to be certified or accredited. Licensure is generally carried out by a state's department of health. State licensure standards strongly emphasize the physical plant's compliance with building codes, fire safety, climate control, space allocations, and sanitation. Minimum standards are also established for equipment and personnel. Generally, state licensure is not directly tied to the quality of care a health care facility actually delivers.

Certification entitles a hospital to participate in Medicare and Medicaid. Legislation in 1972 mandated federal oversight of hospitals if they wished to admit Medicare and Medicaid patients. The Department of Health and Human Services (DHHS) developed standards called ***conditions of participation***. The purpose of the hospital conditions of participation is to protect patient health and safety and help assure that quality care is furnished to all hospital patients. Hospitals must meet the conditions of participation in order to participate in Medicare or Medicaid. Conditions, as currently revised, are intended to focus primarily on the actual quality of care furnished to patients and the outcomes of that care. Actual compliance with the standards is verified through periodic inspections by each state's department of health.

In contrast with licensure and certification, which are government regulatory mechanisms, ***accreditation*** is a private mechanism designed to assure that accredited health care facilities meet certain basic standards. Seeking accreditation is voluntary, but the passage of Medicare in 1965 specified that accredited facilities were eligible for purposes of Medicare reimbursement. Accreditation of a hospital by the Joint Commission on Accreditation of Healthcare Organizations (JCAHO) confers ***deemed status*** on the hospital, meaning the hospital has deemed to have met Medicare and Medicaid certification standards. Thus, an accredited hospital does not need to go through the certification process. Private organizations that have been approved by the Centers for Medicare and Medicaid Services to confer deemed status are said to have "deeming authority." In addition to JCAHO, the American Osteopathic Association also has deeming authority to accredit hospitals.

The American College of Surgeons (ACS) began surveying hospitals in 1918 and established the hospital standardization program after it was recommended that a system of standardization of hospital equipment and hospital wards be developed. Until 1951, the ACS single-handedly worked to improve hospital-based medical practice. This effort evolved into the formation of the Joint Commission on Accreditation of Hospitals, a private nonprofit body formed in 1951 by joint effort of the ACS, the American College of Physicians, the AHA, and the AMA. The organization changed its name in 1987 to the Joint Commission on Accreditation of Healthcare Organizations (JCAHO), which more accurately describes the variety of health facilities it accredits.

The Joint Commission sets standards and accredits most of the nation's hospitals, as well as many of the long-term care facilities, psychiatric hospitals, substance abuse programs, outpatient surgery centers, urgent care clinics, group practices, community health centers, hospices, and home health agencies. Other private organizations also have deeming authority for some of these facilities. Different sets of standards apply to each category of health care organization. Some facilities, such as nursing homes, do not receive deemed status as a result of accreditation, and must also be certified by DHHS to receive Medicare and Medicaid reimbursement. Over the years, JCAHO has refined its accreditation standards and process of verifying compliance. In 2006, JCAHO has moved from scheduled to unannounced inspections with the objective that hospitals will attempt to be in compliance with all the standards all the time.

Ethical and Legal Issues in Patient Care

Ethical issues arise in all types of health services organizations, but the most significant ones occur in acute-care hospitals. Increasing levels of technology create situations requiring decision making under complex circumstances. For example, life-sustaining therapies in intensive care and dealing with life and death issues commonly raise ethical concerns. Ethical issues also arise in health care research and in experimental medicine. In management, ethical conduct becomes important when competition is intense or when cost cutting becomes necessary to save an organization from bankruptcy.

Ethics Principles

Ethics requires judgment. Clear-cut rules are often not available. Hence, medical practitioners and managers generally have to rely on certain well-established principles as guides to ethical decision making.

Four important principles of ethics are respect for others, beneficence, nonmaleficence, and justice. The principle of respect for others has four elements: autonomy, truth-telling, confidentiality, and fidelity. Autonomy allows people to govern themselves by choosing and pursuing a course of action without external coercion. In health care delivery, it refers to patient empowerment: obtain consent for treatment, explain the various treatment alternatives, allow the patient to participate in decision making and selection of treatment options, and treat the patient with respect and dignity. Constant tension exists between autonomy and paternalism, the view that someone else must direct what the patient must undergo without the patient's involvement. Truth-telling requires a caregiver to be honest. This principle often needs to be balanced with nonmaleficence because a tension is created when truth-telling would result in harm to the patient. The principle of confidentiality sometimes comes into conflict when the legal system requires disclosure of patient information. Fidelity means performing one's duty, keeping one's word, and keeping promises.

In a general sense, the principle of beneficence implies that all individuals have some moral obligation to benefit others. A health services organization is ethically obligated to do all it can to alleviate suffering caused by ill health and injury. This obligation includes providing the needy with certain types of services, such as emergency department services.

The principle of nonmaleficence implies that people have a moral obligation not to harm others, but many health care interventions, including certain preventive measures, such as immunization, often carry risks. Hence, in health care, nonmaleficence requires that the potential benefits from medical treatment sufficiently outweigh the potential harm.

The principle of justice encompasses fairness and equality. It denounces discrimination in the delivery of health care.

Legal Rights

Ethical concerns are often triggered in decisions related to informed consent and continuation of life support services to terminally ill patients. One of the most critical decisions relates to patient competency and the right to refuse treatment. Although the right of competent patients to refuse medical care is well established, the desires of incompetent or comatose patients present ethical challenges. Unless such patients have expressed their wishes in advance, family members or legal guardians end up making decisions regarding sustained medical treatment, or state laws may govern such decisions. Medical and legal experts and family members may differ, often bitterly, on the controversial issue of withdrawing nutrition and other life support means for dying patients, as the case of Theresa Schiavo, which made national news in 2004, demonstrated in the state of Florida. However, certain legal mechanisms have been established to deal with the issues of patients' rights.

Bill of Rights and Informed Consent

The Patient Self-Determination Act of 1990 applies to all health care facilities participating in Medicare or Medicaid. The law requires hospitals and other facilities to provide all patients, on admission, with information on patients' rights. Most hospitals and other inpatient institutions have developed what is referred to as the ***patient's bill of rights***. This document reflects the law concerning issues such as confidentiality and consent. Other rights include the right to make decisions regarding medical care, to be informed about diagnosis and treatment, to refuse treatment, and to formulate advance directives.

Based on the principle of autonomy, ***informed consent*** is a fundamental patient right. It refers to the patient's right to make an informed choice regarding medical treatment. The current climate in medical ethics supports honest and complete disclosure of medical information. In 1972, the Board of Trustees of the American Hospital Association affirmed a Patient's Bill of Rights, which states that the patient has the right to obtain from his physician complete current information concerning his diagnosis, treatment, and prognosis in terms the patient can be reasonably expected to understand (Rosner 2004). Informed consent is customarily obtained via a signature on preprinted forms and becomes part of the patient's medical record.

Some of these principles are being incorporated in provider mindsets and organizational culture that has been referred to as ***patient-centered care***. Patients' involvement in their treatment, grounding treatment decisions in patients' preferences, and creating a caregiving environment in which staff solicit patients' inputs and patients' need for information and education collectively promote patient-centered care (Cross 2004).

Advance Directives

Advance directives refer to the patient's wishes regarding continuation or withdrawal of treatment when the patient lacks decision-making capacity. Advance directives are intended to ensure that the patient's end-of-life wishes are carried out.

Three types of advance directives are in common use: do-not-resuscitate orders, living wills, and durable powers of attorney. A ***do-not-resuscitate order*** directs medical caregivers not to administer any artificial means to resuscitate the person when his or her heart or breathing stops. It is based on the theory that a patient may prefer to die rather than live when strong odds are against a good quality of life after cardiopulmonary resuscitation because severe disabilities would likely remain. A ***living will*** communicates a patient's wishes regarding medical treatment when he or she is unable to make decisions due to terminal illness or incapacitation. The main drawback of a living will is that it is general in nature because it cannot possibly cover all possible situations. A ***durable power of attorney*** for health care is a written legal document in which the patient appoints another individual to act as the patient's agent for purposes of health care decision making in the event that the patient is unable or unwilling to make such decisions. Although a durable power of attorney can cover most circumstances, its main drawback is that the appointed person may not act in the same manner in which the patient would have acted had he or she remained competent.

Mechanisms for Ethical Decision Making

Many health care organizations, especially large acute care hospitals, have ***ethics committees*** charged with developing guidelines and standards for ethical decision making in the delivery of health care (Paris 1995). Ethics committees are also responsible for resolving issues related to medical ethics. Such committees are multidisciplinary, involving physicians, nurses, clergy, social workers, legal experts, ethicists, and administrators.

Although physicians and other caregivers have moral responsibilities on the clinical side, the health care executive who leads the health services organization must also assume the role of a moral agent. As a ***moral agent***, the manager morally affects and is morally affected by actions taken. Although executives are entrusted with the fiduciary responsibility to act prudently in managing the affairs of the organization, their responsibilities to patients must take precedence. In governing the affairs of an organization, health care executives must also recognize that ethics is much more than obeying the law. The law represents only the minimum standard of morality established by society. Similarly, health care professionals who deliver care must recognize that even though they are bound by the law, they also have a higher calling, one that includes numerous positive duties to patients and society, and to each other (Darr 1991).

Hospitals and Public Trust

Well-run hospitals are generally regarded with pride by their communities. If a hospital's mission is to benefit the community, then it should be viewed as a community asset regardless of whether it is investor owned or nonprofit. When such a viewpoint is lost, and hospital governance starts placing other priorities ahead of its primary responsibility to serve the community, a breach of public trust can ensue, which sometimes can be irreparable. This balance is one of the greatest challenges hospitals have faced in recent years. As business enterprises, hospitals must respond to economic changes and must maintain their financial and operational integrity. The real danger occurs when these factors are put above a genuine concern for the welfare of the patients and the community. Because hospitals form the institutional hub of health care delivery, their integrity within the system is crucial.

At times, a relentless pursuit of profits and a disconnect from their communities may have blinded management to their institutions' primary mission. For example, a 2004 AHA-sponsored survey found that 60 percent of the people did not completely trust hospitals, and 55 percent feared that they would be harmed during a hospital stay (King 2006). In addition to people's apprehensions about quality of care and patient safety, the public's trust has been eroded by reports of fraud as a number of hospitals and multihospital systems across the country have faced charges of Medicare fraud and abuse because of questionable billing and collection practices. Several hospitals have paid heavy fines, and some hospital executives have served jail sentences for fraud. Although most hospital executives are honest, the wide negative publicity generated by such reports influences the public's perception of hospitals. Rebuilding public trust in the face of scandals and negative press can squander resources that could be used for serving the communities.

Summary

Hospitals are institutions engaged primarily in the delivery of inpatient acute care services. However, they have increasingly branched out to provide postacute and outpatient services. Hospitals developed from the almshouses and pesthouses of the 18th and 19th centuries, and early hospitals mainly served a custodial function and provided services that were more akin to social welfare than to medicine. Taking care of the sick did not develop as a main function of hospitals until the late 19th century, when many of the almshouses were replaced by public hospitals to serve the poor. Voluntary hospitals were developed to serve all classes of people. The growth of medical science and technology made it necessary for physicians to use hospitals as the main venue for the practice of medicine and for training residents. Today, hospitals are at the heart of consolidation and diversification activities that aim to develop a full continuum of health care services.

The growth of hospitals occurred in conjunction with advances in science and medical technology, advances in medical education, the development of professional nursing, and the growth of health insurance. The Hill-Burton Act of 1946 stands as the greatest single factor contributing to the increase in nation's bed supply. The government played an equally important role in reducing inpatient utilization by means of the PPS implemented in 1983. The growth of managed care has been significant in reducing inpatient utilization during the 1990s. Some of the key measures of inpatient utilization are discharges, inpatient days, ALOS, capacity, average daily census, and occupancy rates.

Hospitals can be classified in numerous ways, and the various classification schemes help differentiate one hospital from another. Performance statistics by hospital type can help executives compare their hospital to others in the same category. Although most US hospitals are general community hospitals, various specialty hospitals treat specific types of patients or conditions. Teaching hospitals and academic medical centers play a leading role in graduate medical education. Church-affiliated hospitals are mostly voluntary community hospitals, but they serve a special purpose by emphasizing the sponsoring organization's dietary and spiritual aspects of health care. Osteopathic hospitals are also community general hospitals for the most part, with an emphasis on holistic medicine. Most public and voluntary hospitals are nonprofit. As such, these institutions enjoy some tax advantages. They are expected to provide charity care that is equivalent in value to the tax subsidies received; however, many nonprofit hospitals emulate the behavior of their for-profit counterparts, which has raised some concerns in the US Congress. Some nonprofit hospitals, on the other hand, are beginning to take their mission of service seriously and are finding creative ways to serve their communities.

Hospitals are among the most complex organizations to manage because of the numerous external stakeholders who must be satisfied, and because of hospitals' complex internal governance structure. Hospital organization is represented by a triad in which authority is shared by the board of trustees, the CEO, and the medical staff. The CEO must possess exceptional skills to manage the day-to-day operations while satisfying the demands of the board, the medical staff, and the external stakeholders. Hospital administrators have been under growing pressure to handle the issues of resource allocation, cost containment, and uncompensated care.

A hospital cannot operate unless it is licensed by the state in which it is located. To participate in Medicare and Medicaid, a hospital must also be certified by the DHHS. Certification is maintained by satisfying the conditions of participation. As an alternative to certification, a hospital can voluntarily apply for accreditation by the Joint Commission. Accreditation confers deemed status on a hospital, which exempts the hospital from Medicare and Medicaid certification.

Ethical decision making has been a special area of concern for hospitals. From a medical standpoint, ethical issues often pertain to patient privacy, confidentiality, informed consent, and end-of-life treatment. Bills of rights and advance directives are two of the legal means to address these issues. Active ethics committees must continually address the development of policies and standards for clinicians and administrators. These same multidisciplinary committees also deal with ethical problems as they arise.

Communities usually trust their hospitals, but the behavior of some institutions has called this trust into question. When hospitals fail to be accountable to their communities and when insurance fraud and abuse emerge, the negative repercussions tend to last for years.

Test Your Understanding

Terminology

academic medical center
accreditation
advance directives
average daily census
average length of stay
board of trustees
certification
chief of service
chief of staff
community hospital
conditions of participation
credentials committee
Critical Access Hospital
days of care
deemed status
discharge
do-not-resuscitate orders
durable power of attorney
ethics committee
executive committee
general hospital
hospital
infection control committee
informed consent
inpatient
inpatient day
investor-owned hospital
licensure
living will
long-term care hospital
medical records committee
medical staff committee
moral agent

occupancy rate
osteopathic medicine
patient-centered care
patient's bill of rights
proprietary hospital
public hospital
quality improvement committee
rehabilitation hospital
rural hospital
short-stay hospital
specialty hospital
swing bed
teaching hospital
urban hospital
utilization review committee
voluntary hospital

Review Questions

1. What is the difference between inpatient and outpatient services?
2. As hospitals evolved from rudimentary custodial and quarantine facilities to their current state, how did they change in their purpose and function?
3. What were the main factors responsible for the growth of hospitals until the latter part of the 20th century?
4. Name the three main forces that have been responsible for hospital downsizing. How has each of these forces been responsible for the decline in inpatient hospital utilization?
5. What is a voluntary hospital? Explain. How did voluntary hospitals evolve in the United States?
6. Discuss the role of government in the growth as well as the decline of hospitals in the United States.
7. What are inpatient days? What is the significance of this measure?
8. How does hospital utilization vary according to a person's age, gender, and race?
9. Discuss the different types of public hospitals and the roles they play in the delivery of health care services in the United States.
10. What are some of the differences between voluntary and investor-owned hospitals?
11. What is a long-term care hospital (LTCH)? What role does it play in health care delivery in the United States?
12. The table below gives some operational statistics for two hospitals located in the same community. Answer the questions following the table.

Calendar Year 2006	Nonprofit Community Hospital (A)	Proprietary Community Hospital (B)
Number of beds in operation	320	240
Total discharges	12,051	9,230
Medicare	5,130	3,876
Medicaid	3,565	2,118
Private insurance	3,356	3,236

Calendar Year 2006	Nonprofit Community Hospital (A)	Proprietary Community Hospital (B)
Total hospital days	72,421	51,684
Medicare	36,935	26,359
Medicaid	23,175	12,921
Private insurance	12,311	12,404
Total inpatient revenues	$45,755,000	$35,800,000
Dollar value of charity care	$5,000,000	$3,500,000

(a) Calculate the following measures for each hospital (wherever appropriate, calculate the measure for each pay type). Discuss the meaning and significance of each measure, and point out the differences between the two hospitals.

(1) Hospital capacity

(2) ALOS

(3) Occupancy rate

(b) Operationally, which hospital is performing better? Why?

(c) Do you think the nonprofit hospital is meeting its service obligations to the community in exchange for its tax-exempt status? Please give reasons for your answer.

(d) Do you think the hospitals have a problem with excess capacity? If so, what would you recommend?

13. Why have physicians developed their own specialty hospitals? What legal issues can likely arise when physicians have an ownership interest in a hospital?
14. What criteria does Medicare use to classify a hospital as a rehabilitation hospital?
15. How do you differentiate between a community hospital and a non-community hospital?
16. What is a Critical Access Hospital (CAH)? Why was this designation created?
17. What are some of the main differences between teaching and nonteaching hospitals?
18. Can church-affiliated hospitals be classified as voluntary hospitals? Please explain.
19. Discuss some of the issues relative to the tax-exempt status of nonprofit hospitals. If you were a member of the board of trustees of a nonprofit hospital, what would you recommend such a hospital do to justify its nonprofit status?
20. Why are hospitals among the most complex organizations to manage?
21. Discuss the governance of a modern hospital.
22. In the context of hospitals, what is the difference between licensure, certification, and accreditation?
23. What can a hospital do to address some of the difficult ethical problems relative to end-of-life treatment?
24. What can hospitals do to maintain the public's trust?

REFERENCES

American Hospital Association. 1990. *Hospital statistics 1990–1991 edition*. Chicago.

American Hospital Association. 1994. *AHA guide to the health care field 1994 edition*. Chicago.

Anderson, K., and B. Wootton. 1991. Changes in hospital staffing patterns. *Monthly Labor Review* 114, no. 3: 3–9.

Anonymous. 2002. Nearly half of US public hospitals had negative margins in 2000. *Healthcare Financial Management* 56, no. 9: 22–23.

Appleby, J. 2004. IRS looking closely at what non-profits pay. *USA Today*, September 30, 2004, p. 02b.

Arndt, M., and B. Bigelow. 2006. Toward the creation of an institutional logic for the management of hospitals: Efficiency in the early nineteen hundreds. *Medical Care Research and Review* 63, no. 3: 369–394.

Association of American Medical Colleges (AAMC). 2003. *Teaching hospitals. http://www.aamc.org/teachinghospitals.htm*.

Balotsky, E.R. 2005. Is it resources, habit or both: interpreting twenty years of hospital strategic response to prospective payment. *Health Care Management Review* 30, no. 4: 337–346.

Bazzoli, G.J. et al. 2006. Construction activity in US hospitals. *Health Affairs* 25, no. 3: 783–791.

Bresnohan, J.F., and J.F. Drane. 1986. A challenge to examine the meaning of living and dying. *Health Progress* 67: 32–37, 98.

Clement, J.P., and K.L. Grazier. 2001. HMO penetration: Has it hurt public hospitals? *Journal of Health Care Finance* 28, no. 1: 25–38.

Cross, G.M. 2004. What does patient-centered care mean for the VA? *Forum* (November 2004), Academy Health.

Dalton, M.J. 1995. Inpatient hospital reimbursement. In *Health care administration: Principles, practices, structure, and delivery*. 2nd ed., ed. L.F. Wolper, 166–191. Gaithersburg, MD: Aspen Publishers, Inc.

Darr, K. 1991. *Ethics in health services management*. 2nd ed. Baltimore, MD: Health Professions Press.

D'Cruz, M.J., and T.L. Welter. 2005. No small change: Payment trends call for big preparations for 2006. *Healthcare Financial Management* 59, no. 12: 50–60.

DelliFraine, J.L. 2006. Communities with and without children's hospitals: Where do the sickest children receive care? *Hospital Topics* 84, no. 3: 19–26.

Department of Health and Human Services (DHHS). 1999. *Health, United States, 1999*. Hyattsville, MD.

Department of Health and Human Services (DHHS). 2002. *Health, United States, 2002*. Hyattsville, MD.

Department of Health and Human Services (DHHS). 2006. *Health, United States, 2006*. Hyattsville, MD.

Feldstein, M. 1971. *The rising cost of hospital care*. Washington, DC: Information Resource Press.

Feldstein, P.J. 1993. *Health care economics*. 4th ed. Albany, NY: Delmar Publishers.

Griffith, J.R. 1995. *The well-managed health care organization*. Ann Arbor, MI: AUPHA Press/Health Administration Press.

Grimaldi, P.L. 2002. Inpatient rehabilitation facilities are now paid prospective rates. *Journal of Health Care Finance* 28, no. 3: 32–48.

Guterman, S. 2006. Specialty hospitals: A problem or a symptom? *Health Affairs* 25, no. 1: 95–105.

Haglund, C.L., and W.L. Dowling. 1993. The hospital. In *Introduction to health services*. 4th ed., eds. S.J. Williams and P.R. Torrens, 135–176. Albany, NY: Delmar Publishers.

Harrison, J.P. et al. 2003. A profile of hospital acquisitions. *Journal of Healthcare Management* 48, no. 3: 156–170.

HCIA Inc. and Deloitte & Touche. 1997. *The comparative performance of US hospitals: The sourcebook*. Baltimore, MD: HCIA Inc.

Health Forum. 2001. *AHA guide to the health care field. 2001–2002 edition*. Chicago: Health Forum.

Hoechst Marion Roussel. 1999. *Managed care digest series 1999: Institutional digest*. Kansas City, MO: Hoechst Marion Roussel, Inc.

Iglehart, J.K. 2006. U.S. hospitals: Examining their fraying social contract. *Health Affairs* 25, no. 1: 8–9.

Kahl, A., and D.E. Clark. 1986. Employment in health services: Long-term trends and projections. *Monthly Labor Review*, August, 28.

King, J.G. 2006. Strong public trust is the key to a successful future for every hospital. *AHA News* 42, no. 11: 4–5.

Longest, B.B., and C.J. Lin. 2005. Can nonprofit hospitals do both well and good? *Health Care Management Review* 30, no. 1: 62–68.

Mantone, J. 2005. Critical time at rural hospitals. *Modern Healthcare* 35, no. 10: 22.

Mechanic, D. 1998. Emerging trends in mental health policy and practice. *Health Affairs* 17, no. 6: 82–98.

MedPAC (Medicare Payment Advisory Commission). 2004. *New Approaches in Medicare : Report to the Congress*. Washington DC: Medicare Payment Advisory Commission.

Muller, R.W. 2003. The changing American hospital in the twenty-first century. *Policy Brief No. 26/2003*. Syracuse, NY: Center for Policy Research, Syracuse University.

Newman, J.F. et al. 2001. CEO performance appraisal: Review and recommendations. *Journal of Healthcare Management* 46, no. 1: 21–37.

Nudelman, P.M., and L.M. Andrews. 1996. The "value added" or not-for-profit health plans. *New England Journal of Medicine* 334, no. 16: 1057–1059.

O'Connell, L., and S.L. Brown. 2003. Do nonprofit HMOs eliminate racial disparities in cardiac care? *Journal of Healthcare Finance* 30, no. 2: 84–94.

Owens, B. 2005. The plight of the not-for-profit. *Journal of Healthcare Management* 50, no. 4: 237–250.

Paris, M. 1995. The medical staff. In *Health care administration: Principles, practices, structure, and delivery*. 2nd ed., ed. L.F. Wolper, 32–46. Gaithersburg, MD: Aspen Publishers, Inc.

Patrick, V. et al. 2006. Facilitating discharge in state psychiatric institutions: A group intervention strategy. *Psychiatric Rehabilitation Journal* 29, no. 3: 183–188.

Pfizer Inc. 2003. *Utilization of Veterans Affairs Medical Care Services by United States Veterans*. New York, NY: Pfizer Inc.

Raffel, M.W. 1980. *The US health system: Origins and functions*. New York: John Wiley and Sons.

Raffel, M.W., and N.K. Raffel. 1994. *The US health system: Origins and functions*. 4th ed. Albany, NY: Delmar Publishers.

Rakich, J.S. et al. 1992. *Managing health services organizations*. 3rd ed. Baltimore, MD: Health Professions Press.

Reinhardt, U.E. et al. 2002. Cross-national comparisons of health systems using OECD data, 1999. *Health Affairs* 21, no. 3: 169–181.

Robbins, J.V. 2002. Beyond the walls. *Hospitals & Health Networks* 76, no. 7: 28.

Roemer, M.I. 1961. Bed supply and hospital utilization: A natural experiment. *Hospitals* 35, no. 21: 36–42.

Rosner, F. 2004. Informing the patient about a fatal disease: From paternalism to autonomy—The Jewish view. *Cancer Investigation* 22, no. 6: 949–953.

Safety net in shreds. 2002. *Trustee* (Oct 2002) 55, no. 9: 3.

Sanofi-Aventis. 2007. *Managed care digest series, 2007: Hospital/systems digest*. Bridgewater, NJ: Sanofi-Aventis US, LLC.

Sinay, T. 2005. Cost structure of osteopathic hospitals and their local counterparts in the USA: Are they any different? *Social Science and Medicine* 60, no. 8: 1805–1814.

Sloan, F.A. 1998. Commercialism in nonprofit hospitals. *Journal of Policy Analysis and Management* 17, no. 2: 234–252.

Slusky, R. 2006. An investment in rural hospitals is an investment in healthier communities. *AHA News* 42, no. 5: 4–5.

Snook, I.D. 1981. *Hospitals: What they are and how they work*. Rockville, MD: Aspen Systems Corporation.

Snyder, J. 2003. Specialty hospitals on rise: Facilities source of controversy. *The Arizona Republic*, February 23, 2003.

Stewart, D.A. 1973. The history and status of proprietary hospitals. *Blue Cross Reports—Research Series 9*. Chicago: Blue Cross Association.

Strunk, B.C. et al. 2006. The effect of population aging on future hospital demand. *Health Affairs* 25, no. 3: w141–149.

Stuart, B. et al. 2006. Financial consequences of rural hospital long-term care strategies. *Health Care Management Review* 31, no. 2: 145–155.

Teisberg, E.D. et al. 1991. *The hospital sector in 1992*. Boston: Harvard Business School.

Thorpe, K.E. et al. 2000. Hospital conversions, margins, and the provision of uncompensated care. *Health Affairs* 19, no. 6: 187–194.

US Census Bureau. 2002. *Statistical abstract of the United States, 2002*.

US Census Bureau. 2007. *Statistical abstract of the United States, 2007*.

Vogt, W.B., and R. Town. 2006. *How has hospital consolidation affected the price and quality of hospital care?* Princeton, NJ: The Robert Wood Johnson Foundation.

Williams, S.J. 1995. *Essentials of health services*. Albany, NY: Delmar Publishers.

Wilson, F.A., and D. Neuhauser. 1985. *Health services in the United States*. 2nd ed. Cambridge, MA: Ballinger Publishing Co.

Wolfson, J., and S.L. Hopes. 1994. What makes tax-exempt hospitals special? *Healthcare Financial Management*, July, 56–60.

Zeber, J.E. et al. 2004. Serious mental illness and aging with the veteran population. http://www.hsrd.research.va.gov/meetings/2003/abstracts/2004.htm

Zimmerman, E. 2006. The implications of reimbursement changes for specialty hospitals. *Healthcare Financial Management* 60, no. 7: 42–45.

Chapter 9

Managed Care and Integrated Organizations

Learning Objectives

- To review the link between the development of managed care and earlier organizational entities in the US health care delivery system
- To grasp the basic concepts of managed care and how managed care organizations realize cost savings
- To distinguish between the main types of managed care organizations
- To examine the different models under which health maintenance organizations are organized and to understand the advantages and disadvantages of each model
- To understand the concept of integration and the formation of integrated health care delivery systems
- To explore current trends and issues in managed care and integration of services

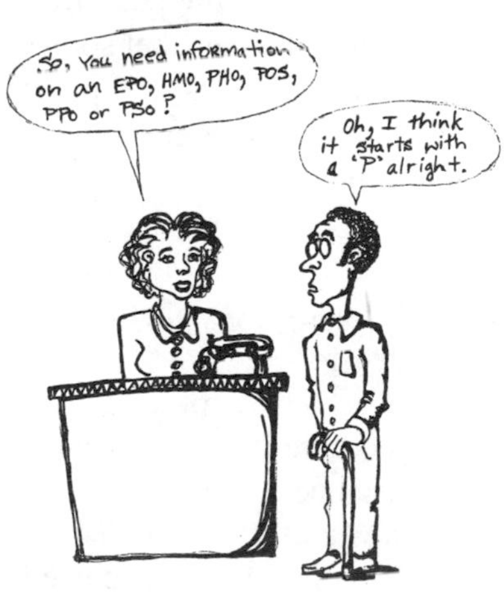
So, You need information on an EPO, HMO, PHO, POS, PPO or PSO?
Oh, I think it starts with a 'P' alright.

Introduction

Managed care has been the single most dominant force that has fundamentally transformed the delivery of health care in the United States since the 1990s. At first, some observers had viewed the managed care phenomenon as an aberration. But, as private employers began to realize cost savings, and public policymakers and administrators saw the opportunity to slow down the growing expense of providing health care through the Medicare and Medicaid programs, they increasingly turned to managed care. For now, managed care has become firmly entrenched in the United States. Health care systems in other countries are also evaluating or adopting certain features of managed care as they reform their own systems of health care delivery.

In the United States, transition to managed care was found necessary as employers grappled with the unaffordable excesses of unrestrained delivery of services that led to spiraling health insurance premiums. In the fee-for-service system that prevailed prior to managed care, insurance companies had no incentive to manage the delivery of services and how the providers should be paid. With no controls on delivery and payment, costs got out of hand. The only way to control runaway costs was to integrate delivery and payment with the other two functions of financing and insurance. This integration of functions was accomplished through managed care. Figure 9–1 illustrates the extent to which employer-sponsored health insurance has shifted from traditional fee-for-service to managed care.

Like any new endeavor, managed care has undergone growing pains. For instance, it has undergone attacks by physicians and consumers. It has faced increasing regulation from policymakers. Consequently, tight controls were relaxed, and recently, there has been a resurgence in the growth of health insurance premiums and health care expenditures in general. Now, the long-term ability of managed care to control health care costs has been called into question. Managed care is facing the challenge of how to further manage cost escalations in hospital care, prescription drugs, and other areas of health care. The US health care delivery system will no doubt continue to evolve, but managed care is likely to remain its central feature.

Professional dominance in health care delivery had long favored the supply side of the market equation. With the growth of managed care, the balance swung toward the demand side. This occurred in two ways: (1) Employers became active purchasers of health insurance with numerous managed care choices available. (2) Managed care, both directly and indirectly, purchased services from providers and wielded enormous buying power. Market forces have attempted to bring about a better equilibrium between health care providers and managed care companies, and have given rise to new organizational arrangements. The many choices in managed care plans and the new types of organizations are commonly recognized by their acronyms, giving rise to a veritable "alphabet soup."

By prompting organizational integration, managed care has literally transformed America's health care delivery landscape. During the 1990s and early 2000s, there was a wave of hospital mergers and acquisitions, a phenomenon that was national in scope. Hospital CEOs generally cited the potential for efficiency gains and strengthening of their financial positions as the main reasons that spurred integration (Williams et al. 2006). This wave of organizational integration occurred simultaneously with the growing power of managed care. True, there

Figure 9–1 Percentage of Enrollment in Managed Care Plans Compared to Traditional Fee-for-Service Plans.

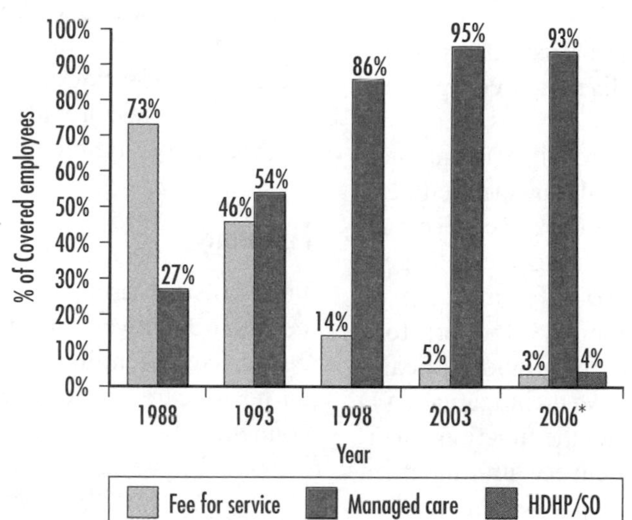

*In 2006, the survey started to include High Deductible Health Plans paired with a savings option (HDHP/SO), [discussed in Chapter 14].

Source: Data from *Employer Health Benefits: 2003 Annual Survey; Employer Health Benefits: 2006 Annual Survey;* The Henry J. Kaiser Family Foundation and Health Research and Educational Trust.

can be numerous reasons why health care organizations have consolidated, such as technology, effects of reimbursement, availability of services in alternative delivery settings, etc. But, the role of managed care cannot be dismissed. For instance, there is some evidence that hospitals gained increased pricing power over managed care organizations subsequent to consolidations (Capps and Dranove 2004). Hence, it can be argued that various types of organizational consolidations were driven at least in part as a response to the growing power of managed care which had a significant negative impact on the utilization of hospital capacity, and consequently, on the financial performance of hospitals. Ginsburg (2005) reached the same conclusion: "Hospitals correctly perceived that by merging with others in the same community, they would increase their leverage with health plans (managed care plans)" (p. 1514).

On the other hand, the managed care industry itself has consolidated by absorbing weaker competitors. The industry now comprises four national plans (United, WellPoint, Aetna, and CIGNA); state-specific Blue Cross and Blue Shield plans; a few regional for-profit plans (such as Humana, HealthNet, and Coventry); and, in some markets, regional nonprofit plans (such as Kaiser Permanente, Tufts Health Plan, and HealthPartners) (Robinson 2006).

Organizational alliances and networks are referred to as integrated delivery systems (IDSs) in this book. These systems are also called "health care systems," "integrated service networks," "integrated health networks," "integrated delivery networks," or "integrated provider networks." Organized networks differ by the degree of integration, but no standard method of classification captures the numerous variations.

What Is Managed Care?

Managed care can be defined as an organized approach to delivering a comprehensive array of health care services to a group of enrolled members through efficient management of services needed by the members, and negotiation of prices or payment arrangements with providers. Managed care is generally discussed in two different contexts. First, and more commonly, it refers to a mechanism or process of providing health care services and has two main features: (1) Managed care integrates the functions of financing, insurance, delivery, and payment within one organizational setting (Figure 9–2). (2) Managed care exercises formal control over utilization. Second, the term "managed care" can refer to a managed care organization (MCO), which can take a variety of forms that are discussed later in this chapter. In this context, managed care is an organization that delivers health care services without using an insurance company to manage risk and without using a third-party administrator to make payments. For the delivery of services, an MCO can use its own staff, outside providers on contract with the MCO, or a combination of the two.

Financing

Premiums are based on contract negotiations between employers and the MCO. Generally, a fixed premium per enrollee includes all health care services provided for in the contract.

Insurance

The MCO functions like an insurance company by assuming all risk. In other words, it takes the financial responsibility if the total cost of services provided exceeds the revenue from fixed premiums. MCOs retain approximately 17 to 20% of the premium dollar

Figure 9–2 Integration of Health Care Delivery Functions through Managed Care.

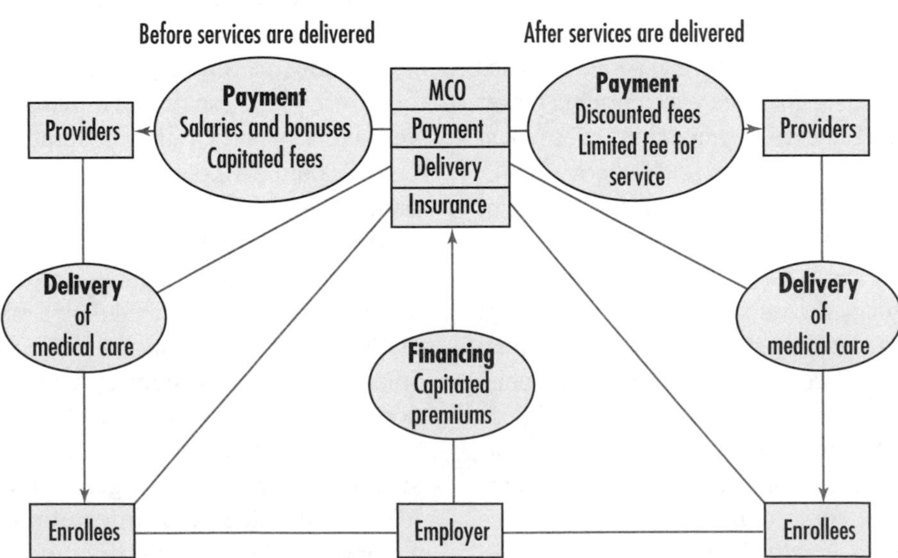

to manage risk and to cover administrative expenses. The rest is spent on health care services (Figure 9–3)* (see medical loss ratio in Chapter 6).

MCOs have successfully competed with traditional insurance plans by offering lower premiums and more comprehensive services. Whereas traditional insurance plans pay for services only when a person becomes sick or develops a condition requiring medical evaluation and treatment, MCOs have generally included regular physical examinations to keep people healthy.

Figure 9–3 Allocation of Premiums for Insurance and Health Services.

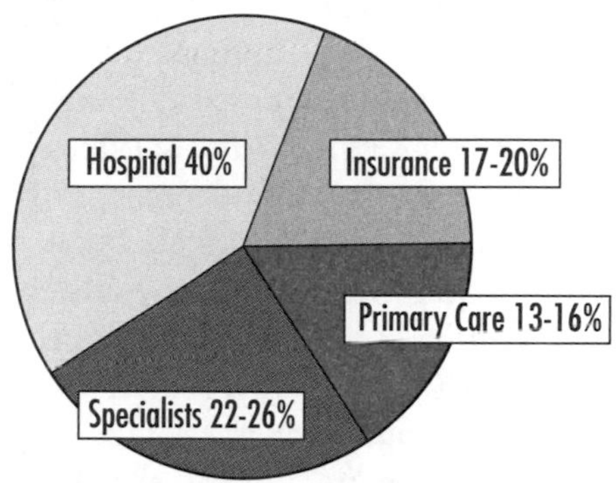

Source: Data from W.A. Zelman, *The Changing Health Care Marketplace: Private Ventures, Public Interests,* p. 55, © 1996, Jossey-Bass Publishers.

Delivery

The MCO promises to provide a comprehensive set of services, including preventive services, ambulatory care, inpatient care, surgery, and rehabilitative services. In an ideal scenario, an MCO would operate its own hospitals and outpatient clinics and employ its own physicians. Many MCOs actually do employ their own physicians on salary. Some large MCOs have concluded mergers with hospitals and/or group practices. Most MCOs, however, have established contracts with physicians, clinics, and hospitals. These providers operate independently but are linked to the MCO through contracts.

MCOs often follow a market strategy of building a broad geographic network in new markets. To enter widespread geographic markets, MCOs must win employer accounts to acquire more enrollees. To serve the medical needs of a geographically diverse population, MCOs contract with local providers already practicing in the various locales where the MCOs have employer contracts.

Payment

MCOs use three main types of payment arrangements with providers: capitation, discounted fees, and salaries. The three methods allow risk sharing in varying degrees between the MCO and the providers. Risk sharing puts the burden on the providers to be cost conscious and to curtail unnecessary utilization. Sometimes, a limited amount of fee-for-service is used for specialized services.

Under ***capitation***, the provider is paid a fixed monthly sum per enrollee, often called per member per month (PMPM) payment. The provider receives the capitated fee per enrollee, regardless of whether the enrollee uses health care services and regardless of the quantity of services used. The provider is responsible for furnishing all needed health care services determined to be medically necessary. Thus, under capitation, risk is shifted from the MCO to the provider. Capitation is the antithesis of fee-for-service,

*Feldstein (1994) provides a rough allocation of 15% for insurance and administration, 40% for facilities (hospitals, outpatient surgery centers, and nursing homes), 40% for physicians, and 5% for pharmacy and ancillary services.

in which the provider can bill separately for each service provided.

The second type of payment arrangement used by MCOs is discounted fees. This arrangement can be regarded as a modified form of fee-for-service. After services have been delivered, the provider can bill the MCO for each service separately but is paid according to a prenegotiated schedule called a ***fee schedule***. In this case, risk is borne by the MCO, but the MCO can lower its costs by paying discounted rates. Providers agree to discount their regular fees in exchange for the volume of business the MCO brings them.

A third method of payment is salaries, which are often coupled with bonuses or withholdings. In this case, the provider is an employee of the MCO. The physicians, for instance, are paid fixed salaries. At the end of the year, a pool of money is distributed among the physicians in the form of bonuses based on various performance measures. From an economic perspective, the physicians are paid only partial compensation up front. The remainder is withheld and is paid on condition that certain performance standards are met. Hence, under this method of payment some risk is shifted from the MCO to the physicians.

It is important to note that cost containment is not the only objective managed care seeks to achieve, although the potential for cost containment has been the driving force behind the phenomenal growth of managed care. A survey of physicians and employers reported consensus of the two groups on seven essential features of managed care (Business Word Inc. 1996): cost containment, accountability for quality and cost, measurement of health outcomes and quality of care, health promotion and disease prevention programs, management of resource consumption, consumer education programs, and continuing quality improvement initiatives.

Evolution of Managed Care

The concept of managed care is not new, even though the widespread adoption of the concept is a more recent phenomenon. The principles on which managed care is based have been around for about a century (the prototypes of managed care are discussed in Chapter 3, and are summarized in the following section). The idea of managed care evolved from what the medical establishment pejoratively referred to as the corporate practice of medicine, referring to contract practice and prepaid group practice discussed in Chapter 3. Even before private health insurance became widespread, these practices were used sporadically as cost-effective means of providing health care services to certain groups of people. The subsequent health insurance model loosely retained the insurance and payment functions but abandoned the delivery function. It let the insured decide where they would receive health services. This fragmentation was strongly influenced by the medical establishment, which preferred the fee-for-service system. Managed care reemerged in the form of Health Maintenance Organizations (HMOs) when the HMO Act of 1973 required employers to offer an HMO alternative to conventional health insurance.

Conceptual Foundations of Managed Care

Private health insurance began as a prepaid plan at the Baylor Hospital in 1929. For a predetermined fixed fee per month, Baylor, and subsequently other hospitals, started providing inpatient services. Thus, the financial structure of the first health insurance plan was based on capitation. Because the hospital bore all risk, it virtually functioned as an insurance company, but hospital accountants were not adept at actuarial determination of risk. Within a few years, the insurance function was taken over by the Blue Cross Commission (which later became the Blue Cross Association). Even though, in this particular case, the idea of combining insurance and delivery under the same organizational entity did not last long, the concept had been born.

Contract practice takes the idea of capitation a step further by incorporating a defined group of enrollees. Here, an employer is the financier who contracts with one or more providers to furnish health care to a group of enrollees—the employees—at a predetermined fee per enrollee. Prepaid group practice goes another step. First, it preserves the principles of capitation, bearing of risk by the provider, and a defined group of enrollees whose health care contract is financed by their employers. It then adds the provision of comprehensive services.

The idea of prepaid group practice was adopted by early MCOs. To achieve greater cost-efficiency, various utilization control measures were adopted. Management of utilization is, in essence, the "managed" part of managed care. Later, MCOs adopted variations in payment and delivery mechanisms that gave rise to different forms of managed care plans and MCOs. The evolution of concepts that later culminated in the development of MCOs is summarized in Figure 9–4.

The First Prepaid Plans and the HMO Act

Prepaid group practice plans first became popular in some selected large urban markets in the United States. The AMA opposed the first plan, the Group Health Association of Washington (started in 1937 in Washington, DC), but the AMA was found guilty of restraint of trade in violating the Sherman Antitrust Act. This verdict may have been crucial in paving the way for the growth of other prepaid group practice plans. Notable among them are the Kaiser-Permanente Medical Care Program, started in 1942; the Group Health Cooperative of Puget Sound, opened in 1947; the Health Insurance Plan of Greater New York, started in 1947; and the Group Health Plan of Minneapolis, started in 1957 (MacLeod and Prussin 1973). The Health Insurance Plan of Greater New York became one of the most successful health insurance programs, providing comprehensive medical services through organized medical groups of family physicians and specialists, but it provided hospital insurance through Blue Cross. Kaiser-Permanente went a few steps further. It exercised control over hospitals by contracting their services; placed considerable emphasis on preventive medicine; and employed mechanisms, such as penalizing physicians, to curtail excessive use of hospital facilities (Mechanic 1972, 107; Raffel 1980, 415). In due course, Kaiser-Permanente became the model for HMOs.

The HMO Act of 1973 was passed during the Nixon administration with the objective of stimulating growth of HMOs by providing federal funds for the establishment and expansion of new HMOs (Wilson and Neuhauser 1985, 206). The underlying reason for supporting the growth of HMOs was the belief that prepaid medical care, as an alternative to traditional fee-for-service practice, would stimulate competition among health plans, enhance efficiency, and slow the rate of increase in health care expenditures. The HMO Act also required employers with 25 or more employees to offer an HMO alternative if one was available in their

Figure 9–4 The Evolution of Managed Care.

Health insurance	Capitation Bearing of risk by providers

Initially, health insurance combined the insurance, delivery, and payment functions of health care, as seen in the Baylor plan, but further evolution of this initial concept was thwarted by organized medicine. Contract practice moved toward the integration of these functions, bypassing the insurance companies.

Contract practice	Defined group of enrollees Capitation or salary Bearing of risk by providers
	↓
Prepaid group practice	Comprehensive services Defined group of enrollees Capitation Bearing of risk by providers
	↓
Managed care	Utilization controls Comprehensive services Defined group of enrollees Capitation, discounted fees, or salary Limited fee for service Limits on choice of providers Sharing of risk with providers Financial incentives to providers Accountability for plan performance

geographic area. The objective was to create 1,700 HMOs to serve 40 million members by 1976 (Iglehart 1994). However, the HMO Act failed to achieve its objective. By 1976, only 174 HMOs had formed, having an enrollment of 6 million (Public Health Service 1995, 242). In 1977, only 4% of those having job-based insurance were enrolled in managed care plans (Gabel 1999). By the end of the 1970s, enrollment in HMOs still remained below 10 million.

Alternative Forms of Managed Care

Competition among MCOs gave rise to new forms of managed care arrangements. Various MCO types resulted from the way they differentiated themselves by offering enrollees greater freedom to choose their providers, adopting variations in the methods of payment to providers, and using creative means of organizing medical care providers. Competition from commercial insurance companies led MCOs to adopt measures that would distinguish them as more cost-efficient. Thus, MCOs adopted various methods to control health care costs, active management of utilization being one such method.

Accreditation of Managed Care Organizations

Managed care has now become the primary vehicle for managing health care for a vast number of Americans. The National Committee for Quality Assurance (NCQA) began accrediting MCOs in 1991. Accreditation began in response to the demand for standardized, objective information about the quality of MCOs. At this point, participation in the accreditation program is voluntary, but about half of the plans are accredited. To be accredited, MCOs must comply with NCQA standards. Compliance is determined by a review process and evaluation by physicians and managed care experts. A national oversight committee of physicians supervises the process. Accreditation is combined with a rating system that has five status categories: excellent, commendable, accredited, provisional, and denied (NCQA 2007). At this point, the effects of accreditation on higher quality in health plans and on gaining market share appear to be mixed (Dean and Epstein 2002).

Growth of Managed Care

As mentioned earlier, the main impetus for managed care's growth was rapid cost escalations during the 1970s and 1980s under the dominant fee-for-service system. For example, in the 1980s, health insurance premiums rose on an average more than 12% annually. Managed care offered relief from a growing cost burden. Some evidence suggests that, at least initially, managed care was also in a position to take advantage of the weakened economic position of health care providers.

Flaws in Fee-for-Service

Uncontrolled Utilization

Under the former dominant fee-for-service practice of medicine, utilization of medical care and payment to providers were practically unrestricted. In a system dominated by specialists and an absence of primary care gatekeeping, patients were free to go to any provider. Care received from specialists and utilization of sophisticated technology gave patients the impression of high quality. Competition was driven by such impressions, rather than by cost. Physicians and hospitals competed for patients by offering the most up-to-date technologies and the most attractive practice settings (Wilkerson et al. 1997). Under the fee-for-service system, providers had an incentive to incur high utilization because they could increase their incomes by providing more services than medically necessary (provider-induced demand).

Uncontrolled Prices and Payment

In traditional health insurance, insurance companies had no responsibility to provide covered health services or to take responsibility for the quality of care and its cost. The insurance company exercised little control over the prices providers charged or patients' use of services. Providers set charges at artificially high levels. The provider billed insurance an item-by-item claim. The insurance company was merely a passive payer of claims—it paid what the providers billed, limited only by what the insurer deemed as usual, customary, and reasonable. The insurance company had little incentive to control costs because it could simply increase the premiums the following year based on utilization during the previous year.

Focus on Illness Rather Than Wellness

Conventional insurance paid for services only when a specific medical diagnosis was reported on the insurance claim. Visits for preventive checkups were not covered. The fee-for-service system presented a second and bigger problem. Traditional insurance provided more thorough coverage when a person was hospitalized. Also, the physician was paid for daily hospital visits when the patient was being treated in the hospital. Thus, it was more lucrative for the physician to put the patient in the hospital, and the patient received more comprehensive care (Mayer and Mayer 1984, 15–16).

Cost Appeal of Managed Care

Mainly due to the flaws in fee-for-service, health care delivery through conventional insurance led to rapid escalation of health care costs. Various methods of cost control were tried during the 1970s and 1980s, but they produced only limited results. At its inception, the concept of managed care was designed to compete against fee-for-service medicine. Up until the 1980s, HMOs were the predominant form of managed care. The price-based competition from HMOs was often referred to as "shadow pricing," in which HMOs would offer more benefits and somewhat lower premiums than fee-for-service plans (Zelman 1996, 2). However, at this stage, managed care plans had limited appeal. Individuals who were covered by insurance plans that allowed them to choose their own physician or hospital saw little benefit in joining a plan that would restrict these choices. Most providers also saw little benefit in joining an MCO that might restrict their potential income or alter their style of practice that would have external controls (Wilkerson et al. 1997). For the most part, employers remained passive.

Between 1980 and 1990, total cost of private health insurance on the average went up at an annual rate of over 12% (Figure 9–5). As premiums escalated unchecked, economic realities forced employers to make the transition from traditional insurance plans to managed care. Among the US population with employer-sponsored health insurance, the proportion of those enrolled in various managed care plans jumped from 27% in 1988 to 86% in 1998 and to 95% in 2003 (see Figure 9–1).

Weakened Economic Position of Providers

Indirectly, excess capacity in the health care delivery system may also have contributed to the growth of managed care (McGuire 1994). This was perhaps true initially because the Medicare prospective payment system, introduced in the mid-1980s, had a marked impact on hospital economics. Left with significant unused capacity in the form of empty beds, the bargaining power of hospitals was substantially weakened. Physicians initially showed great resistance to managed care, but as the financing of health care was quickly shifting toward managed care, they could no longer resist the growing momentum. In most cases, they were left with the choice of participating or being left out completely.

Figure 9–5 Growth in the Cost of Health Insurance (private employers), 1980–1995.

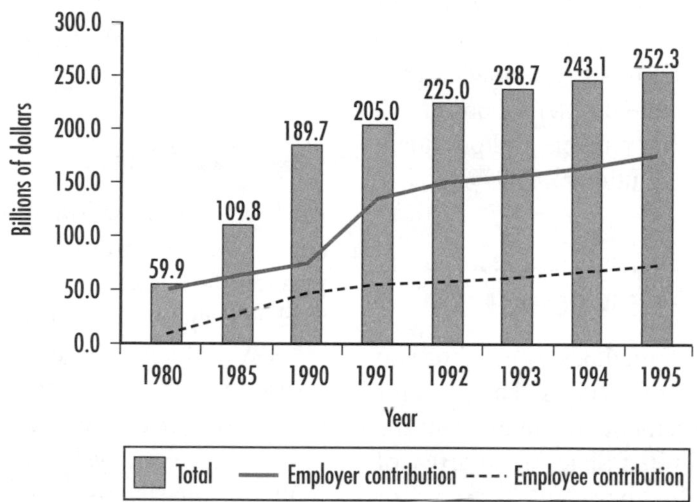

Source: Data from *Health, United States, 1998,* p. 348, National Center for Health Statistics.

Efficiencies and Inefficiencies in Managed Care

Managed care systems offer the potential to control costs by organizing providers into coherent networks and by integrating the financing, insurance, delivery, and payment functions. First, by eliminating insurance and payer intermediaries, MCOs can realize some savings. Second, MCOs control costs by sharing risk with providers or by extracting discounts from providers. Risk sharing promotes delivery of health care that is economically prudent. Hence, risk sharing is an indirect method of utilization control. Third, cost savings are achieved by coordinating a broad range of patient services and by monitoring care to determine that it is appropriate and delivered in the most cost-effective settings (Health Insurance Association of America 1991, 4). For example, by emphasizing outpatient services, MCOs achieved lower rates of hospital utilization. HMOs provide a substantially higher amount of preventive care than traditional insurance plans (Rizzo 2005). Preventive care keeps people healthy and saves money through prevention as well as early detection and treatment of more serious illnesses. Also, some evidence suggests that HMO plans have lower use of costly procedures compared to nonHMO plans (Miller and Luft 1997).

Although many of the cost-control measures adopted by managed care have been applauded, other results have not been so commendable. Most providers find the complexity of having to deal with numerous plans overwhelming. A tremendous amount of inefficiency is created for providers, who must deal with differences in each plan's protocols and procedures. Another problem is that many of the contracts with providers exclude some services. For example, carving out laboratory testing services for outpatients has become a common practice. Many MCOs use one of the large national lab chains, such as Quest Diagnostics or Roche Diagnostics, which may present certain inconveniences for both patients and providers.

A third area of inefficiency is the sometimes lengthy appeals process that patients and providers must go through when a service is denied by an MCO. In short, managed care does not always create the well-coordinated, seamless system that patients and providers would like to see (Southwick 1997).

Cost Control Methods in Managed Care

MCOs use various methods to monitor and control utilization of services. The need for utilization management emanates from the fact that in the United States about 10% of patients—typically those with chronic or complex medical conditions—account for 70% of overall health care spending (Berk and Monheit 2001). Utilization management requires (1) an expert evaluation of which services are medically necessary in a given case. Such an evaluation ensures that unnecessary services are minimized. (2) It requires a determination of how those services can be provided most inexpensively while maintaining acceptable quality standards. (3) It requires a review of the process of care and changes in the patient's condition to revise the course of medical treatment if necessary. Utilization management of institutional inpatient services takes priority because such services account for 40% or more of the total expenses in a managed care plan (Kongstvedt 1995a). The methods commonly used for utilization monitoring and control are:

- Choice restriction
- Gatekeeping
- Case management
- Disease management
- Utilization review
- Practice profiling

Not all MCOs use all of these mechanisms to control utilization. Traditionally, HMOs have employed tighter utilization controls than other managed care plans.

Choice Restriction

As discussed earlier, traditional health insurance gave the insured open access to any provider, whether generalist or specialist. Such indiscretion led to overutilization of services. Most managed care plans impose some restrictions on where, and from whom, the patient will obtain medical care. Patients still have a choice of physicians, but the choice is limited to physicians who are either employees of the MCO or the MCO has established contracts with them. A physician who has formal affiliations with an MCO is said to be on the ***panel*** of the MCO. In a ***closed-panel*** (or closed-access or in-network) plan, services obtained from providers outside the panel are not covered by the plan. By contrast, an ***open-panel*** (or open-access or out-of-network option) plan allows access to providers outside the panel, but enrollees almost always have to pay higher out-of-pocket costs.

Because the MCO has greater control over providers who are on its panel, utilization is better managed under closed-panel plans compared to those that allow access outside the panel. From the enrollees' standpoint, restricted choice of providers is a trade-off for lower out-of-pocket costs; however, lack of physician choice has been strongly associated with consumers' dissatisfaction with their health plans (Berenson 1997).

Gatekeeping

Gatekeeping is a method in which a primary care physician coordinates all health care services needed by an enrollee. It is also a means of controlling utilization. The managed care enrollee chooses a primary care physician who becomes the first contact to deliver basic care and to coordinate all health care services the enrollee may need. The physician often uses nurse practitioners and/or physician assistants to provide comprehensive case management, which may include such services as telephone counseling, reorders for prescriptions, and blood pressure monitoring. Gatekeeping emphasizes preventive care, routine physical examinations, and other primary care services. Secondary care services, such as diagnostic testing, consultation with specialists, and admission to a hospital are provided only when referred by the primary care gatekeeper. Under the gatekeeping method, the primary care physician becomes the portal of entry to the health care delivery system. The primary care physician controls access to higher levels of medical services, hence the appellation, "gatekeeper." Figure 9–6 illustrates the role of primary care gatekeeping.

Case Management

Gatekeeping is a basic type of case management. However, case management takes on added significance when patients have complex, potentially costly problems that require a variety of services from multiple providers over an extended period. Examples include acquired immune deficiency syndrome (AIDS), spinal cord injury, bone marrow transplant, lupus, cystic fibrosis, and severe workplace injuries. These patients may need secondary and tertiary care services more often, whereas primary care may be needed only occasionally. In such circumstances, a primary care gatekeeper cannot adequately coordinate the patient's care. In ***case management***, an experienced health care professional, such as a nurse practitioner, with

Figure 9–6 Care Coordination and Utilization Control through Gatekeeping.

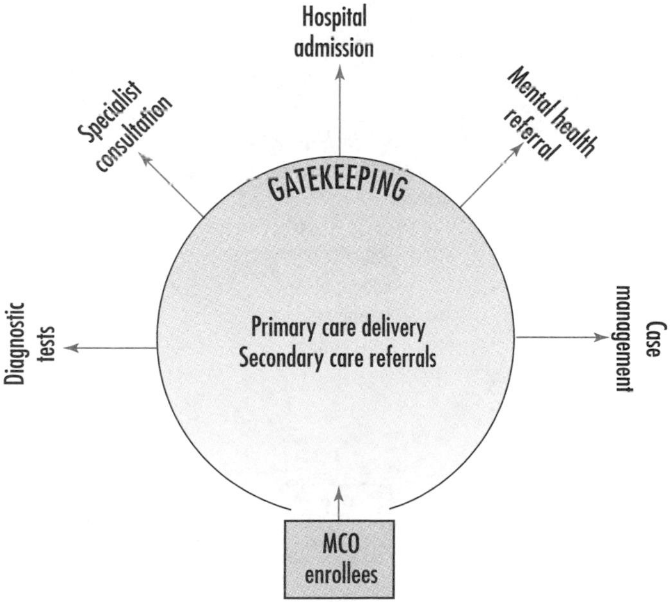

knowledge of available health care resources coordinates an individual's total health care in consultation with primary and secondary care providers. The case manager determines current needs and ensures continuity of care as the patient's needs change over time. The goal of case management is to provide quality health care along a continuous process by arranging the delivery of services in the most appropriate and cost-effective settings. The delivery of services is periodically reviewed to ascertain their appropriateness and efficacy. Case managers are also frequently involved in patient and family support and advocacy. Figure 9–7 illustrates the case management model.

Disease Management

Whereas case management is typically highly individualized, and focuses on coordinating the care of high-risk patients with multiple or complex medical conditions (Short et al. 2003), ***disease management*** is a population-oriented strategy for people with chronic conditions such as diabetes, asthma, depression, and coronary artery disease. Disease management is based on well-established, evidence-based treatment guidelines. After subgroups among all the enrollees in a health plan have been identified according to their specific chronic conditions, disease management focuses on patient education, train-

Figure 9–7 The Case Management Function in Health Services Utilization.

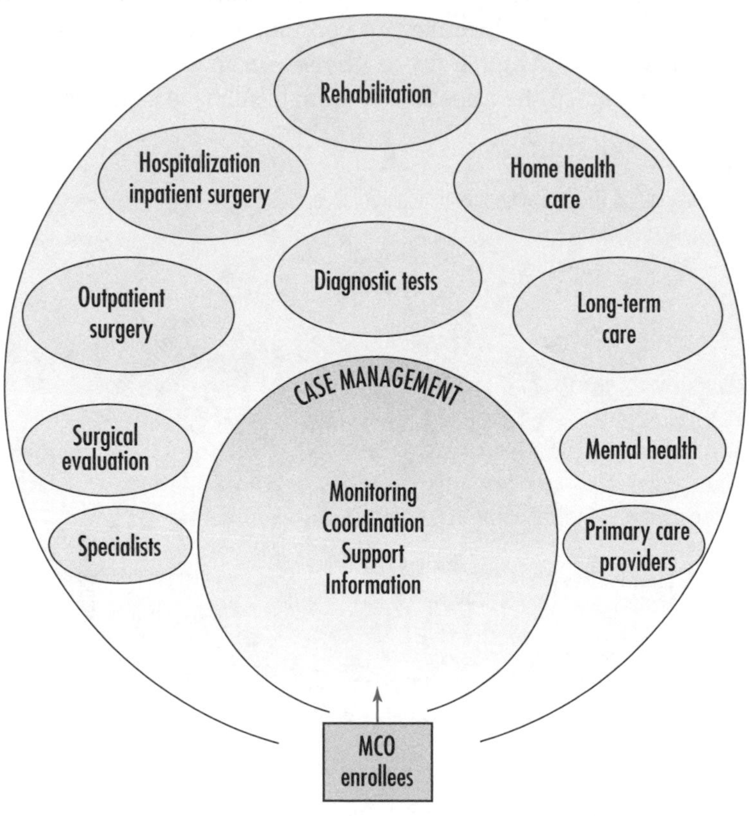

ing in self-management, ongoing monitoring of the disease process, and follow-up to ensure that people are complying with their medical regimens. It is estimated that more than half of health care spending is on behalf of people with multiple chronic conditions (Sipkoff 2003). By preventing or delaying comorbidities and complications arising from uncontrolled chronic conditions, disease management has the potential for increased cost efficiencies (i.e., cost savings and improved quality) because disease management programs can lower emergency room visits and hospitalizations. In at least one large-scale study involving patients served by the Permanente Medical Group in northern California, substantial quality improvements were noted, but not cost savings. The rising costs of improved health care may have offset any cost savings (Fireman et al. 2004).

Utilization Review

Utilization review (UR) is the process of evaluating the appropriateness of services provided by reviewing each case. It is sometimes misunderstood as a mechanism for denying services, but its main objective is to ensure that appropriate level of services are delivered, the care is cost-efficient, and subsequent care is planned. The management of utilization may be broadly divided into three categories: prospective, concurrent, and retrospective.

Prospective Utilization Review

Under this method, appropriateness of utilization is determined before the care is actually delivered. An example of prospective UR is the decision by a primary care gatekeeper to refer or not refer a patient to a specialist. However, not all managed care plans use gatekeepers. Some plans require the enrollee or the provider to call the plan administrators for preauthorization (also called precertification) of services, generally for hospital admissions and surgical procedures. In case of an emergency admission to an inpatient facility, plans generally require notification within 24 hours. Most plans now use preestablished clinical guidelines to determine the appropriateness of services.

One objective of prospective utilization review is to prevent unnecessary or inappropriate institutionalization; however, it also serves other functions. It notifies the concurrent review system that a case will be occurring and allows concurrent review to prepare for discharge planning. In the event of a potentially complex and expensive case, it notifies case management to evaluate and take over the case (Kongstvedt 1995a).

Concurrent Utilization Review

Concurrent UR in a hospital seeks to control primarily the length of stay. It also monitors the use of ancillary services and ensures that the medical treatment is appropriate and necessary. When a patient is hospitalized, a certain number of inpatient days are generally preauthorized. Trained nurses then monitor the patient's status and review the case with a physician if a longer stay is necessary. A decision is made to authorize or deny additional days. The UR nurse also coordinates discharge planning.

Discharge planning is often part of the overall treatment plan from the outset. It includes an estimate of how long the patient will be in the hospital, what the expected outcome is likely to be, whether any special requirements must be met at discharge, and what needs to be facilitated (Kongstvedt 1995a). For example, if a patient is admitted with a fractured hip, it is important to estimate whether a rehabilitation hospital or a skilled nursing facility would be more appropriate for convalescent care. If the patient requires care in a skilled nursing facility, discharge planning must find out whether the appropriate level of rehabilitation services would be available and how long the plan will pay for rehabilitation therapies in a long-term care setting. Discharge planners should involve case managers to plan for subsequent home health services and the need for durable medical equipment. The objective is "to get all the ducks in a row" to provide seamless services at the lowest cost and in the best interest of the patient.

Retrospective Utilization Review

Retrospective UR refers to managing utilization after services have been delivered. The review is based on an examination of medical records to assess the appropriateness of care. Large claims may be reviewed for billing accuracy. Retrospective review may also involve an analysis of utilization data to determine patterns. Such patterns may be provider specific. For example, a particular provider may show patterns of excessive utilization or underutilization compared to his or her peers (Kongstvedt 1995b). Pattern review is often used to furnish feedback to providers. Incentive compensation, such as bonuses, is often tied to pattern reviews in an effort to influence future practice behavior. The analyses may also show plan-wide variations from previous periods or from established medical practice norms. Such statistical data can be helpful for taking corrective action and for monitoring subsequent progress.

Practice Profiling

Also called "profile monitoring," ***practice profiling*** refers to the evaluation of provider-specific practice patterns and the comparison of individual practice patterns to some norm. As previously mentioned, practice profiling may be a by-product of retrospective UR. Mainly, such profiles are used to decide which providers have the right fit with the plan's managed care philosophy and goals. The profile reports are also used to give feedback to providers so they can modify their own behavior of medical practice. Other uses include identifying specialists to whom the plan should refer certain types of cases, detecting fraud and abuse, and determining how to focus the UR program (Kongstvedt 1995c).

Physicians become understandably anxious when their practices are put under scrutiny. They may think that the standards used to evaluate their work do not consider any extenuating circumstances and that their fate may be decided based on sterile reports. For MCOs, the ability to report the behavior of individual physicians provides a powerful tool to discipline nonconforming physicians; however, great care must be exercised when using physician-specific reports. The administrator must look behind the data and investigate reasons for the reported performance. It is necessary to see how the norms for comparisons are established. It is also important to examine provider behavior from the standpoint of total health care resource consumption and outcome, and to employ a variety of performance measures (Kongstvedt 1995c). According to one study, about half of all physicians affected by practice profiling viewed it positively as a useful tool to improve quality and efficiency, but 40% expressed mixed feelings (Reed et al. 2003).

Types of Managed Care Organizations

Three main factors led to the development of different types of managed care plans, the first being choice of providers. HMOs were the most common type of MCOs in the 1970s, but HMO plans employed tight restrictions on the choice of providers. To compete with HMOs, MCO plans that offered a greater freedom of choice were developed. Different ways of arranging the delivery of services also led to different forms of MCOs because there is no single way to arrange providers into a delivery network. Payment and risk sharing make up the third major factor. These variables led to the development of different types of managed care plans and various models of HMOs.

Health Maintenance Organization

Commonly referred to as HMOs, health maintenance organizations were the most common type of MCO until commercial insurance companies developed PPOs to compete with HMOs. An ***HMO*** is distinguished from other types of plans by its focus on wellness care, payment in the form of capitation, use of a closed panel, and accountability:

1. In the traditional system, health insurance pays for medical care only when a person is ill. An HMO not only provides medical care during illness but also offers a variety of services to help people maintain their health. Hence, the name "health maintenance" organization. HMOs place considerable emphasis on preventive services, such as routine checkups.
2. A fixed fee per member per month (PMPM) provides access to a complete range of health care services. The utilization of these services is coordinated and managed by the HMO, mainly through primary care gatekeepers.
3. All health care must be obtained from in-network hospitals, physicians, and other health care providers, although some may allow out-of-network use at a higher out-of-pocket cost. Specialty services, such as mental health and substance abuse treatment, are frequently carved out. A ***carve out*** is a special contract outside regular capitation, which is funded separately by the MCO. Compared to other managed care plans, HMOs are also more likely to use disease management as a means for delivering cost-effective health care.
4. The HMO is responsible for ensuring that services comply with certain established standards of quality.

HMO enrollments grew rapidly in the first half of the 1990s (Figure 9–8). Subsequently, other types of managed care plans—notably PPO and POS plans—gained in popularity. HMOs fell into disfavor with the enrollees because these plans were the most restrictive. The trend since the mid-1990s has been in favor of plans offering the enrollees greater freedom to select their physicians.

Figure 9–8 Percent of Covered Employees Enrolled in HMO Plans (selected years).

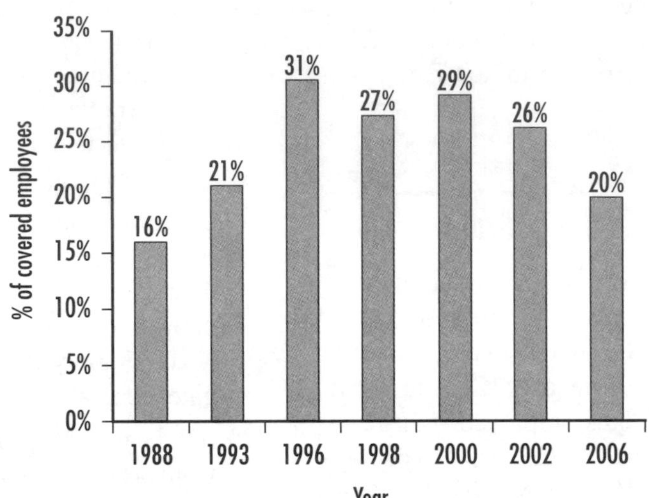

Source: Data from *Employer Health Benefits: 2002 Annual Survey; Employer Health Benefits: 2006 Annual Survey;* The Henry J. Kaiser Family Foundation and Health Research and Educational Trust.

There are four common HMO models—staff, group, network, and IPA—differing primarily in their arrangements with participating physicians. Some HMOs cannot be categorized neatly into any one of the four models because they may use a hybrid arrangement referred to as a ***mixed model***. An example of a mixed model is an HMO that partially employs the staff model, employing its own physicians, and partially relies on the group model by contracting with a group practice.

Staff Model

A ***staff model*** HMO employs its own salaried physicians. Based on the physician's productivity and the HMO's performance, bonuses may be added to salary. Physicians work only for their employer HMO and provide services to that HMO's enrollees (Rakich et al. 1992, 281). Staff model HMOs must employ physicians in all the common specialties to provide for the health care needs of their members. Contracts with selected subspecialties are established for infrequently needed services. The HMO operates one or more ambulatory care facilities that contain physicians' offices, employs support staff, and may have ancillary support facilities, such as a laboratory and radiology departments. In most instances, the HMO contracts with area hospitals for inpatient services (Wagner 1995).

Compared to other HMO models, staff model HMOs can exercise a greater degree of control over the practice patterns of their physicians. Hence, it is easier to monitor utilization. These HMOs also offer the convenience of "one-stop shopping" for their enrollees, because most common services are located in the same clinic (Wagner 1995).

Staff model HMOs also present several disadvantages. The fixed salary expense can be high, requiring these HMOs to have a large number of enrollees to support the operating expenses. Enrollees generally have a limited choice of physicians. Using the staff model concept, expansion into new markets requires heavy capital outlays (Wagner 1995). Because of such disadvantages, the staff model has been the least popular. Nationwide, the number of staff model HMOs has continued to decline, from 30 (3.3% of all HMOs) in 1998 to 13 (3.0% of all HMOs) in 2005 (Aventis Pharmaceuticals/SMG Marketing-Verispan LLC 2002; Sanofi-Aventis 2006a).

Group Model

A ***group model*** HMO contracts with a single multispecialty group practice and separately with one or more hospitals to provide comprehensive services to its members. The physicians in the group practice are employed by the group practice, not the HMO. The HMO generally pays an all-inclusive capitation fee to the group practice to provide physician services to its members. The group practice may be an independent practice, in which case the physicians may also generally treat nonHMO patients. Under a different scenario, the HMO may own the group practice as a separate corporation that is administratively tied to the HMO. In this case, the group practice may provide services exclusively to the HMO's members. An exclusive contract with a group practice enables the HMO to exercise better control over utilization.

Even when it is not an exclusive contract, the HMO brings a block of business to the group practice, which gives the HMO a fair amount of leverage on financial terms and utilization controls. Large groups are usually attractive to HMOs because they deliver a large block of physicians with one contract. However, a large group contract can also be a downside for the HMO. If the contract is lost, the HMO will have difficulties meeting its service obligations. As for other advantages, the HMO is able to avoid large expenditures in fixed salaries and facilities. Affiliation with a reputable multispecialty group practice generally lends the HMO prestige and creates a perception of quality among its enrollees. On the other hand, enrollees may find the choice of physicians limited. In 2005, there were 35 group practice HMOs (7.7% of all HMOs) in the United States (Sanofi-Aventis 2006a).

Network Model

Under the ***network model***, the HMO contracts with more than one medical group practice. This model is specially adaptable to large metropolitan areas and widespread geographic regions where group practices are located. A common arrangement in the network model is to have contracts only with group practices of primary care physicians. Enrollees generally may select physicians from any of these groups. Each group is paid a capitation fee based on the number of enrollees. The group is responsible for providing all physician services. It can make referrals to specialists but is financially responsible for reimbursing them for any referrals it makes. In some cases, the HMO may contract with a panel of specialists, in which case, referrals can be made only to physicians serving on the panel (Wagner 1995). The network model can generally offer a wider choice of physicians than the staff or group model. The main disadvantage is the dilution of utilization control. In 2005, there were 153 network model HMOs (33.6% of all HMOs) in the United States (Sanofi-Aventis 2006a).

Independent Practice Association (IPA) Model

In 1954, a variant of the prepaid group practice plan was established by the San Joaquin

County Foundation for Medical Care in Stockton, California. The plan was a prototype of the ***IPA model*** and was initiated by the San Joaquin County Medical Society (MacColl 1966, 20–24). As a result of political pressures from organized medicine, this form of HMO was specifically included in the HMO Act of 1973 (Mackie and Decker 1981).

An ***independent practice association*** (IPA) is a legal entity separate from the HMO. The IPA contracts with both independent solo practitioners and group practices. In turn, the HMO contracts with the IPA instead of contracting with individual physicians or group practices (Figure 9–9). Hence, the IPA is an intermediary representing a large number of physicians. The IPA is generally paid a capitation amount by the HMO. The IPA retains administrative control over how it pays its physicians. It may reimburse physicians through capitation or some other means, such as a modified fee-for-service. The IPA often shares risk with the physicians and assumes the responsibility for utilization management and quality assessment. The IPA also generally carries stop-loss reinsurance, or the HMO may provide stop-loss coverage to prevent the IPA from going bankrupt (Kongstvedt and Plocher 1995).

Figure 9–9 The IPA-HMO Model.

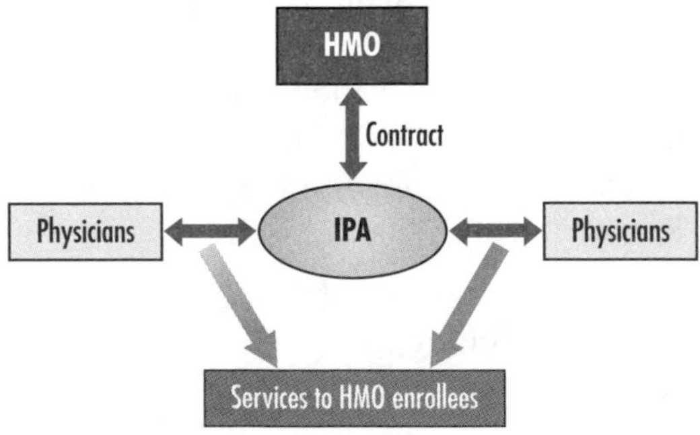

Under the IPA model, the HMO is still responsible for providing health care services to its enrollees, but the logistics of arranging physician services are shifted to the IPA. The HMO is thus relieved of the administrative burden of establishing contracts with numerous providers and controlling utilization. Financial risk is also transferred to the IPA. The IPA model provides an expanded choice of providers to enrollees. It also allows small groups and individual physicians the opportunity to participate in managed care and to get a slice of the revenues. IPAs may be independently established by community physicians, or the HMO may create an IPA and invite community physicians to participate in it. An IPA may also be hospital-based and structured so that only physicians from one or two hospitals are eligible to participate in the IPA (Wagner 1995). One major disadvantage of the IPA model is that if a contract is lost, the HMO loses a large number of participating physicians. The IPA acts as a buffer between the HMO and physicians. Hence, the IPA does not have as much leverage in changing physician behavior as a staff or a group model HMO would have. Finally, many IPAs have a surplus of specialists, which creates some pressures to use their services (Kongstvedt and Plocher 1995). Of the four HMO models, the IPA model has been the most successful in terms of the share of all enrollments over time. Perhaps its success can be attributed to the buffer an IPA creates between the HMO and its practicing physicians. This amounts to less direct HMO control over the providers. In 2005, there were 255 IPA model HMOs (56% of all HMOs) in the United States (Sanofi-Aventis 2006a). Enrollments in all models have been declining in recent years (Figure 9–10).

Figure 9–10 Nationwide Enrollment in HMOs by Model Type, 1993–2005.

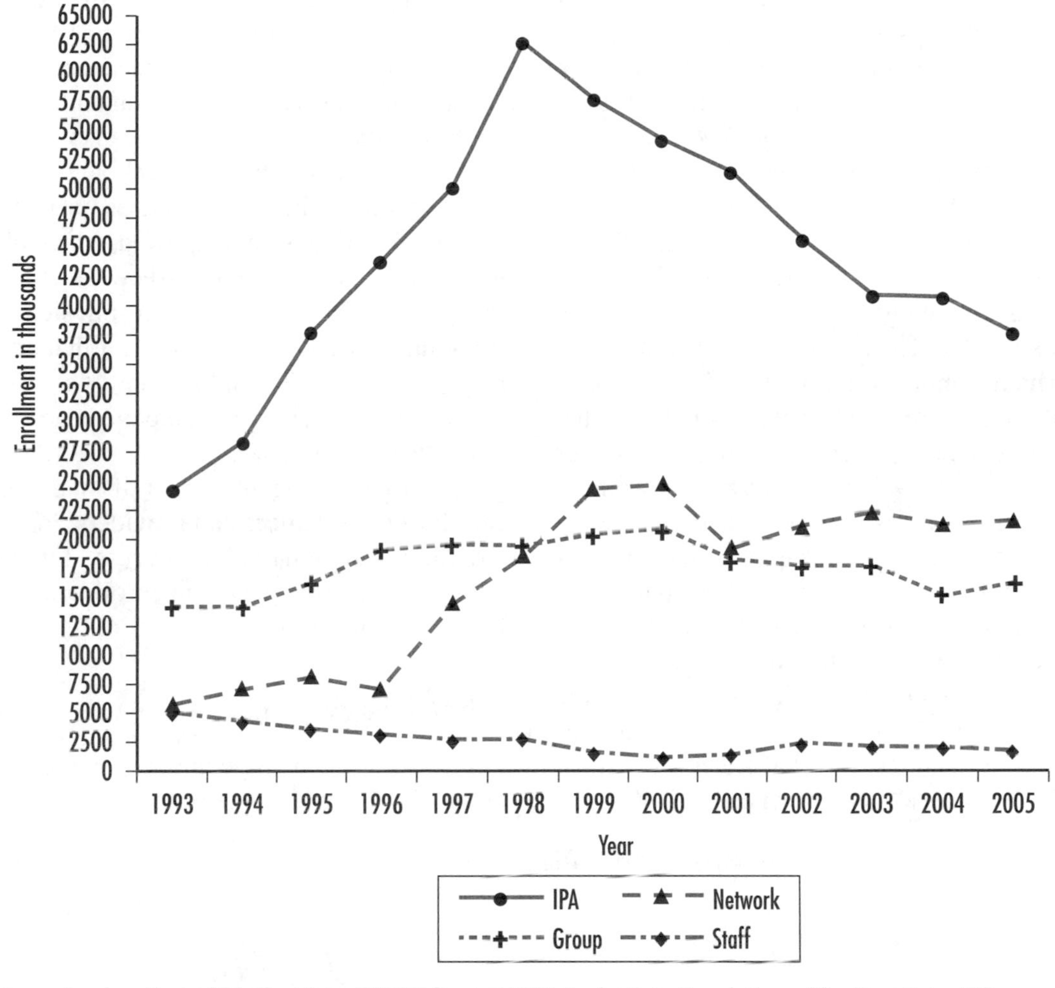

Sources: Data from *Managed Care Digest Series: HMO-PPO Digest,* © 1996, Hoechst Marion Roussel; *Managed Care Digest Series: HMO-PPO/Medicare-Medicaid Digest,* © 1999, Hoechst Marion Roussel; *HMO-PPO/Medicare-Medicaid Digest,* © 2003, Aventis Pharmaceuticals; *HMO-PPO Digest,* © 2006 Sanofi-Aventis.

Preferred Provider Organization

PPOs first appeared in the medical marketplace in the late 1970s as a competitive response by insurance companies to HMOs' growing market share. They differentiated the PPO product by offering open-panel options for enrollees and offering noncapitation payment to providers. The enrollees agree to use a selected set of physicians and hospitals with whom the PPO has contracts. These providers on the PPO's panel are referred to as "preferred providers." The main appeal of PPOs is that they allow patients the choice of using physicians and hospitals outside the panel, for which the patients must pay higher copayments than if they used in-network providers. The additional out-of-pocket expenses act largely as a deterrent to going outside the panel. If a PPO does not provide an out-of-network option, it is referred to as an ***exclusive provider plan***.

Instead of capitation, PPOs make discounted fee arrangements with providers. The discounts can range between 25 and 35% from the provider-established charges. Thus, in paying providers, PPOs substitute discounted fee-for-service for capitation, which is more commonly used by HMOs—although some HMOs also switched to discounted fee-for-service to reduce risk for physicians. Negotiated payment arrangements with hospitals can take any of the forms discussed in Chapter 6, such as payments based on DRGs, bundled charges for certain services, or discounts. Hence, no direct risk sharing with providers is involved.

Insurance companies (including Blue Cross and Blue Shield), independent investors, and hospital alliances own most PPOs. Other PPOs are owned by HMOs, and some are jointly sponsored by a hospital and physicians. Although HMOs have organizational mechanisms to assume corporate responsibility for cost containment and quality assessment, PPOs do not have such intrinsic controls (MacLeod 1995). PPOs also apply fewer restrictions to the care-seeking behavior of enrollees. In most instances, primary care gatekeeping is not employed, which allows enrollees to see specialists without being referred by a primary care physician. Prior authorization (retrospective utilization review) is generally employed only for hospitalization and high-cost outpatient procedures (Robinson 2002).

As a less stringent choice of managed care for both enrollees and providers, PPOs have enjoyed remarkable success. Figure 9–11 illustrates the growth in enrollments in PPO plans over time.

Point-of-Service Plan

Point-of-service plans combine features of classic HMOs with some of the characteris-

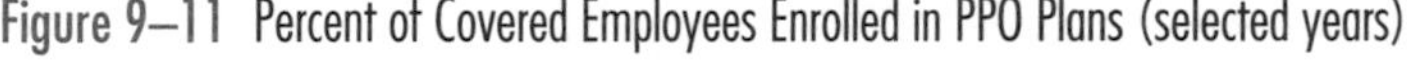
Figure 9–11 Percent of Covered Employees Enrolled in PPO Plans (selected years).

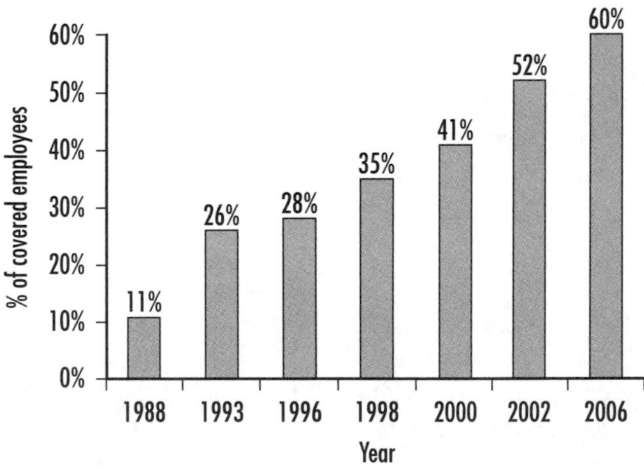

Source: Data from *Employer Health Benefits: 2002 Annual Survey; Employer Health Benefits: 2006 Annual Survey;* The Henry J. Kaiser Family Foundation and Health Research and Educational Trust.

tics of patient choice found in PPOs. Hence, they are sometimes referred to as hybrid plans or open-ended HMOs. These plans have a two-pronged objective: retain the benefits of tight utilization management found in HMOs but offer an alternative to their unpopular feature of restricted choice. The features borrowed from HMOs are capitation or other risk-based provider reimbursement and the gatekeeping method of utilization control. Each enrollee chooses a primary care provider. The feature borrowed from PPOs is the patient's ability to choose a nonparticipating provider at the point (time) of receiving services, hence the name, "point-of-service." Of course, the enrollee has to pay extra for the privilege of using nonparticipating providers because these providers are paid their fee-for-service rates. From the consumer's perspective, free choice of providers is a major selling point for POS plans. They grew in popularity soon after they first emerged in 1988. However, after reaching a peak in popularity in 1998 and 1999, enrollment in POS plans has gradually declined (Figure 9–12), mainly due to the increased out-of-pocket costs enrollees must incur.

Trends in Managed Care

Private Health Insurance Enrollment

Managed care has indeed become a mature industry in the United States. Within a decade, from 1996 to 2006, enrollment in traditional fee-for-service insurance plans declined from 27% to 3% (Figure 9–13). In essence, employer-sponsored private health insurance can now be equated to managed care. Many employers offer their workers a choice of plans with level-dollar employer contribution, meaning workers pay more themselves—in premium contributions, deductibles, and copayments—if they choose a more expensive plan.

For employers, the cost of health insurance remains the biggest economic concern related to employee benefits. Managed care

Figure 9–12 Percent of Covered Employees Enrolled in POS Plans (selected years).

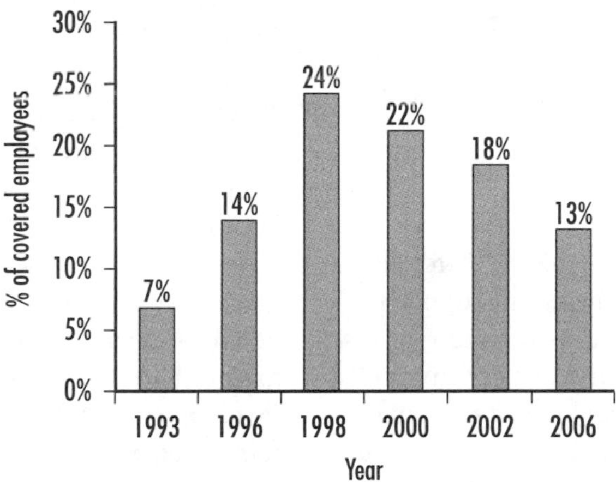

Source: Data from *Employer Health Benefits: 2002 Annual Survey; Employer Health Benefits: 2006 Annual Survey;* The Henry J. Kaiser Family Foundation and Health Research and Educational Trust.

Figure 9–13 Changes in Enrollment in Job-Based Health Plans, 1996 and 2006.

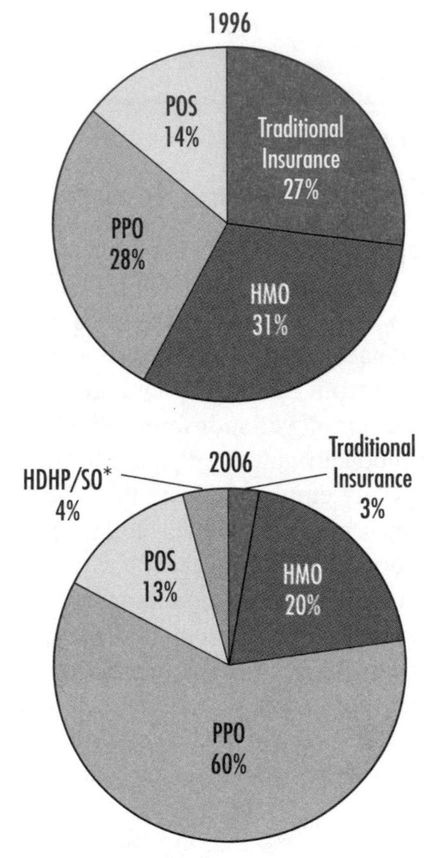

*High Deductible Health Plan paired with a savings options.

Source: Data from *Employer Health Benefits: 2002 Annual Survey; Employer Health Benefits: 2006 Annual Survey;* The Henry J. Kaiser Family Foundation and Health Research and Educational Trust.

received wide acclaim in the 1990s for slowing the growth rate of health insurance premiums, a burden borne mostly by employers. In 1989, health insurance premiums grew 18%. As employers abandoned traditional insurance plans for managed care, the annual rate of increase in premiums dropped to 0.8% in 1996 (Kaiser/HRET 2002). Since then, the rate of increase did pick up, but remained below the rate of general inflation until 1998. However, since 1999, the rate of premium increases has intensified once again. Even though the rise in premiums moderated in 2006 (Figure 9–14), it still remained above general inflation (3.5%) and increase in workers' earnings (3.8%) [Kaiser/HRET 2006]. To cope with the rising premiums, employers are requiring increased cost sharing from covered employees. Another emerging strategy is to offer high-deductible health plans in conjunction with health savings accounts (discussed in Chapter 14). Employers may also resort to changes in benefits, such as moving from defined-benefit plans to defined-contribution plans (discussed in Chapter 14), even though current interest in such options is low.

Medicaid Enrollment

Waivers under the Social Security Act, particularly sections 1115 and 1915(b), allowed states to enroll their Medicaid recipients in managed care plans. The Balanced Budget Act of 1997 gave states the authority to implement mandatory managed care programs without requiring federal waivers (Moscovice et al. 1998). Since then, enrollment of Medicaid beneficiaries into managed care programs has grown rapidly. Over 60% of Medicaid beneficiaries now receive health care services through managed care, which is up from 23.2% a decade ago (Robinson 2006).

Some states have developed a different model of managing health care delivery, particularly in rural areas where managed care has not flourished. ***Primary care case management*** (PCCM), sometimes referred to as integrated case management, uses fee-for-service instead of capitation. It is an open-access delivery system. While Medicaid beneficiaries are required to have a primary care physician for routine care, gatekeeper

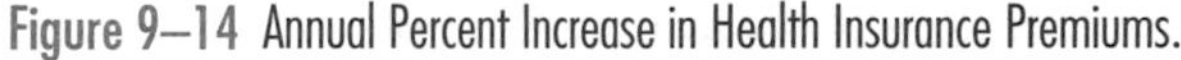
Figure 9–14 Annual Percent Increase in Health Insurance Premiums.

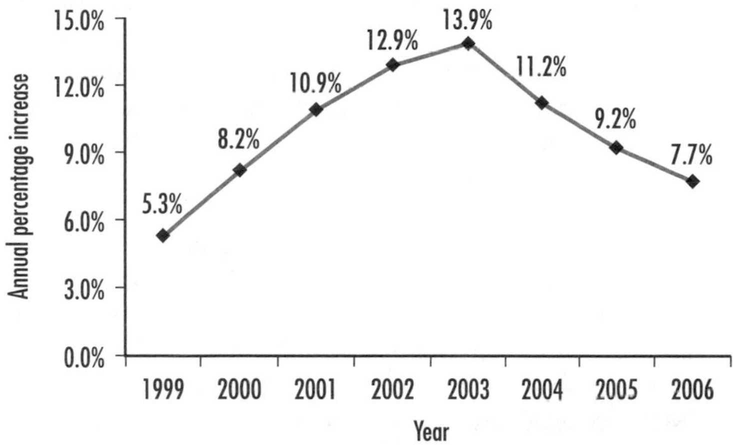

Source: Data from *Employer Health Benefits, 2006 Annual Survey,* The Henry J. Kaiser Family Foundation and Health Research and Educational Trust.

referrals are not necessary. Under this program, states may also contract with a management company to be responsible for network development, utilization review, quality assurance, and case management (Senterfitt 2005).

Medicare Enrollment

Under the provisions of the Tax Equity and Fiscal Responsibility Act (TEFRA) of 1982, Medicare beneficiaries have the option to enroll in managed care or remain in the traditional fee-for-service program. The legislation introduced a full-risk capitation reimbursement to include all covered services. Another program introduced was the Health Care Prepayment Plan (HCPP) for Part B services only. Under this program, MCOs are paid on a reasonable cost basis for outpatient and other services covered under Part B.

Medicare managed care contracts are commonly referred to as ***risk contracts***, in which the MCO is liable for services regardless of their extent, expense, or degree, in exchange for a fixed capitated fee. As an incentive for MCOs to enroll Medicare beneficiaries, generous capitated rates were initially offered. Between 1996 and 2000, Medicare enrollment in managed care had increased from 4.7 million (12% of all beneficiaries) to 6.7 million (17% of all beneficiaries) [Hoechst Marion Roussel 1998; Aventis Pharmaceuticals/SMG Marketing-Verispan LLC 2002]. Then, in 1997, Congress passed the Balanced Budget Act, which created the Medicare+Choice program to keep managed care as an active player in the delivery of health care services, but the legislation also reduced payments to HMOs. As HMOs withdrew from the Medicare program, 800,000 beneficiaries lost their HMO coverage between 2000 and 2001 (Aventis Pharmaceuticals/SMG Marketing-Verispan LLC 2002). Enrollment in Medicare+Choice fell from 6.3 million in December 1999 to 5 million by February 2002, a decline of 21% (Thorpe and Atherly 2002).

In 2003, Medicare+Choice was renamed Medicare Advantage with the passage of the

Medicare Prescription Drug, Improvement, and Modernization Act of 2003 (MMA 2003). The federal government added generous funding for Medicare Advantage as part of the new Part D program, and once again, enrollment of Medicare beneficiaries in managed care plans was on the rise, albeit at a slow pace. Medicare advantage programs are luring Medicare beneficiaries by offering richer benefits at lower costs, and are moving into new markets (Fine 2005). Given the fee-for-service choice, enrollment of the Medicare population stands at around 14%. Perhaps the main reason is that Medicare seniors value unrestricted choice of providers. According to a national study, only 44% of the seniors were willing to trade broad provider choice for lower out-of-pocket costs (Tu 2005a).

Impact on Cost, Access, and Quality

Influence on Cost Containment

Managed care has been widely credited with slowing down the rate of growth in health care expenditures during the 1990s. It is estimated that over a five-year period the cumulative savings in medical spending was between 10 and 15% (Newhouse 2001). Unnecessary hospitalizations and inappropriate surgeries are two areas that were costing the system money without producing better health. However, as discussed later, a subsequent backlash from both enrollees and providers prompted MCOs to back away from aggressive cost control measures. Now, as health care cost inflation has reignited, a greater proportion of consumers indicate that controlling costs should be a major priority for health system reform in the United States. Interestingly, however, people who are the most indifferent to tight cost and utilization controls are the uninsured or the young and healthy, who consume relatively little health care. Both of these groups seemingly have little to lose if tight utilization measures are adopted. Those who have the worst health status do not approve of strategies that might interfere with their ability to obtain health care (Schur et al. 2004). As managed care may have started to refocus on cost containment, current strategies to shift costs to the consumers or to use case management and disease management programs are likely to have only a limited impact on overall cost trends (Mays et al. 2004). Future cost reductions may not be forthcoming without tighter restrictions on utilization, particularly on the use of expensive new technology. At the moment, however, no one is sure how to introduce such explicit rationing into the delivery of health care.

A number of HMOs have been trying to include both conventional and alternative therapies in their range of covered services. Yet the availability and coverage of alternative therapies in HMOs remain quite variable (Meenan and Vuckovic 2004). Effective coordination of complementary and conventional medical services has the potential to save money as well as improve quality. This is because for some chronic problems, conventional medicine offers few proven benefits. Examples include psychosomatic ailments and cases in which patients have recurring complaints of unexplained painful symptoms or spells of dizziness. Such nagging complaints can rack up high costs and compromise an individual's quality of life. Lower cost therapies, such as stress management and meditation classes, can save numerous trips to physicians and costly diagnostic tests. However, alternative medicine is not widely integrated into conventional medical practice because there is inadequate evidence of the former's efficacy and economic potential.

Impact on Access

Managed care enrollees generally have good access to primary and preventive care. For example, Baker and colleagues (2004) found that timely breast cancer screening and cervical cancer screening were twice as likely for women receiving services in geographical areas with greater HMO market share compared to women in areas with low managed care penetration. As people's ability to obtain health care improved between 2001 and 2003, health plan-related barriers that would have led some people to delay care or go without it declined significantly (Strunk and Cunningham 2004). It perhaps reflects relaxed utilization controls adopted by health plans in the years following the bashing of managed care.

On a larger scale, managed care's impact on access is not known. For instance, it is not clear to what extent, during the 1990s, managed care might have enabled small employers to offer employees health insurance coverage by holding down premium increases. Between 1996 and 2000, the proportion of employers offering health insurance benefits increased from 59% to 67% among firms employing between 3 and 199 workers, and the most notable increase was among the smallest firms employing between 3 and 9 workers (Kaiser/HRET 2002). However, this period also saw unprecedented economic growth that may have enabled more employers to add new benefits.

Influence on Quality of Care

During the 1990s, concerns were raised that risk sharing between providers and payers would influence treatment decisions made by physicians, which would result in skimping on necessary services. However, evidence suggests that financial pressures do not lead to significant changes in physician behavior because under capitation a physician takes full responsibility for the patient's overall care (Eikel 2002). This is particularly true for life-saving treatment decisions such as treatment of cancer patients (Bourjolly et al. 2004).

Physicians also feel positively about care-management tools, such as practice guidelines, patient satisfaction surveys, and practice profiling, and believe that overall they positively influence both quality and efficiency. Risk adjustment to reflect greater need for services by people with health problems plays an important role in physicians' view of care management (Reed et al. 2003).

Despite anecdotes, individual perceptions, and isolated stories propagated by the news media, no comprehensive research to date has clearly demonstrated that managed care's growth has been at the cost of quality in health care. Actually, available evidence points to the contrary. Quality of health care provided by MCOs has improved over time (Hofmann 2002). Early detection and treatment is more likely in a managed care plan than in a traditional fee-for-service plan (Riley et al. 1999). Higher managed care penetration was associated with increased quality in hospitals when such indicators as inappropriate utilization, wound infections, and iatrogenic complications were used to assess quality (Sari 2002). Studies measuring health outcomes show little or no measurable difference between managed care and traditional fee-for-service care. A comprehensive review of the literature by Miller and Luft (2002) concluded that HMO and nonHMO plans provided roughly equal quality of care as measured by a wide range of conditions, diseases, and interventions. At the same time, HMOs lower the use of hospitals and other expensive resources. Hence, medical care delivered through managed care plans has been cost effective.

Even in the case of vulnerable populations, such as the poor insured by Medicaid, managed care plans provide similar quality of care as commercial plans do serving the same population (Bruce et al. 1999). Concerns about disparities in quality of care based on race and socioeconomic status are also largely unfounded (DeFrancesco 2002). An examination of diabetes care in managed care settings showed that most quality indicators and intermediate outcomes were comparable across race/ethnicity and socioeconomic status (Brown et al. 2005). The authors of this study concluded that social disparities in health might actually be reduced in managed care settings. There is further confirmation that, in terms of benefits and costs, being white or a member of a minority class makes no difference for Medicare enrollees regardless of whether they are enrolled in Medicare managed care or in the traditional fee-for-service program (Balsa et al. 2007).

In the delivery of mental health, earlier reports had suggested poorer outcomes in managed care plans (Rogers et al. 1993; Wells et al. 1989). However, more recent investigations conclude otherwise. Examining both qualitative and quantitative aspects of specialty managed outpatient mental health treatment, managed care was found to achieve cost savings, but not at the expense of quality of care (Goldman et al. 2003). On the other hand, there is evidence that quality of care may be lower in for-profit health plans compared to nonprofit plans (Himmelstein et al. 1999; Schneider et al. 2005).

Managed Care Backlash, Regulation, and the Aftermath

The large-scale transition of health care delivery to the managed care system in the 1990s was met with widespread criticism, which turned into a backlash from consumers, physicians, and legislators. There were three main reasons behind the discontent, and widespread media reports further shaped unsympathetic public opinion toward managed care. (1) To restrain the spiraling costs of health insurance premiums, employers around the country switched to managed care by dropping, in many instances, traditional health insurance plans that offered choice of physicians and hospitals. A large number of employees experienced at least some loss of freedom and, to some extent, faced barriers to free access. (2) Generally, people did not see a reduction in their own share of the premium costs or a drop in their out-of-pocket expenses when they received health care. (3) In reaction to tight utilization management and lower reimbursement from MCOs, physicians became openly hostile toward managed care. Actually, in national surveys, managed care penetration continues to be negatively correlated with physicians' satisfaction (Landon et al. 2003). Much of this discontent arises from pressures to change the way physicians had traditionally practiced medicine with no accountability for appropriateness of utilization and costs. Physicians' vocal discontent no doubt also helped shape patients' views about managed care. Both physicians and patients perceived that managed care would drive a wedge between the patient-provider relationships. However, as the momentum continued to shift toward enrollment in managed care, physicians had little choice but to contract with managed care or lose patients; employees had little choice but to enroll in managed care plans or personally bear significantly higher premium costs, or go without health insurance altogether. As this drama was unfolding, employers largely remained passive as their main objective of sharp reductions in premium costs was being attained.

Regulation of Managed Care

In response to widespread complaints and negative publicity against managed care, legislators across the states were prompted to take action. This is because the state governments are primarily responsible for overseeing issues pertaining to health insurance. Hence, states passed an extensive array of anti-managed care legislation. On the other hand, proposed federal legislation, commonly referred to as the patients' bill of rights, failed to pass. The US Congress did pass the Newborns' and Mothers' Health Protection Act of 1996, although numerous states already had laws against "drive-through deliveries." The federal law prohibits a health plan to offer less than a 48-hour inpatient maternity coverage for a mother and her child following a normal vaginal delivery, and less than a 96-hour coverage following a caesarean section. Most states have adopted legislation to limit financial incentives to physicians for curtailing utilization, to expand the rights of health care professionals, to promote continuity of care, and to give patients the right to an expeditious appeals process to review denial of services, including mandatory external reviews. States have also continued to mandate that certain benefits be included in the health plans. Some examples include chiropractic services, women's health screening, diabetic supplies, and obesity care. Increasingly, state legislation also includes provisions for insurer liability, which gives enrollees the right to seek civil remedy in the courts for negligent actions of health plans, including the denial of services (Hurley and Draper 2002). While managed care legislation provides both consumers and providers certain protections, it also has negative implications of increasing costs.

The Aftermath

The backlash and anti-managed care laws seem to have produced their intended effects. MCOs have taken significant steps to develop better relationships with physicians and other providers. MCOs have also relaxed tight controls on utilization. Yet 40% of privately insured Americans continue to believe their doctor is strongly influenced by health plan rules when deciding about their care (Reed and Trude 2002). Enthoven (2001) demonstrated that choice restriction was a main cause of the managed care consumer backlash. Satisfaction increases as employers offer more choices among plans. In response, several employers have started to offer choices among HMO, PPO, and POS plans. On the other hand, the proportion of working-age Americans willing to limit their choice of health care providers to save on out-of-pocket medical costs grew significantly between 2001 and 2003 (Tu 2005b).

However, managed care now stands at the crossroads of its past successes and future abilities to control mounting costs. As rising premiums increasingly shift the burden to employees, a greater differentiation among plans will again become necessary and this differentiation, on a continuum of tight controls to more relaxed management, will have to be reflected in the level of premiums. Employees can then evaluate for themselves each plan's benefits against its costs and make choices that best suit their individual needs. Such a trend is perhaps already visible in a drop in POS enrollments (see Figure 9–12), which offer the greatest choice but are also the most expensive managed care option. Defined contribution plans and the emerging high deductible plans are also pointing in this direction. These trends would culminate in a greater choice of plans, but at greater individual responsibility. For now, managed care is the established delivery system, and health care in America will be managed by all three parties in the health care delivery equation—employers, employees, and MCOs.

Consolidation, Expansion, Diversification, and Integration

Consolidation, diversification, and other forms of organizational integration have occurred in response to cost pressures, development of new alternatives for the delivery of health care, concentration of power on the demand side because of managed care, and the need to provide services more efficiently to populations spread over large geographic areas. Consolidation, expansion, diversification, and integration are different types of growth strategies used by health services organizations.

Although in previous discussions these terms have been used rather loosely, they do carry specific meanings. ***Consolidation*** refers to a concentration of control by a few organizations over other organizations through a consolidation of existing facility assets. Acquisitions, mergers, alliances, and the formation of contractual networks are examples of consolidation. ***Expansion*** is another growth strategy in which an organization adds new services or services similar to those it has offered before, but there is one difference. Whereas consolidation is achieved through the integration of existing facilities, expansion involves the building of new ones. Examples include expansion of a nursing home by adding more beds, a multifacility corporation building new facilities to expand into new markets, and a hospital adding a women's health center to its existing services. ***Diversification*** refers to addition of new services that the organization has not offered before. Diversification can be achieved through consolidation or expansion, but it can also be achieved without the two growth strategies. For example, a hospital may acquire an existing long-term care facility (diversification through consolidation). As a second option, the hospital may diversify into long-term care by converting an unused acute care wing into a long-term care facility (diversification not involving consolidation or expansion but the use of existing idle resources). As a third option, the hospital may build a long-term care facility (diversification through expansion). In each instance, the hospital has realized its strategy of diversification through different means. The term ***integration***—more specifically, organizational integration—is commonly used as a catch-all expression that may refer to certain consolidations, expansions, or diversifications that generally involve new products or services. In other words, integration can be achieved via any of the strategies discussed above. The ultimate aim of integration is to provide a seamless array of services around a hospital, which functions as the central core. Such an organization would be a veritable health system capable of fulfilling most of a community's health care needs. Figure 9–15 illustrates the various integration strategies.

Integration adds complexity to an organization's size and management. It can also present obstacles for customers. Many frail and sick people may find it difficult to navigate a large and complicated delivery sys-

Figure 9–15 Organizational Integration Strategies.

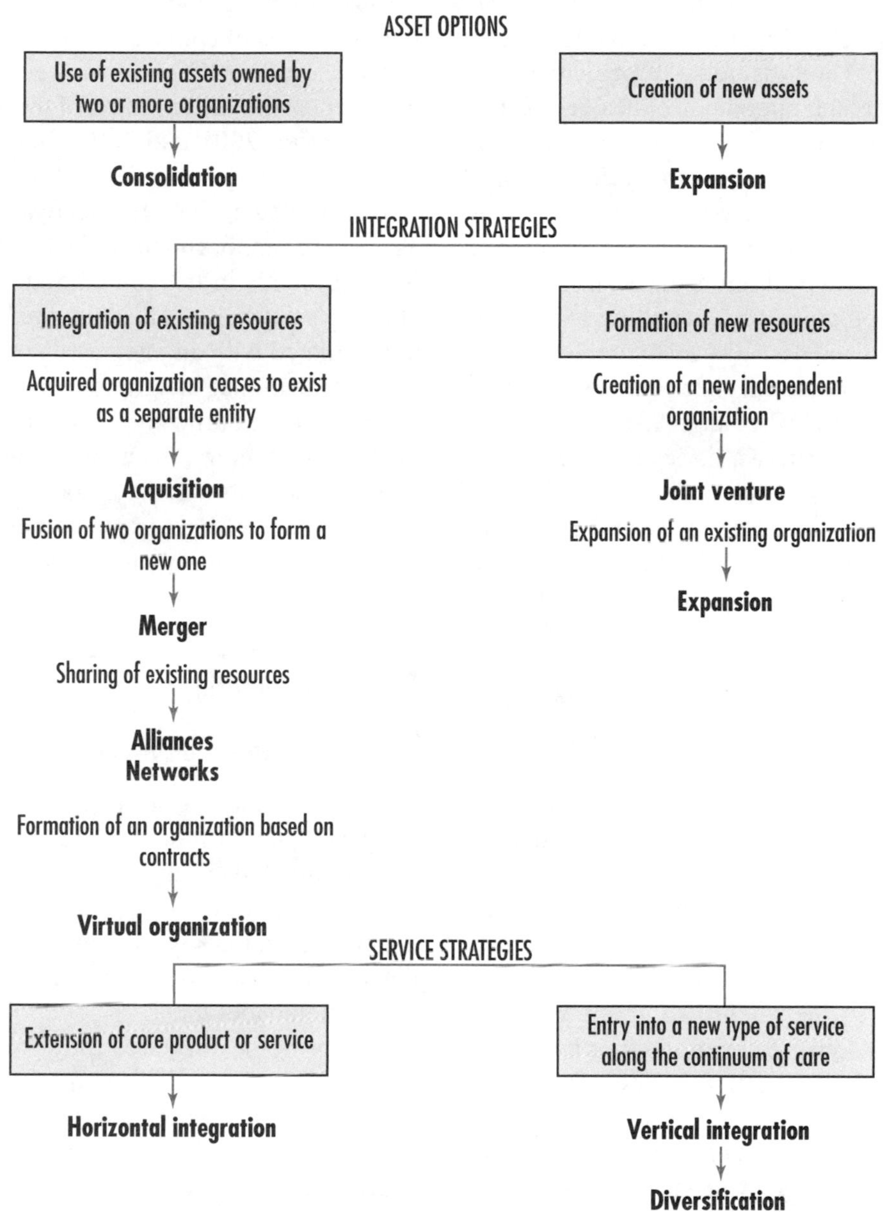

tem. Many of these systems have also failed to live up to their potential to deliver cost-efficient care, and many have experienced significant financial distress (Nader and Walston 2005).

Integrated Delivery Systems

For over a decade, the US health care industry has been consolidating and expanding to form what is now commonly referred to as integrated delivery systems (IDSs). An IDS represents various forms of ownership and other strategic linkages among hospitals, physicians, and insurers. Its objective is to achieve greater integration of health care services along a continuum of care (Shortell and Hull 1996). An ***integrated delivery system*** may be defined as a network of organizations that provides or arranges to provide a coordinated continuum of services to a defined population, and is willing to be held clinically and fiscally accountable for the outcomes and health status of the population serviced (Shortell et al. 1993). Not all integrated organizations, however, have arrived at this stage of maturity.

Integration of services and providers into coordinated systems of care occurred partly because of the growth of managed care. Market domination by managed care prompted providers to integrate for three main reasons. (1) For MCOs, it is more cost-effective to contract with organizations that offer comprehensive services to ensure a full spectrum of services to the MCO's enrollees. Various integrated systems developed so as not to be left out of the expanding managed care market. (2) Managed care also seeks providers who can render services in a cost-efficient manner and who will take responsibility for the quality of those services. Providers seek greater efficiencies by joining with other organizations or by diversifying into providing new services. Large organizations are in a better position to acquire up-to-date management and information systems to monitor their operations and address inefficiencies successfully. (3) Hospitals, physicians, and other providers have been concerned with protecting their autonomy. They found the growing power of managed care invading their turf when they were isolated. By forging linkages, they have strengthened their bargaining power in dealing with MCOs. Merging with an MCO gives providers the best of both worlds. They can have a say in how the MCO is run and get referrals of patients who are enrollees of the MCO.

Between 2001 and 2004, 304 mergers and acquisitions involving 695 hospitals were completed (Galloro and Evans 2005). There are approximately 580 integrated health systems in the United States (Evans 2005). Nearly half of all acute care hospitals are affiliated with an integrated system. After organizational integration went through a frenzied pace during the 1990s and the start of the 21th century, the activity has slowed down considerably. Perhaps not accidentally, the slow pace of integration coincides with the maturation of the managed care industry.

Types of Integration

Integration Based on Major Participants

From the standpoint of integration, the major participants in the health care delivery system are physicians, hospitals, and insurers. A variety of configurations can emerge depending on the key strategic position that physicians, hospitals, or insurers hold in the integration endeavor.

Many of the integrated entities discussed in this section actually became risk-bearing organizations. However, during the period of managed care bashing, earlier promises of success for some of these entities waned away. In a dynamic health care environment, we are likely to see new configurations emerge whereas others will disappear while the basic forms of consolidation and expansion are likely to remain intact provided they continue to successfully address changing demands in cost, access, and quality.

Physicians

Group practices (discussed in Chapter 7) and IPAs, discussed earlier in this chapter, are two types of organizations that integrate individual physicians into operating setups that provide practical advantages in contracting with HMOs. Physicians have increasingly recognized that they need management expertise to survive in the complex health care environment that requires contracts and other affiliations. Various types of arrangements known as management services organizations (***MSOs***) bring to physician group practices management expertise and, in some instances, capital for expansion. MSO services are often needed by smaller group practices because they find it uneconomical to employ full-time managers. The services provided by MSOs include billing and collection, administrative support, and others, such as managed care contracting. In more complex arrangements, the MSO may actually purchase many of the assets of the physicians' practices—for example, the office space and equipment. The MSO may also employ the office support staff for the physician. Other services offered by the MSO may include utilization management, quality assessment, provider relations, and services for the enrollees, such as health bulletins and 24-hour telephone access. Private entrepreneurs, a hospital, or a group of physicians may develop an MSO. Equity-based MSOs provide capital and management expertise. A variation of this MSO model, in which the management company uses venture capital and sale of stock to actually buy physician practices and integrate them into a network, is referred to as a physician practice management (***PPM***) company.

A later addition to the array of MCOs and integrated organizations is the provider-sponsored organization (***PSO***), which emerged in the 1990s. PSOs are risk-bearing entities sponsored by physicians, hospitals, or jointly by physicians and hospitals, to compete with regular MCOs by agreeing to provide health care to a defined group of enrollees under capitation. They bypass MCOs by contracting directly with employers and public insurers. When formed jointly by physicians and hospitals, PSOs do not differ much from a physician-hospital organization (PHO), discussed in the following section. PSOs gained national attention in 1996 when the US Congress proposed that PSOs could legitimately participate in Medicare risk contracts. Then, the Balanced Budget Act of 1997 opened up the Medicare market to PSOs as an option to HMOs under the Medicare +Choice program. At first, PSOs had been left largely unregulated. Later, the Balanced Budget Act required these entities to carry adequate coverage for risk protection. The initial appeal of PSOs was that they would deal with patients directly, rather than through contracted arrangements, as an HMO normally would do. However, after they suffered financial losses, PSOs failed in large numbers. In many instances, PSOs were acquired by larger HMOs. One major reason for PSO failures is their lack of experience with risk management (the insurance function).

Hospitals

A physician-hospital organization (***PHO***) is a legal entity that forms an alliance between a hospital and local physicians. Apart from contracting with MCOs, if a PHO is large enough, it can also contract its services directly to employers while engaging a third-party administrator to process claims. A large number of physicians allied with a hospital can provide one-stop shopping for enrollees. PHOs are often initiated by the hospital, but the PHO is unlikely to succeed without the participation of the medical staff leaders. PHOs provide the benefits of integration while preserving the independence and autonomy of physicians. For this reason, coupled with the relatively loose structure of PHOs, it can be difficult to affect provider behavior when cost containment and utilization management are important to the organization (Kongstvedt and Plocher 1995).

Other types of hospital-physician alliances include nonprofit foundations and health systems that employ physicians directly. It is important to keep in mind that hospital-physician alliances can have legal ramifications. In the case of physicians holding equity in a hospital as shareholders, problems with Medicare and Medicaid fraud and abuse can potentially arise (Kongstvedt and Plocher 1995). This issue stems from the Medicare and Medicaid antikickback statute that prohibits payments for patient referrals.

Between 1998 and 2000, the number of hospitals associated with PHOs more than doubled. However, the number of these organizations has been steadily declining since. Many failed because of poor management, undercapitalization, and federal antitrust scrutiny.

Insurance

PHOs and MSOs can contract out insurance and payment functions to third-party administrators. The true need for insurance is actually minimal when these organizations contract with self-insured employers. In other cases, a commercial insurance company can buy or have shared ownership with a hospital and one or more physician group practices. In this case, the entity would function as an MCO.

Integration Based on Degree of Ownership

Organizational consolidation or expansion can take various forms. Ownership involves the purchase of a controlling interest in another company, which can be accomplished through a merger or acquisition. Ownership does not have to be an all-or-nothing deal. Joint ventures allow two or more entities to participate in joint ownership of a new entity. A third approach, which can take various forms, does not involve ownership of another company's assets. In principle, it may simply involve cooperative arrangements and joint responsibilities. There may just be sharing of existing resources among two or more organizations, or formation of an organization based on contracts.

Mergers and Acquisitions

Mergers and acquisitions involve integration of existing assets. ***Acquisition*** refers to the purchase of one organization by another. The acquired company ceases to exist as a separate entity and is absorbed into the purchasing corporation. A ***merger*** involves a mutual agreement to unify two or more organizations into a single entity. The separate assets of two organizations are brought together, typically under a new name. Both entities cease to exist, and a new corporation is formed. A merger requires the willingness of all parties. All partners in the merger must assess the advantages and disadvantages of joining together (Carson et al. 1995, 209, 222).

Small hospitals may merge to gain efficiencies by eliminating duplication of services. A large hospital may acquire smaller hospitals to serve as satellites in a major metropolitan area with sprawling suburbs. A regional health care system may be formed after a large hospital has acquired smaller hospitals and certain providers of long-term care, outpatient care, and rehabilitation to diversify its services. Multifacility nursing home chains and home health firms often acquire other facilities to enter new geographic markets.

Joint Ventures

A ***joint venture*** results when two or more institutions share resources to create a new organization to pursue a common purpose (Pelfrey and Theisen 1989). Each partner in a joint venture continues to conduct business independently. The new company created by the partners also remains independent. Joint ventures are often used to diversify when the new service can benefit all the partners and when competing against each other for that service would be undesirable. Hospitals in a given region may engage in a joint venture to form a home health agency that benefits all partners. An acute care hospital, a multispecialty physician group practice, a skilled nursing facility, and an insurer may join to offer a managed care plan (Carson et al. 1995, 209). Each participant would continue to operate its own business, and they all would have a common stake in the new MCO.

Alliances

In one respect, the health care industry is unique because organizations often develop cooperative arrangements with rival providers. Cooperation instead of competition, in some situations, eliminates duplication of services while ensuring that all the health needs of the community are fulfilled (Carson et al. 1995, 217). An ***alliance*** is an agreement between two organizations to share their resources without joint ownership of assets. A PHO, for example, can be formed through a merger, a joint venture, or an alliance. Each type of integration determines the extent to which the hospital controls the assets owned by the physicians or group practices.

The main advantages of alliances are: (1) They are relatively simple to form. (2) They provide the opportunity to evaluate financial and legal ramifications before a potential "marriage" takes place. Forming an alliance gives organizations the opportunity to evaluate the advantages of an eventual merger. (3) Alliances require little financial commitment and can be easily dissolved, similar to an engagement prior to a marriage.

Networks

A network is formed through alliances with numerous providers. Generally, it is built around a core organization, such as an MCO. Although networks are often sponsored by an MCO, hospitals, physicians, and other organizations, such as an IPA, may form networks. A PHO, for example, may simply be a network, or it may result from a joint venture, a merger, or an acquisition.

Virtual Organizations

Alliances and networks often involve resource-sharing arrangements between organizations. However, when contractual arrangements between organizations form a new organization, it is referred to as a virtual organization or organization without walls. The formation of networks based on contractual arrangements is called ***virtual integration***. IPAs are prime examples of virtual organizations. A PHO may also be a virtual organization. The main advantage of virtual organizations is that they require less capital to enter new geographic or service markets (Gabel 1997). They also help bring together scattered entities under one mutually cooperative arrangement.

Integration Based on Service Consolidation

Horizontal and/or vertical integration is almost always necessary for the creation of a continuum of integrated services. Of the two strategies, only vertical integration results in diversification (see Figure 9–15).

Horizontal Integration

Horizontal integration is a growth strategy in which a health care delivery organization extends its core product or service. Commonly, the services are similar or may be substitutes for existing services. Horizontal integration may be achieved through internal development, acquisition, or merger. Horizontally linked organizations may be closely coupled through ownership consolidation or loosely coupled through alliances. The main objective of horizontal integration is to control the geographic distribution of a certain type of health care service. Multihospital chains, nursing facility chains, or a chain of drugstores, all under the same management, with member facilities offering the same core services or products, are horizontally integrated. Diversification into new products and/or services is not achieved through horizontal integration.

Vertical Integration

Vertical integration links services at different stages in the production process of health care—for example, organization of preventive services, primary care, acute care, and postacute service delivery around a hospital. The main objective of vertical integration is to increase the comprehensiveness and continuity of care across a continuum of health care services. Hence, vertical integration is a diversification strategy.

Vertical integration may be achieved through ownership consolidation, expansion into new services, joint ventures, or alliances. Formation of networks and virtual organizations can also involve vertical integration. Large hospital systems are particularly attracted to group practices in the interest of vertical integration because group practices can give them a large slice of the patient market. In essence, this kind of integration extends a hospital's control over the delivery of health services to the outpatient setting (Goldfarb 1993). Vertically integrated regional health systems may be the best positioned organizations to become the providers of choice for managed care or for direct contracting with self-insured employers (Brown 1996).

Issues Related to Integration

Economies of Scale

In terms of efficiency and the overall effectiveness of the health care delivery system, integration is a positive development, at least from a theoretical standpoint. Fragmentation is often inefficient. Among the nation's over 580 integrated delivery systems, many are highly efficient. Successfully integrated organizations find cost-control opportunities and an increased ability to reach a larger population with their range of services. These organizations are able to transition patients smoothly from their inpatient facilities to less costly outpatient and long-term care settings. Many of these systems are also collaborating with independent facilities or other integrated systems to broaden the geographic reach and scope of medical services (Survey identifies top IHNs 2004), but research on the results of integration is mixed. There is some consensus that integrated systems do not produce internal or external efficiencies. Studies during the 1980s and 1990s generally did not support the idea that system integration resulted in any marked improvements in organizations' internal productivity or profitability. These studies also suggested that in terms of external efficiencies, there was no evidence that integration had led to better health for the populations served, more charity care, or better patient outcomes (Burns and Pauly 2002). More recent evidence, however, gives a more favorable view of internal organizational performance (Wang et al. 2001; Wan et al. 2002). Industry trends support these analyses. Highly integrated systems that include a hospital, a physician component, and at least one systemwide contract with a payer have been on the rise for quite some time. For example, the number of hospitals that were part of a highly integrated system increased by 7% between 2003 and 2005. In the same period, the number of HMOs and PPOs affiliated with integrated systems climbed nearly 20% (Sanofi-Aventis 2006b). On the other hand, questions still linger as to whether external efficiencies create value for patients.

Competition and Antitrust

A side effect of integration is limitation of choice for physicians and patients. Some concern exists that the wave of integration activity may produce a few dominant companies that can squeeze out competition. Erosion of competition can compromise consumer access to affordable quality care (Alpha Center 1997).

Laws have been designed, however, as a check against anticompetitive behavior. If an IDS is formed primarily to stifle competition, it may be found in violation of antitrust legislation (Kongstvedt and Plocher 1995). ***Antitrust*** policy consists of federal and state laws that make certain types of business practices illegal. The business practices prohibited or regulated by antitrust laws include price fixing, price discrimination, exclusive contracting arrangements, and mergers among competitors. The purpose of antitrust policy is to ensure the competitiveness, and thus the efficiency, of economic markets. Despite antitrust laws, however, large medical systems have come to dominate the health care landscape in some parts of the country, creating virtual monopolies as smaller players have been bought out because of economic pressures.

Role of Physicians

Physicians have resented the dominance of managed care and IDSs. Berenson (1997) cogently remarked that physicians are generally individualistic and strive for personal achievement. They resist management techniques that reduce their authority and autonomy. Because physicians are not upset about the cost or quality of care, they are not interested in remaking the health care system. Regardless of which direction the structure of the health care delivery system takes, however, physicians are likely to remain critical players. To avoid being left out of the market, they may have been forced by economic necessities to join the integrated organizations, but their participation remains important. In the long run, integrated systems will be better served if physicians and other direct caregivers can participate in organizational policy setting and decision making. Physicians possess the knowledge necessary to make the system more efficient in its use of resources and more effective in producing desirable health outcomes (Zwanziger and Melnick 1996). For their part, physicians will have to reexamine their attitudes toward working in organizational settings. In particular, physicians need to develop greater sensitivity to the cost of providing health care.

Need for Up-to-Date Information Systems

The need for well-organized information systems (discussed in Chapter 5) presents a critical challenge to MCOs and IDSs. Well-designed information systems strengthen internal planning and quality control to enhance management and clinical functions. Information technology is also critical to providing timely and accurate information for external reporting. Typically, an MCO has to provide periodic reports to multiple external constituencies, which include the National Committee for Quality Assurance and the state governments (in the case of Medicaid 1115 Waivers). However, most MCOs do not have well-organized information systems. The problem is especially serious in newly emerging MCOs, which typically target Medicaid populations. Another pressing issue concerns IDSs. It is how to upgrade and integrate information systems across separate facilities that have become part of an integrated delivery network. Attention and spending in information technology are moving from hardware and software applications toward connectivity, networking, data architecture, and other labor-based services requiring highly skilled personnel in the application of information technology.

Summary

Managed care has evolved through an integration of the insurance function with the concepts of contract practice and prepaid group practice of the late 19th and early 20th centuries. Hallmarks of managed care are fixed premiums, risk-sharing with providers, comprehensive services, emphasis on primary care, and utilization management. Over time, various MCO types have evolved, particularly to fill consumer desires for a greater choice of providers. Private employers have made almost a complete transition to managed care plans, and the government-sponsored Medicaid program has shown increased enrollments in managed care. The Medicare program, however, remains almost completely under the fee-for-service system, despite the benefits offered by the Medicare Advantage option.

Evidence suggests that managed care has slowed the rate of growth in health care expenditures. Fears of lower quality have been largely unwarranted. Managed care has also suffered from negative public opinions, only some of which are justified. Legislation enacted to restrain abuses has been on the rise, although federal legislation in the form of a patient's bill of rights has failed to pass. Taken to an extreme, however, unrelenting bashing of managed care would likely jeopardize the potential for cost savings that are essential in the face of rising health care expenditures. On the other hand, recent increases in premiums have raised questions about managed care's ability to control future costs. However, this does not imply that something else will soon replace managed care. It does mean increased cost shifting from employers to employees, and greater differentiation in health plans so employees can choose what is best for them individually, based on each plan's benefits and costs.

Managed care's growth is one force that has led to consolidation and diversification in the health care industry. Although consolidations are theoretically beneficial, taken to extremes they could limit future competition. Erosion of competition will have negative effects on access, cost, and quality. Antitrust policy is designed to provide some safeguards. Nevertheless, various kinds of consolidation concentrate power on the supply side.

Test Your Understanding

Terminology

acquisition
alliance
antitrust
capitation
carve out
case management
closed-panel
consolidation
discharge planning
disease management
diversification
exclusive provider plan
expansion
fee schedule
group model
Health maintenance organization (HMO)
horizontal integration
independent practice association (IPA)
integrated delivery system
integration
IPA model
joint venture
merger
mixed model
MSOs
network model
open panel
panel
physician-hospital organization (PHO)
point-of-service plan
PPM
practice profiling
preferred provider organization (PPO)
primary care case management (PCCM)
PSO
risk contract
staff model
utilization review (UR)
vertical integration
virtual integration

Review Questions

1. What are some of the key differences between traditional health insurance and managed care?
2. Explain how the fee-for-service practice of medicine led to increased health care costs.
3. Despite increasing health care costs, why did the Health Maintenance Organization Act of 1973 fail to achieve its objectives?
4. What are the three main payment mechanisms managed care uses? In each mechanism, who bears the risk?

5. What three main avenues have been used by MCOs to achieve cost efficiencies?
6. What are some of the inefficiencies that have resulted from numerous health plans in the managed care system?
7. Discuss the concept of utilization monitoring and control.
8. What are the various mechanisms used by MCOs to monitor and control utilization? Briefly discuss each mechanism.
9. Describe the three utilization review methods, giving appropriate examples. Discuss the benefits of each type of utilization review.
10. How does case management achieve efficiencies in the delivery of health care?
11. How do case management and disease management differ?
12. What is an HMO? How does it differ from a PPO?
13. Briefly explain the four main models for organizing an HMO. Discuss the advantages and disadvantages of each model.
14. What is a point-of-service plan? Why did it grow in popularity? What caused its subsequent decline?
15. What strategies are employers using to cope with the rising cost of health insurance premiums?
16. Why has managed care enrollment among Medicare beneficiaries remained low despite the creation of Medicare Advantage?
17. To what extent has managed care been successful in containing health care costs?
18. Has the quality of health care gone down as a result of managed care? Explain.
19. What is organizational integration? What is the purpose of integration in health care delivery? What are its drawbacks?
20. Explain how managed care has contributed to the development of integrated delivery systems.
21. What are the different types of services provided by a management services organization (MSO)?
22. What is the difference between a merger and an acquisition? What is the purpose of these organizational consolidations? Give examples.
23. When would a joint venture be considered a preferable integration strategy?
24. What is the main advantage of two organizations forming an alliance?
25. State the main strategic objectives of horizontal and vertical integration.
26. What is antitrust policy? Which business practices does antitrust law prohibit? Why do antitrust laws exist?

REFERENCES

Alpha Center. 1997. Hospital mergers reduce acute care beds but overcapacity remains an issue. *Health Care Financing and Organization Findings Brief*, June, 1.

Aventis Pharmaceuticals/SMG Marketing-Verispan LLC. 2002. Managed care digest series: HMO-PPO/Medicare-Medicaid digest. Bridgewater, NJ: Aventis Pharmaceuticals.

Baker, L. et al. 2004. The effect of area HMO market share on cancer screening. *Health Services Research* 39, no. 6: 1751–1772.

Balsa, A. et al. 2007. Does managed health care reduce health care disparities between minorities and Whites? *Journal of Health Economics* 26, no. 1: 101–121.

Berenson, R.A. 1997. Beyond competition. *Health Affairs* 16, no. 2: 171–180.

Berk, M.L., and A.C. Monheit. 2001. The concentration of health expenditures revisited. *Health Affairs* 20, 2: 9–18.

Bourjolly, J.N. et al. 2004. The impact of managed health care in the United States on women with breast cancer and the providers who treat them. *Cancer Nursing* 27, no. 1: 45–54.

Brown, A.F. et al. 2005. Race, ethnicity, socioeconomic position, and quality of care for adults with diabetes enrolled in managed care. *Diabetes Care* 28, no. 12: 2864–2870.

Brown, M. 1996. Mergers, networking, and vertical integration: Managed care and investor-owned hospitals. *Health Care Management Review* 21, no. 1: 29–37.

Burns, L.R., and M.V. Pauly. 2002. Integrated delivery networks: A detour on the road to integrated health care? *Health Affairs* 21, no. 4: 128–143.

Business World Inc. 1996. Physicians and employers identify seven essentials of managed care. *Health Care Strategic Management* 14, no. 12: 4.

Capps, C., and D. Dranove. 2004. Hospital consolidation and negotiated PPO prices. *Health Affairs* 23, no. 2: 175–181.

Carson, K.D. et al. 1995. *Management of healthcare organizations*. Cincinnati, OH: South-Western College Publishing.

Dean, B.N., and A.M. Epstein. 2002. National Committee on Quality Assurance health-plan accreditation: Predictors, correlates of performance, and market impact. *Medical Care* 40, no. 4: 325–337.

DeFrancesco, L.B. 2002. HMO enrollees experience fewer disparities than older insured populations. *Findings Brief: Health Care Financing & Organization* 5, no. 2: 1–2.

Eikel, C.V. 2002. Fewer patient visits under capitation offset by improved quality of care: Study brings evidence to debate over physician payment methods. *Findings Brief: Health Care Financing & Organization* 5, no. 3: 1–2.

Enthoven, A.C. 2001. Consumer choice and the managed care backlash. *American Journal of Law & Medicine* 27, no. 1: 1–14.

Evans, M. 2005. Experts at integration. *Modern Healthcare* 35, no. 5: 24–25.

Feldstein, P.J. 1994. *Health policy issues: An economic perspective on health reform*. Ann Arbor, MI: AUPHA Press/Health Administration Press.

Fine, A. 2005. Medicare managed care plans grow. *Managed Care Quarterly* 13, no. 4: 26–27.

Fireman, B. et al. 2004. Can disease management reduce health care costs by improving quality? *Health Affairs* 23, no. 6: 63–75.

Gabel, J. 1997. Ten ways HMOs have changed during the 1990s. *Health Affairs* 16, no. 3: 134–145.

Gabel, J.R. 1999. Job-based health insurance, 1977–1998: The accidental system under scrutiny. *Health Affairs* 18, no. 6: 62–74.

Galloro, V., and M. Evans. 2005. 2005 mergers and acquisitions report: The surge to merge. *Modern Healthcare* 35, no. 4: 20–29.

Ginsburg, P.B. 2005. Competition in health care: Its evolution over the past decade. *Health Affairs* 24, no. 6: 1512–1522.

Goldfarb, B. 1993. Corporate health care mergers. *Medical World News* 34, no. 2: 26–34.

Goldman, W. et al. 2003. A four-year study of enhancing outpatient psychotherapy in managed care. *Psychiatric Services* 54, no. 1: 41–49.

Health Insurance Association of America. 1991. *Source book of health insurance data*. Washington, DC.

Henry J. Kaiser Family Foundation/Health Research and Educational Trust (Kaiser/HRET). 2002. *Employer health benefits: 2002 annual survey*. Menlo Park, CA: Kaiser Family Foundation.

Henry J. Kaiser Family Foundation/Health Research and Educational Trust (Kaiser/HRET). 2006. *Employer health benefits: 2006 annual survey*. Menlo Park, CA: Kaiser Family Foundation.

Himmelstein, D. et al. 1999. Quality of care in investor-owned vs. not-for-profit HMOs. *Journal of the American Medical Association* 282, no. 2: 159–163.

Hoechst Marion Roussel. 1998. *Managed care digest series: HMO-PPO/Medicare Medicaid digest*. Kansas City, MO: Hoechst Marion Roussel, Inc.

Hofmann, M.A. 2002. Quality of health care improving. *Business Insurance* 36, no. 38: 1–2.

Hurley, R.E., and D.A. Draper. 2002. Health plan responses to managed care regulation. *Managed Care Quarterly* 10, no. 4: 30–42.

Iglehart, J.K. 1994. The American health care system: Managed care. In *The nation's health*. 4th ed., eds. P.R. Lee and C.L. Estes, 231–237. Boston: Jones & Bartlett Publishers.

Kongstvedt, P.R. 1995a. Managing hospital utilization. In *Essentials of managed health care*, ed. P.R. Kongstvedt, 121–135. Gaithersburg, MD: Aspen Publishers, Inc.

Kongstvedt, P.R. 1995b. Managed health care. In *Health care administration: Principles, practices, structure, and delivery*. 2nd ed., ed. L.F. Wolper, 627–642. Gaithersburg, MD: Aspen Publishers, Inc.

Kongstvedt, P.R. 1995c. Use of data and reports in medical management. In *Essentials of managed health care*, ed. P.R. Kongstvedt, 173–181. Gaithersburg, MD: Aspen Publishers, Inc.

Kongstvedt, P.R., and D.W. Plocher. 1995. Integrated health care delivery systems. In *Essentials of managed health care*, ed. P.R. Kongstvedt, 35–49. Gaithersburg, MD: Aspen Publishers, Inc.

Landon, B.E., and A.M. Epstein. 1999. Quality management practices in Medicaid managed care: A national survey of Medicaid and commercial health plans participating in the Medicaid program. *Journal of the American Medical Association* 282, no. 18: 1769–1775.

Landon, B.E. et al. 2003. Changes in career satisfaction among primary care and specialist physicians, 1997–2001. *Journal of the American Medical Association* 289, no. 4: 442–449.

MacColl, W.A. 1966. *Group practice and prepayment of medical care*. Washington, DC: Public Affairs Press.

Mackie, D.L., and D.K. Decker. 1981. *Group and IPA HMOs*. Gaithersburg, MD: Aspen Publishers, Inc.

MacLeod, G.K. 1995. An overview of managed health care. In *Essentials of Managed Health Care*, ed. P.R. Kongstvedt, 1–9. Gaithersburg, MD: Aspen Publishers, Inc.

MacLeod, G.K., and J.A. Prussin. 1973. The continuing evolution of health maintenance organizations. *New England Journal of Medicine* 288, no. 9: 439–443.

Mayer, T.R., and G.G. Mayer. 1984. *The health insurance alternative: A complete guide to health maintenance organizations*. New York: Perigee Books.

Mays, G.P. et al. 2004. Managed care rebound? Recent changes in health plans' cost containment strategies. *Health Affairs (Supplement 2)* 23: 427–437.

McGuire, J.P. 1994. The growth of managed care. *Health Care Financial Management* 48, no. 8: 10.

Mechanic, D. 1972. *Public expectations and health care*. New York: John Wiley & Sons.

Meenan, R.T., and N. Vuckovic. 2004. On the integration of complementary and conventional medicine within health maintenance organizations. *Journal of Ambulatory Care Management* 27, no. 1: 43–52.

Miller, R.H., and H.S. Luft. 1997. Does managed care lead to better or worse quality of care? *Health Affairs* 16, no. 5: 7–26.

Miller, R.H., and H.S. Luft. 2002. HMO plan performance update: An analysis of the literature, 1997–2001. *Health Affairs* 21, no. 4: 63–86.

Moscovice, I. et al. 1998. Expanding rural managed care: Enrollment patterns and prospectives. *Health Affairs* 17, no. 1: 172–179.

Nader, R., and S. Walston. 2005. Transfer pricing and integrated delivery systems: The effects of interdependence and risk. *Managed Care Quarterly* 13, no. 4: 1–8.

National Committee for Quality Assurance (NCQA). 2007. What accreditation levels can a plan achieve? *http://web.ncqa.org/tabid/197/Default.aspx*.

Newhouse, J.P. 2001. Lessons from the medical marketplace. In *Governance amid bigger, better markets*, eds. J.S. Nye and J.D. Donahue. Washington, DC: Brookings Institution Press.

Pelfrey, S., and B.A. Theisen. 1989. Joint venture in health care. *Journal of Nursing Administration* 19, no. 4: 39–42.

Public Health Service. 1995. *Health United States*, 1994. Washington, DC: Government Printing Office.

Raffel, M.W. 1980. *The US health system: Origins and functions*. New York: John Wiley & Sons.

Raffel, M.W., and N.K. Raffel. 1994. *The US health system: Origins and functions*. 4th ed. Albany, NY: Delmar Publishers.

Rakich, J.S. et al. 1992. *Managing health services organizations*. 3rd ed. Baltimore, MD: Health Professions Press.

Reed, M. et al. 2003. Physicians and care management: more acceptance than you think. *Issue brief* [Center for the Study of Health System Change], January (60): 1–4.

Reed, M.C., and S. Trude. 2002. Who do you trust? Americans' perspectives on health care, 1997–2001. *Tracking report* [electronic resource] August (3): 1–4.

Riley, G.F. et al. 1999. Stage at diagnosis and treatment patterns among older women with breast cancer. *Journal of the American Medical Association* 281: 720–726.

Rizzo, J.A. 2005. Are HMOs bad for health maintenance? *Health Economics* 14, no. 11: 1117–1131.

Robinson, J.C. 2002. Renewed emphasis on consumer cost sharing in health insurance benefit design. *Health Affairs Web Exclusives 2002:* W139–W154.

Robinson, J.C. 2006. The commercial health insurance industry in an era of eroding employer coverage. *Health Affairs* 25, no. 6: 1475–1486.

Rogers, W.H. et al. 1993. Outcomes for adult outpatients with depression under prepaid or fee-for-service care: Results from the Medical Outcomes Study. *Archives of General Psychiatry* 50, no. 7: 517–525.

Sanofi-Aventis. 2006a. *Managed care digest series, 2006: HMO-PPO digest*. Bridgewater, NJ: Sanofi-Aventis US, LLC.

Sanofi-Aventis. 2006b. Integrated health systems afterword. *http://www.managedcaredigest.com/edigests/hosp2006/Keys.jsp#.*

Sari, N. 2002. Do competition and managed care improve quality? *Health Economics* 11, no. 7: 571–584.

Schneider, E.C. et al. 2005. Quality of care in for-profit and not-for-profit health plans enrolling Medicare beneficiaries. *American Journal of Medicine* 118, no. 12: 1392–1400.

Schur, C.L. et al. 2004. Public perceptions of cost containment strategies: Mixed signals for managed care. *Health Affairs (Supplement 2)* 23: 513–525.

Senterfitt, B. 2005. Managed care experiments with new Medicaid model. *Managed Healthcare Executive* 15, no. 7: 13.

Short, A.C. et al. 2003. Disease management: A leap of faith to lower-cost, higher-quality health care. *Issue Brief No. 69 (October 2003)*. Washington, DC: Center for Studying Health System Change.

Shortell, S.M. et al. 1993. Creating organized delivery systems: The barriers and facilitators. *Hospital and Health Services Administration* 38, no. 4: 447–466.

Shortell, S.M., and K.E. Hull. 1996. The new organization of the health care delivery system. In *Strategic choices for a changing health care system*, eds. S.H. Altman and U.E. Reinhardt. Chicago: Health Administration Press.

Sipkoff, M. 2003. Health plans begin to address chronic care management. *Managed Care Magazine. http://www.managedcaremag.com/archives/0312/0312.kaiserchronic.html.*

Southwick, K. 1997. Case study: How United HealthCare and two contracting hospitals address cost and quality in era of hyper-competition. *Strategies for Healthcare Excellence* (COR Healthcare Resources) 10, no. 8 (August): 1–9.

Strunk, B.C. and P.J. Cunningham. 2004. Trends in Americans' access to needed medical care, 2001–2003. Tracking Report No. 10 (August 2004). Washington, DC: Center for Studying Health System Change.

Survey identifies top IHNs, indicates stabilized growth. 2004. *Healthcare Financial Management* 58, no. 3: 25.

Thorpe, K.E., and A. Atherly. 2002. Medicare+Choice: Current role and near-term prospects. *Health Affairs Web Exclusives 2002:* W242–W252.

Tu, H.T. 2005a. Medicare seniors much less willing to limit physician-hospital choice for lower costs. *Issue Brief No. 96 (June 2005)*. Washington, DC: Center for Studying Health System Change.

Tu, H.T. 2005b. More Americans willing to limit physician-hospital choice for lower medical costs. *Issue Brief No. 94 (March 2005)*. Washington, DC: Center for Studying Health System Change.

Wagner, E.R. 1995. Types of managed care organizations. In *Essentials of managed health care*, ed. P.R. Kongstvedt, 24–34. Gaithersburg, MD: Aspen Publishers, Inc.

Wan, T.T. et al. 2002. Integration mechanisms and hospital efficiency in integrated health care delivery systems. *Journal of Medical Systems* 26, no. 2: 127–143.

Wang, B.B. et al. 2001. Managed care, vertical integration strategies and hospital performance. *Health Care Management Science* 4, no. 3: 181–191.

Wells, K.B. et al. 1989. Detection of depressive disorder for patients receiving prepaid or fee-for-service care: Results from the Medical Outcomes Study. *Journal of the American Medical Association* 262, no. 23: 3298–3302.

Wilkerson, J.D. et al. 1997. The emerging competitive managed care marketplace. In *Competitive managed care: The emerging health care system*, eds. J.D. Wilkerson et al., 3–29. San Francisco: Jossey-Bass Publishers.

Williams, C.H. et al. 2006. How has hospital consolidation affected the price and quality of hospital care? *Policy Brief* No. 9 (February 2006). Princeton, NJ: The Robert Wood Johnson Foundation.

Wilson, F.A., and D. Neuhauser. 1985. *Health services in the United States*. 2nd ed. Cambridge, MA: Ballinger Publishing Co.

Zelman, W.A. 1996. *The changing health care marketplace*. San Francisco: Jossey-Bass Publishers.

Zwanziger, J., and G.A. Melnick. 1996. Can managed care plans control health care costs? *Health Affairs* 15, no. 2: 185–199.

Chapter 10

Long-Term Care

Learning Objectives

- To comprehend the concept of long-term care and its main features
- To get an overview of the main types of services encompassed in the delivery of long-term care
- To discover who needs long-term care and why
- To become familiar with the large variety of community-based long-term care services and who pays for these services
- To learn about the various types of long-term care institutions and the levels of services they provide
- To get an overview of specialized long-term care facilities
- To get acquainted with the main aspects of the nursing home industry and the patients it serves
- To learn about the main sources of nursing home financing
- To survey the requirements for participation in the Medicare and Medicaid programs

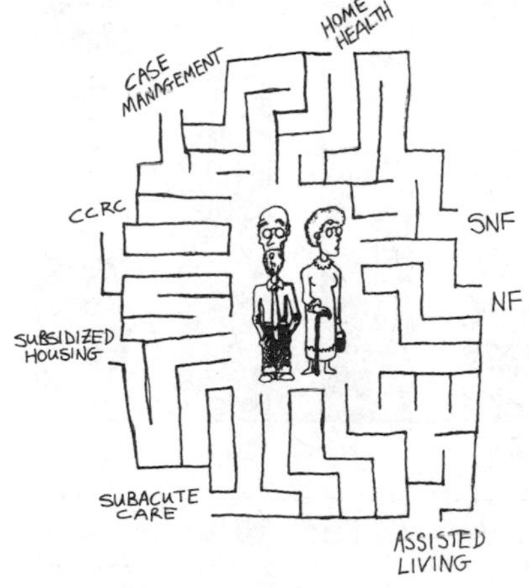

"Now, honey, where are we supposed to go from here?"

Introduction

Long-term care (LTC) is often associated with care provided in nursing homes, but that is a rather narrow view of LTC. Several types of noninstitutional LTC services are provided in a variety of community-based settings. These services include informal care provided by family and surrogates, home health services brought into a person's own home, home delivered meals, and personal assistance provided in residential settings, such as foster care homes and board-and-care facilities. Older Americans overwhelmingly show a strong desire to remain in their own homes. In one study, 73% of Americans aged 55 and older expected to always live in their current residences (Hoffman 2001). It is also important to note that LTC is not confined to the elderly, although the elderly are the predominant users of these services, and most LTC services have been designed with the elderly patient in mind.

This chapter focuses on the elderly as the primary recipients of LTC, but this does not mean that most elderly people are in need of such care. To the contrary, most elderly people are physically and mentally healthy enough to function independently. In 2003, 92% of elderly Americans lived either alone (19%) or with a spouse (73%) (Federal Interagency Forum 2004). Also, over 73% of adults aged 65 and over assessed their own health status as good, very good, or excellent (Figure 10–1), although 59% of elderly blacks compared to 76% of elderly non-Hispanic whites assessed their health status this positively. Nevertheless, the aging process leads

Figure 10–1 Respondant Assessed Health Status for Adults 65 Years and Over (age adjusted), 2005 (percentage distribution).

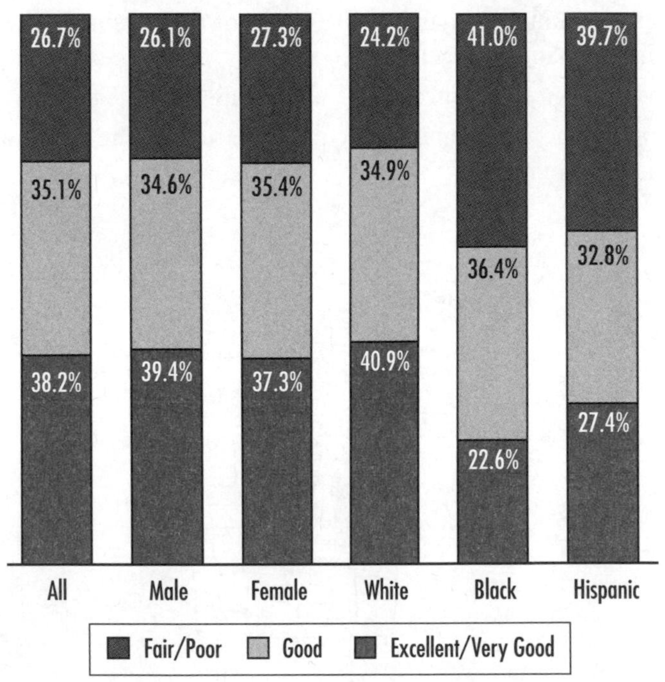

Source: Data from *Trends in Health and Aging,* National Center for Health Statisitcs, US Department of Health and Human Services, http://209.217.72.34/aging/ReportFolders/ReportFolders.aspx?CS_referer=&CS_ChosenLang=en.

to chronic, degenerative conditions that resist cure. Services that enable people with chronic conditions to live independently for as long as possible are often those that emphasize assistance and caring, rather than curing. However, the clients of LTC need a variety of health care services over time. Hence, long-term care cannot be an isolated component of the health care delivery system. The LTC system must be closely integrated with the rest of the system. Here, integration refers to the ease of transition among various types of health care settings and services.

Although medical care provided in hospitals is generally associated with acute episodes, LTC is often associated with chronic conditions. Chronic conditions are the leading causes of illness, disability, and death in the United States today. ***Chronic conditions*** are characterized by persistent and recurring health consequences lasting over a long period. In order of their prevalence among the aged population, the most common chronic conditions are hypertension, arthritis, heart disease, cancers, and diabetes (Federal Interagency Forum 2004). Also common among the elderly are hearing and vision impairments, cognitive loss, and depressive symptoms. Both low cognitive functioning and depressive symptoms are associated with a high risk for functional decline (Mehta et al. 2002). Serious illness or injury can also lead to a rapid decline in one's health and further limit one's ability to do things for oneself.

Disability and functional limitations rise dramatically among those who have multiple chronic conditions (Figure 10–2). As the elderly population in the United States continues to grow, between 2000 and 2020, the number of Americans with chronic conditions is projected to increase from 125 million (45% of the population) to 157 million (Figure 10–3). Moreover, approximately 57 million Americans (22% of the population) suffer from multiple chronic conditions. This number will rise to 81 million (25% of the population) by 2020 (Anderson 2003). It is also estimated that direct medical costs for chronic conditions will rise from $510 billion in 2000 to $1,070 billion by 2020

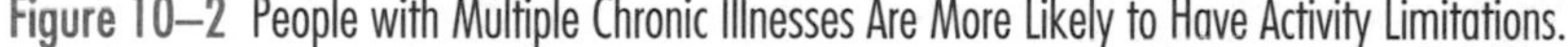

Figure 10–2 People with Multiple Chronic Illnesses Are More Likely to Have Activity Limitations.

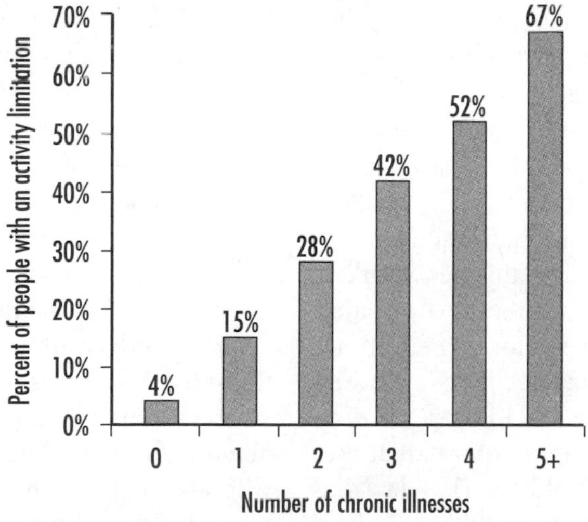

Source: Chronic Conditions: Making the Case for Ongoing Care, Partnership for Solutions, Johns Hopkins University, December 2002, p.12.

Figure 10–3 The Number of People with Chronic Conditions.

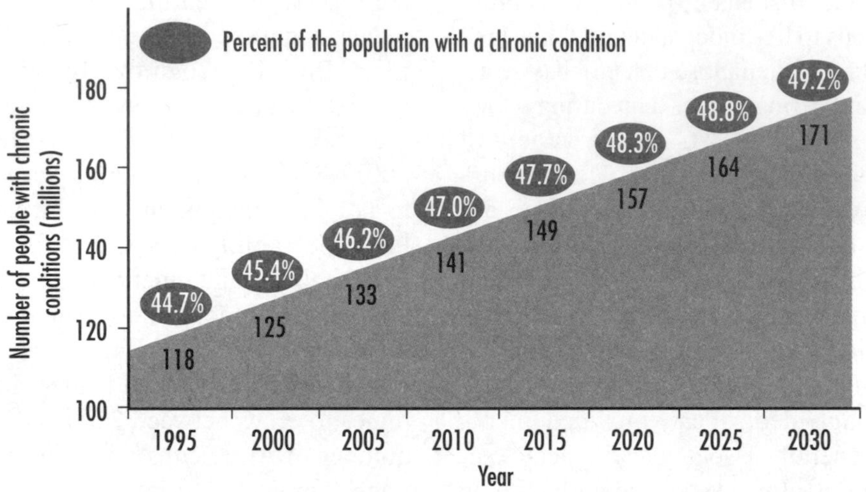

Source: Chronic Conditions: Making the Case for Ongoing Care, Partnership for Solutions, Johns Hopkins University, December 2002.

(Partnership for Solutions 2002). The number of people 70 and older needing LTC will increase from 10 million in 2000 to 15 million in 2020 and to 21 million in 2030 (National Academy on an Aging Society 2000). Further, a 2003 analysis suggests that the future demand for nursing home use will be greater than what may be apparent from simple extrapolations of past declines in disability. (Declines in disability among the elderly during the 1980s and 1990s were noted by preliminary investigations of the National Long-Term Care Survey. A number of issues with this initial conclusion were brought to light by Wolf et al. 2005.) Although the rate of institutionalization among the elderly has been falling, this trend is likely to reverse itself within the next decade, pointing to a growing need for nursing home care in the future. This is due to rising levels of obesity and diabetes, and increases in disability among the younger cohorts that are beginning to approach old age (Lakdawalla et al. 2003; Goldman et al. 2005). Studies show that other health problems, such as osteoporosis, hip fractures, stroke, cancer, heart disease, arthritis, and glaucoma, have also increased among the older population (see, for example, Crimmins 2004).

The rest of the developed world also faces aging-related problems and challenges in providing adequate LTC services very similar to those in the United States. Actually, the elderly population as a proportion of the total population in other developed countries such as Japan, Germany, France, and Great Britain is already higher than it is in the United States.

This chapter presents a comprehensive view of LTC, its main clients, various types of community-based and institution-based services, and how these services are financed. Both community-based and institution-based services form a continuum of services demanded by the varied needs of a heterogeneous population. Even the elderly, who are the predominant users of LTC services, are not a homogeneous group.

The Nature of Long-Term Care

Long-term care can be defined as a variety of individualized, well-coordinated services that are designed to promote the maximum possible independence for people with functional limitations, and these services are provided over an extended period of time to meet the patients' physical, mental, social, and spiritual needs while maximizing their quality of life (Singh 2005). The seven components of LTC apply to both institutional and community-based LTC services.

Variety of Services

A variety of services is necessary because individual needs, as determined by health status, finances, and other factors, vary greatly among people who require LTC services. Also, individual needs often change over time and call for different services and settings. The variety of services also depends on where the services are provided, who provides the services, and the level of care provided. Accordingly, LTC services can be institutional versus community-based, formal versus informal, and light versus intense.

Individualized Services

LTC services are individually tailored based primarily on an assessment of the individual's current physical, mental, and emotional condition. Other factors used for this purpose include past history of the patient's medical and psychosocial conditions, a social history of family relationships, former occupation, leisure activities, and cultural factors. Services are provided according to an individualized plan of care that addresses each type of need through customized interventions.

Well-Coordinated Total Care

LTC providers are responsible for managing the total health care needs of an individual client. ***Total care*** requires that any health care need is recognized, evaluated, and addressed by appropriate clinical professionals (Singh 2005). For example, a patient may need to be referred to a dentist, optometrist, podiatrist, or mental health professional or transferred to an acute care hospital. Hence, LTC often overlaps with non-LTC services. The LTC delivery system cannot function independently of other health care services. Patients needing LTC often require coordination among many services because as needs change over time, these patients may have to transition among different types of services. Hence, the LTC system must be rationally linked to the rest of the health care delivery system (Figure 10–4). In a well-integrated system, patients should be able to move with relative ease between needed services.

Promotion of Functional Independence

A key determinant of the need for LTC is the degree to which an individual is unable to independently perform certain common tasks of daily living. Different indicators can be used to assess these limitations, including impairment in activities of daily living (ADLs) or instrumental activities of daily living (IADLs) (see Chapter 2 for a description of ADLs and IADLs), and other measures of physical, cognitive, and social functioning. The goal of LTC is to enable the individual to maintain functional independence to the maximum level that is practicable. For example, some people can continue to perform certain daily living tasks in spite of their disability by using adaptive devices such as

Figure 10–4 Key Characteristics of a Well-Designed LTC System.

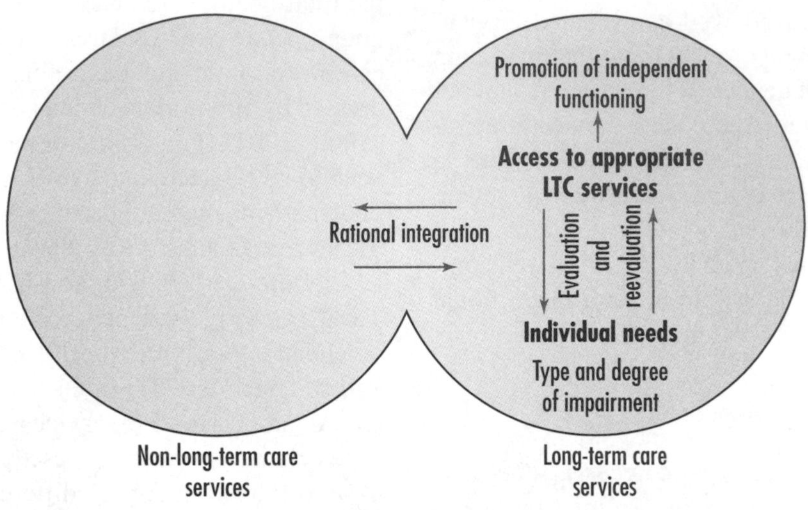

KEY CHARACTERISTICS

1. The LTC system is rationally integrated with the rest of the health care delivery system. This rational integration facilitates easy access to services between the two components of the health care delivery system.
2. Appropriate placement of the patient within the LTC system is based on an assessment of individual needs. For example, individual needs determine whether and when institutionalization may be necessary.
3. The LTC system accommodates changes in individual needs by providing access to appropriate LTC services as determined by a reevaluation of needs.
4. LTC services are designed to compensate for existing impairment and have the objective of promoting independence to the extent possible.

walkers and wheelchairs for mobility, adaptive utensils for eating, and portable oxygen devices for breathing. Modification of the physical environment is another way to enhance the functional capacity of individuals. Examples of modifications are ramps that provide access to buildings, extra-wide doors and corridors, grab bars in bathrooms, and adequate lighting. Caregiving staff should concentrate on maintaining whatever ability to function the patient still has and on preventing further decline of that ability.

Extended Period of Care

For most LTC clients, the delivery of various services extends over a relatively long period because most recipients of care will at least require ongoing monitoring to note any deterioration in their health and to address any emerging needs. Certain types of services, such as rehabilitation therapies, postacute convalescence, or stabilization may be needed for a relatively short duration, generally less than 90 days. The patient subsequently returns to independent living. On the other hand, the need for LTC may necessitate long-range confinement to a nursing care facility. For example, postacute medical complications may occur, leading to a rapid decline in a patient's health, or certain postacute conditions may remain unstable.

Holistic Care

As discussed in Chapter 2, the holistic model of health proposes that a person's health care needs extend beyond the physical and mental domains; they emphasize well-being in every aspect of what makes a person whole and complete. In holistic care, a patient's physical, mental, social, and spiritual needs and preferences should be incorporated into medical care delivery.

Quality of Life

A sense of satisfaction, fulfillment, and self-worth is regarded as a critical patient outcome in any health care delivery setting. It takes added significance in LTC because (1) a loss of self-worth often accompanies disability, and (2) patients remain in LTC settings for relatively long periods with little hope of full recovery in most instances.

Quality of life is a multifaceted concept that recognizes at least five factors: lifestyle pursuits, living environment, clinical palliation, human factors, and personal choices.

- Lifestyle factors are associated with personal enrichment and making one's life meaningful through activities one enjoys. Many older people still enjoy pursuing their former leisure activities, such as woodworking, crocheting, knitting, gardening, and fishing. People also want to engage in spiritual pursuits, or spend some time alone. Even those whose functioning has decreased to a vegetative or comatose state must be engaged in something that promotes sensory awakening through visual, auditory, olfactory, and tactile stimulation.
- The living environment must be comfortable, safe, and appealing to the senses. Cleanliness, décor, furnishings, and other aesthetic features are important.
- Clinical ***palliation*** should be available for relief from unpleasant symptoms such as pain or nausea, for instance, when a patient is undergoing chemotherapy.
- Human factors refer to caregiver attitudes and practices that emphasize caring, compassion, respect, and preservation of human dignity for the patient. Institutionalized patients generally find it disconcerting to have lost their autonomy and independence. Quality of life is enhanced when patients residing in a long-term care facility, who are often referred to as residents, have some latitude to govern their own lives. Residents also desire an environment that gives them adequate privacy.
- Being able to make personal choices is important to most people. In nursing facilities, for example, food is often the primary area of discontentment, which can be addressed by offering a selection of menu choices. Also, the ability to set one's own schedule is important to most people. Many elderly resent being awakened early in the morning when caregivers begin their responsibilities to care for patients' hygiene, bathing, and grooming.

Long-Term Care Services

LTC services are an amalgam of medical care, mental health services, social support, housing, and end-of-life care. There is no standard way to classify the large variety of LTC services. However, one way to better understand the complex array of these services is to view them from different perspectives:

- Medical care
- Mental health services
- Social support
- Preventive and therapeutic long-term care
- Informal and formal care
- Community-based and institutional services
- Levels of intensity
- Housing
- End-of-life care

Medical Care

Medical care in the LTC environment generally focuses on three main areas: (1) post-acute continuity of care, (2) clinical management of chronic illness and comorbidity, and (3) the treatment of physical and mental dysfunction. LTC generally becomes necessary after the treatment of an acute episode in a hospital. However, patients in LTC settings also encounter acute episodes, such as pneumonia, bone fracture, or stroke, and require admission to a general hospital. For the same medical conditions, the elderly are more prone to be hospitalized compared to younger age groups who may be treated as outpatients. Hence, the overall utilization of acute care is higher among the elderly. Medical care in LTC settings is typically provided by nurses, rehabilitation therapists, nutritionists, and other professionals under the direction of a physician. Preventing complications from chronic conditions is an important aspect of LTC.

Mental Health Services

It is erroneous to believe that mental disorders are a normal part of aging. Nevertheless, mental disorders affect about 20% of the elderly population (Rouse 1995). Hence, LTC patients often suffer from mental conditions, most notably anxiety disorders, depression, delirium, and dementia. Dementias are prevalent among 5% of the elderly population and have an unexplained predominance in women (Ritchie and Lovestone 2002). Psychiatric symptoms and cognitive decline are particularly common among nursing home residents (Scocco et al. 2006). Mental disorders range in severity from problematic, to disabling, to fatal. Yet, major barriers must be overcome in the delivery of mental health care. In general, assessing psychiatric illness in geriatric patients can be difficult for a variety of reasons, especially since medical comorbidity may obscure the diagnosis. For example, the patient with multiple chronic illnesses can often have symptoms of either dementia or depression attributed to the primary medical condition rather than to an underlying psychiatric illness (Tune 2001). Hence, elderly people with mental disorders are less likely than younger adults to be diagnosed and to receive needed mental health care.

Social Support

LTC clients need social and emotional support to help cope with changing life events that may cause stress, frustration, anger, fear, or depression. Adaptation to new surroundings is often necessary. Social support is also needed when problems and issues arise in the transactions among people within social systems. For example, conflicts may arise between what a patient wants for himself or herself and what the family may think is best for the patient. Conflicts also arise between patients and caregivers. Social services are also necessary to facilitate the coordination of total care services. Examples include transportation services, information, counseling, recreation, and spiritual support. LTC facilities should also establish linkages with the community through a variety of volunteer programs in which community members can participate. Remaining connected with the community and the outside world is an important aspect of social support for many people.

Preventive and Therapeutic Long-Term Care

One important question pertaining to LTC is how best to prevent and postpone disease and disability and maintain the health, independence, and mobility of an aging population (Satariano 1997). The primary goal is to prevent or delay institutionalization in LTC facilities. Preventive measures call for ensuring that the elderly receive good nutrition and have access to services such as vaccinations, flu shots, and routine medical care.

Certain community-based social support programs also serve a preventive function. Programs such as homemaker, chore, and handyman services can assist with a variety of tasks that older adults may no longer be able to perform. Examples are shopping, light cleaning, general errands, lawn maintenance, and minor home repairs.

In the initial stages of institutionalization, an emphasis on restorative therapies may be important. The objective is to curtail the need for long-range institutionalization and to return the patient to the community as soon as possible. Examples include admission to a nursing facility after orthopedic surgery or an episode of cardiovascular accident (CVA—stroke). Intensive rehabilitation therapies can often restore functioning to the extent that the patient can return home and continue to live independently with short-term or intermittent LTC services, such as home health care.

Informal and Formal Care

Contrary to popular belief, most LTC services in the United States are provided informally by family and friends who receive no payment (donated care). It is estimated that there are somewhere between 27 and 31 million informal caregivers in the United States who provide some assistance to a chronically ill or disabled individual. The monetary value of this care may be as high as $483 billion (Arno 2004). Donated care is also the largest source of financing for LTC costs (Holtz-Eakin 2005). Particularly men, minorities, married individuals, and those with less education are more likely to receive care from family and friends only, and are less likely to receive care in a nursing facility (Alecxih 2001). Adult children and spouses constitute roughly 70% of the caregivers. On the other hand, about one third of the elderly who live in the community have unmet needs with their functional impairments (National Academy on an Aging Society 2000).

Informal care reduces the use of formal home health care and delays nursing home entry (Van Houtven and Norton 2004). Older people who have close access to family or surrogates (neighbors, friends, and church or other community organizations) often continue to live in the community much longer than those who do not have such support. However, the pool of informal caregivers in relation to the growing elderly population needing LTC is going to shrink rather dramatically in the future (Robert Wood Johnson Foundation 1996). The number of older people who are divorced, unmarried, or without children has been increasing (Boaz and Hu 1997).

Family caregivers often experience a range of physical, emotional, social, and financial problems. Negative feelings such as anger, dissatisfaction, guilt, frustration, tension, and family conflict are some common issues these caregivers face. In general, these caregivers have poorer health and quality of life than non-caregivers (Schofield et al. 1998; Broe and Jorm 1999). Under these circumstances, caregivers experience stress and burnout. ***Respite care*** is the most frequently suggested intervention to address family caregivers' feeling of stress and burden. The objective is to provide relief or assistance to caregivers for limited periods to allow them some free time without neglecting the patient. Respite care can include any kind of LTC service, such as adult day care, home health care, or temporary institutionalization.

Community-Based and Institutional Services

For those who do not have adequate means of informal support, the availability of community-based services provided by formal agencies becomes an important factor in living independently. Services are brought to the patient's home or delivered in a community-based location. Most people have a strong preference for receiving LTC services at home rather than in an institution, which is generally viewed as an avenue of last resort. Various types of community-based services as well as different types of LTC institutions are discussed later in this chapter, and are illustrated in Figure 10–5.

Institutionalization generally becomes necessary when ADL impairments become high or behavioral problems develop as a result of cognitive impairment (McFall and Miller 1992). Compared to the elderly who can live in the community on their own or with assistance from informal or formal sources of LTC, those in need of institutionalization are more often frail, vulnerable, terminally ill, or functionally and/or cognitively impaired. These individuals are likely to remain in a nursing facility for a long time, perhaps indefinitely. The main objective of LTC in these situations is to manage chronic functional disability in two specific areas. The facility must (1) provide professional help for ADL functions that the patient cannot perform and (2) implement measures to prevent further degeneration of remaining function—a form of tertiary prevention (see Chapter 2). The latter includes exercises for range of motion, ambulation of wheelchair-bound patients, prevention of contractures, programs for preventing falls, frequent turning of bedbound patients to prevent pressure sores, and, if needed, bowel and bladder training. Reality orientation and validation therapy are examples of cognitive stimulation for demented patients. In addition to the two objectives discussed here, which are fundamental to LTC, any chronic health problems must be actively treated. Pharmaceutical and diet regimens are an important part of the treatment plan. Trained staff must also watch for any deterioration in existing conditions and for the onset of any acute problems.

Most care in LTC institutions is provided by nonphysician staff, such as nurses, nursing assistants, dietitians, social workers, and therapists. Personnel who provide basic ADL services and/or assist licensed and professional staff are technically referred to as

Figure 10–5 Interlinkages between Services for Those in Need of Long-Term Care.

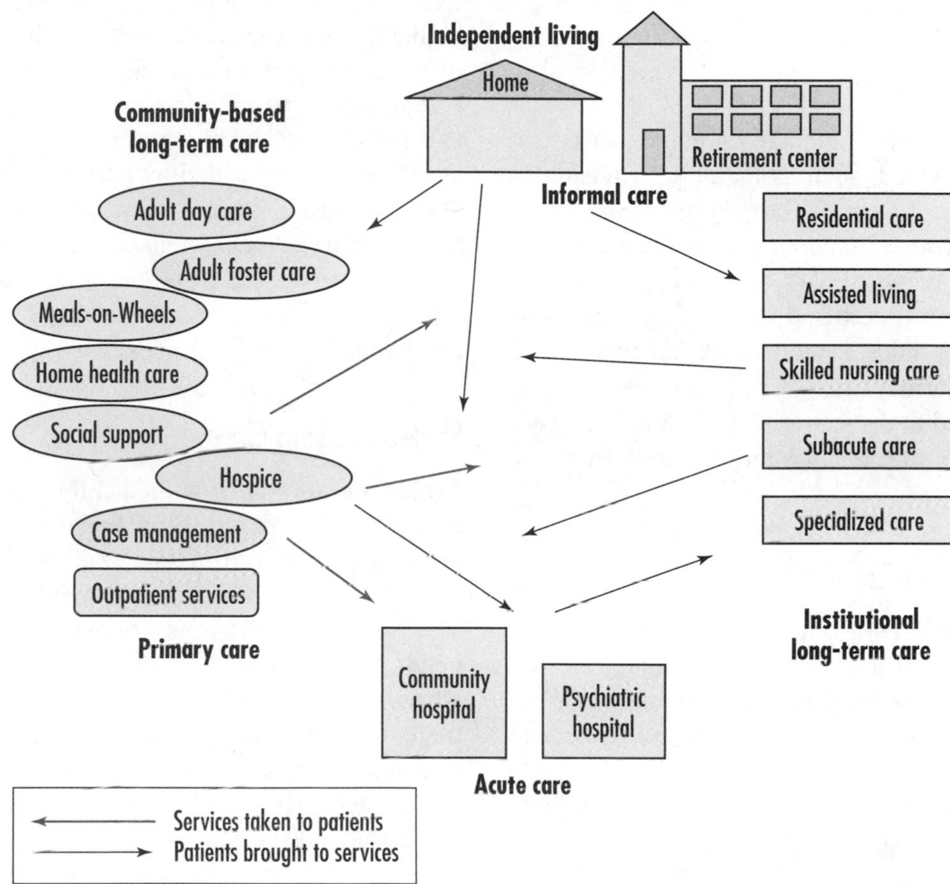

Source: Adapted with permission from D.A. Singh, *Nursing Home Administrators: Their Influence on Quality of Care,* p. 15, © 1997, Garland Publishing, Inc.

paraprofessionals. Examples of paraprofessionals are certified nursing assistants and therapy aides.

Residents have the right to be treated by a physician of their choice, who should make regular rounds to visit the patients. Between rounds, the professional nursing staff should communicate with the physician, especially when changes in a patient's condition are noticed or treatment orders are not producing the desired results. A transfer agreement with a local hospital must be in place to facilitate transition between the acute care and LTC facilities. At the onset of an acute episode, such as pneumonia or severe injury from a fall, the patient is hospitalized.

Levels of Intensity

As mentioned earlier, a variety of services are now available to address the varied requirements of a heterogeneous population in need of LTC. This has given rise to a continuum of clinical categories ranging from basic personal care to the more specialized subacute care.

Personal Care

Personal care refers to light assistance with basic ADLs, such as bathing. Provision of these services is largely the domain of paraprofessionals, such as home health aides, personal care attendants, transportation aides, certified nursing assistants, and therapy aides. Personal care can be provided by informal caregivers, home health agencies, adult day care (ADC), adult foster care (AFC), and residential and assisted living facilities.

Custodial Care

Custodial care is non-medical care provided to support and generally maintain the patient's condition and the essentials of daily living. It generally requires no active medical or nursing treatments. The focus is on providing routine assistance with ADLs. Services provided are designed to maintain rather than restore functioning. The emphasis is on preventing further deterioration. In contrast to restorative services, custodial care is generally longer term. It is often continued after the prognosis for restoration shows no potential for improvement or when the patient cannot participate in restorative therapies. The settings in which custodial care is provided resemble those for personal care.

Restorative Care

Restorative care or rehabilitation is based on the philosophy of caregiving in which patients are viewed as participants who can reach their maximum potential in physical and mental functioning. Restorative services include but go beyond the typical rehabilitative therapies (physical therapy, occupational therapy, and speech therapy). Restoration of functioning is integrated into the daily care routine. Examples are range-of-motion exercises, bowel and bladder training, and assisted walking provided by paraprofessionals. Restorative care is often provided by home health agencies, rehabilitation hospitals, outpatient rehabilitation clinics, adult day care centers, and assisted living and skilled nursing facilities (SNFs).

Skilled Nursing Care

Skilled nursing care is medically oriented care provided mainly by a licensed nurse under the overall direction of a physician. Delivery of care includes assessment and reassessment to determine the patient's care needs, monitoring of acute and unstable chronic conditions, and a variety of treatments that may include wound care, tube care management, intravenous therapy, oncology care, HIV/AIDS care, management of neurological conditions, and phlebotomy. Rehabilitation therapies often form an important component of skilled nursing care. Skilled nursing care is provided by home health agencies and SNFs.

Subacute Care

Subacute care is often required during the postacute phase of an acute episode. Although postacute recovery often requires nothing more than skilled nursing care, the term "subacute care" is used for technically complex services that are beyond traditional skilled nursing care. Hence, subacute care is appropriate for patients who remain critically ill during the postacute phase of illness or injury, or who have actively complex conditions that require ongoing monitoring and treatment or intense rehabilitation. Subacute care includes various medical, surgical, oncological, rehabilitation, and other intensive services. Micheletti and Shlala (1995) suggested four levels of subacute care services, which are illustrated in Table 10–1. Depending on their complexity, these services can be provided in long-term care hospitals (LTCHs—described in Chapter 8), transitional care (or extended care) units in hospitals, skilled nursing or subacute care facilities, or by home health agencies.

Housing

Housing is a key social aspect of LTC because health and housing concerns of the elderly and disabled are often interrelated. The physical features of housing affect the ability of frail older people and young disabled individuals to care for themselves and maintain their independence. Congregate housing—multi-unit housing with support services—is an option for seniors and disabled adults who do not want to live alone. Congregate housing combines privacy and

Table 10–1 Scope of Subacute Care Services

Level	Description	Services
I.	**Extensive Care**	• Parenteral feedings • Suctioning • Tracheostomy with continuous mechanical ventilation • Tracheostomy with suctioning
II.	**Special Care**	• Postburn care • Pressure sores • IV therapy • Radiation therapy after care • Dialysis • Transfusions • Inhalation therapy on all shifts • Gastrostomy/nasogastric tube feedings
III.	**Clinically Complex**	• Wound care other than decubitus • Terminal illness • Multiple illness • Postsurgical aftercare
IV.	**Rehabilitation**	• Physical therapy, occupational therapy, speech therapy: two hours per day, five days a week

Source: Adapted from J.A. Micheletti and T.J. Shiala. "Understanding and Operationalizing Subacute Services," *Nursing Management,* Vol. 26, No. 6, pp. 49–56, © 1995.

companionship, by offering each resident a private bedroom or apartment, and shared living space. Support services may include meals, transportation, housekeeping, building security, and social activities.

Section 202 of the National Affordable Housing Act of 1990 is administered by the Department of Housing and Urban Development (HUD). The program provides federal funds to construct supportive housing designed specifically for the low-income elderly. The program also provides rent subsidies to make such housing more affordable.

End-of-Life Care

Dealing with death and dying is very much a part of LTC. End-of-life care deals with preventing needless pain and distress for terminally ill patients and their families. High emphasis is placed on the patient's dignity and comfort.

Roughly three fourths of all deaths occur at 65 years of age or older. Among the elderly, 35% of all deaths are related to heart disease and 22% are related to cancer. Other diseases often fatal to the elderly are cerebrovascular disease (stroke), chronic obstructive pulmonary disease, diabetes, pneumonia, and influenza (Sahyoun et al. 2001). Care professionals seem to be well positioned to provide end-of-life care in some LTC settings. In others, terminal patients are referred to a hospice. Regardless of the LTC setting, patients who suffer pain or dyspnea are more likely to be referred to a hospice (Munn et al. 2006).

The Clients of Long-Term Care

Nearly 10 million Americans need help with ADLs and IADLs. Among those who need LTC services, more than 80% use community-based services and 17% are in nursing homes. Nearly 36% of the LTC clients are under the age of 65 (Burke et al. 2005).

LTC clients can be classified into five main categories:

- Older adults
- Children and adolescents
- Young adults
- People with HIV/AIDS
- People requiring subacute or specialized care

Older Adults

At the beginning of the 20th century, persons 65 years of age and older constituted just 4% of the population in the United States, and numbered 3.1 million. Today, just over 100 years later, roughly 12.5% of the population, numbering 36 million, falls in that age group. For some time now, the over-85 age group, referred to as the "oldest old," has been the most rapidly growing sector of the US population. It is growing at an average annual rate of over 3%, compared to a little over 1% for the entire population. By 2030, when all of the "baby boom generation" will have reached retirement age, the elderly are expected to constitute 20% of the population, 13% of whom are projected to be 85 years of age and older according to the latest projections by the US Census Bureau (Figure 10–6).

As mentioned earlier, the prevalence of chronic conditions and associated disabilities is expected to rise as the population ages (Figure 10–3). Table 10–2 provides data on activity limitations caused by chronic conditions among the elderly. Although a person's age or the mere presence of chronic conditions by itself does not predict the need for

Figure 10–6 Growth of Older Population According to Age Groups.

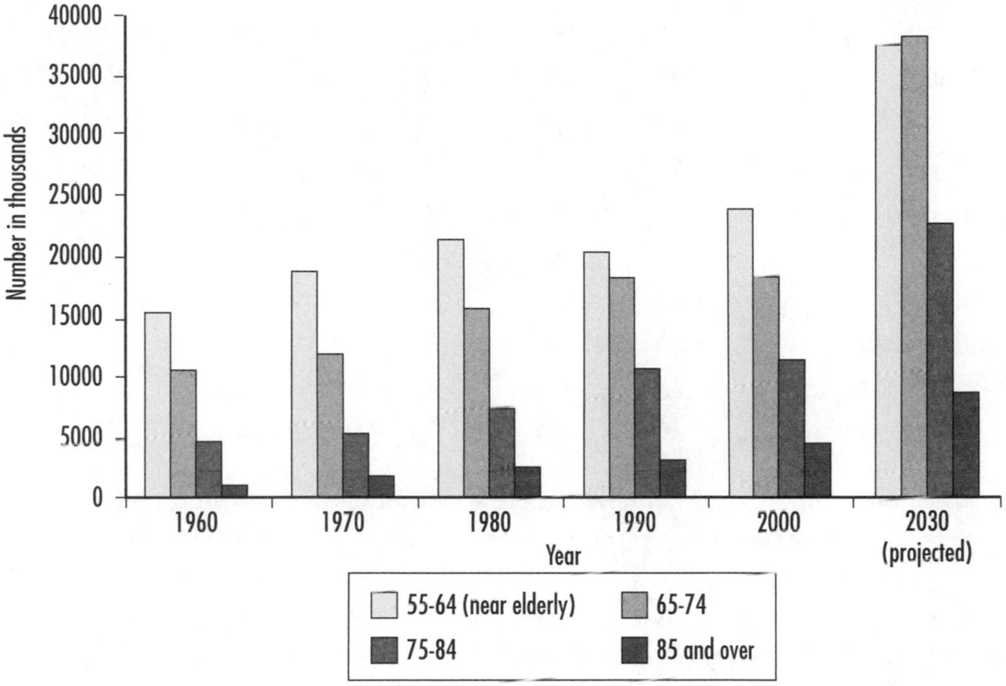

Source: Data from *Health, United States, 2002,* p. 79. National Center for Health Statistics, US Department of Health and Human Services.

LTC, aging, chronic ailments, comorbidity, disability, and dependency for common daily functions can follow each other, increasing the likelihood that an elderly person would need LTC services. Even though only about 4.3% of the total elderly population resides in US nursing homes (DHHS 2005, 339), many more require assistance at home or in less clinical institutional settings. The demographic trends have serious implications for the financing and delivery of LTC services. It is widely believed that a growing elderly population will put severe financial strains on a shrinking cohort of working taxpayers. Elderly in the lowest socioeconomic status are at the greatest risk of need for LTC (see Table 10–2) and are also the least able to pay for such services.

Children and Adolescents

In children, functional impairments are often birth related, such as brain damage, which can occur before or during childbirth. Examples of birth-related disorders include cerebral palsy, autism, spina bifida, and epilepsy. These children grow up with physical disability and need help with ADLs. The term ***developmental disability*** describes the general physical incapacity such children may face at a very early age. Those who acquire such dysfunctions are referred to as developmentally disabled, or DD for short. ***Mental retardation*** (MR), that is, below-average intellectual functioning, also leads to DD in most cases. Down's syndrome is the most common cause of MR in America. DD and

Table 10–2 Persons 65 Years Old and Over with Limitation of Activity Caused by Chronic Conditions: 1997 to 2004

	Percent with ADL limitation			Percent with IADL limitation		
Characteristic	1997	2000	2004	1997	2000	2004
Total	**6.7**	**6.3**	**6.1**	**13.7**	**12.7**	**11.5**
65 to 74 years	3.4	3.3	2.9	6.9	6.6	5.5
75 years and over	10.4	9.5	9.5	21.2	19.3	18.1
Male	5.2	5.1	4.8	9.1	9.2	8.4
Female	7.7	7.0	6.9	16.9	15.1	13.6
Below 100% poverty	12.5	9.6	10.1	25.3	20.2	20.9
100 – < 200% poverty	7.4	7.1	6.7	15.8	15.3	13.3
200% or above poverty	5.3	5.2	5.2	10.4	9.4	9.1

Source: Data from *Health, United States, 2002,* p. 190; *Health, United States, 2006,* p. 256, National Center for Health Statistics.

MR can occur separately, but about 52% of persons with DD also have MR (Braddock 2001).

The close association between the two is reflected in the term MR/DD, which is short for mentally retarded/developmentally disabled. About 6 to 7.5 million mentally retarded individuals live in the United States (Ford-Martin 2003). Most of these people are only mildly retarded, but those with severe retardation and/or DD usually require institutional care in specialized facilities. LTC services for children and adolescents are generally available in special pediatric LTC and MR/DD facilities.

Young Adults

Permanent disability among young adults commonly stems from neurological malfunctions, degenerative conditions, traumatic injury, or post-surgical complications. For example, multiple sclerosis is potentially the most common cause of neurological disability in young adults (Compston and Coles 2002). Severe injury to the head, spinal cord, or limbs can occur in victims of vehicle crashes, sports mishaps, or industrial accidents. Other serious diseases, injuries, and respiratory or heart problems following surgery can make it difficult, or even impossible, for a patient to breathe naturally. Such individuals, who cannot breathe (or ventilate) on their own, require a ventilator. A ventilator is a small machine that takes over the breathing function by automatically moving air into and out of the patient's lungs. Ventilator-dependent patients also require total assistance with their ADLs.

MR/DD is no longer merely a pediatric diagnosis, as was the case in the past. Today, the average life expectancy of those with MR approaches 66 years (Fisher and Kettl 2005). The aging process begins earlier in people with MR, and the age of 50 has been suggested to demarcate the elderly segment in this population (Altman 1995). This population confronts the same chronic illnesses—

cardiovascular disease, cancer, diabetes, and dementia—as the general aging population.

Before 1970s, MR/DD populations were housed in state-operated institutions. Since then, a serious effort began to move the residents out of state institutions into community-based settings such as foster care homes. According to a June 1999 US Supreme Court ruling, states must provide community-based services for MR/DD patients if treatment professionals determine that such services are appropriate and the affected individuals do not object to such placement, provided the states have the resources to provide such services. Also, states must develop a comprehensive working plan to place qualified MR/DD people in less restrictive settings.

Evidence suggests that MR/DD patients may function better in community-based residential settings than in traditional nursing homes. Studies of patients who had moved out of nursing homes to community settings demonstrated that these patients had higher levels of adaptive behavior, lifestyle satisfaction, and community integration than residents who remained in nursing homes (Heller et al. 1998; Spreat et al. 1998).

People with HIV/AIDS

When it was first discovered, AIDS was a fatal disease that resulted in a relatively painful death shortly after HIV infection developed into AIDS. In recent years, the introduction of protease inhibitors, antiretroviral therapy, and antibiotics for the treatment of AIDS-related infections has vastly improved the health condition of HIV/AIDS patients. These treatments have slowed the progression of the disease from the appearance of first symptoms to death. Consequently, AIDS has evolved from an end-stage terminal illness into a chronic condition. With reduced mortality, the prevalence of HIV in the population has actually increased, including among the elderly.

Over a period of time, people with AIDS are subject to a number of debilitating conditions, creating the need for assistance. For instance, nervous system disorders are common in AIDS patients even though they may survive for several years. Infections of the nervous system, such as cytomegalovirus, can cause blindness and dementia. The accompanying disabilities, in spite of the advanced treatments just mentioned, have actually increased the demand for LTC as dictated by the patient's changing health condition over time (Montoya et al. 1996). An increasing number of AIDS patients are receiving care in nursing facilities.

Care of HIV/AIDS patients presents special challenges, especially since this population has characteristics that are quite dissimilar to the rest of the LTC population. In LTC facilities, HIV/AIDS patients are likely to be younger than 60 years, male, and black or Hispanic (Shin et al. 2002). They have a significantly higher prevalence of depression, other psychiatric disorders, and dementia associated with AIDS. HIV/AIDS patients also have a significantly higher prevalence of weight loss and incontinence of bladder and bowel (Shin et al. 2002).

People Requiring Subacute or Specialized Care

A growing number of nursing facilities have developed subacute and other specialized services. Subacute care was discussed in a previous section. Other specialized services include ventilator care, and specialized care for head trauma victims, comatose patients, and those with progressive Alzheimer's disease.

Types of Community-Based Long-Term Care Services

Community-based LTC services have a fourfold objective:

1. To deliver LTC in the most economical and least restrictive setting whenever appropriate for the patient's health care needs,
2. To supplement informal caregiving when more advanced skills are needed than what family members or surrogates can provide to address the patients' needs,
3. To provide temporary respite to family from caregiving stress, and
4. To delay or prevent institutionalization by meeting the needs of the most vulnerable elderly in community settings.

Financing for community-based services comes from a variety of sources. Although the monetary value of donated care is the most significant, private out-of-pocket payments, private long-term care insurance, Medicaid, Medicare, and other public sources of funds cover formal services.

Title III of the Older Americans Act of 1965 (most recently reauthorized in 2006) grants funds to states for community planning, advocacy, service development, information, training of family caregivers, and respite care. Americans aged 60 years and older, particularly those with social or economic need, can receive services funded under the act. Provisions of the act are carried out through an administrative network that includes the Federal Administration on Aging, State Units on Aging, and Area Agencies on Aging. Nationally, approximately 670 Area Agencies on Aging administer funds and programs funded by the Older Americans Act. Federal appropriations generally cover a portion of the costs. State and local government funds, individual savings, and private donations cover the remainder.

Some federal funding available to the states under Title XX Social Services Block Grants from the Department of Health and Human Services may be used for community-based LTC services when such services prevent or reduce inappropriate institutionalization. Federal funding is also available to the states under Section 1915(c) of the Social Security Act of 1981, commonly known as the Home and Community Based Waiver (HCBW) programs. Under this program, services are available to those Medicaid beneficiaries who would otherwise require institutional care. The program can serve the elderly, and people with physical disabilities, DD, MR, and mental illness. States may also target programs by specific illness or conditions, such as technology-assisted children or individuals with AIDS. Some states also provide limited assistance with ADLs in a person's home under the Medicaid Personal Care Services program. Both public demand and the 1999 *Olmstead v. L.C. and E.W.* Supreme Court decision have called on states to expand community-based programs.

Home Health Care

Home health care, discussed in Chapter 7, refers to health care provided in the home of the patient by health care professionals. The organizational setup commonly requires a community- or hospital-based home health agency that sends health care professionals and paraprofessionals to patients' homes to deliver services approved by a physician. The number of persons under the care of home health agencies nearly doubled between 1992 and 1996. Subsequent utilization has declined as the Balanced Budget Act of 1997 imposed restrictions on home health coverage for Medicare beneficiaries (Figure 10–7). The new regulatory requirements provided incentives for agencies to deliver care more efficiently, and to rein in the use of home care services for long-term personal care (McCall et al. 2001). Medicare specifies the use of home health benefits for skilled nursing care only. To control costs further, the balanced budget legislation also required discontinuation of cost-based reimbursement and the development of a prospective payment system for home health services (see Chapter 6). As a result of these changes, home health services have become more medically oriented, and utilization has declined.

Home health care services are provided mainly to the elderly. In 2000, 70.5% of home health care patients were 65 years of age or older (DHHS 2002, 248). Figure 10–8 provides information on ADL and IADL assistance required by all home care patients. As Figure 10–9 points out, skilled nursing care is the most common service provided to the patients receiving home health care. Eligibility requirements for home health care under Medicare are discussed in Chapter 7 (see "Home Health Care"). Medicaid pays for home health care for the poor and medically indigent.

Figure 10–7 Change in Home Health Utilization (persons enrolled in home health agencies on the day before the date of survey).

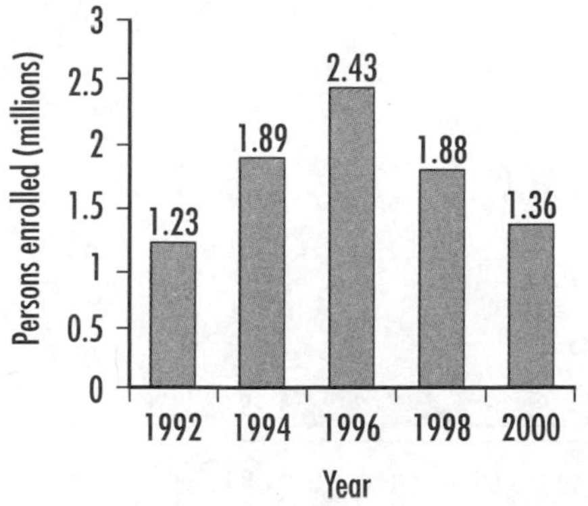

Source: Data from *Health, United States, 2002,* p. 248, National Center for Health Statistics.

Adult Day Care

Adult day care (ADC), also referred to as "adult day service," is a daytime program of nursing care, rehabilitation therapies, supervision, and socialization that enables frail (usually elderly) people to remain in the community. The National Adult Day Services Association (NADSA) defined ADC as a community-based group program designed to meet the needs of functionally and/or cognitively impaired adults through an individual plan of care. This structured, comprehensive program provides a variety of health, social, and other related support services in a protective setting during any part of a day, but less than 24-hour care. Adult day centers generally operate programs during normal business hours five days a week. Some programs offer evening and weekend services (NADSA 2003). An estimated 3,500 ADC programs are operating in all 50 states and the District of Columbia.

ADC is designed for people who, because of physical or mental conditions, cannot remain alone during the day, but who have family members to take care of them. ADC is an important respite program because it enables family caregivers to work during the day or allows informal caregivers

Figure 10–8 The Most Common Types of ADL and IADL Assistance Provided to All Patients Receiving Home Health Care, 2000.

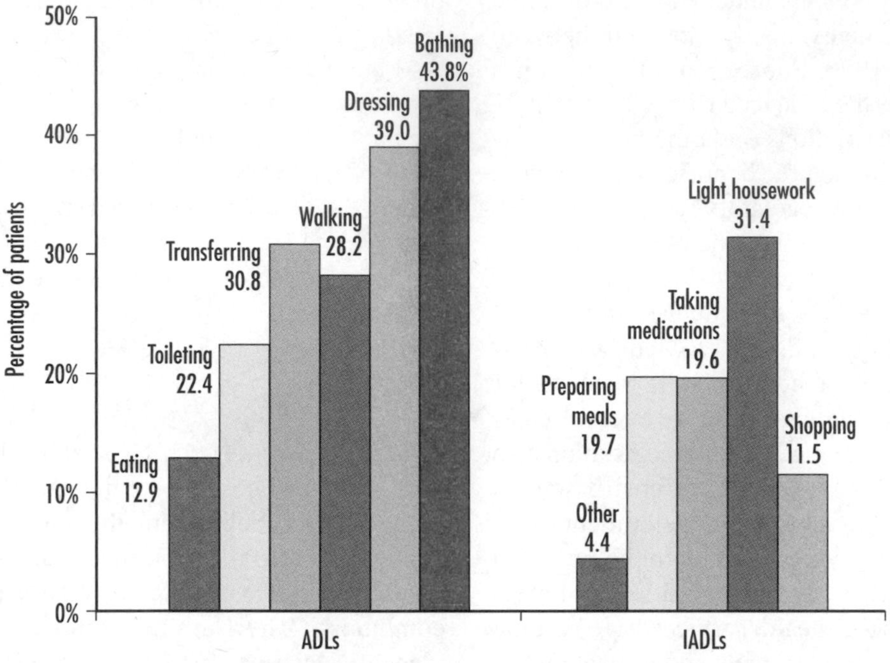

Source: Data from *Current Home Health Care Patients* (Table 8, February 2004), National Home and Hospice Care Survey 2000, National Center for Health Statistics.

Figure 10–9 Most Frequently Provided Services to All Home Health Care Patients, 2000.

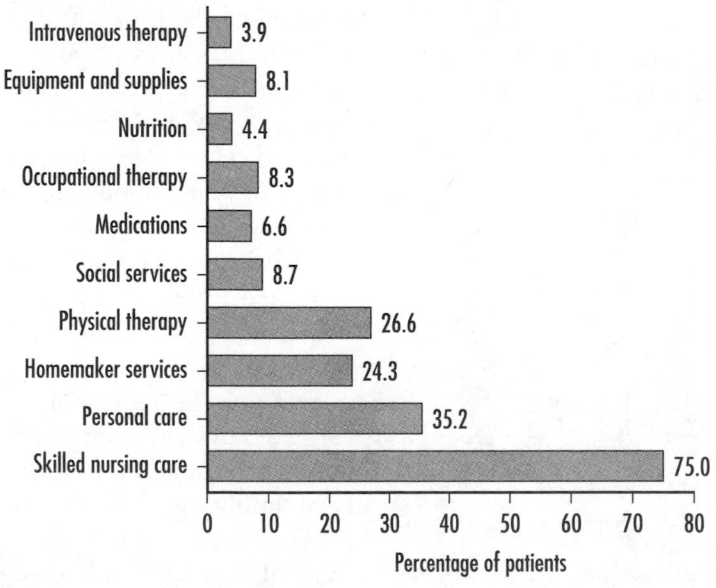

Source: Data from *Current Home Health Care Patients* (Table 6, February 2004), National Home and Hospice Care Survey 2000, National Center for Health Statistics.

to pursue other responsibilities of life. The program is also cost-effective compared to other formal services. Hence, Section 703 of the Medicare Prescription Drug, Improvement, and Modernization Act of 2003 has authorized the Medicare program to begin a demonstration project in which some home health agencies will partner with medical adult day care facilities to substitute a portion of the home health services by adult day care.

Three models of ADC are commonly recognized: (1) the health-rehabilitative model, (2) the health-maintenance model, and (3) the social-psychological model. All of these programs generally provide personal care (help with ADLs), midday meals, social services, and transportation. Many programs provide a mix of medical, maintenance, and social/psychological services. Group socialization and therapeutic recreational activities are also important parts of all three models.

Programs based on the health-rehabilitative model offer more intense medical, nursing, and therapy services compared to the other two models. Participants in this group may be recovering from various acute episodes, such as stroke or heart attack, or may have late stages of chronic disabling or degenerative conditions, such as arthritis or Parkinson's disease (Kirwin 1991, 55; Tedesco 1996). These programs generally have formal procedures for evaluating and addressing the participants' medical condition, rehabilitation goals, and nutritional status. An individualized plan of care is based on this evaluation. The need for ADC is often discontinued once a participant can function independently. This model is the most appropriate for clients who may be candidates for placement in a nursing home.

Programs using the health-maintenance model focus on participants' physical and psychological needs. The programs are designed to focus on the maintenance of health and function. Hence, they are preventive—and generally last longer than the health-rehabilitative programs (Dychtwald et al. 1990, 83).

The social-psychological model is best suited for individuals who suffer from dementia, such as Alzheimer's disease. As such, these programs address special concerns, in addition to providing basic services similar to those found in the other models.

The primary sources of funding for ADC are Medicaid and private out-of-pocket payments. Medicaid provides some funding under waiver programs that support community-based alternatives to institutional LTC. Medicare does not pay for ADC but may cover rehabilitation services through Part B.

Adult Foster Care

Adult foster care (AFC) is a service characterized by small, family-run homes providing room, board, and varying levels of supervision, oversight, and personal care to nonrelated adults who are unable to care for themselves (AARP Studies Adult Foster Care 1996). Foster care generally provides services in a community-based dwelling in an environment that promotes the feeling of being part of a family unit (Stahl 1997). Participants in the program are elderly or disabled individuals who have a current medical diagnosis, a psychiatric diagnosis, or a need for assistance with at least one ADL. Typically, the caregiving family resides in part of the home. To maintain the family environment, most states license fewer than 10 beds per family unit; however, many people have made a business of AFC by buying several houses and hiring families to live in them to care for functionally impaired and elderly people (Fein 1994).

The program differs widely from state to state and goes by several names, including adult family care, community residential care, and domiciliary care. Each state has established its own standards for the licensing of foster care homes. Funding for AFCs typically comes from Medicaid, private insurance, or personal sources. It is estimated that the cost of care averages about one third of that in nursing homes (Fein 1994), mainly because services in AFC are primarily designed to focus on room and board, supervision, and light assistance with ADLs. Medicare does not pay for AFC but may cover rehabilitation services under Part B.

Senior Centers

Senior centers are local community centers for older adults where seniors can congregate and socialize. Many centers offer one or more meals daily. Others sponsor wellness programs, health education, counseling services, recreational activities, information and referrals, and limited health care services, including health screening, especially for glaucoma and hypertension. Nearly all senior centers receive some public funding. Other common revenue sources are United Way and private donations.

Home-Delivered and Congregate Meals

The elderly nutrition program (ENP) is the nation's oldest framework for providing community- and home-based preventive nutrition in the United States. The program generally provides a hot noon meal five days a week to Americans 60 years of age and older (and their spouses) who cannot prepare a nutritionally balanced noon meal for themselves. Home-delivered meals for homebound persons are commonly referred to as ***meals on wheels***. Ambulatory clients are encouraged to get their meals at senior centers or other congregate settings where they also get the opportunity to socialize.

The ENP program was authorized under the Older Americans Act which also provides the majority of the funding. Additional funds are provided through Title XX block grants, 1915(c) waivers, and private donations. The ENP program currently provides congregate and home-delivered meals to about 7% of the nation's older population, including an estimated 20% of the nation's poor elders. Compared with nonparticipants, both ambulatory and homebound ENP clients are better nourished (Millen et al. 2002). However, the demand for services far exceeds the current capacity. The elderly often have to be on waiting lists to participate in the program.

It is a common practice for the Area Agency on Aging to contract out the preparation and delivery of meals to local nursing homes, hospitals, or religious organizations. In the meals-on-wheels program, volunteers carry the meals to homebound participants. Congregate meals may be served on the premises of participating facilities, such as hospitals and nursing homes, or at local senior centers or religious establishments.

Homemaker Services

Some older adults are relatively healthy but cannot carry out a few simple tasks necessary for independent living. These tasks may be as urgent as repairing a burst pipe or as mundane as cleaning the house. Some tasks, such as grocery shopping, must be performed often, whereas others, such as replacing storm windows, require attention just once or twice a year. Homemaker, chore, and handyman services can assist older adults with a variety of these tasks, including shopping, light cleaning, general errands, and minor home repairs. Homemaker programs may be staffed largely or entirely by volunteers. The Medicaid program may pay for some homemaker services, or these services may be funded through the local seniors programs under Title XX Social Services Block Grants or the Older Americans Act.

Emergency Response and Telephone Reassurance

Many of the frail elderly living alone do not need medical or supportive care, but they may nonetheless be vulnerable in an emergency. Other patients, after returning home from hospitals and nursing homes, are plagued by anxiety about relapses or accidents because people are often unprepared to manage themselves after returning home. Personal emergency response systems (PERS), also referred to as medical emergency response systems, address these needs. A ***PERS*** provides a cost-effective mechanism that enables at-risk elderly persons to summon help in an emergency. Usually, these people wear or carry a transmitter unit with which they can send a medical alert to a local 24-hour monitoring and response center.

A telephone reassurance program consists of friendly calls provided by agencies or volunteers to check up on and offer reassurance, contact, and socialization to elderly people at a scheduled time each day. If the person does not answer, an appropriate dispatch is sent to check on the individual.

Case Management

The term "case management" can have different meanings, but in the context of LTC it assumes a centralized coordinating function. As pointed out in this chapter, the myriad of LTC services, eligibility requirements, and financing can be overwhelming both for individuals who may need LTC and their families. The essential need for case management is recognized as a community-based covered service in 1915(c) waiver programs. Although there is no standard definition for ***case management***, at a fundamental level it refers to the process of matching client needs with available services that are likely to best address those needs. Case-management services are designed to assess the special needs of older adults, to prepare a care plan to address those needs, to specify services that are most appropriate, to determine eligibility for services, to make referrals and coordinate delivery of care, to arrange for financing, to ensure that clients are receiving services, and to reevaluate needs as circumstances change over time.

Although efficiency and cost containment have been the primary motivations behind case management, the service has proven to be immensely valuable to the elderly and their adult children. For example, many families live far from their older relatives. A case-management program can take responsibility for assessing needs and coordinating all care, saving the adult child or the older parent from relocating (Dychtwald et al. 1990, 105).

Three traditional models of case management in LTC have been identified: brokerage model, managed care model, and integrated care model (Scharlach et al. 2001).

Brokerage Model

In the ***brokerage model***, once needs have been independently assessed, case managers arrange services through other providers. The case manager is usually a freestanding agent who is mainly responsible for linking the client with other organizations, agencies, and service providers, with no formal administrative or financial relationship with these entities. Need assessment, development of a service plan, and making referrals are the main functions of case management in this model. There is minimal coordination and monitoring of services. Although private geriatric case managers provide case-management services, in the public domain, most states have implemented ***preadmission screening*** rules for need assessment and referral for community-based or institutional services. Also, federal regulations mandate a Preadmission Screening and Resident Review (PASRR) process for individuals with serious mental illness or mental retardation who apply to or reside in Medicaid-certified nursing facilities regardless of the source of payment.

Managed Care Model

This model is offered through a managed care organization (MCO), and it involves capitated financing which places the MCO at financial risk. Professionally trained nurses and social workers are typically the case managers who are likely to be more closely involved in the monitoring and coordination of services than is the case in the brokerage model (Scharlach et al. 2001). Delivery of services is arranged through a social health maintenance organization (***S/HMO***) which coordinates acute, chronic, LTC, and social services to address a patient's comprehensive needs. One primary goal is to prevent or delay placement in a nursing home. Hence, preventive and supportive services are strongly emphasized. There is some evidence that S/HMOs may help at-risk elderly postpone long-term nursing home placement (Fischer 2003). The S/HMO model has so far existed in the form of Medicare demonstration projects in which Medicare beneficiaries have to voluntarily enroll. Once enrolled, the beneficiaries have to obtain all covered services through the MCO. Perhaps for this reason, the model has not gained wide acceptance.

Integrated Care Model

This model exists within an interdisciplinary organizational structure that strives to provide all necessary services the clients may need. Services include medical and social services that include counseling, advocacy, and ongoing coordination and monitoring. The goal is ongoing prevention of the progression of disability (Scharlach et al. 2001). Similar to the managed care model, capitation is used, for which funding comes from both Medicare and Medicaid programs. Services are delivered through a nonprofit health care organization. At the core of the program is adult day care, augmented by home care and meals at home (Gross et al. 2004).

The Program of All-inclusive Care for the Elderly (***PACE***), which was discussed in Chapter 6, is an example of integrated case management. The PACE program was authorized under the Balanced Budget Act of 1997 after the On Lok project in San Francisco demonstrated that, in many instances, LTC institutionalization could be prevented through appropriate case management. The PACE program focuses on frail elderly who have already been certified for nursing home placement under Medicare and/or Medicaid.

Hospice Care

For an introduction to hospice care, see Chapter 7. The elderly constitute nearly three quarters of all hospice patients. In addition to typical hospice care, homemaker services and social services, such as finalization of wills and estate planning, are often important for dying older adults.

The availability of Medicare and Medicaid benefits for hospice care encourages providers and patients to consider palliative care as an alternative to more aggressive treatment. Medicare and Medicaid cover a substantial list of hospice benefits, including physician services, nursing care, medical supplies, prescription drugs, home health aide, physical therapy, counseling, social work services, and short-term inpatient and respite care. These services are provided under a plan of care established by the hospice and the patient's attending physician (Vladeck 1995). Figure 10–10 illustrates trends in hospice care utilization.

Hospice care is particularly cost-effective because cost savings are realized by foregoing aggressive medical treatment. Otherwise, medical expenditures during the last year of life for persons 65 years of age and older are estimated to be five times greater than during nonterminal years. One study estimated that last year of life expenses constitute approximately 22% of all medical expenditures in a given year (Hoover et al. 2002).

Figure 10–10 Hospice Patients, 1992–2000.

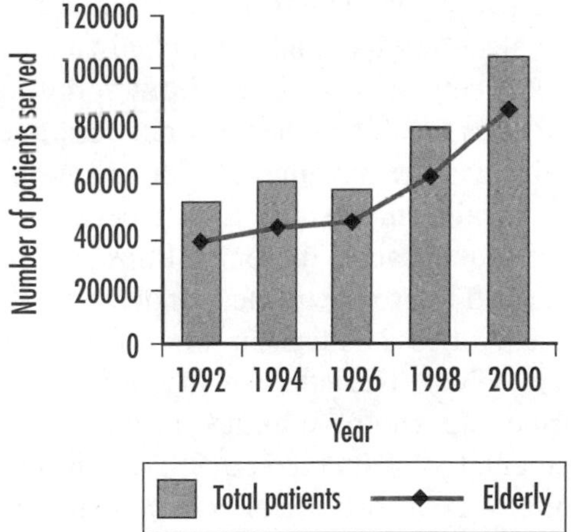

Source: Data from *Health, United States, 2002,* p. 249, National Center for Health Statistics.

Institutional Long-Term Care

Given the continuum of LTC services available, institutional LTC is more appropriate for patients whose needs cannot be adequately met in a less acute, community-based setting. The institutional sector of LTC also provides a continuum of services (Figure 10–5) according to the patient's level of acuity and dependency for care.

The generic term "nursing home" encompasses a wide spectrum of facilities. All of these facilities provide room and board in addition to varying levels of nursing and medical care. Various alternative living arrangements now address a variety of care needs that have gradually filled the gap between living in one's own home and living in a typical skilled nursing care facility. Retirement living, for instance, offers the most independence and provides no nursing or medical services. Residential care generally offers some additional services, such as meals, assistance with taking medications, and basic supervision. Assisted living goes a step further in providing most services associated with the ADLs and management of light incontinence. However, the distinction between some of these alternatives often blurs. Hence, facility labels do not always clearly define the levels of care.

Unless a resident has a drastic deterioration in health status that necessitates specialized services, such as those offered in an SNF or an acute care hospital, the changing health care needs of residents are generally accommodated in the existing setting instead of making frequent transfers between facilities (Singh 1997).

Institutional LTC may be categorized in five distinct groups, based on the level of services: independent or retirement living centers, residential or personal care facilities, assisted living facilities, SNFs, and subacute care facilities. In all states, facilities must be licensed by the state to handle medications and to provide assistance with ADLs. Hence, all the aforementioned facilities, except independent and retirement living centers, are licensed facilities in most states. Further, Medicare and Medicaid funding involves certification of facilities by the federal government.

Independent or Retirement Living Centers

As the name suggests, these facilities essentially meet the housing needs of older adults. They are not LTC institutions in the true sense because they do not deliver clinical services. Residents maintain their own independent lifestyles. The main advantage of special elderly housing, in contrast to ordinary housing, is found in its physical features and amenities that are adapted to the needs of the physically disabled and create a supportive environment to promote independence. Examples of adaptations are railings in hallways, extra-large bathrooms that facilitate wheelchair negotiation, grab bars in bathrooms, and pull cords to summon help in an emergency. In addition, such facilities often provide transportation for shopping and outings, and many facilities organize regular recreational activities and social events to promote an active lifestyle. Others provide one or two meals a day in a congregate setting. Although these facilities do not provide personal or custodial care, occasional needs for LTC services are met by obtaining home health care services through an outside agency.

Depending on the type of housing, independent living arrangements include congregate housing in multiunit rental complexes providing self-contained apartments. Upscale retirement communities sell individual apartments and generally require monthly maintenance fees, all to be paid out of private funds. More modest housing complexes provide government-assisted subsidized housing for low income, frail older people, based on their incomes.

Residential or Personal Care Facilities

These facilities are also known as "domiciliary care facilities" or "board-and-care homes." Sometimes AFC homes (discussed earlier) are included in this category. Others have called them "sheltered care facilities." These facilities provide physically supportive dwelling units, monitoring and/or assistance with medications, oversight, and light care with certain ADLs that do not involve nursing services. They all generally store medications and provide assistance with drug-use management. To maintain a residential rather than an institutional environment, many such facilities limit admitting residents who use wheelchairs. Others requiring assistance with ADLs, or having cognitive impairments, are also generally not admitted because these facilities are not equipped to provide professional care.

Facilities can range anywhere from spartan to deluxe. The latter are often private pay. For people who have limited incomes, Supplemental Security Income (SSI) can be used along with other types of government assistance funds. Services generally include meals, housekeeping and laundry services, and social and recreational activities. Transportation is an important support service that allows people to live independently. Minimal staffing is provided 24 hours a day for supervision and assistive purposes. Beyond the very basic nursing care, more advanced services can be arranged through an external home health agency, when needed.

Assisted Living Facilities

An ***assisted living facility*** (ALF) can be described as a residential setting that provides personal care services, 24-hour supervision, scheduled and unscheduled assistance, social activities, and some health care services (Citro and Hermanson 1999). Assisted living and personal care are not clearly distinct, except that assisted living centers generally have licensed nurses, and sometimes therapists, to provide some basic nursing and rehabilitation services in addition to assistance with ADLs.

During the past few years, assisted living facilities have burgeoned in popularity as an alternative to the traditional nursing home. The services are specially designed for people who cannot function independently, and therefore cannot be accommodated in a residential care setting, but do not require skilled nursing care. Intermittent skilled nursing care can be arranged through a home health agency, if needed. Compared to skilled nursing facilities (discussed in the next section), the environment in ALFs is less clinical and more homelike. Hence, people generally prefer to be in ALFs than in skilled nursing facilities, provided their needs can be adequately met in ALFs.

Regulation of assisted living facilities is mainly at the state level through the licensing process. These regulations continue to evolve in response to the rising acuity levels of residents. For example, facilities that serve Alzheimer's or dementia patients face increased oversight in some states. Some states have started to require resident assessment, plan of care, and staff training.

The absence of a common definition for assisted living makes it difficult to pinpoint the number of residences in the United States. However, best estimates suggest that approximately 33,000 assisted living residences, housing about 800,000 people, are in operation. In 2006, the average age of an assisted living resident was 85 years. The typical resident is mobile but needs assistance with two ADLs. The most common areas of ADL assistance are bathing, dressing, and toileting. Also, the majority of residents require help with medications. Approximately one third of the residents are discharged because they need a higher level of services in a nursing facility; another one third pass away (National Center for Assisted Living 2006).

Assisted living is primarily paid for privately. The average monthly fees are about $2,000, but costs vary widely according to amenities, room size and type (e.g., shared versus private), and the services the resident requires. Most facilities charge a basic monthly rate that covers rent and utilities, and then charge separately for services. Many facilities also charge a one-time entrance fee. For people who have limited assets and income, in most states, assisted living care is covered under the Medicaid program for SSI recipients and through Title XX Social Services Block Grants. However, such funds are limited.

Skilled Nursing Facilities

Skilled nursing facilities are heavily regulated through licensure and certification requirements. All facilities in a particular state must be licensed and, therefore, must comply with the licensing regulations, which differ considerably from state to state. Most licensing regulations establish minimum qualifications required for administrators and other staff, prescribe minimum staffing levels, establish standards for building construction, and require compliance with the national fire and safety codes. To admit patients covered under the Medicaid and/or Medicare programs, nursing homes must also be certified and must demonstrate compliance with the federal certification standards enforced by the Centers for Medicare and Medicaid Services (CMS).

Until 1989, federal statutes classified nursing homes into two types: skilled nursing facilities (SNFs) for Medicare and/or Medicaid residents, and intermediate care facilities (ICFs) for those covered by Medicaid only. Patients needing a higher level of care were eligible for admission to an SNF, which was required to have a licensed nurse on duty 24 hours a day and a registered nurse (RN) on the day shift. By contrast, ICFs had to have a licensed nurse on duty only on the day shift.

From a clinical standpoint, the Nursing Home Reform Act, passed in 1987, removed the differences between ICFs and SNFs. The new law created two categories for certification purposes. A nursing home certified to admit Medicare patients is now called a skilled nursing facility (***SNF***). This facility can be freestanding or a ***distinct part***, that is, a section of a nursing home that is distinctly separate and distinguishable from the rest of the facility. When SNF certification applies to a distinct part, Medicare patients can be admitted only to that section. A nursing home certified for Medicaid only (but not for Medicare) is called a nursing facility (***NF***). A facility may be dually certified, as an SNF and an NF. Facilities having ***dual certification*** can admit Medicare and/or Medicaid patients to any part of the facility. The federal certification standards governing SNFs and NFs are essentially the same.

The labels of SNF and NF represent only two types of certifications, often for facilities providing similar levels of care. Thus, the term "skilled nursing facility" has both a regulatory as well as a clinical meaning. The SNF and NF categories have been created for the two distinct sources of funding. Medicare and Medicaid patients generally do not receive two different levels of services, although Medicare patients who receive postacute services may have a little higher acuity level. From a clinical standpoint, as well as from the standpoint of the institutional continuum, an SNF is a geriatric nursing home providing skilled nursing care services that are described earlier in this chapter. The term "facility" does not necessarily mean a separate physical structure. The term can be used for the facility as a whole or, within the context of licensure and certification, it may apply more specifically to different sections or units of a building (distinct parts) with different certifications or no certification.

A small proportion of facilities have elected not to participate in the Medicaid and/or Medicare programs. They can admit only patients who have a private funding source for nursing home care. These facilities are ***noncertified***; however, they must be licensed under the state licensure regulations. ***Private pay patients***—those not covered by either Medicare or Medicaid for long-term nursing home care—are not restricted to noncertified facilities. These patients also may be admitted to SNF or NF certified beds. The restriction applies to Medicare and Medicaid patients who cannot be admitted to noncertified facilities. By now, it should be clear that all facilities must be licensed, but a licensed facility may or may not be certified. Figure 10–11 illustrates the concepts discussed in this section.

Subacute Care Facilities

As a level of LTC service, subacute care was discussed in an earlier section of this chapter. It became a prominent service after acute care hospitals were brought under the prospective payment system (PPS) in the 1980s.

Subacute services are generally found in three types of institutional locations: (1) LTC units of acute care hospitals may provide subacute care. These hospital-based subacute units are also referred to as ***transitional care units*** (TCUs) or extended care units (ECUs). These hospital-based facilities are certified as SNFs. (2) Nursing homes can open subacute units by raising the staff skill mix to provide services that exceed the general skilled nursing care level. (3) Long-term care hospitals (LTCHs), discussed in Chapter 8, provide subacute care. An LTCH must be certified as an acute care hospital.

Quality and level of services is likely to vary in the different settings. Selection of a setting is governed by numerous factors, both clinical and nonclinical. One main nonclinical factor is the availability of subacute care services in a given location (Buntin et al. 2005). Costs also vary rather considerably among the various settings. LTCHs are the most expensive. SNFs are often a more cost-effective alternative to LTCHs, and at least some physicians think that the level and intensity of care in the two settings is comparable (MedPAC 2004).

Postacute needs can vary widely among patients, but there is no uniform system of clinical assessment and payment for subacute care. Medicare uses different payment methodologies for the different settings. SNF payments are based on RUG categories (discussed later in this chapter). Before 2003, LTCHs were paid on a cost-plus basis. Lured by cost-plus reimbursement, the number of LTCHs grew from 105 in 1993 to 318 in

Figure 10–11 Distinctly Certified Units in a Nursing Home.

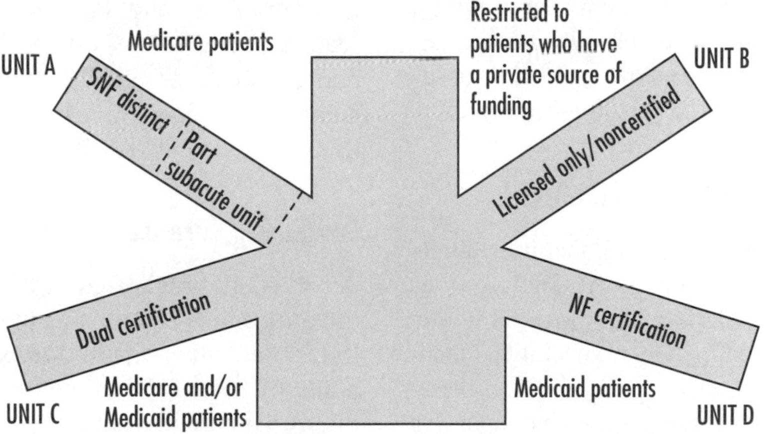

2003 (MedPAC 2004). However, in 2003, a PPS reimbursement program was implemented for LTCHs. Only time will tell whether LTCHs will continue to thrive or whether other more cost-effective alternatives will end up providing the bulk of subacute services in the future. Apart from assessment and reimbursement issues, a uniform evaluation of quality has been difficult among the varied settings. Bryant and colleagues (2004) recommended that a single core set of measures applicable to all settings would be useful for assessing quality and for facilitating transfers between providers.

Specialized Facilities

Specialized facilities generally provide special services for individuals with distinct medical needs. For example, inpatient rehabilitation facilities (IRFs) provide intense therapies, an intermediate care facility for the mentally retarded (ICF/MR) has specialized programs for the MR and/or DD populations, and Alzheimer's facilities have developed a specialized niche within the institutional continuum of LTC. Full-service continuing care retirement communities (CCRCs) provide several levels of care along the entire continuum of institution-based LTC discussed in the previous section.

Inpatient Rehabilitation Facilities

IRFs are either freestanding facilities, sometimes called rehabilitation hospitals, or they may be rehabilitation units located within acute care hospitals. These specialized facilities provide intensive rehabilitation therapies that can last three hours or more per day, five days per week. The most common rehabilitation diagnoses include spinal cord and traumatic brain injuries, orthopedic conditions, stroke, and complex arthritis-related conditions. Medicare has developed a separate IRF prospective payment system that was implemented in 2002. It pays a per discharge prospective rate.

Intermediate Care Facility for the Mentally Retarded

Federal regulations provide a separate certification category for LTC facilities classified as ICF/MRs. In 1971, Public Law 92–223 authorized Medicaid coverage for care in ICF/MR facilities. States have been required to provide appropriate services to each person with MR/DD in an ICF/MR or in a community-based setting outside of institutional care.

Alzheimer's Facilities

Alzheimer's disease is a progressive degenerative disease of the brain, producing memory loss, confusion, irritability, and severe functional decline. The disease becomes progressively worse and eventually results in death. Alzheimer's facilities provide special programming, and have special security features because the residents tend to wander. Carefully designed lighting, color, and signage are used to orient the residents (Skaggs and Hawkins 1994).

Continuing Care Retirement Communities

A ***CCRC*** is specialized in the sense that it integrates and coordinates the independent living and other institution-based components of the LTC continuum illustrated in Figure 10–5. Different levels of services are generally housed in separate buildings, all located on one campus. The range of services is based on the concept of aging in place, and yet accommodates the changing needs of older adults. The range of services includes housing, health care, and social services. Residents generally choose to enter these communities when they are still relatively healthy. The residents' independence is preserved, but assistance and nursing care are provided when needed. A CCRC commonly has these characteristics (Aaronson 1996):

- It provides independent living units, which may be in the form of cottages or apartments. Generally, various size options are available. The facility has carports and/or garages. Each apartment may have a kitchenette and other facilities to support independence. A congregate dining room provides one or more meals a day. Recreational and social programs are designed to promote an active lifestyle.
- Residential and assisted living are available in an adjoining facility. These services represent a midpoint between independent living and nursing care. Tenants living in such units receive some monitoring and assistance with ADLs.
- An SNF generally provides intermittent as well as permanent accommodations to residents of the CCRC. SNFs serve the same function for the CCRC that nursing homes serve for the general community.
- A CCRC requires some form of prepayment, generally an entrance fee and/or monthly fees.
- A contract that lasts for more than one year and that describes the service obligations of the CCRC and the financial obligations of the resident must be signed.

CCRCs, for the most part, require private financing, with the exception of services delivered in a Medicare-certified SNF. Entrance and monthly fees vary considerably, depending on which services are included. The services are directed at middle- and upper-middle-income clientele using a strong customer-oriented marketing approach. The most important reason clients give for joining a CCRC is guaranteed access to institutional LTC services when they are needed (Cohen et al. 1988).

Nursing Home Industry and Patient Demographics

Industry Overview

In 2004, over 16,000 nursing homes were providing services to almost 1.5 million individuals (Table 10–3). Between 1999 and 2004, the number of nursing homes in the United States declined by a little over 10%, and nationally, bed capacity declined by almost 8%. This represents a decline from 52 beds to 48 beds per 1,000 elderly persons in the United States. The decline in the supply of nursing home beds is primarily due to ongoing emphasis on community-based alternatives to nursing home care. Consequently, there has been an increase in the number of home care agencies and assisted-living facilities.

Between 1999 and 2004, the proportion of dually certified nursing home beds increased from approximately 87% to 93%, and the proportion of beds with NF certification decreased from 9% to 4.4%. This trend has been mainly triggered by low Medicaid reimbursement. Only a little over 200 facilities nationwide are noncertified and, therefore, can admit only private pay patients.

Table 10–3 Number and Percentage Distribution of Nursing Homes, Number of Beds and Beds per Home, and Selected Facility Characteristics, 2004

	Nursing Homes		Beds			Current Residents	
Facility Characteristic	Number	% Distribution	Number (1,000)	Distribution %	Beds per Nursing Home	Number (1,000)	Occupancy Rate (%)
All facilities	16,100		1,730	100	107.6	1,492	86.3
Ownership:							
Proprietary	9,900	61.5	1,074	62.1	108.6	918	85.5
Voluntary nonprofit	5,000	30.8	504	29.1	101.6	440	87.4
Government and other	1,200	7.7	152	8.8	123.6	134	88.0
Certification:							
Medicare and Medicaid certified (SNF/NF)	14,100	87.6	1,600	92.5	113.5	1,380	86.3
Medicare only (SNF)	700	4.1	33	1.9	50.6	28	85.0
Medicaid only (NF)	1,100	6.9	76	4.4	69.0	68	89.1
Bed size:							
Fewer than 50 beds	2,200	13.9	76	4.4	33.8	62	82.1
50–99 beds	6,000	37.3	455	26.3	75.7	423	92.9
100–199 beds	6,800	42.5	903	52.2	132.0	789	87.3
200 beds or more	1,000	6.2	296	17.1	298.2	219	73.9
Region:							
Northeast	2,800	17.4	382	22.1	136.0	331	86.8
Midwest	5,300	33.0	527	30.4	99.4	448	85.1
South	5,400	33.6	586	33.8	108.3	502	85.6
West	2,600	16.0	236	13.7	92.1	211	89.5
Affiliation:							
Chain	8,700	54.2	939	54.3	107.9	813	86.5
Independent	7,400	45.8	791	45.7	107.2	680	86.0

Source: Data from *Nursing Home Facilities* (Table 1, December 2006), National Nursing Home Survey 2004, National Center for Health Statistics.

The nursing home industry is dominated by the proprietary for-profit sector. Nationally, the average nursing home had 107.6 beds and maintained an occupancy rate of over 86%. Most of the nursing homes are operated by multifacility chains. The 10 largest chains have at least 90 nursing homes each and together operate 14% of the national bed capacity (Table 10–4).

Services and Patients Served

At least 90% of all nursing home residents are 65 years of age and older. Trends also show a nursing home population that has aged and has become more racially diverse. Over 80% of the residents are dependent for their mobility, 66% are incontinent, and 47% require assistance with eating; 37% are dependent in all three areas (DHHS 2006, 352).

Most nursing homes provide a variety of services to fit the varied needs of their patient populations. Restorative care, treatment of skin wounds, and dementia care are the most commonly available services (Table 10–5). The three most common conditions that patients in nursing homes suffer from are bladder incontinence, Alzheimer's disease, and bowel incontinence. The prevalence of these and other conditions is shown in Figure 10–12. A relatively large percentage of nursing home residents (over 63%)

Table 10–4 The Nation's 10 Largest Nursing Home Chains

Chain/Headquarters	Total Facilities	Total Beds	Avg. Beds/ Facility	# of States
1. Beverly Enterprises (Fort Smith, AR)	335	34,292	102.4	23
2. Manor Care (Toledo, OH)	284	37,882	133.4	30
3. Sava Senior Care (Atlanta, GA)	256	30,617	119.6	23
4. Kindred Healthcare (Louisville, KY)	247	33,050	133.8	29
5. Life Care Centers of America (Cleveland, TN)	224	29,092	129.9	28
6. The Evangelical Luth. Good Samaritan Soc. (Sioux Falls, SD)	192	14,886	77.5	24
7. Genesis Eldercare (Kennett Square, PA)	171	22,549	131.9	12
8. Extendicare Health Services (Milwaukee, WI)	147	15,018	102.2	11
9. Trans Healthcare Inc. (Sparks, MD)	98	10,895	111.2	16
10. Sun Healthcare Group (Albuquerque, NM)	92	9,916	107.8	14

Note: All but No. 6 are for-profit.

Source: Data from *Managed Care Digest Series—Senior Care Digest*, 2006. Bridgewater, NJ: Sanofi-Aventis US, UC.

Table 10–5 Percentage of Nursing Homes by Availability of Special Programs, 2004

	Type of Program							
	Hospice End of Life	Palliative Care	Dementia Care	Restorative Care	Behavior Problems	Pain Management	Continence Management	Skin Wounds
All facilities	18.8	16.7	31.5	68.9	23.8	25.6	21.7	53.5
Ownership								
Proprietary	16.7	14.6	28.5	71.8	23.8	23.3	22.6	54.0
Voluntary nonprofit and other	22.3	20.1	36.4	64.3	23.8	29.3	20.4	52.7
Beds								
Fewer than 50 beds	*	*	*	45.2	*	18.1	*	35.6
50–99 beds	17.6	14.3	25.0	70.6	25.2	24.4	22.5	50.2
100 beds or more	21.3	19.6	41.2	74.3	25.9	28.6	23.9	61.1

Source: Data from *Nursing Home Facilities* (Table 18, December 2006), National Nursing Home Survey 2004, National Center for Health Statistics.

Figure 10–12 Percentage of Nursing Home Residents with Various Conditions, 2005.

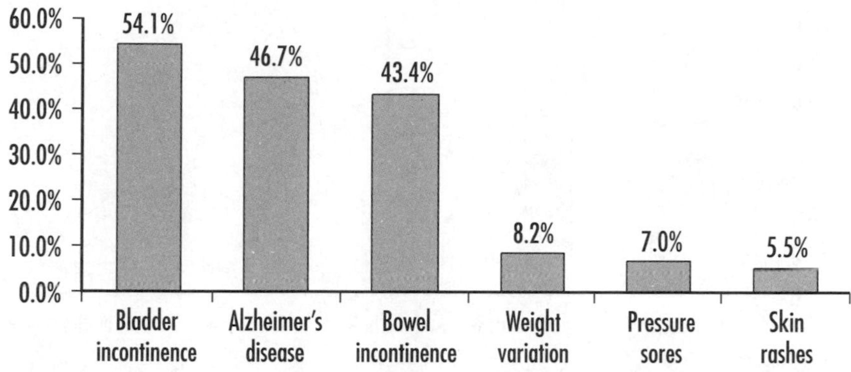

Source: Data from *Managed Care Digest Series—Senior Care Digest*, 2006. Bridgewater, NJ: Sanofi-Aventis US, LLC.

use psychoactive medications. These are prescription drugs that alter brain function, resulting in temporary changes in perception, mood, consciousness, and behavior. A little less than half of the residents use antidepressants (Figure 10–13).

Staffing

Staffing ratios for nursing staff are recorded in Table 10–6. For-profit facilities have the lowest staffing ratios in relation to patients (per patient per day—PPD), with the exception of LPN staffing. RN staffing PPD is the highest in the smallest facilities.

Table 10–6 Nursing Home Staffing Ratios per Patient per Day (PPD) by Facility Ownership and Size, 2005

	Nursing Staff Categories		
	Registered Nurse (RN)	Licensed Practical Nurse (LPN)	Certified Nursing Assistant (CNA)
Ownership			
Overall average	**.54**	**.72**	**2.32**
Government	.60	.72	2.57
Church-related	.64	.71	2.53
Other nonprofit	.65	.73	2.47
For-profit	.51	.72	2.25
Facility size (beds)			
Overall average	**.54**	**.72**	
< 50	.78	.71	
50–100	.54	.69	
101–150	.50	.75	
151–200	.51	.78	
201+	.53	.71	

Source: Data from *Managed Care Digest Series—Senior Care Digest*, 2006. Bridgewater, NJ: Sanofi-Aventis US, LLC.

Financing

Figure 10–14 provides a comparison of total expenditures for the delivery of hospital care, nursing home care, physician services, prescription drugs, and other personal health care (dental services, home health care, drugs, durable medical equipment, vision care, other professional services, etc.). National expenditures for nursing home care have been much lower than those in other sectors of health care delivery. Also, they have not

Figure 10–13 Percentage of Nursing Home Residents Receiving Various Medications, 2005.

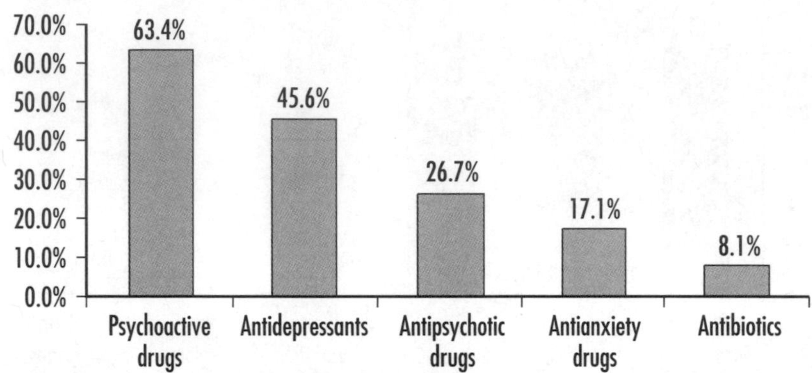

Source: Data from *Managed Care Digest Series—Senior Care Digest*, 2006. Bridgewater, NJ: Sanofi-Aventis US, LLC.

Figure 10–14 Distribution of Personal Health Care Expenditures.

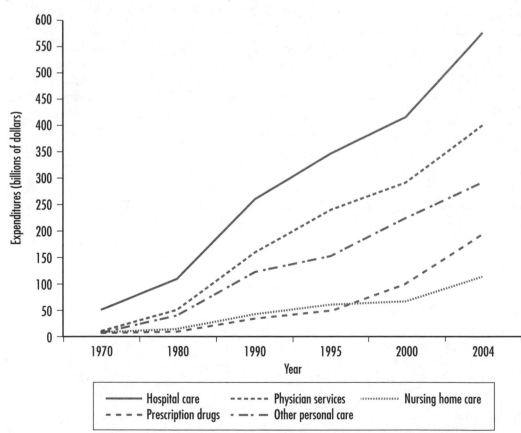

Source: Data from *Health, United States, 2002*, pp. 293, 294; *Health, United States, 2006*, pp. 379, 380, National Center for Health Statistics.

increased as fast as they have in the other sectors of the US health care delivery system. For a number of years now, expenditures on prescription drugs have exceeded the dollars spent on nursing home care. Most nursing home care is financed by Medicaid (Figure 10–15), but private sources (out of pocket, private insurance, and other private) also cover a sizable portion of nursing home expenses.

Medicare

Even though Medicare is the primary payer for health care services for the elderly, in 2004 it covered only 13.9% of the cost of care in nonhospital nursing homes. This is because Medicare provides for only limited benefits for nursing home care. However, Medicare's share of expenditures has consistently risen since 1990. Declines have occurred in private financing except that private insurance has been relatively stable in recent years. Figure 10–16 illustrates the trends in financing from the four main sources.

SNF care is covered under Part A of Medicare. To be eligible for coverage, a patient must be admitted to the SNF within 30 days of an inpatient hospital stay of three or more days; however, coverage is not automatic. The patient's physician must certify that the patient requires skilled nursing care. The maximum benefit is 100 days per benefit period. Medicare pays 100% for the first 20 days. A copayment is required from days 21 through 100 ($124.00 per day in 2007), but few patients qualify for the full 100 days of coverage. In recent years, Medicare has paid for an average of about 35 days of care per covered admission (Longtermcare.com 2003).

Medicaid

Of the 52 million Medicaid beneficiaries, only 3.3% received services in nursing fa-

Figure 10–15 Sources of Funding for Nursing Home Care (non-hospital affiliated), 2004.

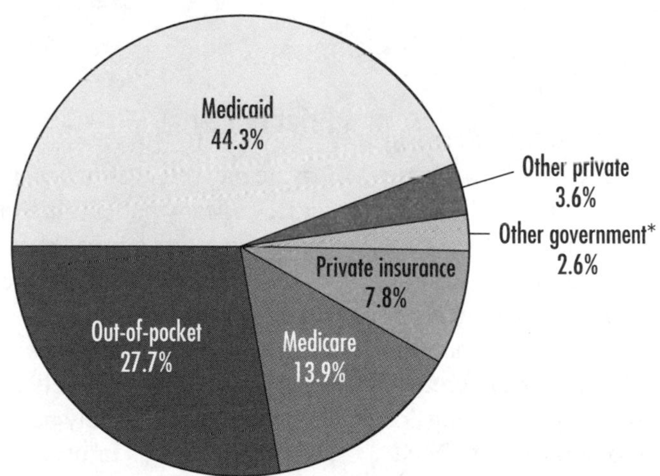

*Other government expenditures include, for example, care funded by the Department of Veterans Affairs.

Source: Data from *Health, United States, 2006*, p. 379, National Center for Health Statistics.

Figure 10–16 Main Sources of Financing Nursing Home Care (non-hospital affiliated facilities).

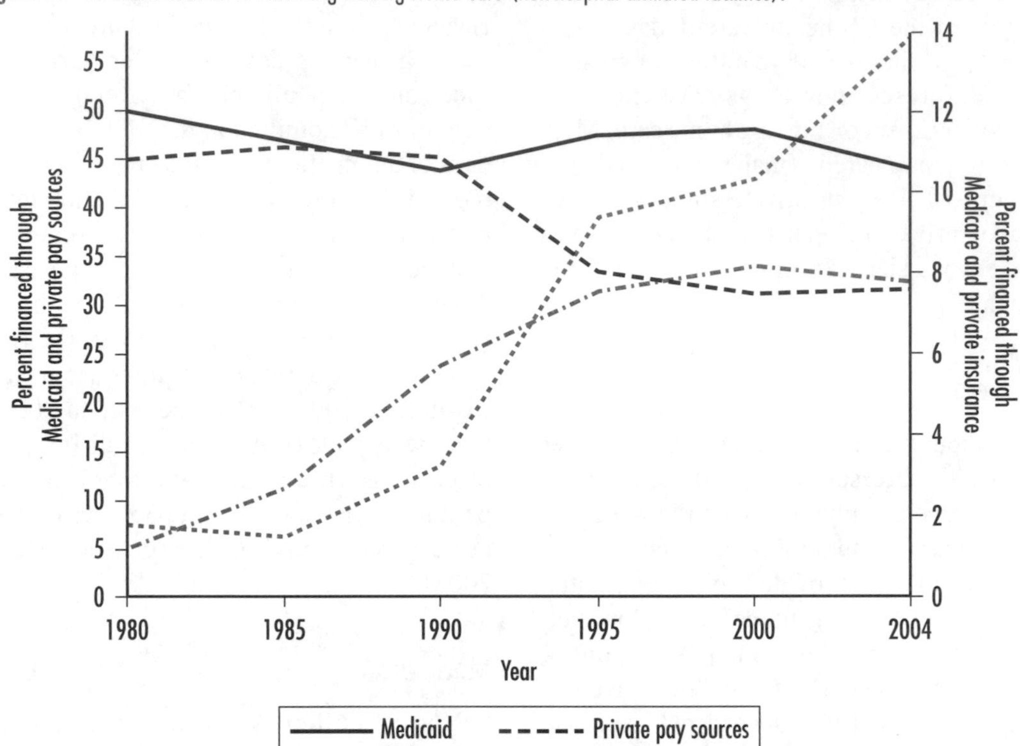

Source: Data from *Health, United States, 1999,* p. 289; *Health, United States, 2006,* p. 379; National Center for Health Statistics, Department of Health and Human Services.

cilities, and another 0.2% received care in ICF/MRs in 2003 (DHHS 2006, 410). These facilities consumed 22% of total Medicaid expenditures, far more than what Medicaid spent on any other service (Figure 10–17). The share of expenditures has either decreased or remained constant for the four services shown in Figure 10–17. The decreases were made up by increases in spending for prescription drugs and other services. Medicaid and private pay patients may receive rehabilitation therapies under Medicare Part B, provided those services are certified as medically necessary.

Private Pay

Private pay refers to out-of-pocket financing for LTC. Many patients are initially admitted to a facility with a private pay source of funding. When private funds are exhausted, these patients generally become eligible for Medicaid assistance. The term ***spend-down*** refers to exhausting one's assets and one's annual income to the medically needy levels to qualify for Medicaid. In other words, if the income and resources of a medically needy individual are above a state-prescribed level, the individual must first incur a certain amount of medical expenses to lower the

Figure 10–17 Trends in the Distribution of Medicaid Expenditures among Selected Services.

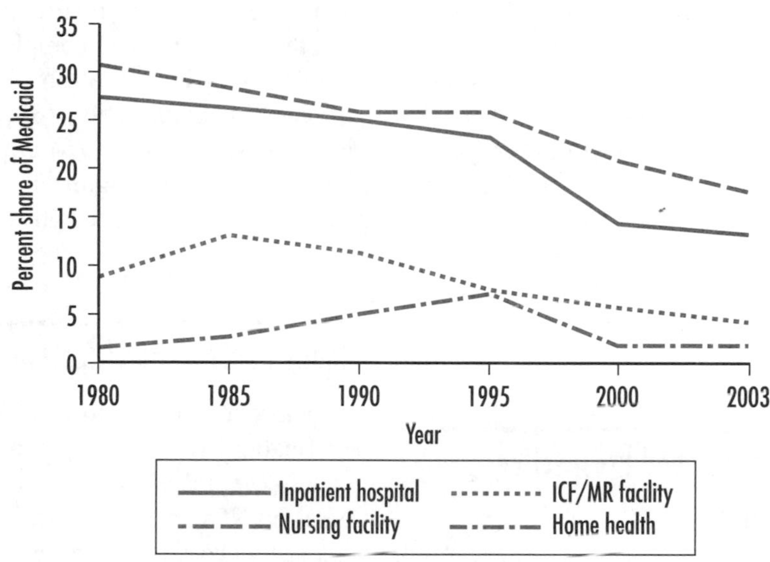

Source: Data from *Health, United States, 2002,* p. 328; *Health, United States, 2006,* p. 410, National Center for Health Statistics.

income and assets to the medically needy level established by the state (Burwell et al. 1996). In the case of married couples, when one spouse requires nursing home care and the other remains in the community, Medicaid rules are intended to prevent the impoverishment of the spouse remaining in the community.

Private Long-Term Care Insurance

Private LTC insurance is available in a wide range of choices in services covered and prices. In addition to nursing home care, private insurance also generally covers community-based services such as home health care or adult day care. In 2004, private LTC insurance covered 7.8% of nursing home expenditures, a figure that has remained relatively constant for several years.

Private LTC insurance has been growing, but rather slowly. There are two main problems. (1) There is a wide range of policies to choose from, and trying to decide the right coverage can be a daunting task. (2) For most people, the premiums are unaffordable. The costs vary substantially depending on the type of coverage, which can have options such as the daily or monthly benefit amount the insurer would pay, a waiting period before benefit payments will begin, the number of years over which benefits will be paid, and inflation protection to cover rising future costs of LTC. LTC insurance policies are particularly expensive if a plan is purchased in later years of one's life. People in younger age groups, for whom the cost of LTC insurance would be more affordable, generally face other financial priorities, such as saving for retirement, children's college education, life insurance, and buying a home. The need for LTC in the distant future is often seen as a much lower priority. However, people are learning about the catastrophic financial risks posed by a long stay in a nursing home, and a number of states now offer tax incentives for purchasing LTC policies. In 2004, 104 companies sold more than 900,000 policies. Through the end of 2002, approximately 9.2 million Americans had purchased LTC insurance. The market for private LTC insurance grew an average of 18% annually between 1987 and 2002 (America's Health Insurance Plans 2004). However, risk selection is a problem. For example, about 15% of applicants are denied coverage because of their health.

Patient Assessment and Prospective Payment for SNFs

As discussed in Chapter 6, in 1998, Medicare implemented the PPS program to replace cost-based reimbursement for SNFs. The prospective reimbursement is based on case mix. Patients who are more seriously ill require more intensive use of resources and incur greater costs to the facility. Therefore, a higher case mix calls for greater reimbursement.

Patient assessment plays a critical role in prospective reimbursement because it is used to determine the case mix. A trained RN in the facility oversees the assessment process for which a standardized resident assessment instrument (RAI) called the ***minimum data set*** (MDS) is used. The MDS contains over 100 assessment items that provide extensive information on the resident's nursing care needs, ADL impairments, cognitive status, behavioral problems, and medical diagnoses.

The facility's case mix is derived from a patient-classification system called ***Resource Utilization Groups***, version 3 (RUG-III). The MDS data provide the input for classifying each patient in one of the 44 RUG-III categories, which are mutually exclusive. The 44 RUG categories are part of eight major classification groups, listed here from the most clinically complex to the least complex: (1) rehabilitation plus extensive services, (2) rehabilitation, (3) extensive services, (4) special care, (5) clinically complex, (6) impaired cognition, (7) behavior problems, and (8) reduced physical function.

Requirements of Participation

As mentioned earlier, to qualify for federal certification, which enables nursing homes to admit Medicare and/or Medicaid patients, SNFs and NFs must comply with established standards. These standards are referred to as Requirements of Participation (in the Medicare and Medicaid programs), and were authorized under the Omnibus Budget Reconciliation Act of 1987 (OBRA-87). The standards are also widely regarded as minimum standards of quality for nursing homes. Roughly 185 different standards are classified under 17 major categories (DHHS 1995):

1. Resident rights. These rights include the right to choose a physician, to be fully informed of one's medical condition and treatments, to authorize the facility to manage personal funds and require accounting for the funds, the right to personal privacy and confidentiality, and the right to voice grievances without fear of retaliation.
2. Admission, transfer, and discharge rights. These rights provide residents certain safeguards against transfer or discharge from a facility and allow one to return to the same facility after brief periods of hospitalization or therapeutic leave.

3. Resident behavior and facility practices. This limits the facility's use of physical and chemical restraints, and prohibits mistreatment, neglect, or abuse of residents.
4. Quality of life. It promotes recognition of the patient's individuality, dignity, and respect. It allows them to exercise choice and self-determination. For example, residents have the right to smoke in specially designated lounge areas. Residents can organize resident and family groups for mutual support and planned activities. The facility must make reasonable accommodation for individual preferences, such as meals and roommates. The standard also requires a clean, safe, comfortable, and homelike environment.
5. Resident assessment. Initially on admission and periodically thereafter, the facility must undertake a comprehensive assessment of each patient's functional capacity and medical needs. Based on the needs assessment, the facility must develop a comprehensive plan of care and provide the necessary services.
6. Quality of care. Each resident must receive, and the facility must provide, the necessary care and services to attain or maintain the highest practicable physical, mental, and psychosocial well-being. The facility must provide access to vision and hearing services, adopt measures to prevent pressure sores, provide appropriate treatment for pressure sores, ensure adequate nutrition and hydration, provide special treatments as necessary, and manage the administration of prescribed medications. The standards also address appropriate use of urinary catheters and nasogastric tubes.
7. Nursing services. The facility must have sufficient nursing staff to provide necessary care.
8. Dietary services. The facility must provide a nourishing, palatable, and well-balanced diet that meets the daily nutritional and special dietary needs of each resident.
9. Physician services. A physician must approve each admission, and each resident must remain under the care of a physician.
10. Rehabilitation services. The facility must provide specialized rehabilitative therapies when needed.
11. Dental services. The facility must assist residents in obtaining needed dental services.
12. Pharmacy services. The facility must provide pharmaceutical services with consultation from a licensed pharmacist.
13. Infection control. The facility must have an infection-control program and maintain records of incidents and corrective actions.
14. Physical environment. The facility must comply with the Life Safety Code of the National Fire Protection Association. The facility should provide for emergency electrical power in case of power failure. The building must have adequate space and equipment for dining, health services, and recreation. Resident rooms must meet certain requirements for size and furnishings.

15. Administration. The facility must operate in compliance with all applicable federal, state, and local regulations and must be licensed by the state. The governing body has legal responsibility for the management and operation of the facility. The governing body must appoint a licensed nursing home administrator to manage the facility. Nurses' aides working at the facility must receive required training, a competency evaluation, periodic performance review, and needed inservice education. The facility must also designate a physician to serve as medical director.
16. Laboratory services. The facility must provide or obtain needed laboratory services.
17. Other services. These include maintenance of clinical records, disaster and emergency preparedness, and transfer agreement with a hospital.

Summary

LTC includes medical care, social services, and housing alternatives. Hence, it involves a range of services that can vary according to individual needs. The prevalence of chronic conditions sometimes leads to physical and/or mental disability. These disabilities may impair the performance of ADL and/or IADL functions. LTC services often complement what people with impaired functioning can do for themselves. Informal caregivers provide the bulk of LTC services in the United States. Respite care can provide family members temporary relief from the burden of caregiving. When the required intensity of care exceeds the capabilities of informal caregivers, available alternatives include professional community-based services to supplement informal care or admission to an LTC facility. Services vary from basic personal assistance to more complex skilled nursing care and subacute care. Some patients may require long-range custodial care without the prognosis of a cure. Others may require short-term postacute convalescence and therapy. Still others may need end-of-life care through a hospice program.

Community-based LTC services include home health care, adult day care, adult foster care, meals on wheels, congregate dining and nutritional assistance, homemaker services, case management, personal emergency response systems, and telephone reassurance programs. The various LTC institutions include independent and retirement living centers, residential or personal care facilities, assisted living facilities, and SNFs. The latter may also provide subacute care. A CCRC generally offers a full continuum of independent living and institution-based LTC services. Specialized institutions accommodate people with severe MR and/or DD. Some facilities specialize in Alzheimer's care. LTC facilities can be proprietary, private nonprofit, or government owned. They may be independent or affiliated with a multifacility chain. The average size of a nursing home in the United States is a little more than 100 beds. Nursing homes require federal certification as SNFs to admit Medicare patients. NF certification is needed to admit Medicaid patients. Most facility beds in the United States are dually certified as both SNF and NF. Medicaid is the most common source of funding for nursing home care.

LTC services may be appropriate for people of any age, but most of these services are used by the elderly because aging often brings on chronic conditions, multiple illnesses, physical disability, and decreased mental capacity. When such health problems limit a person's ability to function independently, LTC becomes necessary. LTC must be viewed not as an isolated component of the health care delivery system but as a continuum of both community-based and institution-based services that must be rationally linked to the rest of the system. The LTC system can be like a maze. Many people find the various aspects of LTC, such as levels of care, appropriateness of services, and financing, to be overwhelming. A critical need exists for coordination and integration of services through case management.

Test Your Understanding

Terminology

adult day care (ADC)
adult foster care
Alzheimer's disease
assisted living facility
brokerage model
case management
CCRC
chronic condition
custodial care
developmental disability
distinct part
dual certification
long-term care
meals on wheels
mental retardation
minimum data set (MDS)
noncertified
nursing facility (NF)
PACE
palliation
paraprofessionals
PERS
personal care
preadmission screening
private pay patients
quality of life
Resource Utilization Groups
respite care
restorative care
senior centers
S/HMO
skilled nursing care
skilled nursing facility (SNF)
spend-down
subacute care
total care
transitional care units

Review Questions

1. Long-term care services must be individualized, integrated, and coordinated. Elaborate on this statement, pointing out why these elements are essential in the delivery of LTC.
2. Age is not the primary determinant for long-term care. Comment on this statement, explaining why this is or is not true.
3. What is meant by "quality of life"? Briefly discuss the five main features of this multifaceted concept.
4. What are some of the challenges in the delivery of mental health services for the elderly?
5. Discuss the preventive and therapeutic aspects of long-term care.

6. How do formal and informal long-term care differ? What is the importance of informal care in LTC delivery?
7. What are the main goals of community-based and institution-based long-term care services?
8. What implications does an aging population have for long-term care services?
9. Why is it that some children and adolescents may need long-term care?
10. Why has long-term care become an important service for people with HIV/AIDS?
11. Discuss the three different models of adult day care. Which services are common to all three models?
12. Enumerate the main functions of long-term care case management.
13. Briefly discuss the three main models of case management in the delivery of long-term care.
14. What are the similarities and differences between the S/HMO and PACE models?
15. Briefly discuss the continuum of institutional long-term care services.
16. What is the difference between licensure and certification? What are the two types of certifications? What purpose does each serve from (1) a clinical standpoint and (2) a financial standpoint?
17. What are the main institutional settings for the delivery of subacute care?
18. Which services does a CCRC provide?
19. Even though the elderly are the primary users of nursing homes and, generally speaking, Medicare is the primary source of payment for health care services provided to the elderly, why does Medicare pay only a small fraction of the cost of nursing home care?
20. Why has private long-term care insurance not gained popularity with the consumers?
21. What is the relationship between patient assessment and reimbursement for SNF certified facilities?

REFERENCES

Aaronson, W. 1996. Financing the continuum of care: A disintegrating past and an integrating future. In *The continuum of long-term care: An integrated systems approach*, ed. C.J. Evashwick, 223–252. Albany, NY: Delmar Publishers.

AARP studies adult foster care for the elderly. 1996. *Public Health Reports* 111, no. 4: 295.

Alecxih, L. 2001. The Impact of Sociodemographic Change on the Future of Long-Term Care. *Generations* 25, no. 1: 7–11.

Altman, B.M. 1995. *Elderly persons with developmental disabilities in long-term care facilities.* AHCPR Pub. No. 95–0084. Rockville, MD: Agency for Health Care Policy and Research, July.

American Hospital Association (AHA). 1990. *Health care for older adults: Management advisory*. Chicago.

America's Health Insurance Plans. 2004. *Long term care insurance in 2002: Research findings*. Washington, DC: AHIP.

Anderson, G.F. 2003. Physician, public, and policymaker perspectives on chronic conditions. *Archives of Internal Medicine* 163, no. 4: 437–442.

Arno, P.S. 2004. *Economic value of informal caregiving: 2004*. Presentation at the Care Coordination and the Caregiver Forum, Department of Veteran's Affairs, Bethesda, MD, January 2006.

Bassuk, S.S., and T.A. Glass. 1999. Social disengagement and incident cognitive decline in community-dwelling elderly persons. *Annals of Internal Medicine* 131, no. 3: 165–174.

Bertoti, D.B. 1994. Physical therapy for the child with mental retardation. In *Pediatric physical therapy*. 2nd ed., ed. J.S. Tecklin, 237–261. Philadelphia: J.B. Lippincott Co.

Boaz, R.F., and J. Hu. 1997. Determining the amount of help used by disabled elderly persons at home: The role of coping resources. *Journal of Gerontology: Social Sciences* 52B, no. 6: S317–S324.

Braddock, D. 2001. Expert witness report of David Braddock, Ph.D. for the United States District Court Northern District of Illinois in *Boudreau v. Ryan*, Case Number 00 C 5392. *http://www.iacdd.org/braddock.html.*

Bryant, L.L. et al. 2004. Measuring healthcare outcomes to improve quality of care across post-acute care provider settings. *Journal of Nursing Care Quality* 19, no. 4: 368–376.

Broe, G., and A. Jorm. 1999. Carer distress in the general population: Results from the Sydney Older Persons Study. *Age and Ageing* 28, no. 3: 307–311.

Buntin, M.B. et al. 2005. How much is postacute care use affected by its availability? *Health Services Research* 40, no. 2: 413–434.

Burke, S.P. et al. 2005. *Developing a better long-term care policy: A vision and strategy for America's future*. Washington, DC: National Academy of Social Insurance.

Burwell, B. et al. 1996. Financing long-term care. In *The continuum of long-term care: An integrated systems approach*, ed. C.J. Evashwick, 193–221. Albany, NY: Delmar Publishers.

Citro, J., and S. Hermanson 1999. *Fact sheet: Assisted living in the United States*. Washington, DC: American Association of Retired Persons.

Cohen, M.A. et al. 1988. Attitudes toward joining continuing care retirement communities. *The Gerontologist* 28, no. 5: 637–643.

Compston, A., and A. Coles. 2002. Multiple sclerosis. *Lancet* 359, no. 9313: 1221–1231.

Crimmins, E.M. 2004. Trends in the health of the elderly. *Annual Review of Public Health* 25, no. 1: 79–98.

Department of Health and Human Services (DHHS). 1995. *Standards and Certification*. Hyattsville, MD: Department of Health and Human Services.

Department of Health and Human Services (DHHS). 2002. *Health, United States, 2002*. Hyattsville, MD: Department of Health and Human Services.

Department of Health and Human Services (DHHS). 2005. *Health, United States, 2005*. Hyattsville, MD: Department of Health and Human Services.

Department of Health and Human Services (DHHS). 2006. *Health, United States, 2006*. Hyattsville, MD: Department of Health and Human Services.

Dychtwald, K. et al. 1990. *Implementing eldercare services: Strategies that work*. New York: McGraw-Hill.

Evashwick, C.J., and L.G. Branch. 1996. Clients of the continuum. In *The continuum of long-term care: An integrated systems approach*, ed. C.J. Evashwick, 13–22. Albany, NY: Delmar Publishers.

Federal Interagency Forum on Aging-Related Statistics. 2004. *Older Americans 2004: Key indicators of well-being*. Washington, DC: US Government Printing Office.

Fein, E.B. 1994. *Foster care for elderly: Like a new home. New York Times*, 8 March, A1.

Fischer, L.R. 2003. Community-based care and risk of nursing home placement. *Medical Care* 41, no. 12: 1407–1416.

Fisher, K., and P. Kettl. 2005. Aging with mental retardation. *Geriatrics* 60, no. 4: 26–29.

Ford-Martin, P.A. 2003. Mental retardation. Encyclopedia. HealthAtoZ.com. *http://www.healthatoz.com/healthatoz/Atoz/common/standard/transform.jsp?requestURI=/healthatoz/Atoz/ency/mental_retardation.jsp*.

Goldman, D.P. et al. 2005. Consequences of health trends and medical innovation for the future elderly. *Health Affairs-Web Exclusive* 24, supp. 2: W5–R5.

Gross, D.L. et al. 2004. The growing pains of integrated health care for the elderly: Lessons from the expansion of PACE. *The Milbank Quarterly* 82, no. 2: 257–282.

Guerrero, J.L. et al. 1999. The prevalence of disability from chronic conditions due to injury among adults ages 18–69 years: United States, 1994. *Disability and Rehabilitation* 21, no. 4: 187–192.

Heller, T. et al. 1998. Impact of age and transitions out of nursing homes for adults with developmental disabilities. *American Journal of Mental Retardation* 103, no. 3: 236–248.

Hoffman, E. 2001. When the old age home is your own. *Business Week* (December 10): 94–96.

Holtz-Eakin, D. 2005. *CBO testimony: The cost of financing of long-term care services*. Before the Subcommittee on Health Committee on Energy and Commerce. US House of Representatives. April 27, 2005.

Hoover, D.R. et al. 2002. Medical expenditures during the last year of life: Findings from the 1992–1996 Medicare current beneficiary survey. *Health Services Research* 37, no. 6: 1625–1642.

Kirwin, P.M. 1991. *Adult day care: The relationship of formal and informal systems of care*. New York: Garland Publishing.

Lakdawalla, D. et al. 2003. Forecasting the nursing home population. *Medical Care* 41, no. 1: 8–20.

Longtermcare.com. 2003. We hear so much about the cost of long term care. *http://www.longtermcare.com/cost_of_care.htm*.

Luckasson, R.A. et al. 1992. *Mental retardation: Definition, classification, and systems of support*. 9th ed. Washington, DC: American Association on Mental Retardation.

McCall, N. et al. 2001. Medicare home health before and after the BBA. *Health Affairs* 20, no. 3: 189–198.

McFall, S., and B. Miller. 1992. Caregiver burden and nursing home admission of frail elderly persons. *Journal of Gerontology* 47, no. 2: S73–S79.

MedPAC (Medicare Payment Advisory Commission). 2004. *New approaches in Medicare: Report to the Congress*. Washington, DC: Medicare Payment Advisory Commission.

Mehta, K.M. et al. 2002. Cognitive impairment, depressive symptoms, and functional decline in older people. *Journal of the American Geriatric Society* 50, no. 6: 1045–1050.

Micheletti, J.A., and T.J. Shlala. 1995. Understanding and operationalizing subacute services. *Nursing Management* 26, no. 6: 49–56.

Millen, B.E. et al. 2002. The elderly nutrition program: An effective national framework for preventive nutrition interventions. *Journal of the American Dietetic Association* 102, no. 2: 234–240.

Montoya, V.L. et al. 1996. Drug abuse, AIDS, and the coming crisis in long-term care. *Journal of Nursing Management* 4, no. 3: 151–162.

Munn, J.C. et al. 2006. Is hospice associated with improved end-of-life care in nursing homes and assisted living facilities? *Journal of the American Geriatrics Society* 54, no. 3: 490–495.

National Academy on an Aging Society. 2000. *Caregiving: Helping the elderly with activity limitations*. Washington, DC: National Academy on an Aging Society.

National Adult Day Services Association (NADSA). 2003. *http://www.nadsa.org*.

National Center for Assisted Living. 2006. Assisted living resident profile. *http://www.ncal.org*.

Ostir, G.V. et al. 1999.Disability in older adults 1: prevalence, causes, and consequences. *Behavioral Medicine* 24, no. 4: 147–156.

Partnership for Solutions. 2002. *Chronic conditions: Making the case for ongoing care*. Baltimore, MD: Partnership for Solutions.

Ritchie, K., and S. Lovestone. 2002. The dementias. *Lancet* 360, no. 9347: 1759–1766.

Robert Wood Johnson Foundation. 1996. *Chronic care in America: A 21st century challenge*. Princeton, NJ.

Rouse, B. A. 1995. *Substance abuse and mental health statistics sourcebook*. DHHS Publication No. (SMA) 953064. Washington, DC: Government Printing Office.

Sahyoun, N.R. et al. 2001. Trends in causes of death among the elderly. *Aging Trends, No. 1* (March 2001), Centers for Disease Control and Prevention, National Center for Health Statistics.

Satariano, W.A. 1997. Editorial: The disabilities of aging—Looking to the physical environment. *American Journal of Public Health* 87, no. 3: 331–332.

Scharlach, A.E. et al. 2001. *Case management in long-term care integration: An overview of current programs and evaluations*. Center for the Advanced Study of Aging Services, University of California, Berkeley, November 2001.

Schofield H. et al. 1998. *Family caregivers: Disability, illness and ageing*. Sydney: Allen & Unwin.

Scocco, P. et al. 2006. Nursing home institutionalization: A source of eustress or distress for the elderly. *International Journal of Geriatric Psychiatry* 21, no. 3: 281–287.

Sebelist, R.M. 1983. Mental retardation. In *Willard and Spackman's occupational therapy*. 6th ed., eds. H.L. Hopkins and H.D. Smith, 335–351. Philadelphia: J.B. Lippincott Co.

Shin, J.K. et al. 2002. Quality of care measurement in nursing home AIDS care: a pilot study. *Journal of the Association of Nurses in AIDS Care* 13, no. 2: 70–76.

Singh, D.A. 1997. *Nursing home administrators: Their influence on quality of care*. New York: Garland Publishing.

Singh, D.A. 2005. *Effective management of long-term care facilities*. Boston: Jones and Bartlett Publishers.

Skaggs, R.L., and H.R. Hawkins. 1994. Architecture for long-term care facilities. In *Essentials of long-term care administration*, ed. S.B. Goldsmith, 254–284. Gaithersburg, MD: Aspen Publishers, Inc.

Spreat, S. et al. 1998. Improve quality in nursing homes or institute community placement? Implementation of OBRA for individuals with mental retardation. *Research in Developmental Disabilities* 19, no. 6: 507–518.

Stahl, C. 1997. Adult foster care: An alternative to SNFs? *ADVANCE for Occupational Therapists*, 29 September, 18.

Tedesco, J. 1996. Adult day care. In *The continuum of long-term care: An integrated systems approach*, ed. C.J. Evashwick. Albany, NY: Delmar Publishers.

Tune, L. 2001. Assessing psychiatric illness in geriatric patients. *Clinical Cornerstone* 3, no. 3: 23–36.

Van Houtven, C.H., and E. Norton. 2004. Informal care and health care use of older adults. *Journal of Health Economics* 23, no. 6: 1159–1180.

Verbrugge, L.M., and A.M. Jette. 1994. The disablement process. *Social Science Medicine* 38, no. 1: 1–14.

Vladeck, B.C. 1995. End-of-life care. *Journal of the American Medical Association* 274, no. 6: 449.

Wolf, D.A. et al. 2005. Perspectives on the recent decline in disability at older ages. *The Milbank Quarterly* 83, no. 3: 365–395.

Chapter 11

Health Services for Special Populations

Learning Objectives

- To learn about population groups facing greater challenges and barriers in accessing health care services
- To understand the racial and ethnic disparities in health status
- To get acquainted with the health concerns of America's children and the health services available to them
- To learn about the health concerns of America's women and health services available to them
- To appreciate the challenges faced in rural health and to learn about measures taken to improve access to care
- To learn about the characteristics and health concerns of the homeless population
- To understand the nation's mental health system
- To understand the AIDS epidemic in America, the population groups affected by it, and the services available to HIV/AIDS patients

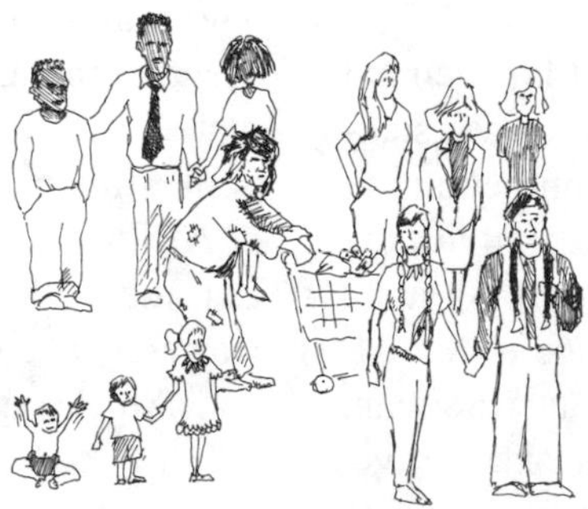

They all have something in common.

Introduction

Certain population groups in the United States face greater challenges than the general population in accessing timely and needed health care services (Lurie 1997; Shortell et al. 1996). They are at greater risk of poor physical, psychological, and/or social health (Aday 1994). Various terms are used to describe these populations, such as "underserved populations," "medically underserved," "medically disadvantaged," "underprivileged," and "American underclasses." The causes of their vulnerability are largely attributable to unequal social, economic, health, and geographic conditions. These population groups consist of racial and ethnic minorities, uninsured children, women, those living in rural areas, the homeless, the mentally ill, the chronically ill and disabled, and those with human immunodeficiency virus (HIV)/acquired immune deficiency syndrome (AIDS). These population groups are more vulnerable than the general population and experience greater barriers in access to care, financing of care, and racial or cultural acceptance. This chapter defines these population groups, describes their health needs, and summarizes the major challenges they face.

Racial/Ethnic Minorities

In October 1997, the Office of Management and Budget (OMB) announced revised standards for federal data on race and ethnicity to better reflect the growing diversity in the country (US Census Bureau 2000). As such, the minimum categories for race in the US population are Black or African American, Asian, American Indian or Alaska Native, Native Hawaiian or Other Pacific Islander, and White. Instead of allowing a multiracial category as was originally suggested in public and congressional hearings, the OMB adopted the Interagency Committee's recommendation to allow respondents to select one or more races when they self-identify. With the OMB's approval, the Census 2000 questionnaires also included a sixth racial category: Some Other Race. Effective January 1, 2003, the seven official racial categories are White alone, Black or African American alone, American Indian and Alaska Native alone, Asian alone, Native Hawaiian and Other Pacific Islander alone, Some Other Race alone, and Two or More Races.

Two minimum categories for ethnicity were also created: Hispanic or Latino and Not Hispanic or Latino. Hispanic or Latino Americans include Mexicans, Puerto Ricans, Central or South Americans, Cubans, and persons from other Spanish cultures or origins. Asian Americans include persons originating from the Far East, Southeast Asia, or the Indian subcontinent including, for example, Cambodia, China, India, Japan, Korea, Malaysia, Pakistan, the Philippine Islands, Thailand, and Vietnam. Native Hawaiians or Other Pacific Islanders include persons originating from Hawaii, Guam, Samoa or other Pacific Islands. American Indian or Alaskan Natives include persons originating from North and South America (including Central America) who maintain tribal affiliation or community attachment. The US Census Bureau estimated that in 2005, over 30% of the US population was made up of minorities: Black or African Americans (12.8%), Hispanics or Latinos (14.4%), Asians (4.3%), Native Hawaiian and Other Pacific Islanders (0.2%), and American Indian and Alaska Natives (1%). In addition, 1.5% identified as two or more races (US Census Bureau 2007).

Significant differences exist across the various racial/ethnic groups on health-related lifestyles and health status. For example, in 2004, the percentage of live births weighing less than 2,500 grams (low birth weight) is greatest among Blacks, followed by Asians or Pacific Islanders, American Indians or Native Americans, Whites, and Hispanics (Figure 11–1). White mothers are more likely to begin prenatal care during their first trimester, followed by Asian and Pacific Islanders, Hispanics, Blacks, and American Indians or Alaskan Natives (Table 11–1). Mothers of Asian and Pacific Islander origin are least likely to smoke cigarettes during pregnancy, followed by Hispanics, Blacks, and Whites (Figure 11–2). The White adult population is more likely to consume alcohol than other races (Figure 11–3). Among women 40 years of age and older, utilization of mammography is the highest among Whites and lowest among Hispanics (Figure 11–4).

Black Americans

Black Americans are more likely to be economically disadvantaged than Whites. Likewise, they fall behind in health status despite progress made during the past few decades. Blacks have shorter life expectancies than Whites (Figure 11–5); higher age-adjusted death rates for leading causes of death (Table 11–2); higher age-adjusted maternal mortality rates (Figure 11–6); and higher infant, neonatal, and postneonatal mortality rates (Table 11–3). On self-reported measures of health status, Blacks are more likely to report fair or poor health status than Whites (Figure 11–7). In terms of behavioral risks, Black males are slightly more likely to smoke cigarettes than White males (23.5% versus 23%), but White females are more likely to smoke than Black females (19.5% versus 16.9%) (Figure 11–8), although smoking among Black females has increased. On the

Figure 11–1 Percentage of Live Births Weighing Less Than 2,500 Grams by Mother's Detailed Race.

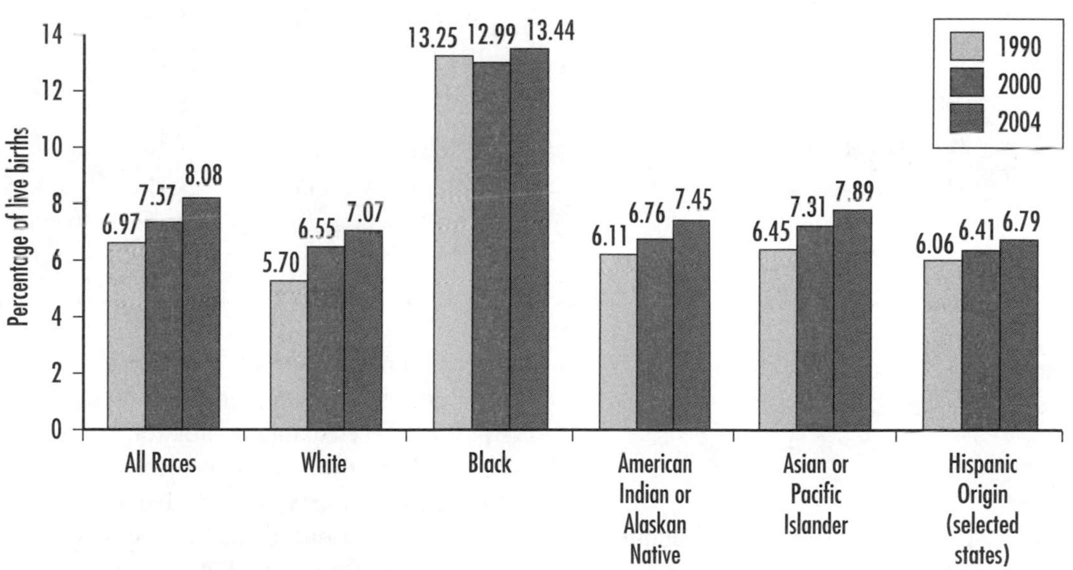

Source: Data from *Health, United States, 2006*, p. 148.

Table 11–1 Characteristics of Mothers by Race/Ethnicity

Item	1970	1980	1990	2000	2002
Prenatal care began during 1st trimester					
All mothers	68.0	76.3	75.8	83.2	83.7
White	72.3	79.2	79.2	85.0	85.4
Black	44.2	62.4	60.6	74.3	75.2
American Indian or Alaskan native	38.2	55.8	57.9	69.3	69.8
Asian or Pacific Islander	—	73.7	75.1	84.0	84.8
Hispanic origin	—	60.2	60.2	74.4	76.7
Education of mother 16 years or more					
All mothers	8.6	14.0	17.5	24.7	25.9
White	9.6	15.5	19.3	26.3	27.3
Black	2.8	6.2	7.2	11.7	12.7
American Indian or Alaskan native	2.7	3.5	4.4	7.8	8.7
Asian or Pacific Islander	—	30.8	31.0	42.8	45.7
Hispanic origin	—	4.2	5.1	7.6	8.3
Low birthweight (less than 2,500 grams)					
All mothers	7.93	6.84	6.97	7.57	7.82
White	6.85	5.72	5.70	6.55	6.80
Black	13.90	12.69	13.25	12.99	13.29
American Indian or Alaskan native	7.97	6.44	6.11	6.76	7.23
Asian or Pacific Islander	—	6.68	6.45	7.31	7.78
Hispanic origin (selected states)	—	6.12	6.06	6.41	6.55

Source: Data from *Health, United States, 2006*, pp. 140, 146, 148.

other hand, Blacks have lower levels of serum cholesterol than Whites (Table 11–4).

Hispanic Americans

The Hispanic segment of the US population is growing at a significantly higher rate than other population segments. Between 2000 and 2005, the Hispanic segment increased by 20.9% compared to a 5.3% increase in the total population (US Census Bureau 2007). In 2005, the Hispanic population numbered nearly 43 million and is projected to reach 53 million by the year 2015. Hispanic Americans are also one of the youngest groups among Americans. In 2005, the median age among Hispanic Americans was 27.2 years (compared to 40.3 years for non-Hispanic

Figure 11–2 Percentage of Mothers Who Smoked Cigarettes during Pregnancy According to Mother's Race.

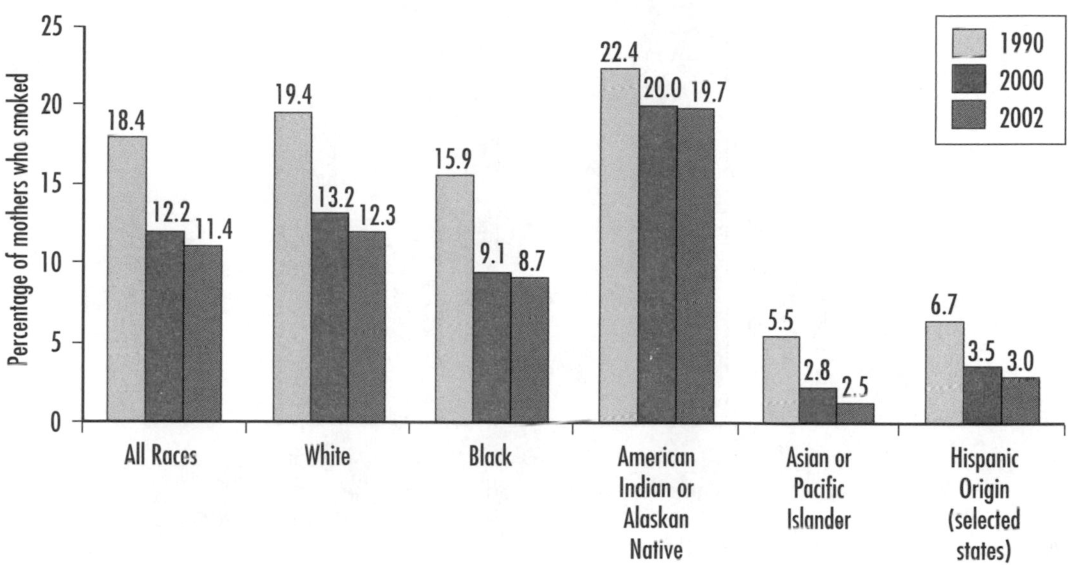

Source: Data from *Health, United States, 2006,* p. 147.

Figure 11–3 Alcohol Consumption by Persons 18 Years of Age and Over.

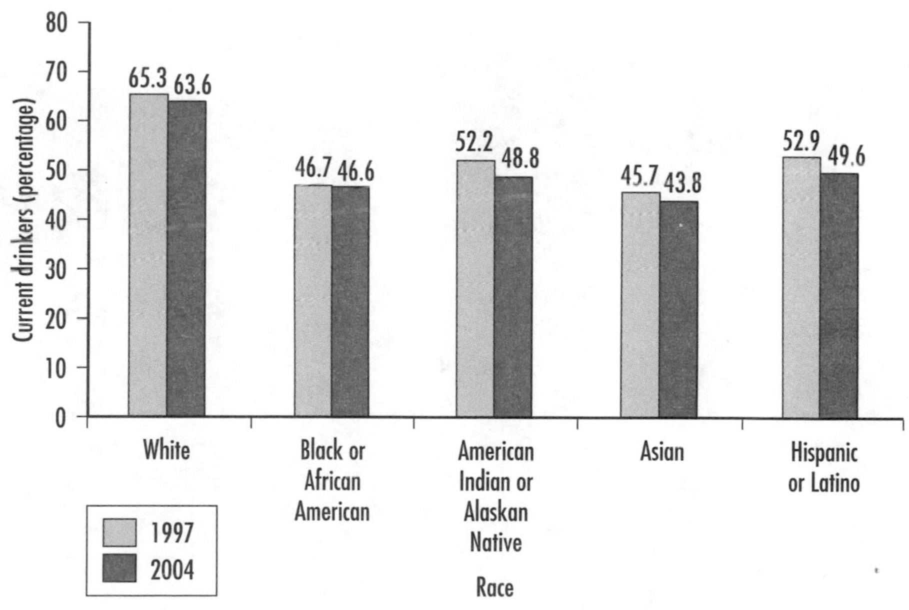

Source: Data from *Health, United States, 2006,* p. 276.

Figure 11–4 Use of Mammography by Women 40 Years of Age and Over, 2003.

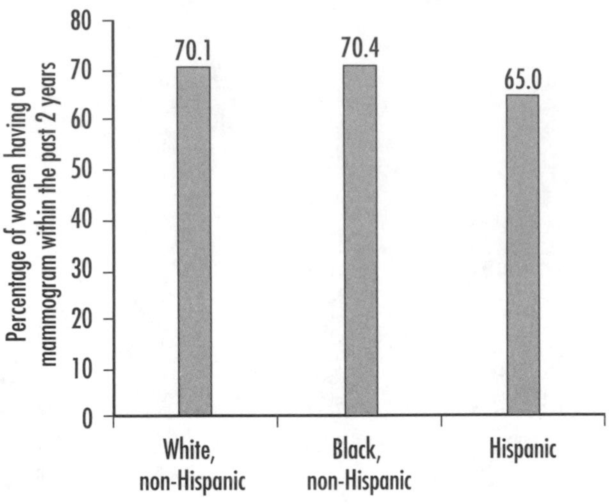

Source: Data from *Health, United States, 2006*, p. 313.

Figure 11–5 Life Expectancy at Birth, 1970–2003.

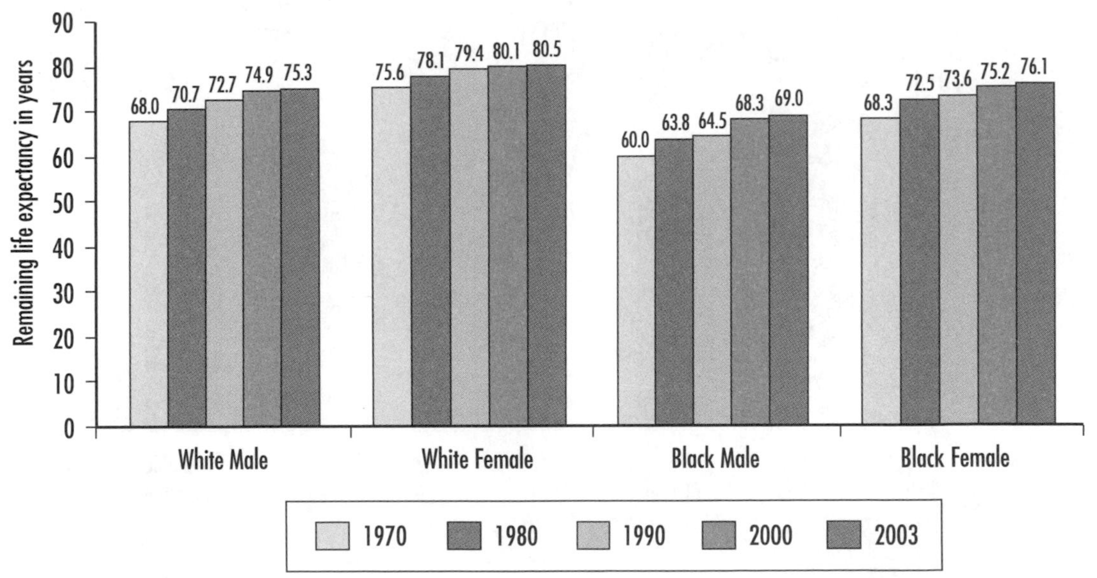

Source: Data from *Health, United States, 2006*, p. 176.

Table 11–2 Age-Adjusted Death Rates for Selected Causes of Death (1970–2003)

Race and Cause of Death	1970	1980	1990	2000	2003
	Deaths per 100,000 standard population				
All persons					
All causes	1,222.6	1,039.1	938.7	869.0	832.7
Diseases of the heart	492.7	412.1	321.8	257.6	232.3
Ischemic heart disease	—	345.2	249.6	186.8	162.9
Cerebrovascular diseases	147.7	96.2	65.3	60.9	53.5
Malignant neoplasms	198.6	207.9	216.0	199.6	190.1
Chronic lower respiratory diseases	21.3	28.3	37.2	44.2	43.3
Influenza and pneumonia	41.7	31.4	36.8	23.7	22.0
Chronic liver disease and cirrhosis	17.8	15.1	11.1	9.5	9.3
Diabetes mellitus	24.3	18.1	20.7	25.0	25.3
Human immunodeficiency virus (HIV) disease	—	—	10.2	5.2	4.7
Unintentional injuries	60.1	46.4	36.3	34.9	37.3
Motor vehicle-related injuries	27.6	22.3	18.5	15.4	15.3
Suicide	13.1	12.2	12.5	10.4	10.8
Homicide	8.8	10.4	9.4	5.9	6.0
White					
All causes	1,193.3	1,012.7	909.8	849.8	817.0
Diseases of the heart	492.2	409.4	317.0	253.4	228.2
Ischemic heart disease	—	347.6	249.7	185.6	161.7
Cerebrovascular diseases	143.5	93.2	62.8	58.8	51.4
Malignant neoplasms	196.7	204.2	211.6	197.2	188.5
Chronic lower respiratory diseases	21.8	29.3	38.3	46.0	45.4
Influenza and pneumonia	39.8	30.9	36.4	23.5	21.9
Chronic liver disease and cirrhosis	16.6	13.9	10.5	9.6	9.5
Diabetes mellitus	22.9	16.7	18.8	22.8	23.0
Human immunodeficiency virus (HIV) disease	—	—	8.3	2.8	2.5
Unintentional injuries	57.8	45.3	35.5	35.1	38.2
Motor vehicle-related injuries	27.1	22.6	18.5	15.6	15.7
Suicide	13.8	13.0	13.4	11.3	11.8
Homicide	4.7	6.7	5.5	3.6	3.7

continues

Table 11–2 Age-Adjusted Death Rates for Selected Causes of Death (1970–2003) *(continued)*

Race and Cause of Death	1970	1980	1990	2000	2003
Black					
All causes	1,518.1	1,314.8	1,250.3	1,121.4	1,065.9
Diseases of the heart	512.0	455.3	391.5	324.8	300.2
Ischemic heart disease	—	334.5	267.0	218.3	195.0
Cerebrovascular diseases	197.1	129.1	91.6	81.9	74.3
Malignant neoplasms	225.3	256.4	279.5	248.5	233.3
Chronic lower respiratory diseases	16.2	19.2	28.1	31.6	30.1
Influenza and pneumonia	57.2	34.4	39.4	25.6	23.3
Chronic liver disease and cirrhosis	28.1	25.0	16.5	9.4	8.4
Diabetes mellitus	38.8	32.7	40.5	49.5	49.2
Human immunodeficiency virus (HIV) disease	—	—	26.7	23.3	21.3
Unintentional injuries	78.3	57.6	43.8	37.7	36.1
Motor vehicle-related injuries	31.1	20.2	18.8	15.7	14.9
Suicide	6.2	6.5	7.1	5.5	5.2
Homicide	44.0	39.0	36.3	20.5	21.0

Source: Data from *Health, United States, 2006*, pp. 179–180, Centers for Disease Control and Prevention, National Center for Health Statistics.

Figure 11–6 Age-Adjusted Maternal Mortality Rates.

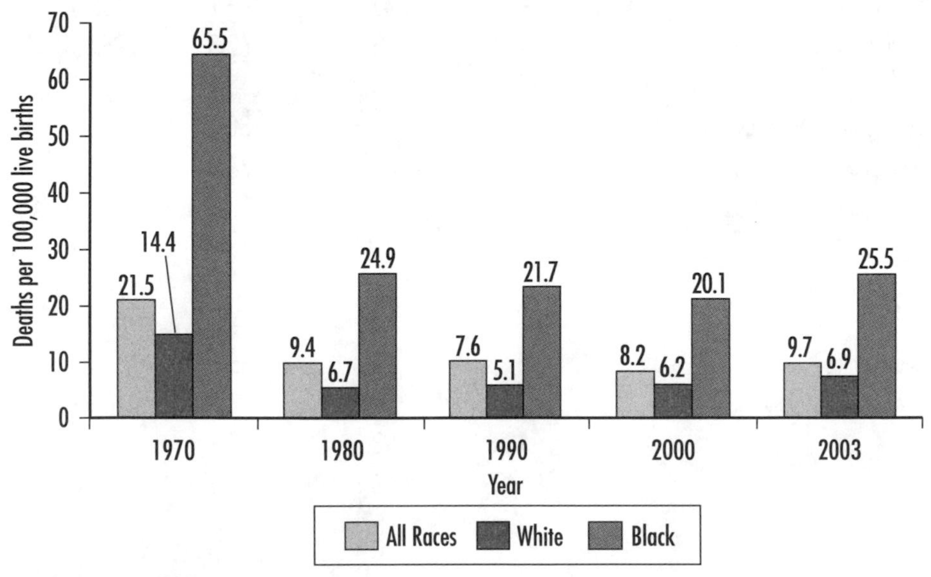

Source: Data from *Health, United States, 2006*, p. 222.

Table 11–3 Infant, Neonatal, and Postneonatal Mortality Rates by Mother's Race (per 1,000 live births)

	Infant Deaths				Neonatal Deaths				Postneonatal Deaths			
Race of Mother	1983	1990	2000	2003	1983	1990	2000	2003	1983	1990	2000	2003
All mothers	10.9	8.9	6.9	6.8	7.1	5.7	4.6	4.6	3.8	3.2	2.3	2.2
White	9.3	7.3	5.7	5.7	6.1	4.6	3.8	3.9	3.2	2.7	1.9	1.9
Black	19.2	16.9	13.5	13.5	12.5	11.1	9.1	9.2	6.7	5.9	4.3	4.3
American Indian or Alaskan native	15.2	13.1	8.3	8.7	7.5	6.1	4.4	4.5	7.7	7.0	3.9	4.2
Asian or Pacific Islander	8.3	6.6	4.9	4.8	5.2	3.9	3.4	3.4	3.1	2.7	1.4	1.4
Hispanic origin (selected states)	9.5	7.5	5.6	5.6	6.2	4.8	3.8	3.9	3.3	2.9	1.8	1.7

Source: Data from *Health, United States, 2006,* p. 160.

Figure 11–7 Respondent-Assessed Health Status.

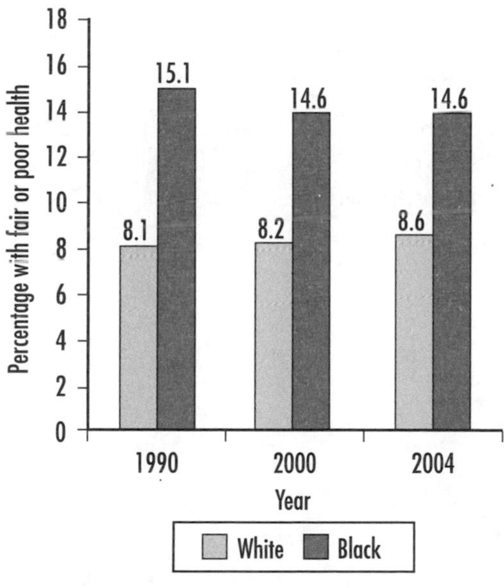

Source: Data from *Health, United States, 1995,* p. 172, Centers for Disease Control and Prevention, National Center for Health Statistics, 1996, and *Health, United States 2006,* p. 260.

Figure 11–8 Current Cigarette Smoking by Persons 18 Years of Age and Over, Age-Adjusted, 2004.

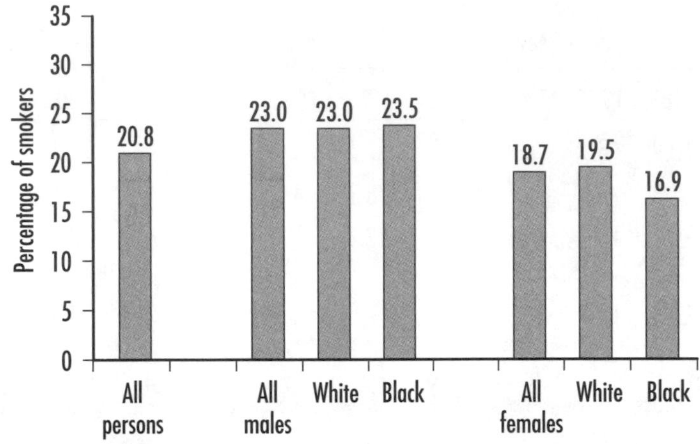

Source: Data from *Health, United States, 2006,* p. 266, Centers for Disease Control and Prevention, National Center for Health Statistics, 2006.

Whites), and 10.6% are below age 5 (compared to 5.7% of non-Hispanic Whites) (US Census Bureau 2007). As of 2005, 58.5% of Hispanic Americans age 25 and older had completed high school (compared to 87.5% of Whites), and 12% of Hispanic Americans age 25 and older had completed college (compared to 28% of Whites) (US Census Bureau 2007). In 2004, about 20% of Hispanic persons lived below the federal poverty line (compared to 6.5% of non-Hispanic White persons) (US Census Bureau 2007).

Table 11–4 Serum Cholesterol Levels among Persons 20 Years and Older, 2001–2004

Sex and Race*	Percentage of Persons 20 Years of Age of Age and Over with Hypertension	Mean Serum Cholesterol Level (mg/dl) of Persons 20 Years of Age and Over	Percentage of Overweight Persons 20 Years of Age and Over
Both sexes	29.7	202	66.0
White			
Male	26.8	201	71.0
Female	28.5	203	57.6
Black			
Male	41.6	198	67.0
Female	44.7	199	79.6

*20–74 years, age adjusted.

Source: Data from *Health, United States, 2006,* pp. 279, 282, 287, Centers for Disease Control and Prevention, National Center for Health Statistics, Division of Health Examination Statistics, 2006.

Many Hispanic Americans experience significant barriers in accessing medical care. Many Hispanic families who immigrated to the United States may not qualify for Medicaid (Rosenbaum and Darnell 1997). This represents a greater problem for those from Central America (79% foreign born) and South America (75% foreign born) than those from Spain (17% foreign born) or Mexico (28% foreign born). Place of birth is also related to Hispanic people's inability to speak English, which is another factor associated with reduced access to medical services (Solis et al. 1990).

Low education is related to employment and occupational status. Hispanic Americans have higher unemployment rates than non-Hispanic Whites (4.8% versus 3.5% in 2005) and are more likely to be employed in semiskilled, nonprofessional occupations (US Census Bureau 2007). Due to the close association between employment status and health insurance, Hispanic Americans are more likely to be uninsured and underinsured than non-Hispanic Whites. In 2004, 34.4% of Hispanic persons were uninsured, compared to 12% of non-Hispanic Whites and 17.3% of non-Hispanic Blacks or African Americans (National Center for Health Statistics 2006). Among Hispanics, 37.6% of Mexican Americans were uninsured, followed by 22.8% of Cubans, 20.4% of Puerto Ricans, and 32.3% of other Hispanics (National Center for Health Statistics 2006).

Homicide was the sixth leading cause of death for Hispanic males in 2003. They have the highest ranking, along with Blacks, for this cause of death (National Center for Health Statistics 2006).

Hispanic Americans are less likely to take advantage of preventive care than non-Hispanic Whites and certain other races. Hispanic women 40 years of age or older were least likely to use mammography (65% versus 70.1% for non-Hispanic Whites and 70.4% for non-Hispanic Blacks; see Figure 11–4). In 2002, fewer Hispanic mothers begin their prenatal care during the first trimester than mothers of some other ethnic origins (76.7% for Hispanic mothers versus 85.4% for White mothers and 84.8% for Asian and Pacific Islander mothers; see Table 11–1). Hispanic children have lower vaccination rates than White and Asian children. In 2004, 81% of Hispanic children aged 19–35 months had received the combined series vaccines (4:3:1:3) compared to 85% of White children, 84% of Asian children, 76% of Black children, and 75% of American Indian and Alaskan Native children (National Center for Health Statistics 2006). Among Hispanics aged two and older in 2004, 52.7% had at least one dental visit during a year compared to 67.1% for non-Hispanic Whites (National Center for Health Statistics 2006).

People of Hispanic origin also experience greater behavioral risks than Whites and certain other racial/ethnic groups. For example, among individuals 18 years of age or older in 2004, a higher proportion of Hispanics are current drinkers than people of other ethnic origins (49.6% for Hispanics versus 46.6% for Blacks and 43.8% of Asians; see Figure 11–3). However, fewer Hispanics smoke compared to people of other ethnicities. In 2004, 20.1% of Hispanic males 18 years of age and older identified themselves as "current smokers," compared to 24.8% of non-Hispanic White males and 25.1% of non-Hispanic Black males (National Center for Health Statistics 2006). Among female adults, 10.6% of Hispanics smoked in 2004, compared to 21.9% of non-Hispanic Whites and 17.8% of non-Hispanic Blacks (National Center for Health Statistics 2006).

Asian Americans

Minority health epidemiology has typically focused on Blacks, Hispanics, and American Indians or Alaskan Natives because Asian Americans (AAs) have relatively small numbers. In the reporting of comparative research data, AAs have generally appeared in a category labeled "other," a category that is meaningless, but changing demographics are expanding these categories. The 2000 US Census made a distinction between Asian Americans and Native Hawaiians/Other Pacific Islanders. The term "Asian" refers to persons originating from the Far East, Southeast Asia, or the Indian subcontinent (e.g., Cambodia, China, India, Japan, Korea, Malaysia, Pakistan, the Philippine Islands, Thailand, and Vietnam). The National Center for Health Statistics has now expanded the race codes to include nine categories: White, Black, Native American, Chinese, Japanese, Hawaiian, Filipino, Other Asian/Pacific Islanders, and other races. But even the category of "Other Asian/Pacific Islander" is extremely heterogeneous, encompassing 21 subgroups with different health profiles. The 1990 census described the Asian American and Pacific Islander (AAPI) population as originating from at least 29 Asian countries and 20 Pacific Island cultures found in the Far East, Southeast Asia, the Indian subcontinent, and the Pacific Islands. Therefore, since 1992, the National Center for Health Statistics has been using a new race code for AAPIs in the National Health Interview Survey that includes the following subcategories: Chinese, Filipino, Hawaiian, Korean, Vietnamese, Japanese, Asian Indian, Samoan, Guamanian, and Other Asian Pacific Islander. Use of these subcategories accounts for about 90% of the AAPI population (Kuo and Porter 1998). In 2005, Asians accounted for 4.3% of the US population and numbered 12.7 million (US Census Bureau 2007).

AAs constitute one of the fastest-growing population segments in the United States. The percent change in the Asian population was 19.8% between 2000 and 2005, compared to 5.3% for the population as a whole (US Census Bureau 2007). The US Census Bureau projects the AA population will reach 16.1 million by 2015 (2007).

In education, income, and health, Asian Americans and Pacific Islanders are very diverse. In 2005, 87.6% of AAPIs 25 years of age or older had at least four years of high school education, compared with 85.7% of non-Hispanic Whites; in addition, the percentage of AAPIs with a bachelor's degree or higher was 50.1%, compared to 28% for non-Hispanic Whites (US Census Bureau 2007). Educational attainment varies greatly among the subgroups. For example, in 1990, 88% of the adults of Japanese descent had graduated from high school, among Vietnamese it was 61% and only 31% of Hmong adults (Kuo and Porter 1998). In 2004, the median income for Asian males (age 15 years and older) was $32,866, compared to $33,652 for non-Hispanic White males (US Census Bureau 2007). In addition, in 2004, a smaller percentage of Asians (9.8%) lived below the federal poverty level, compared to Whites (10.8%), Blacks (24.7%), and Hispanics (21.9%) (US Census Bureau 2007).

The heterogeneity of the AAPI population is reflected in the various indicators of health status. For instance, a greater percentage of Vietnamese and Korean (17.2% and 12.8%, respectively) people assess their own health status as fair or poor compared to people of Chinese, Filipino, and Japanese descent (6.1 to 7.4%) (Kuo and Porter 1998). The incidence of low birth weight babies varies greatly, from 4.5% among Chinese to 7% among Filipinos. Cambodian refugees have extremely high rates of posttraumatic stress disorder, dissociation, depression, and anxiety. Although US smoking rates are reported to be lowest among AAPIs, 92% of Laotians, 71% of Cambodians, and 65% of Vietnamese are smokers (Yoon and Chien 1996). Compared with Whites, Korean-American men have a fivefold incidence of stomach cancer and an eightfold incidence of liver cancer. Cultural practices and attitudes may prevent AAPI women from receiving adequate breast cancer screening and prenatal care. A study analyzing National Health Interview Survey data from 1997–2000 found Chinese, Asian Indian, Filipino, and other AAPI children were more likely to be without contact with a health professional within the past 12 months, compared to non-Hispanic white children. Citizenship/nativity status, maternal education attainment, and poverty status were all significant independent risk factors for health care access and utilization (Yu 2004). Ignorance of this bipolar distribution contributes to the myth of a minority population that is both healthy and economically successful. For example, the 1985 DHHS Task Force Report on Black and Minority Health stated that, as a group, the AAPI population in the United States is at lower risk of early death than the White population. Such a misunderstanding demonstrates an essential need for more in-depth, ethnic-specific health research.

American Indians and Alaskan Natives

In 2005, 2.9 million people identified their race as American Indian or Alaskan Native alone, and nearly 4.2 million people identified themselves American Indian or Alaskan Native in combination with other races (US Census Bureau 2007). More than one-half live in urban areas (Nolan et al. 1996). According to the Census Bureau, this subpopulation is growing at a rate of 2.5% per year (IHS 2001). Concomitantly, demand for expanded health care has been on the increase for several decades and is becoming more acute. The incidence and prevalence of certain diseases and conditions, such as diabetes, hypertension, infant mortality and morbidity, chemical dependency, and AIDS- and HIV-related morbidity, are all high enough to be matters of prime concern. Compared to the general US population, Native Americans also have much higher death rates from alcoholism, tuberculosis, diabetes, injuries, suicide, and homicide (IHS 2001).

It is also no secret that Native Americans continue to occupy the bottom of the socioeconomic strata. American Indians/Alaskan Natives are approximately twice as likely to be poor, to be unemployed, and to not have a college degree, compared to the general populations of the areas in which they live (Castor 2006). A strong positive association exists between socioeconomic status and health status. For example, poverty, not cultural factors, has been found to be associated with the high injury-related mortality rate among Indian children. The effects of Indian poverty are exacerbated by an acute political disempowerment.

The health status of American Indian people appears to be improving, yet it significantly lags behind the health status of the population at large. In the years 1972 to 1974, the mortality rate among Native American expectant mothers was 27.7 per 100,000 live births (Pleasant 2003, 94). By 1994 to 1996, the occurrence rate was only 6.1%—a 78% drop. Infant mortality also declined by 58% from 22.2 per 1,000 births in 1972 to 1974 to 9.3 per 1,000 births in 1994 to 1996.

Still, Native Americans experience significant health disparities when compared to the general US population. Native Americans see seven times more death due to alcohol and 3.5 times more death due to suicide (Pleasant 2003, 95). In some reservation communities, health conditions have been found to be as bad as they are in some of the worst urban slums (Gray 1996). A new emphasis is being placed on the problems of American Indians because they are diverse, hard to reach, and afflicted with many of the problems of America's urban poor (Nolan et al. 1996).

The provision of health services to American Indians by the federal government was first negotiated in 1832 as partial compensation for land cessions. Subsequent laws have expanded the scope of services and allowed American Indians greater autonomy in planning, developing, and administering their own health care programs. These laws explicitly permit the practice of traditional as well as Western medicine.

Indian Health Care Improvement Act

The Indian Health Care Improvement Act was enacted in 1976. This law, and later amendments in 1980, outlined a seven-year effort to help bring American Indian health to a level of parity with the general population. Although appropriations were significantly increased to improve or develop sanitation services, health care programs, and medical facilities, limited fiscal support undermined the act's goal of achieving health parity for American Indians. Other features of the act provided for specific funding for programs to improve access to health care for urban Indians and educational scholarships to increase the number of Indian health care professionals. Thus, the Indian Health Care Improvement Act has at least been successful in minimizing prejudice, building trust, and putting responsibility back into the hands of American Indians.

Indian Health Service

The Indian Health Service (IHS), a federal agency responsible for American Indian health since 1955, operates 49 hospitals and over 600 other facilities (IHS 2006a). The goal of IHS is to assure that Native Americans and Alaskan Natives are provided with comprehensive and culturally acceptable health services (Pleasant 2003). The IHS serves the members and descendants of more than 560 federally recognized American Indian and Alaskan Native tribes (IHS 2006a); however, the health care needs of a rapidly expanding American Indian population are quickly outweighing the available resources.

In the three decades from 1955 to 1985, the IHS estimated a tenfold increase in its service population (Rhodes 1987). During this period, the number of physicians rose from 125 to 770, dentists from 40 to 250, and registered nurses from 780 to 2,000. Other additions to personnel included a number of health-related specialists, such as dietitians, licensed practical nurses, and dental assistants (IHS 1987). Currently, the IHS staff has grown to approximately 2,700 nurses, 900 physicians, 400 engineers, 500 pharmacists, 300 dentists, and 150 sanitarians (IHS 2006b).

The IHS is centrally administered through its headquarters in Rockville, Maryland. Nationally, it is divided into 12 area offices each responsible for program operations in a particular geographic area. Each area office is composed of branches dealing with various administrative and health-related services. Delivery of health services is the responsibility of 164 tribally-managed service units operating at the local level (IHS 2006c).

Over the years, the IHS system has evolved to include not only primary care services but also preventive strategies (Rhodes 1987). Within these environmental, educational, and outreach preventive strategies are special initiatives that focus on areas such as injury control, alcoholism, diabetes, mental health, women's health, Indian youth and children, and elder care (IHS 1999b). One of the more successful features of the IHS system is its Community Health Representative Program. Since its inception, the Community Health Representative Program continues to fulfill a vital role in patient care (Mail 1988). The IHS mandate has been made particularly difficult because the locations of Indian reservation communities are among the least geographically accessible (Burks 1992; Kozoll 1986). Relative isolation and impassable roads continue to present unique challenges to the IHS commitment.

Despite the IHS expansion of services, most American Indian communities continue to be medically underserved. As services have been expanded and medical professionals added, the already meager fiscal support for IHS has become increasingly strained. The IHS is said to be "underfunded and understaffed" (Pevar 1992). The IHS is certainly no exception to limited financial resources and spiraling health care costs. As a result, the IHS has experienced increasing difficulties in meeting the needs of its beneficiaries. The FY 2005 IHS budget appropriation was $3 billion and third-party collections totaled $533 million. This translates to a per capita personal health expenditure of $2,133 for IHS patients, compared to $5,518 for the total US population (IHS 2006c). Despite these constraints, the IHS continues to make positive alterations to its programs. The most notable recent developments include an enhanced commitment to prevention. Programs have been established for AIDS, maternal and child health, otitis media, nursing, aging, and health care database management. Additional proposals include a focus on traditional medicine, domestic violence and child abuse, oral health, sanitation, and new initiatives to improve advocacy for Indian health interests (IHS 1999a). On the other hand, despite limitations in the IHS's scope of service, many American Indian people do not avail themselves of the system's services. Thus, while the IHS remains the largest and most well-established of health care systems designed to meet the specific needs of American Indian people, not all American Indian people are actually using it.

The Uninsured

The uninsured represent a large and growing segment of Americans. The number of uninsured Americans under age 65 increased by 1.3 million between 2004 and 2005, currently affecting approximately 46 million of the nonelderly population (Kaiser Commission on Medicaid and the Uninsured 2006). In 1999 and 2000, a robust economy and expanded public coverage led to the first slight decrease in the number of uninsured in over a decade. However, an economic downturn in 2001 led to an increase in the number of uninsured once again. Among working Americans between the ages of 19 and 64 years, the proportion of those without any health insurance coverage rose from 15.1% in 1979 to 23.3% in 1995. The latter figure remained relatively stable during the period 1992 to 1995 (Kronick and Gilmer 1999); however, with population growth, the actual number of Americans without health insurance has gradually risen. According to 1999 estimates, a little more than 16% of civilian, noninstitutionalized Americans were without health care coverage (National Center for Health Statistics 1999, 319), despite a robust national economy. By 2005, the percentage of Americans without health insurance had increased to approximately 18% (Kaiser Commission on Medicaid and the Uninsured 2006).

For the most part, the uninsured tend to be poor, less educated, working in part-time jobs, and/or employed by small firms. They also tend to be younger (25 to 40) because most of the elderly (65 years of age or older) are covered by Medicare. Ethnic minorities are also more likely to lack health insurance. The US Census Bureau estimates that in 2004, 32.7% of Hispanic residents were uninsured, compared with 19.7% of Blacks, 16.8% of Asian-Americans, and 14.9% of Whites (2007).

Although poorer people are less likely to have insurance, most of the uninsured are neither unemployed nor poor enough to qualify them for federal programs, such as Medicaid or other types of state welfare assistance (Schroeder et al. 1997). It is also important to dispel the myth that the uninsured simply choose to remain without health insurance. Estimates say that only about one in ten uninsured persons lacks insurance by personal choice (Bennefield 1995). Instead, most medically uninsured adults are employed but are not covered because (a) their employer does not offer health benefits, (b) they do not qualify because they do not work an adequate number of hours or have not been with the employer long enough, or (c) they cannot afford to pay their portion of the premium or purchase insurance on their own (Bennefield 1995). Despite recent policies designed to increase health insurance for children (such as the State Children's Health Insurance Program [SCHIP]), an estimated 20% of the uninsured are children under the age of 18 (Kaiser Commission on Medicaid and the Uninsured 2006).

Lack of insurance has a negative effect on the health status of the uninsured. Numerous studies have shown that the uninsured use fewer health services than the insured (Freeman and Corey 1993). Decreased utilization of health services is not because the uninsured are healthier than those with health insurance are. In fact, they usually have poorer health than the general population (Donelan et al. 1996). Nor do the uninsured simply have different health care preferences. Instead, the uninsured face systematic barriers to accessing health care (Schroeder et al. 1997). In 2003, 42% of uninsured people reported having no regular source of health care, compared to 9% of insured people (Kaiser Commission on Medicaid and the Uninsured 2006). Even when the uninsured can access health care, they often have serious problems paying medical bills. While it used to be a common practice for teaching hospitals, private physicians, and community clinics to provide discounted or even free medical care to the uninsured, managed care practices have seriously reduced the ability of this social safety net to provide care for the uninsured (Donelan et al. 1996). In 2003, 47% of uninsured people postponed seeking medical care because of cost, compared to 15% of insured people (Kaiser Commission on Medicaid and the Uninsured 2006).

The plight of the uninsured affects those who have insurance. Medical expenditures for uncompensated care to the uninsured was estimated to be $41 million in 2004 (Kaiser Commission on Medicaid and the Uninsured 2006). Much of this cost is shared by Medicaid, federal grants to nonprofit hospitals, and charitable organizations. If the level of uncompensated care remains at the current levels, these costs are likely to be at least partly passed on to the US public at large. Decreased access to health care can result in higher prevalence of ill health and mortality among the uninsured and their families. Lack of insurance can result in decreased utilization of lower cost preventive services, can ultimately result in an increased need for (and decreased ability to pay for) more expensive emergency health care, and can even contribute to the spread of infectious diseases, such as tuberculosis.

Children

Many children lack adequate health care, as documented by the growing number of children not covered by employer-sponsored insurance. According to the National Center for Health Statistics, the number of children under age 18 without health insurance was between 9.2 and 9.7 million in 2004 (2006). Dwindling federal support for Medicaid translates into fewer low-income households qualifying for health care assistance. Currently, about 26% of children under age 18 are covered under Medicaid and 59% under private insurance (National Center for Health Statistics 2006).

Vaccinations of children for selected diseases differ by race, poverty status, and area of residence (Table 11–5). White children have greater vaccination rates for DTP, polio, measles, HIB, and combined series than Blacks. Children who come from families with incomes below the federal poverty line or who live in central city areas have lower vaccination rates than those at or above poverty or who live in non-inner city areas.

Table 11–5 Vaccinations of Children 19–35 Months of Age for Selected Diseases According to Race, Poverty Status, and Residence in a Metropolitan Statistical Area, 2004 (%)

	Race			Poverty Status		Inside MSA	
Vaccination	Total	White	Black	Below Poverty	At or Above Poverty	Central City	Remaining Areas
DTP[1]	86	88	80	81	87	84	87
Polio[2]	92	92	90	90	92	91	92
Measles-containing (MMR)[3]	93	94	91	91	94	93	94
HIB[4]	94	95	91	92	94	93	94
Combined series[5]	83	85	76	78	85	81	84

[1]Diphtheria-tetanus-pertussis, four doses or more.

[2]Three doses or more.

[3]Respondents were asked about measles-containing or MMR (measles-mumps-rubella) vaccines.

[4]Haemophilus B, three doses or more.

[5]The combined series consists of four doses of DTP vaccine, three doses of polio vaccine, and one dose of measles-containing vaccine (4 : 4 : 1 : 3).

Source: Data from *Health, United States, 2006*, p. 306.

As a result of inadequate health care, children's ability to learn is compromised. Some children stay home and miss school for long periods when they do not receive needed medical care. In addition, delayed access to medical care may result in more serious and expensive illnesses. Some sick children go to school because of unavailability of sick child care or lack of leave benefits for working parents. Once in school, they face not only a diminished learning capacity, but they may also expose other children to contagious illnesses (Wenzel 1996).

Everyone, including children, has human rights. Because they are young, less assertive, and not as well informed as adults, children are more likely to have their rights ignored. Children are not active voters, hence, they do not have their voices represented in the political process. As a result, their plight has been almost ignored in health policy decisions. However, the Balanced Budget Act of 1997, a landmark initiative, created SCHIP (see Chapter 6). It allocated $24 billion in federal matching funds to help the states extend health care to an estimated 10 million uninsured children (King 1997). Ironically, though, issues of poverty and access to health care do not even cross the minds of most Americans when they are asked about the most pressing problems confronting children today. Some fear exists that the initiative could fizzle out because of a lack of public support (APHA 1998). Thus, the root cause of children's health problems may remain unaddressed.

To protect children's rights, the United Nations drew up an international agreement, the UN Convention on the Rights of the Child, in 1992. This agreement is an important step forward in promoting children's rights. The document acknowledges that children are especially vulnerable and have a right to expect special consideration. Similar to the Children Act of 1989, its ethos underscores the importance of acknowledging and respecting children's special needs. In 2007, the United Nations published *The State of the World's Children*, which ties children's health and rights to women's health and rights. This report, which displays child health indicators for every member nation of the UN, maintains that greater gender equality will lead to profound and positive impacts on children's well-being and development (UN 2007).

Children's health has certain unique aspects in the delivery of health care. Among these are children's developmental vulnerability, dependency, and differential patterns of morbidity and mortality. ***Developmental vulnerability*** refers to the rapid and cumulative physical and emotional changes that characterize childhood and the potential impact that illness, injury, or disruptive family and social circumstances can have on a child's life-course trajectory. ***Dependency*** refers to children's special circumstances that require adults to take responsibility for recognizing and responding to their health needs. Children depend on their parents, school officials, caregivers, and sometimes neighbors to discover their need for health care, seek health care services on their behalf, authorize treatment, and comply with recommended treatment regimens. These dependency relationships can be complex and often change over time. These relationships can affect the utilization of health services by children.

Children increasingly are affected by a broad and complex array of conditions collectively referred to as "new morbidities." ***New morbidities*** include drug and alcohol abuse, family and neighborhood violence, emotional disorders, and learning problems from which older generations do not suffer.

These dysfunctions originate in complex family or socioeconomic conditions rather than biological causes exclusively. Hence, they cannot be adequately addressed by traditional medical services alone. Instead, these conditions require a continuum of comprehensive services that include multidisciplinary assessment, treatment, and rehabilitation, as well as community-based prevention strategies.

Serious chronic medical conditions leading to disabling conditions are less prevalent in children. Estimates of the total number of young people with disabilities range from 5% to 20% of the child population. By the most conservative estimates, at least 3 million children age 18 and under are disabled, and 1 million children in the United States have a severe chronic illness. Medical problems in children are usually related to birth or congenital conditions rather than degenerative conditions that affect adults. These differences call for an approach to the delivery of health care that is uniquely designed to address the needs of children.

Children and the US Health Care System

In the United States, the delivery of health care to children is characterized as a patchwork of disconnected programs. Each program has distinct eligibility, administrative, and funding criteria. The different programs can be categorized into three broad sectors: the personal medical and preventive services sector, the population-based community health services sector, and the health-related support services sector.

Personal medical and preventive health services include primary and specialty medical services, which are generally delivered in private and public medical offices, hospitals, and laboratories. Personal medical services are principally funded by private insurance and health plans, Medicaid, and by families' out-of-pocket payments.

The population-based community health services include communitywide health promotion and disease prevention services. Examples are immunization delivery and monitoring programs, lead screening and abatement programs, and child abuse and neglect prevention. Other health services include special child abuse treatment programs and rehabilitative services for children with complex congenital conditions or other chronic and debilitating diseases. Community-based programs also provide assurance and coordination functions, such as case management and referral programs for children with chronic diseases and early interventions and monitoring for infants at risk for developmental disabilities. Funding for this sector comes from federal programs, such as Medicaid's Early Periodic Screening, Diagnosis, and Treatment (EPSDT) program; Title V (Maternal and Child Health) of the Social Security Act; and other categorical programs.

The health-related support services sector includes such services as nutrition education, early intervention, rehabilitation, and family support programs. An example of a rehabilitation service is education and psychotherapy for children with HIV. Family support services include parent education and skill building in families with infants at risk for developmental delay because of physiological or social conditions (such as low birth weight or very low income). Funding for these services comes from diverse agencies, such as the Department of Agriculture, which funds the Supplemental Food Program for Women, Infants, and Children (WIC); and the Department of Education, which funds the Individuals with Disabilities Education Act (IDEA).

Part of the difficulty in integrating health services comes from the sheer volume of categorical programs as well as the scope of eligibility and financial constraints that inhibit greater coordination. Expansion of health insurance coverage and system reorganization based on managed care cannot guarantee children's access to comprehensive and coordinated services. However, the principles of comprehensive, continuous, and coordinated care originally embodied in Medicaid's EPSDT program, and reinforced in the 1989 amendments to Title XIX, recognize that access to basic ambulatory medical care will not suffice to meet the needs of children with complex health conditions and environmental risks. For these children, screening, diagnostic, and treatment services must be supplemented with a constellation of support services, including outreach, comprehensive case management, home visitation, and family counseling services.

Women

Women are playing an increasingly important role in the delivery of health care. Not only do women remain the leading providers of care in the nursing profession, but they are also well represented in other major health professions, including allopathic and osteopathic medicine, dentistry, podiatry, and optometry (Figure 11–9).

Women in the United States can now expect to live almost eight years longer than men, but they suffer greater morbidity and poorer health outcomes. They also have a higher prevalence of certain health problems than men do over the course of their lifetimes (Sechzer et al. 1996). Compared to men of comparable age, women develop more acute and chronic illnesses, resulting in a greater number of short- and long-term disabilities (NIH 1992; Kaiser Family Foundation 2005). Heart disease and stroke account for a higher percentage of deaths among women than men at all stages of life. In contrast to 24% of men, 42% of women who have heart attacks die within a year (OWH 2001).

Even when reproductive conditions are statistically controlled, research has demonstrated that health problems restrict women's activities by 25% more days each year than they do men's. Women are bedridden 35% more days than men are each year because of infectious or parasitic diseases, respiratory diseases, digestive system conditions, injuries, and other acute conditions (Regier et al. 1988). Across all age, race, and ethnic groups, notable differences are present between men and women. Whether it is heart disease, cancer, HIV, substance abuse, or depression, the onset and progress of illness differs between men and women. The differences extend beyond the course of disease to functions that are necessary to address the distinctive health care needs of women, such as research, prevention, treatment, and education.

The differences between men and women are equally pronounced for mental illness. For example, anxiety disorders and major depression affect two to three times as many women as men (OWH 2001; Kaiser Family Foundation 2005). Clinical depression is a major mental health problem for both men and women; however, an estimated 12% of women in the United States, compared with 7% of men, will suffer from major depression during their lifetime (OWH 2001). Certain other mental disorders also affect more women at different stages of life. During their lives, about one in five women experience a significant depressive episode, which is about 1.5 times more than the rate for men,

Figure 11–9 Percentage of Female Students of Total Enrollment in Schools for Selected Health Occupations, 2003–2004.

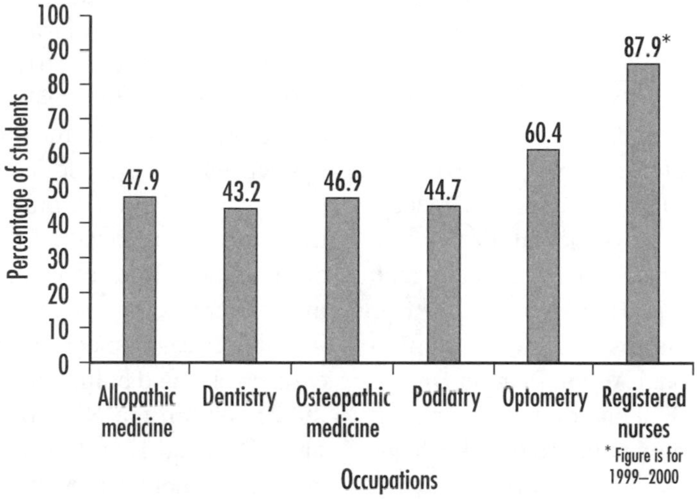

Source: Data from *Health, United States, 2006,* p. 363.

and more than one-third of women experience an anxiety disorder (Misra 2001).

Eating disorders are among the illnesses predominantly affecting women and have been the subject of relatively little rigorous study to date. The incidence rate has doubled over the past two decades and is rising. Up to 3% of women are affected by eating disorders (i.e., anorexia nervosa and bulimia) according to the clinical definitions of these diagnoses, although between 29% and 38% of women report dieting at any given time (Misra 2001). At least 90% of all eating disorder cases occur in young women, and eating disorders account for the highest mortality rates among all mental disorders (OWH 2001; Weissman and Klerman 1977).

Some disorders once thought to primarily affect men are now affecting women in increasing numbers. For example, death rates among women who abuse alcohol are 50% to 100% higher than rates for men who abuse alcohol (OWH 2001). Compared to older men, older women are at substantially greater risk of Alzheimer's disease, a disease responsible for 60% to 70% of all cases of dementia and one of the leading causes of nursing home placement for older adults (Herzog and Copeland 1985).

Office on Women's Health

The Public Health Service's Office on Women's Health (OWH) is dedicated to the achievement of a series of specific goals that span the spectrum of disease and disability. These goals range across the life cycle and address cultural and ethnic differences among women. The OWH stimulates, coordinates, and implements a comprehensive women's health agenda on research, service delivery, and education across the agencies of the Public Health Service (PHS). PHS agencies include the National Institutes of Health (NIH), the Centers for Disease Control and Prevention (CDC), the Food and Drug Administration (FDA), the Health Resources and Services Administration (HRSA), the Agency for Health Research and Quality (AHRQ), the Substance Abuse and Mental Health Services Administration (SAMHSA), and the IHS. The OWH also serves as a link across the country's PHS regions and with other government agencies, including the Department of Defense (DoD), Department of Veterans Affairs (VA), Central Intelligence Agency (CIA), Environmental Protection Agency (EPA), and National Aeronautic and Space Administration (NASA).

The OWH was responsible for implementing the National Action Plan on Breast Cancer (NAPBC), a major public-private partnership dedicated to improving the diagnosis, treatment, and prevention of breast cancer through research, service delivery, and education. The OWH also worked to implement measures to prevent physical and sexual abuse against women, as delineated in the Violence Against Women Act of 1994. Currently, the OWH is active in projects promoting breastfeeding, women's health education and research, girl and adolescent health, and heart health. The OWH also sponsors several awareness days and conferences, including the National Women and Girls HIV/AIDS Awareness Day, a National Women's Health Week, a Rural Women's Health Conference, and a Minority Women's Health Summit (OWH 2007).

Several important women's health initiatives are also breaking new ground (Alcohol, Drug Abuse, and Mental Health Administration 1992). Within SAMHSA, the Office for Women's Services has targeted six areas for special attention: physical and sexual abuse of women; women as caregivers; women with mental and addictive disorders; women with HIV infection or AIDS, sexually transmitted diseases, and/or tuberculosis; older women; and women detained in the criminal justice system. The Women's Health Initiative, supported by the NIH, took place in more than 50 centers across the country. It was the largest clinical trial conducted in US history, involving over 161,000 women (NIH 2002). It focused on diseases that are the major causes of death and disability among women—heart disease, cancer, and osteoporosis. In 2002, the Women's Health Initiative published a groundbreaking study finding detrimental effects of postmenopausal hormone therapy on women's development of invasive breast cancer, coronary heart disease, stroke, and pulmonary embolism (NIH 2002). Within the NIH, the National Institute of Mental Health has issued a specific program announcement to broaden the full spectrum of research on issues pertinent to women's health. Both the National Institute on Drug Abuse (NIDA) and the National Institute of Alcohol Abuse and Alcoholism (NIAAA), also within the NIH, support research related to women's health.

Women and the US Health Care System

Women have a large stake in how health care services are financed and delivered. They are the principal users of the health care system, both for themselves and as the coordinators of care for their families.

Until the oldest age groups, 65 to 74, and 75 and older, they have higher physician utilization rates than men (Misra 2001). Rates of hospitalization are comparable for men and women (0.17 for women and 0.19 for men) (Misra 2001, 177).

The main source of insurance coverage for women and men is through employment. This relationship places women at a distinct disadvantage because they have less attachment to the labor market than men do. In other words, women are more likely than men to work part time, receive lower wages, and have interruptions in their work histories. All these factors reduce their likelihood of receiving employment-based health insurance coverage. Hence, women are at a higher risk of being uninsured. Women are more likely to be covered as dependents under their husbands' plans. Women must also place greater reliance on Medicaid for their health care coverage. Prior to 1996, women were twice as likely as men to be covered under Medicaid because the program was linked to Aid to Families with Dependent Children (AFDC). In August 1996, Congress passed welfare reform legislation abolishing AFDC in favor of Temporary Assistance to Needy Families (TANF), a block grant that passes funds to the states to provide welfare assistance through state-designed programs. At this time, Medicaid and TANF were separated such that qualifying for one program did not automatically enroll the applicant in the other program.

Even among women who have health insurance, gaps in benefit coverage discourage them from seeking medical and preventive services. Women are more likely than men to use contraceptives (Figure 11–10), but contraceptive services are not well funded. In fact, contraceptives are among the most poorly covered reproductive health care service in the United States. As of September 2004, 21 states required private health insurance plans to cover prescription contraceptives if they cover other prescription drugs; however, these laws did not affect workers who are in self-funded plans (Kaiser Family Foundation 2004). Many nonsurgical contraceptors, such as diaphragms, Norplant implants, intrauterine devices (IUDs), and oral contraceptives, are either not covered or inadequately covered. One half of all health insurance plans provide no coverage for these reversible contraceptives. According to one source, about 87% of employers with HMO

Figure 11–10 Percentage of Contracepting Women 15–44 Years Old, 2002.

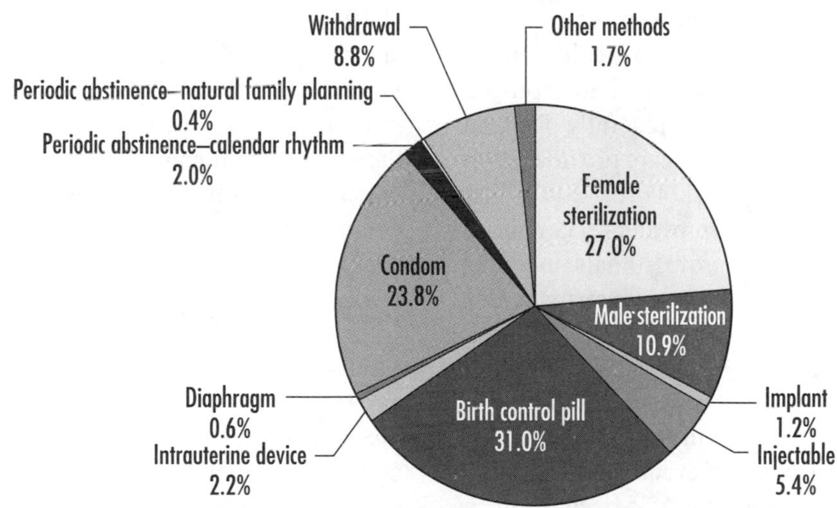

Source: Data from *Health, United States, 2006,* pp. 155–156.

plans include coverage for oral contraceptives; however, coverage drops to as low as 60% among firms with other types of health insurance (Appleby 2000). Oral contraceptives, the most widely used form of reversible contraception, are covered by 78% of employer-based insurance (Kaiser Family Foundation 2002).

Rural Health

Poverty is a consistent dimension of life. Poor economic conditions are often reflected in diminished access to health care and poor health of rural citizens (Cohen et al. 1994). Access to health care is affected by poverty, long distances, rural topography, weather conditions, and limited availability of personal transportation.

Geographic maldistribution that creates a shortage of health care professionals in rural settings is another dimension of poor health care delivery (see Chapter 4). About 20% of the US population resides in areas where primary care health professionals are in short supply (Bureau of Health Professions 2002). An estimated 22 million-plus rural Americans live in a federally designated area of primary health care provider shortages (HHS Rural Task Force 2002). The scarcity of health care providers encompasses a broad spectrum of professionals, including pediatricians, obstetricians, internists, dentists, nurses, and allied health professionals (Patton and Puskin 1990). Additionally, rural hospitals tend to be smaller and provide fewer services than urban hospitals. The health care financing crisis has been especially keen in rural hospitals because of the large number of poor, uninsured, and underinsured patients served. Thus, the closing of rural hospitals has further diminished access to health care. Rural residents, especially poor ones, seek health care services less frequently throughout their lives than do urban residents (Stratton et al. 1993).

Low population density makes it difficult for communities to attract physicians and for physicians to establish financially viable practices. Physicians are often geographically isolated, which makes it more difficult for them to obtain consultations and backup coverage. As a result, rural populations face greater barriers in access to care. Various measures have been taken to improve access in rural America, including the promotion of the National Health Service Corps (NHSC), the designation of Health Professional Shortage Areas (HPSAs) and Medically Underserved Areas (MUAs), the development of Community and Migrant Health Centers (C/MHCs), and the enactment of the Rural Health Clinics Act. In addition, the Office of Rural Health Policy, within the Health Resources and Services Administration of the US Department of Health and Human Services, was established in 1987 to promote better health care in rural America (HRSA Office of Rural Health Policy 2007). As managed care has become more pervasive nationally, rural areas face the pressing challenge of adapting this mechanism of health care delivery to fit their communities.

The National Health Service Corps

The NHSC was created in 1970 to recruit and retain physicians to provide needed services in physician shortage areas (the Emergency Health Personnel Act, P.L. 91–623). A scholarship program, amended to the Corps legislation in 1972, required that the Corps placements be targeted to the HPSAs (P.L. 92–582). The scholarship and loan repayment program applies to doctors, dentists, nurse practitioners, midwives, and mental health professionals who serve a minimum of two years in underserved areas. Since 1972, over 27,000 health professionals have been placed in medically underserved communities in hospitals and clinics, such as community health centers, migrant centers, Indian health facilities, and small group practice clinics (HRSA Bureau of Health Professions 2003). President Bush's 2002 budget included $191.5 million—a $44 million increase—to strengthen the NHSC. With the increased funding, the NHSC was expected to provide scholarships or loan assistance to about 1,800 professionals practicing in underserved areas—an increase of about 500 participants. In FY 2005, the NHSC awarded a record 1,223 loan repayment contracts to health professionals (HRSA Bureau of Health Professions 2007a).

Health Professional Shortage Areas

The Health Professions Educational Assistance Act of 1976 (P.L. 94–484) provided the designation criteria for Health Manpower Shortage Areas, later renamed Health Professional Shortage Areas (Fitzwilliams 1977; HRSA Bureau of Health Professions 2007b). The act provided that three different types of health professional shortage areas (HPSA) could be designated: geographic areas, population groups, and medical facilities. A geographic area must meet the following three criteria for designation as a primary care HPSA: (1) The geographic area involved must be rational for the delivery of health services; (2) one of the following conditions must prevail in the area: a) the area has a population to full-time-equivalent primary care physician ratio of at least 3,500:1; or b) the area has a population to full-time-equivalent primary care physician ratio of less than 3,500:1 but greater than 3,000:1 and has unusually high needs for primary care services or insufficient capacity of existing primary care providers; and 3) primary medical care professionals in contiguous areas are overutilized, excessively distant, or inaccessible to the population of the area under consideration (HRSA Bureau of Health Professions 2007c).

A population group can be designated as an HPSA for primary care if it can be demonstrated that access barriers prevent members of the group from using local providers. In addition, medium- and maximum-security federal and state correctional institutions and public or nonprofit private residential facilities can also be designated as facility-based HPSAs. HPSAs are classified on a scale from one to four with one or two signifying areas of greatest need.

Medically Underserved Areas

The MUAs concept was developed to support the federal Health Maintenance Organization (HMO) grant program. Congress included in the 1973 HMO Act (P.L. 93–222) a requirement that federal support for HMOs be targeted to applicants with at least 30% of their membership in MUAs; however, the primary purpose of the MUA-designated process was to target the community health center and rural health clinic programs.

The statute required that several factors be considered in designating MUAs, such as available health resources in relation to area size and population, health indices, and care and demographic factors affecting the need for care. To meet this mandate, the Index of Medical Underservice was developed, comprising four variables: (1) percentage of population below poverty income levels, (2) percentage of population 65 years of age and older, (3) infant mortality rate, and (4) primary care physicians per 1,000 population. The index yields a single numerical value on a scale from 0 to 100; any area with a value less than 62 (the median of all counties) is designated an MUA. Only one-half of the MUA population lives in a physician shortage area.

Community and Migrant Health Centers

C/MHCs provide services to low-income populations on a sliding-fee scale, thereby addressing both geographic and financial barriers to access. Health centers serve more than 16 million patients annually, including 1 in 10 rural Americans (NACHC 2006). The patients are drawn principally from minority groups: 22% Black, 34% Hispanic, and 4% other minorities (Shi 2007). For more than four decades, C/MHCs have provided primary care and preventive health services to populations in designated MUAs. These designated areas receive national priority in meeting their health care needs and are targeted for special federal health initiative programs. Traditionally, these areas have had trouble attracting private physicians, particularly in primary care specialties. As a result, C/MHCs rely heavily on nonphysician providers for the delivery of services. The migrant program supports 134 grantees, who run approximately 400 clinics in 40 states and Puerto Rico (HRSA Bureau of Primary Health Care 2007a). They serve approximately 727,000 migrants and seasonal farm workers (HRSA Bureau of Primary Health Care 2007b). Although community health centers must be located in areas designated as MUAs, migrant centers must be located in "high-impact" areas, defined as areas that serve at least 4,000 migrant and/or seasonal farm workers for at least two months per year.

The Rural Health Clinics Act

The Rural Health Clinics Act (P.L. 95–210) was developed to respond to the concern that isolated rural communities could not generate sufficient revenue to support the services of a physician. In many cases, the only source of primary care or emergency services was midlevel practitioners who were ineligible at that time for Medicare or Medicaid reimbursement. The Act is a reimbursement mechanism that strengthens the financial viability of eligible entities by increasing the opportunities for Medicare and Medicaid reimbursement. The Act permitted physician assistants, nurse practitioners, and certified nurse midwives associated with rural clinics to practice without the direct supervision of a physician; enabled rural health clinics (but not midlevel practitioners) to be reimbursed by Medicare and Medicaid for their services; and tied the level of Medicaid payment to the level established by Medicare. To be designated as a rural health clinic, a public or private sector physician practice, clinic, or hospital must meet several criteria, including location in an MUA, geographic HPSA, or a population-based HPSA. Over 3,000 rural health clinics are currently operating, providing primary care services for over 7 million people in 47 states (NARHC 2007).

Rural Managed Care

Managed care plans can improve the conditions of rural medical practice by providing practitioners with consultation opportunities, continuing education, and coverage for time off. These plans can improve the quality of care by subjecting providers to consistent, tested medical practice guidelines and by establishing referral relationships for secondary and tertiary care.

Rural managed care faces demographic, geographic, and infrastructure challenges. The demographic and geographic characteristics of rural communities pose important barriers to managed care. Some rural communities do not have a big enough population to support the array of practitioners and services necessary to provide cost-efficient health care. At the same time, health care needs in rural areas are as great as or greater than those in urban areas because of high rates of chronic disease and other unmet needs. Moreover, rural incomes remain low, making it difficult for managed care plans to generate the revenues that comparable resources might generate in an urban area.

Rural infrastructure also presents serious challenges. The health care infrastructure includes physicians, hospitals, and community leadership and governance. All of these factors influence the success of managed care plans in rural areas. Physicians and hospitals are generally in short supply in rural areas. Some rural physicians cannot meet board certification or eligibility requirements imposed by managed care plans. Physician attitudes can impair the acceptance of managed care plans. Many physicians practicing in rural areas may find the corporate culture of managed care plans alien. The isolation of rural practice can attract individualistic practitioners who are used to making independent decisions and who are unwilling to be held accountable to a managed care organization.

The Homeless

Although an exact number is unknown, an estimated 3.5 million people, 1.35 million of them children, are likely to experience homelessness in a given year (National Coalition for the Homeless 2006a). Nationally, approximately 26 million people (14% of the US population) are homeless at some point in their lives. Although most homeless persons live in major urban areas, a surprising 19% live in rural areas.

The homeless population of today includes 43% single men, 17% single women, and 39% children under age 18 (National Coalition for the Homeless 2006b). About 33% of the homeless population is families with children (National Coalition for the Homeless 2006b). About 40% of all homeless men are veterans of war (National Coalition for the Homeless 2006b).

Homeless women in particular face major difficulties: economic and housing needs and special gender-related issues that include pregnancy, child care responsibilities, family violence, fragmented family support, job discrimination, and wage discrepancies. Homeless women, regardless of parenting status, should be linked with social services, family support, self-help, and housing resources. Mentally ill women caring for children need additional consideration, with an emphasis on parenting skills and special services for children. Thus, homelessness is a multifaceted problem related to personal, social, and economic factors.

The economic picture of homeless persons is dismal, as would be expected, and suggests that they are severely lacking in the financial and educational resources necessary to access health care. Further, almost one-half of homeless people have not graduated from high school and, on average, they have been unemployed for four years. Despite these figures, only 20% receive income maintenance, and only 26% have health insurance. These numbers remain low because of federal restrictions that prohibit federal help to those without a physical street address.

The shortage of adequate low-income housing is the major precipitating factor for homelessness. Unemployment, personal or family life crises, rent increases that are out of proportion to inflation, and reduction in public benefits can also directly result in the loss of a home. Illness, on the other hand, tends to result in the loss of a home in a more indirect way. Other indirect causes of homelessness include deinstitutionalization from public mental hospitals, substance abuse programs, and overcrowded prisons and jails.

Community-based residential alternatives for mentally ill individuals vary from independent apartments to group homes staffed by paid caregivers. Independent living may involve either separate apartments or single-room occupancy units (SROs) in large hotels, whereas group homes are staffed during at least a portion of the day and traditionally provide some on-site mental health services (Schutt and Goldfinger 1996).

The homeless, adults and children, have a high prevalence of untreated acute and chronic medical, mental health, and substance abuse problems. Why this is true has been the subject of much debate. Some argue that people may become homeless because of a physical or mental illness. Others argue that homelessness itself may lead to the development of physical and mental disability because homelessness produces risk factors, which include excessive use of alcohol, illegal drugs, and cigarettes; sleeping in an upright position, which results in venous stasis and its consequences; extensive walking in poorly fitting shoes; and grossly inadequate nutrition.

Homeless persons are also at a greater risk of assault and victimization, as well as exposure to harsh weather. Homeless people are at an increased risk of being victimized because of lack of personal security, regardless of whether they live in a shelter or outdoors. The homeless are also exposed to illness because of overcrowding in shelters and overexposure to extreme heat and cold.

Barriers to Health Care

The homeless population encounters many barriers to health care services. The patterns of health services utilization by the homeless suggest that health care resources are utilized inappropriately. The homeless face barriers to ambulatory services but incur high rates of hospitalization. A high use of inpatient services in this manner amounts to the substitution of inpatient care for outpatient services. Both individual factors (competing needs, substance dependence, and mental illness) and system factors (availability, cost, convenience, and appropriateness of care) account for the barriers to adequate ambulatory services. On the other hand, compared to the general population, the homeless consume more outpatient services, despite higher rates of hospitalization. Thus, higher rates of morbidity in this population result in greater utilization of both inpatient and outpatient services.

The homeless face several barriers to adequate and appropriate health care. They have financial barriers and problems in satisfying eligibility requirements for health insurance. Accessible transportation to medical facilities is often unavailable to this population. The homeless have competing needs, and they place a greater priority on basic needs for food, shelter, and income than on obtaining needed health services or following through with a prescribed treatment plan. Homeless individuals who experience psychological distress and disabling mental illness may be in the greatest need of health services and yet may be the least able to obtain them. This inability to obtain health care may be attributable to such individual traits of mental illness as paranoia, disorientation, unconventional health beliefs, lack of social support, lack of organizational skills to gain access to needed services, or fear of authority figures and institutions resulting from previous institutionalization. The social conditions of street life affect compliance with medical care. The homeless usually lack proper sanitation and a stable place to store medications safely and are unable to obtain proper food for a medically indicated diet necessary for conditions like diabetes mellitus or hypertension.

Federal efforts to provide medical services to the homeless population are primarily conducted by the Health Care for the Homeless (HCH) program. Community health centers supported by the 1985 Robert Wood Johnson Foundation/Pew Memorial Trust HCH program (subsequently covered by the 1987 McKinney Homeless Assistance Act) have addressed many of the access and quality-of-care issues faced by the homeless. In 2004, community health centers served approximately 703,000 homeless patients (HRSA Bureau of Primary Health Care 2007b).

A critical aspect of these programs is outreach, in which teams of health care professionals bring a wide range of services to homeless persons in shelters, hotels, soup lines, beaches and parks, train and bus stations, religious facilities, and other places where homeless people may gather. Such programs help overcome some of the barriers to care, such as lack of transportation, lack of information about available facilities, and psychological problems. Outreach teams are typically based in health care centers, to which clinicians can refer homeless patients who need additional medical attention. In addition, a walk-in appointment system reduces access barriers at these medical facilities. Medical care, routine laboratory tests, substance abuse counseling, and some medications are provided free of charge to eliminate financial barriers.

The Mental Health Services for the Homeless Block Grant program sets aside funds for states to implement services for homeless persons with mental illness. These services include outreach services; community mental health services; rehabilitation; referrals to inpatient treatment, primary care, and substance abuse services; case management services; and supportive services in residential settings.

The Homeless Families Program, a national demonstration program in nine cities cosponsored by the Robert Wood Johnson (RWJ) Foundation and the Department of Housing and Urban Development, awarded its first grants in 1990. This program provided housing combined with appropriately designed health and support services for homeless families. The program was discontinued in 1998.

Services for homeless veterans are provided through the VA. The Homeless Chronically Mentally Ill Veterans Program provides outreach, case management services, and psychiatric residential treatment for homeless mentally ill veterans in community-based facilities in 45 US cities. The Domiciliary Care for Homeless Veterans Program addresses the health needs of veterans who have psychiatric illnesses or alcohol or drug abuse problems, operating 1,800 beds at 31 sites across the country (US Dept of Veterans Affairs 2006).

The Salvation Army also provides a variety of social, rehabilitation, and support services for homeless persons. Its centers include adult rehabilitation and food programs, and permanent and transitional housing.

Mental Health

In December 1999, David Satcher, the US Surgeon General, released a groundbreaking report on the extent of mental illness in the United States and unveiled a plan to tackle this formidable challenge. According to the report, the burden of mental illness on health and productivity in the United States has long been underestimated. Mental illness ranks second, after ischemic heart disease, as a burden on health and productivity. Surveys indicate that one in five Americans has a mental disorder in any one year (Satcher 1999). Treatments for mental illnesses also consume a fair portion of the US health care budget. In 1996, treatment of mental disorders, substance abuse, and Alzheimer's disease cost the United States $99 billion. Between 1993 and 2003, state mental health agency per capita expenditures for mental health services increased from $54 to $92 (National Center for Health Statistics 2006) According to Satcher (1999):

> Even more than other areas of health and medicine, the mental health field is plagued by disparities in the availability of and access to its services. These disparities are viewed readily through the lenses of racial and cultural diversity, age, and gender. A key disparity often hinges on a person's financial status; formidable financial barriers block off needed mental health care from too many people regardless of whether one has health insurance with inadequate mental health benefits, or is one of the 44 million Americans who lack any insurance. We have allowed stigma and a now unwarranted sense of hopelessness about the opportunities for recovery from mental illness to erect these barriers. It is time to take them down.

The report suggests that promoting mental health for all Americans will require increased scientific research as well as extensive public education to help confront the attitudes, fear, and misunderstanding that remain associated with mental illness. The proposed plan of action consists of eight main points: (1) continue to build the science base; (2) overcome stigma; (3) improve public awareness of effective treatment; (4) ensure the supply of mental health services and providers; (5) ensure delivery of state-of-the-art treatments; (6) tailor treatment to age, gender, race, and culture; (7) facilitate entry into treatment; and (8) reduce financial barriers to treatment. One of the key means to improve access will be to insist on parity; that is, to ensure that managed care and other health plans treat mental illnesses similarly to other chronic health conditions.

Mental disorders are common psychiatric illnesses affecting adults and present a serious public health problem in the United States (Barker et al. 1989; Klerman and Weisman 1989; Myers et al. 1984; Regier et al. 1988; Romanoski et al. 1992). About one in four adults, or 57.7 million people, suffer from a diagnosable mental disorder every year (NIMH 2007). Mental disorders are the leading cause of disability for people aged 15–44 (NIMH 2007). Mental illness is a risk factor for death from suicide, cardiovascular disease, and cancer.

Mental health disorders can be either psychological or biological in nature. Many mental health diseases, including mental retardation, developmental disabilities, and schizophrenia, are now known to be biological in origin. Other behaviors, including those related to personality disorders and neurotic behaviors, are still subject to interpretation and professional judgment. Defining what is and is not normal in a population is difficult and often raises far-reaching moral and ethical issues (Williams 1995).

National studies have concluded that the most common mental disorders include phobias, substance abuse (including alcohol and drug dependence), and affective disorders (including depression). Schizophrenia is considerably less common, affecting an estimated 1.1% of the population (NIMH 2006).

Most mental health services are provided in the general medical sector—a concept first described by Regier and colleagues (1988) as the de facto mental health service system—rather than through formal mental health specialist services. The de facto system combines specialty mental health services with general counseling services, such as those provided in primary care settings, nursing homes, and community health centers by ministers, counselors, self-help groups, families, and friends. Specifically, mental health services are provided through public and private resources in both inpatient and outpatient facilities. These facilities include state and county mental hospitals, private psychiatric hospitals, nonfederal general hospital psychiatric services, VA psychiatric services, residential treatment centers, and freestanding psychiatric outpatient clinics (Table 11–6). The nation's ***mental health system*** is composed of two subsystems, one primarily for individuals with insurance coverage or private funds, and the other for those without private coverage.

Table 11–6 Mental Health Organizations (numbers in thousands), 2002

Service and Organization	Number of MH Organizations
All organizations	4,301
State and county mental hospitals	222
Private psychiatric hospitals	253
Nonfederal general hospital psychiatric services	1,285
Department of Veterans Affairs medical centers	140
Residential treatment centers for emotionally disturbed children	508
All other	1,893

Source: Data from *Health, United States, 2006,* p. 365.

The Uninsured

Patients without insurance coverage or personal financial resources are treated in state and county mental health hospitals and in community mental health clinics. Care is also provided in short-term, acute care hospitals and emergency departments. Local governments are the providers of last resort with the ultimate responsibility to provide somatic and mental health services for all citizens regardless of ability to pay.

The Insured

For patients with financial resources, including insurance coverage and the personal ability to pay, availability of both inpatient and ambulatory mental health care has expanded tremendously. Inpatient mental health services for patients with insurance are usually provided through private psychiatric hospitals. These hospitals can be operated on either a nonprofit or a for-profit basis. National chains of for-profit mental health hospitals have expanded immensely over the past 20 years. Patients with insurance coverage are also more likely to be provided care through the offices of private psychiatrists, clinical psychologists, and licensed social workers. Mental health services are also provided by the VA and by the military health care system; however, access to these services is limited by eligibility.

Managed Care

Managed care is also expanding its services into mental health. As part of comprehensive health care, managed care plans generally include limited mental health benefits. Psychiatrists and other mental health providers also contract with insurers, employers, and managed care plans to provide mental health services for enrolled populations, often based on capitation payments. The ability of managed care plans to provide comprehensive services and to meet the full range of patient needs, given the constraints of these contracts, is an open question at the present time.

Similar to other physicians who have confronted the new imperatives of managed care, providers of mental health and substance-abuse services (behavioral health care) are no longer simply advocates for the patient; they must satisfy multiple payers, insurance plan managers, and other consumers (Iglehart 1996). State and local governments are also moving rapidly to contract with managed care organizations to manage the mental health and substance-abuse services covered by Medicaid, one of the major public programs funding services of this type.

Many HMOs contract with specialized companies that provide managed behavioral health care, in part because they lack the in-house capacity to provide treatment. Using case managers and reviewers, most of whom are psychiatric nurses, social workers, and psychologists, these specialized companies oversee and authorize the use of mental health and substance abuse services. The case reviewers, using clinical protocols to guide them, assign patients to the least expensive appropriate treatment, emphasizing outpatient alternatives over inpatient care.

Working with computerized databases, a reviewer studies a patient's particular problem and then usually authorizes an appointment with an appropriate provider in the company's selective network. On average, psychiatrists constitute about 20% of any given provider network, psychologists constitute 40%, and psychiatric social workers constitute another 40%. Although the nature of contracts with providers varies widely, most practitioners are paid a discounted fee.

Most corporations now assign (or carve out) their behavioral health coverage by contracting with these specialized companies. Whereas private payers have been attracted to these specialized providers of managed behavioral health care because of their desire to reduce their mental health and substance abuse expenses, psychiatrists have reservations about the emergence of this market-driven phenomenon. The application of managed care principles to mental health and substance abuse services has provoked unprecedented turmoil in the profession by eroding the autonomy of practitioners, squeezing their incomes, and forcing them into constricted new roles.

Historically, state mental health authorities have operated with categorical program budgets (with a strong emphasis on inpatient care) derived from an appropriation of public funds for the mentally ill. Now, these authorities manage a complex array of services funded by a variety of federal, state, and sometimes local sources. The single largest payer for state-financed mental health care is Medicaid. With the mounting pressure on all levels of government to reduce expenditures, state mental health authorities have begun to pursue the adoption of managed care techniques and to sign contracts with behavioral health care companies.

Mental Health Professionals

Mental health services are provided by a variety of professionals (Table 11–7) that includes, but is not limited to, ***psychiatrists***, psychologists, social workers, nurses, counselors, and therapists.

Psychiatry is the branch of medicine that specializes in mental disorders. Psychiatrists are physicians who receive postgraduate specialty training in mental health after completing medical school. Psychiatric residencies cover medical as well as behavioral diagnosis and treatments. A relatively small proportion of the total mental health workforce consists of psychiatrists. Psychiatrists exert disproportionate power in the system because they are physicians and can prescribe drugs and admit patients to hospitals. The increasing use of psychotropic drugs to treat mental disorders is likely to give psychiatrists even greater power in the future.

Psychologists usually hold a doctoral degree, although some hold master's degrees. They are trained in interpreting and changing the behavior of people. Psychologists cannot prescribe drugs; however, they provide a wide range of services to patients with neurotic and behavioral problems. Psychologists use such techniques as psychotherapy and counseling, which psychiatrists typically do not engage in. Psychoanalysis is a subspecialty in mental health that involves the use of intensive treatment by both psychiatrists and psychologists.

Social workers receive training in various aspects of mental health services, particularly counseling. Social workers are generally trained at the master's level. They also compete with psychologists and, to a lesser extent, psychiatrists for patients.

Nurses are involved in mental health through the subspecialty of psychiatric nursing. Specialty training for nurses had its origins in the latter part of the 1800s. Nurses provide a wide range of mental health services.

Many other health care professionals contribute to the array of available services,

Table 11–7 Full-Time Equivalent Patient Care Staff in Mental Health Organizations, 1998

Staff Discipline	Number	Percentage
All patient care staff	531,532	78.1
Professional patient care staff	304,449	44.8
Psychiatrists	28,374	4.2
Other physicians	3,561	0.5
Psychologists	28,729	4.2
Social workers	72,367	10.6
Registered nurses	78,562	11.5
Other mental health professionals	78,854	11.6
Physical health professionals and assistants	14,002	2.1
Other mental health workers	130,551	33.4

Source: Section VI, Chapter 18, Table 7, *Mental Health, United States, 2002*. Ed. Ronald W. Manderscheid, Marilyn J. Henderson, US Department of Health and Human Services, Substance Abuse and Mental Health Services Administration, Center for Mental Health Services, Rockville, MD.

including marriage and family counselors, recreational therapists, and vocational counselors. Numerous people work in related areas, such as adult day care, alcohol and drug abuse counseling, and as psychiatric aides in institutional settings.

Depression

Major depressive disorder is one of the most common illnesses among primary care patients, affecting approximately 14.8 million adults in the United States each year (NIMH 2006). The risk of a depressive episode reaches its peak in women between 35 and 45 years of age, whereas in men, it usually occurs after age 55. A typical episode of depression lasts approximately 9 months, with a range of 6 to 12 months (Salazar 1996).

Depressed persons are more likely to experience disability and more severe medical illness than nondepressed patients. Risk factors for depression are history of depression, family history, stressful life events, lack of social support, history of anxiety, postpartum period, substance abuse, medical comorbidity, being single, old age, low socioeconomic status, and female gender.

The most common consequences of unrecognized and untreated depression are economic costs (estimated by Greenberg et al. as $83 billion in 2000), work absenteeism, decreased productivity, unemployment, high health care costs, high expenditure of clinician time, and institutionalization, especially among the elderly. From the patient's perspective, there is increased risk of suicide, alcoholism, drug abuse, and comorbid medical and psychiatric conditions.

A structured, consistent approach to the depressed patient is essential and should include patient education; eliciting information about symptoms, history of previous psychiatric episodes, and family history of affective disorders; clinical observation and examination; history from relatives, other providers, or other clinics, if necessary; aggressive use of medication alone or in combination with psychotherapeutic techniques; and appropriate referral.

The Chronically Ill and Disabled

Every person is vulnerable to chronic illness and/or disability during his or her life. Indeed, chronic conditions are the major cause of illness, disability, and death in the United States. Chronic illness and disability also pose unique challenges to a health care system that is primarily oriented toward treating acute illness. More resources and research must be devoted to such issues because chronic illness and disability are on the rise (see Figures 10–2 and 10–3). In 2005, more than 90 million Americans lived with chronic conditions, with 11.9% having limitations in their ability to perform certain daily activities (National Center for Chronic Disease Prevention and Health Promotion 2005; National Center for Health Statistics 2006). By 2010, it is projected that 141 million Americans will have a chronic condition (Figure 10–3). Furthermore, the loss in human potential and work days notwithstanding, chronic disease is expensive, incurring more than 75% of the total medical expenditure ($1.4 trillion annually) (National Center for Chronic Disease Prevention and Health Promotion 2005). The disabled also tend to be covered by public sources (30% by Medicare and 10% by Medicaid) versus those who have no disabilities, who are more likely to pay for care with private coverage (Kraus et al. 1996, 28). Overall, chronic disease is responsible for 7 out of 10 deaths (totaling 1.7 million Americans) and is largely attributable to preventable chronic illnesses (National Center for Chronic Disease Prevention and Health Promotion 2005). Tobacco use, lack of physical activity, poor nutrition, and lack of regular screening for cancers of the breast, cervix, colon, and rectum contribute to the major chronic-disease killers—cardiovascular disease, cancer, diabetes, and chronic obstructive pulmonary disease (National Center for Chronic Disease Prevention and Health Promotion 2005).

Chronic illness can often lead to disability. Indeed, in the elderly, disability is primarily caused by chronic disease, although disability can also result from acute disease (Ostir et al. 1999, 148, 151). The level of disability can wax and wane during the course of chronic disease, which also can increase and decrease over time (The Robert Wood Johnson Foundation 1996). Furthermore, for some illnesses, disability can further exacerbate disease. For instance, not being able to care for oneself can cause complications in diabetics, and people who are physically disabled double their risk for coronary heart disease (Ostir et al. 1999, 152). The chronic conditions most responsible for disabilities are arthritis, heart disease, back problems, asthma, and diabetes (Kraus et al. 1996, 26)

An illness is considered ***chronic*** if a disease or injury with long-term conditions or symptoms is observed for three months or more. Other illnesses—namely, congenital anomalies, asthma, diabetes, and heart disease—have been specifically classified as chronic by the National Center for Health Statistics, regardless of duration (Benson and Marano 1998; Kraus et al. 1996, 59; Newacheck and Halfon 1998, 610).

Generally, the concept of ***disability*** centers around a person's short-term or long-term limitation or inability to perform particular tasks or roles that previously could be accomplished unaided; a gap exists between what the task requires and what the person can now do (National Center for Health Statistics 2005; Kraus et al. 1996, 60; Ostir et al. 1999, 148). Furthermore, disability can be categorized as mental, physical, or social; tests of disability tend to be more sensitive to some categories than others. Physical disability usually addresses one's mobility and other basic activities performed in daily life; mental disability involves both the cognitive and emotional states; and social disability is considered the most severe disability because management of social roles requires both physical and mental well-being (Ostir et al. 1999, 149). About 19.4% of the noninstitutionalized US population, or 48.9 millions Americans, have a disability (Kraus et al. 1996, 4).

Disability is measured in terms of a person's inability to perform certain functions called activities of daily living (ADLs) and instrumental activities of daily living (IADLs) (see Chapter 2). Because IADLs require more cognitive skill, it is assumed that if someone has limitations with ADLs, they will also need help with IADLs. Another tool for assessing disability is the Survey of Income and Program Participation (SIPP), which measures disability by asking participants about functional limitations (difficulty in performing activities such as seeing, hearing, walking, having one's speech understood, etc.), but ADL and IADL scales are more widely used. In 2004, an estimated 6.1% of all Americans age 65 and older had an ADL limitation, and 11.5% of this same group had an IADL limitation (National Center for Health Statistics 2006).

Despite the availability of community-based and institutional long-term care services for people with functional limitations, many people are not getting the help they need with the basic tasks of personal care. It is estimated that more than one-third of people with chronic conditions do not receive assistance with ADLs (such as bathing, eating, transferring, using the toilet, and dressing). Consequently, these people do not bathe or shower because of a fear of falling, are unable to follow a dietary regimen, and sustain falls. Ultimately, unmet needs lead to exacerbated health problems, costly treatments, and unnecessary pain and suffering (The Robert Wood Johnson Foundation 1996).

HIV/AIDS

In July 1982, acquired immune deficiency syndrome (***AIDS***) was officially named a disease. Figure 11–11 illustrates trends in AIDS reporting. The number of AIDS cases reported increased between 1987 and 1993, decreased between 1994 and 1999, and then increased again between 2000 and 2004 (US Census Bureau, Statistical Abstracts of the United States 2007).

Deaths from AIDS have been in decline since 1998 and decreased 4% between 2001 and 2005, from 17,726 to 17,011 (CDC 2006). Declines in reported AIDS cases between 1994 and 1999 were ascribed to new treatments; decreasing death rates may reflect the fact that benefits from new treatments are being fully realized. Meanwhile, the number of people living with AIDS continues to increase. In 2005, 425,910 people were living with AIDS; in 2001, the figure was 341,332 (CDC 2006).

AIDS is believed to be caused by the human immunodeficiency virus (***HIV***). HIV is an unusual type of virus, called a retrovirus, which causes the immune system suppression leading to AIDS. Individuals infected with HIV generally develop antibodies within a short period but may exhibit no symptoms for many years. Typically, the immune system weakens gradually and the blood level of CD4 cells (a type of white blood cell known as a T-helper/inducer lymphocyte) drops below the normal level of between 1,200 and 1,400/mm. Persons with few CD4 cells are prone to opportunistic infections. Symptoms such as persistent fever, night sweats, and weight loss begin to occur more often when the CD4 count drops below 500/mm. The development of AIDS is estimated to occur at 11 years on average from the time of HIV infection.

Certain widely recognized risk factors promote the transmission of HIV, including male-to-male sexual contact, male-to-female sexual contact, injection drug use (IDU), blood product exposure, and perinatal transmission from mother to infant—during pregnancy, delivery, or possibly during breastfeeding (Table 11–8).

Most individuals infected with HIV produce antibodies within six to nine months of exposure, although some people do not form antibodies until two to three years after exposure to HIV. Consequently, an individual can be exposed to HIV and not develop the antibodies for several years. Further, people may transmit HIV before they know they have been exposed, making transmission unsuspecting. HIV infection was the sixth leading cause of death among persons 25 to 44 years of age in 2003 (CDC 2006).

For Blacks, Hispanics, and minority women, AIDS/HIV is still a major public health concern. In 2004, males and Blacks continued to have significantly higher rates of HIV/AIDS than females and Whites (Table 11–9). Also, only in the Black and Hispanic male populations is HIV infection a leading

Figure 11–11 AIDS Cases Reported, 1987–2004.

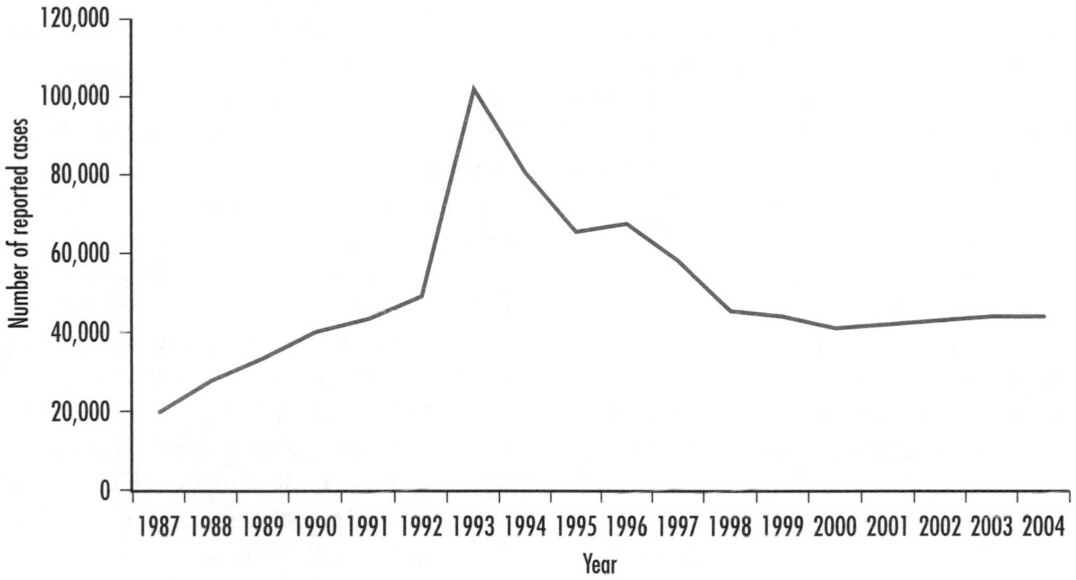

Source: Reprinted from US Centers for Disease Control and Prevention, *Statistical Abstracts of the United States, 2001,* p. 119; and *Statistical Abstracts of the United States, 2007,* p. 120.

Table 11–8 Reports of All AIDS Cases: All Years through 2004

Sex and Diagnosis	Percentage Distribution	Number of Reported Cases
All races	100.0	908,905
Men who have sex with men	44.3	402,722
Injecting drug use	24.1	219,053
Men who have sex with men and injecting drug use	6.6	60,038
Hemophilia/coagulation disorder	0.6	5,427
Heterosexual contact	13.0	117,887
Sex with injecting drug use	0	35,616
Transfusion	1.0	9,274
Undetermined	10.4	94,504

Source: Data from *Statistical Abstract of the United States, 2007,* p. 121.

cause of death (National Center for Health Statistics 2006). In 2005, rates of AIDS cases per 100,000 people were 59.0 in the Black population, 19.8 in the Hispanic population, 8.0 in the American Indian/Alaskan Native population, 6.3 in the White population, and 4.0 in the Asian/Pacific Islander population (CDC 2006). Blacks accounted for 49% of all HIV/AIDS cases diagnosed in 2005 (CDC 2006). Racial differences in HIV/AIDS infection probably reflect social, economic, behavioral, and other factors associated with HIV transmission risks.

New York leads the states in the proportion of individuals afflicted with AIDS at 39.5 cases per 100,000 population (Table 11–10). The state of Montana has the lowest AIDS rate at 0.9 per 100,000 population. New York has more reported AIDS cases than any other state, followed by Florida, California, Texas, and New Jersey. Wyoming has the smallest number of reported AIDS cases, followed by South Dakota and Vermont (US Census Bureau, Statistical Abstract of the US 2007).

HIV infection has risen to the level of a global pandemic and has become the world's modern-day plague. At the end of 2006, 39.5 million people were estimated to be living with HIV worldwide (WHO 2006). An estimated 4.3 million people acquired HIV in 2006, including 3.8 million adults and 530,000 children younger than 15 years of age (WHO 2006). AIDS caused the deaths of an estimated 2.9 million people, including 2.6 million adults and 380,000 children younger than 15 years of age (WHO 2006). These figures represent a decrease over previous years, but the global HIV/AIDS epidemic is far from under control, particularly

Table 11–9 AIDS Cases Reported through 2004

	All Years		2004	
Characteristic	Number	Percentage	Number	Percentage
Total	944,306	100.0	42,514	100.0
Sex				
Male (13 and over)	756,399	80.1	31,024	73.0
Female (13 and over)	178,463	18.9	11,442	26.9
Children under 13 years	9,443	1.0	48	0.1
Race/ethnic group				
White	375,155	39.8	12,013	28.4
Black	379,278	40.3	20,965	49.5
Hispanic	177,164	18.8	8,672	20.5
Asian/Pacific Islander	7,317	0.8	488	1.2
American Indian/Alaskan Native	3,084	0.3	193	0.5

Source: Data from *Health, United States, 2006,* p. 242.

Table 11–10 Top and Bottom 10 States for AIDS, According to Cases per 100,000 Population, 2004

Top States	Reported Cases	Cases per 100,000 Population	Bottom States	Reported Cases	Cases per 100,000 Population
New York	7,624	39.5	Iowa	64	2.2
Florida	5,869	33.8	Maine	60	4.6
California	4,764	13.3	Alaska	55	8.4
Texas	3,307	14.7	New Hampshire	45	3.5
New Jersey	1,849	21.3	Wyoming	21	4.2
Illinois	1,702	13.4	Idaho	20	1.4
Georgia	1,682	18.9	North Dakota	18	2.8
Pennsylvania	1,663	13.4	Vermont	17	2.7
Maryland	1,453	26.1	South Dakota	12	1.6
North Carolina	1,152	13.5	Montana	8	0.9

Source: Data from *Statistical Abstract of the United States, 2007,* pp. 120, 20.

in sub-Saharan Africa, where 24.7 million of the world's 39.5 million cases of people living with HIV reside (WHO 2006).

Many public health experts believe that cases of AIDS still remain underreported. The reasons for such underreporting include poor reporting standards in US health departments (Selike et al. 1993), physicians desiring to protect the confidentiality of their patients because of the stigma of HIV/AIDS (AIDS Forecasting 1989), lack of physician knowledge about the diagnosis of AIDS (Anonymous 1988), patients' denial of the risk behaviors that are likely to transmit HIV, and the absence of, or decreased access to, health care (Robertson et al. 1974), which prevents the diagnosis of HIV. With the advent of combination antiretroviral therapy, AIDS surveillance data no longer reflect trends in HIV transmission because this therapy has effectively delayed the progression of HIV to AIDS (CDC 1999a).

HIV testing is anonymous or confidential. In anonymous HIV testing, patient-identifying information or other locating information is not linked to the HIV test, whereas in confidential HIV testing, the test result is linked (CDC 1999c). In September 2006, CDC released new recommendations for HIV testing, which called for routine HIV screening of adults, adolescents, and pregnant women in health care settings in the United States (Branson 2006).

The implementation of rapid HIV testing in recent years—versus the previous method, ELISA (enzyme-linked immunosorbent assay)—makes it possible to get early results, permitting the initiation of combined antiretroviral therapy earlier in the disease process. Furthermore, the rapid HIV test may improve the outreach at clinics where testing and counseling are offered together.

Both the rapid HIV test and ELISA require a second testing, using a Western blot or an immunofluorescence assay (IFA), to confirm positive test results. The ELISA test (also known as enzyme immunoassays or EIAs) required special equipment. Blood samples had to be sent to laboratories and test results were not available for one or two weeks, requiring the clients to make a second visit to the testing site. Many people did not return for their results. The CDC estimates that in 2000, 31% of patients who tested positive for HIV at public-sector testing points did not return to get their results (Greenwald 2006). With rapid HIV testing, results are available in 5 to 30 minutes, and the test is as accurate as the ELISA. Thus, testing and counseling can be available during the same visit.

Current treatment for HIV/AIDS centers on therapies for slowing the progress of HIV and preventing ***opportunistic infections*** (OI), thereby reducing the number of people with HIV who develop and die from AIDS. For example, medications such as oral antibiotics are often used to prevent a common pneumonia (pneumocystis carinii or PCP), an OI that often develops in persons with AIDS. Other OIs include tuberculosis, toxoplasmosis, and mycobacterium avium complex (MAC). Opportunistic infections occur when organisms naturally present in the body get out of control and cause health problems due to a weakened immune system. Protease inhibitors, a combination of new, more effective drugs, are now taken in conjunction with antiretrovirals, the initial drugs used in AIDS/HIV therapy. Combination drug therapy—known as highly active antiretroviral therapy (HAART) or "drug cocktail"—has been more effective because it can reduce the viral load (level of HIV particles circulating in the blood) to extremely low levels; however, the long-term effectiveness of HAART is unknown, and it is extremely expensive. The cost of $12,000 or more per year makes the treatment unavailable to many patients in the United States, and keeps it out of reach in developing countries where more than 90% of the new HIV infections occur. Also, the complicated drug regimen requires coordination of many pills and doses, which makes it easier to skip medications or doses so that some patients temporarily stop treatment. This lack of regimen adherence not only makes the treatment less effective but also increases the chance of developing a drug-resistant strain of HIV. It is suspected that HIV will eventually develop multidrug resistance. After experiencing improvements in one's condition, complacency may lead to relaxed preventive behavior, which would risk spreading a potential drug-resistant strain of HIV (CDC 1998, 1999b).

HIV and Urban Home Health Care

In 1981, the predominant provider of health care for persons infected with HIV was the acute care facility (Ungvarski 1996). Because most individuals were diagnosed only in the last stages of the disease and no testing methods were available to identify the presence of infection, many patients never left the hospital after the initial diagnosis. As clinicians rapidly gained experience in treating the manifestations of the disease, however, the need for postacute care services rapidly escalated. Gaps in appropriate care after hospital discharge soon became apparent. Although patients had high-level nursing needs, skilled nursing facilities were extremely reluctant to admit persons diagnosed with HIV. Moreover, because of the complex issues associated with providing health care to people with HIV, such as fear of contracting the virus and attitudes about caring for homosexual men and those who used intravenous (IV) drugs, most services in home care agencies were provided by staff who volunteered to care for this specific client population.

The challenges for home care nurses in urban areas in caring for persons with HIV disease are varied and complex. First, those people increasingly affected by this disease are the poor and disenfranchised in society. Often, they are the most difficult groups to work with because of other social, economic, and emotional issues. Families are often plagued by challenging behaviors that immediately become obvious to home care nurses when performing the initial case assessment.

HIV Infection in Rural Communities

Recognition of the spread of HIV into rural communities in the United States is growing. CDC reported 23,615 new cases of AIDS in nonmetropolitan areas of the United States between March 1994 and February 1995 (CDC 1995b). In 1999, 7% of cumulative adult/adolescent AIDS cases were reported from nonmetropolitan areas (CDC 2001).

Rural persons with HIV and AIDS are more likely to be young, non-White, and female, and to have acquired their infection through heterosexual contact. Additionally, a growing number of these HIV-infected persons live in the rural South, a region historically characterized by a disproportionate number of poor and minority persons, strong religious beliefs and sanctions, and decreased access to comprehensive health services (DHHS, Office of Minority Health 2003; CDC 1995a, 1995b; Morrison 1993). Trends in new cases of HIV and AIDS in rural areas indicate that poor and non-White residents are disproportionately affected (Aday 1993; Lam and Liu 1994; Rumby et al. 1991).

HIV in Children

In the absence of specific therapy to interrupt transmission of HIV, an infected woman has a 25% chance of having a child born with HIV. Therefore, in 1994 and 1995, the US Public Health Service (PHS) began recommending that pregnant women be counseled and voluntarily tested for HIV and that zidovudine (AZT) be given to infected women during pregnancy and delivery, and to the infant after delivery. The drop in perinatal transmission rates has been attributed to this strategy, and in one study, perinatal transmission rates dropped from 21% to 11% after use of AZT according to PHS guidelines. The number of children with a diagnosis of AIDS who had been perinatally exposed to HIV declined from 122 in 2000 to 47 in 2004 (CDC 2005). The importance of preventing perinatal transmission is underscored by the fact that 91% of all AIDS cases among US children are caused by mother-to-child transmission in pregnancy, labor, delivery, or breastfeeding (CDC 1999d, 1999f). The earliest and most common symptom in HIV-positive children is enlarged lymph nodes, which are often associated with an enlarged spleen (Johnson and Vink 1992). HIV-infected children also have severe and persistent skin infections. Children who are born with AIDS suffer from failure to thrive, the inability to grow and develop as healthy children. Without intervention, this failure to thrive may lead to developmental delays that can have negative lifetime consequences for the child and his or her family.

HIV infection causes morbidity in two different but equally destructive ways. First, viruses like HIV cause illness by direct infection of cells; HIV can infect every organ system in the body and has a particular affinity for cells of the nervous system. Second, as HIV infects and destroys CD4 cells and weakens the immune system, the child becomes increasingly susceptible to various illnesses (O'Hara and D'Orlando 1996).

Family-centered care provides care and support to all immediate family members of children with HIV. It allows health care providers to develop and implement an interdisciplinary treatment plan to manage HIV infection for all children regardless of how they acquired the infection. For example, as the child becomes symptomatic, health care providers may add new therapies to the already prescribed medication regimen. Providers may also perform numerous diagnostic procedures to rule out potential problems or to diagnose a particular disease process to reduce pain and suffering.

The family must be involved in treatment planning if medical and social services interventions are to be effective. Families are the best source of information for health care providers and can indicate when and why a particular treatment plan does not work. Finally, the family decides whether to trust the regimen prescribed by the medical team and whether to adhere to its protocols.

The school nurse can play an important role in caring for HIV-infected children. With educational training in science, health, psychology, and child development, the nurse can ensure that the child has a positive school experience. Children with HIV infection attend day care, preschool programs, and schools in communities throughout the country. The knowledgeable school nurse can make an impact on HIV disease in communities by educating child care providers, supporting parents who are adapting to child care programs, acting as a liaison between child care providers and agencies, educating children and child care and school staff about health behaviors and HIV prevention, and caring and advocating for HIV-infected children and their families (Gross and Larkin 1996).

HIV in Women

Women are a rapidly growing proportion of the population with HIV/AIDS. In 2004, women made up approximately half of HIV/AIDS cases worldwide (WHO 2004). For US women 25 to 44 years of age, HIV/AIDS is a leading cause of death. Furthermore, in 2000, women accounted for 30% of adult cases of HIV infection reported in that time, and a study showed that females constituted nearly one-half (47%) of HIV cases in the 13- to 24-year-old age group. From 1985 to 1999, the proportion of AIDS cases among adult and adolescent females increased from 7% to 25%, more than tripling (CDC 2002). Between 2001 and 2005, the estimated number of AIDS cases increased 17% for women and 16% for men (CDC 2006). For women, heterosexual exposure to HIV, followed by IDU, are the greatest causes for exposure. Aside from the inherent risks in IDU, drug use overall contributes to a higher risk of contracting HIV if heterosexual sex with an IDU user occurs or when sex is traded for drugs or money (CDC 2002).

Black and Hispanic minority women are at particular risk. Despite representing less than one-fourth of the total US female population, Black and Hispanic women represent more than three-fourths (79%) of all AIDS cases in women (National Institute of Allergy and Infectious Diseases 2006). Also, for Black women 25 to 44 years of age, AIDS is the leading cause of death (National Institute of Allergy and Infectious Diseases 2002).

It is common for women to face the triple burden of racism, classism, and sexism (Priscilla et al. 1996). Many women of color come from economically disadvantaged backgrounds, further compounding the impact of HIV/AIDS on them and their families. Poor families are often unjustly labeled dysfunctional because they are disadvantaged. Many disadvantaged families cope creatively with the challenge of HIV despite their limited resources.

Because of women's position in society, HIV-positive women face many problems not confronted by men with HIV. For instance, the social expectation is that women are the caregivers for those who are ill in the family. As a result, women with HIV often care for their partner or children when they are ill themselves. Domestic violence has been increasingly identified among women living with HIV.

HIV/AIDS-Related Issues

Need for Research

HIV-related research seeks to develop a vaccine to prevent HIV-negative people from acquiring HIV. Researchers are also seeking to develop a therapeutic vaccine to prevent HIV-positive people from developing symptoms of AIDS.

People with HIV/AIDS often belong to groups that differ from each other. For example, women with AIDS may have different concerns than adolescents with AIDS. People with HIV/AIDS represent a broad spectrum of social classes, races, ethnicities, sexual orientations, and genders. Behavioral intervention research, therefore, should focus particularly on populations that are most vulnerable to HIV infection and are in urgent need of preventive interventions. These populations include gay youth and young adults (especially Black and Hispanic), disenfranchised and impoverished women, heterosexual men (again, Black and Hispanic in particular), inner city youth, and out-of-treatment substance abusers and their sexual partners. Research should be aimed not only at the individual but also at the impact of broader interventions (e.g., among drug users or those involved in sexual networks or communitywide groups) that change behavioral norms and, consequently, affect individual behavior (Merson 1996).

Public Health Concerns

AIDS underscores the synergy between poverty and IV drug use. The despair commonly caused by poverty is often mitigated only by addictions, such as drug use. Further, control of the HIV epidemic among the poor is hampered by their preoccupation with other problems related to survival, such as homelessness, crime, and lack of access to adequate health care.

Additionally, a relationship exists between the current tuberculosis epidemic and HIV. Indeed, tuberculosis, an opportunistic infection, is the worldwide leading cause of death among HIV-infected people. Tuberculosis in HIV-infected persons is also a particular public health concern because HIV persons are at greater risk of developing multidrug-resistant tuberculosis. Multidrug-resistant tuberculosis is understandably difficult to treat and can be fatal (CDC 1999e, 1999g).

Reducing the spread of AIDS requires the understanding and acceptance of a variety of sexual issues, ranging from the likelihood that even heterosexual men may engage in anonymous homosexual intercourse to the difficulty that adolescents may have controlling their sexual urges. Prejudice against gays and lesbians is manifested as ***homophobia***, a fear and/or hatred of these individuals. Homophobia explains the initial slow policy-related response to the HIV epidemic. Historically, powerful social institutions, such as religions, the law, the medical profession, and the media, have supported homophobia.

A variety of traditional public health measures have been used during the HIV crisis to reduce the spread of HIV, from mass testing for HIV to subjecting the exposed to lifelong quarantine—although quarantine has rarely been used. For several reasons, these traditional measures are much less effective when applied to HIV/AIDS as opposed to sexually transmitted diseases (STDs), such as gonorrhea or syphilis. The primary purpose for testing for STDs is to limit their spread. This goal is easily accomplished because the symptoms of STDs appear early and are generally treatable and curable. Testing for the presence of HIV, however, may not limit its spread because many people who learn their HIV status do not change the behaviors that contribute to its spread. Further, HIV has no cure. Current treatments do not affect the transmissibility of HIV, and some treatments are of questionable use for treatment of the symptoms of AIDS. Quarantine has generally not been used to contain the spread of HIV. Current legal standards require that quarantine be of limited duration and through the least restrictive means possible. Because HIV-positive people can transmit HIV throughout their lives, lifetime quarantine is not only legally impossible but also economically unfeasible.

Criminal law has also been used to contain the spread of HIV and to protect public health. For example, several laws nationwide require that those convicted of sex offenses be tested for HIV. Most of these laws, however, are disproportionately enforced against prostitutes. These laws suggest that those who test HIV-positive may receive greater prison sentences; however, it is questionable whether this type of punishment actually reduces the spread of HIV. Rather, it seems to promote scapegoating of some groups as opposed to others that may be just as likely to spread HIV.

Health promotion efforts, including those used to reduce the transmission of HIV, are often hamstrung by many psychosocial factors and other systematic factors. Some of the psychosocial factors include the fact that human beings have a hard time changing their behavior. People have a tendency to justify it. Further, much human behavior is associated with functional needs (e.g., unsafe sex might fulfill a need for intimacy). Because of the strength of these psychosocial factors, knowledge about how HIV is actually transmitted may be too weakly correlated with behavior change. The social learning theory explains that behavior change first requires knowledge, followed by a change of attitude or perspective.

Discrimination

HIV-positive people face many legal problems, including discrimination in employment, insurance, and access to health care. The federal Americans with Disabilities Act (ADA) prohibits employment discrimination against HIV-positive people; however, such discrimination is often difficult to prove. HIV-positive individuals cannot be fired or demoted if they can perform the essential duties of their job with reasonable accommodations. The largest barrier in any HIV-related employment discrimination case is proving that the employer knows or perceives that the employee is HIV-positive. Difficulty also arises because HIV-positive status is an invisible disability, not a visible trait like other disabilities, such as polio.

Insurance discrimination against people with HIV/AIDS has included denial of coverage through redlining, by both ZIP code and occupation, and based on an apparent preexisting condition. Although the latter is true in many other conditions, such as Down's syndrome, cancer, and so on, denial of insurance coverage to HIV-infected individuals is less discreet.

Discrimination also exists in access to health care and ranges from refusal of treatment to breach of confidentiality. Even though HIV is difficult to transmit through casual contact, some health care workers often refuse to treat HIV-positive people. Some providers fear losing other patients. A physician who becomes HIV-positive would almost certainly lose patients in his or her practice. Many health care workers simply do not like homosexuals and IV drug users because they do not accept their behavior. Again, the ADA legislation intends to prevent health care providers from discriminating against HIV-positive individuals based on their HIV status. Although physicians may refuse to treat patients covered under Medicaid, they cannot refuse to treat patients solely because of their HIV status.

The policies of various government agencies intended to help have also had a discriminatory impact on people with HIV/AIDS. For example, the Social Security Administration has not historically considered many of the HIV-related symptoms of women and IV drug users in adjudicating disability claims. The policies of the Immigration and Naturalization Service (INS) specifically exclude HIV-positive people unless, for example, they can prove that they would face religious or political persecution in their own country. Although the Department of Defense provides adequate medical care to individuals who acquire HIV in the military, recruits who test HIV-positive cannot join the military.

Provider Training

In a study of the HIV-related training needs of health care providers, medical information was identified as the primary training need. Patients with HIV, on the other hand, emphasized that their health care providers needed psychosocial skills, cultural competency, and sensitivity in addition to medical proficiency. According to HIV patients, the criteria for appropriate care should include providers' attitudes toward patients (body language denoting respect, treating the consumer as an equal partner in decision making about care) and providers' concern about nonmedical aspects of consumer quality of life (e.g., child care, transportation, and emotional well-being).

Increased knowledge about HIV and personal contact with people who have HIV have been shown to improve the attitudes of health care providers toward individuals with HIV and to contribute to their willingness to care for people with HIV. Training should encompass not only medical and treatment-related information but also a range of competencies related to interpersonal interaction.

In the area of psychosocial skills, the following characteristics are essential for an effectively trained provider: good communication skills (ability to establish rapport, ask questions, and listen), positive attitudes (respect, empowerment, trust), and an approach that incorporates principles of holistic care. In the area of cultural competence, essential elements include understanding of, and respect for, the person's specific culture; understanding that racial and ethnic minorities have important and multiple subdivisions or functional units; acknowledging the issues of gender and sexual orientation within the context of cultural competence; and respecting the customs, including modes of communication, of the person's culture. In the area of substance abuse, the following key elements are essential for primary care providers: understanding the complex medical picture presented by a person who suffers both from HIV and addiction; understanding the complicated psychosocial, ethical, and legal issues related to care of addicted persons; and being aware of the personal attitudes about addiction that may impair the providers' ability to give care objectively and nonjudgmentally (e.g., in the administration of pain medication) (Gross and Larkin 1996).

The risk of transmission of HIV from an infected health care worker to a patient lies somewhere between 1 in 4,000 and 1 in 40,000 (Pell et al. 1996). Guidelines adopted in the United Kingdom on the management of HIV-infected health care workers encompass three main principles: a duty to protect patients, a duty of confidentiality toward infected health care workers, and the concept that the risk of HIV transmission is restricted to certain exposure-prone procedures from which infected staff should refrain (Pell et al. 1996, 1,151):

- Infected health care workers should stop performing exposure-prone procedures immediately after diagnosis.
- Patients who have undergone an exposure-prone procedure when the infected health care worker was the sole or main operator should be notified of this situation, offered reassurance and counseling, and administered an HIV test if requested.
- If possible, letters to patients should be sent so that they arrive before or on the day of the planned press statement.
- A dedicated local telephone helpline should be established as soon as possible.
- Health care workers have a right to confidentiality, which can be breached only in exceptional circumstances when required in the public interest.

Cost of HIV/AIDS

Medical care for an HIV/AIDS patient is extremely expensive. Pharmaceutical companies claim that the high prices they charge for AIDS drugs are related to their extensive investment in research and development of drugs. At least for HIV/AIDS-related drugs, the government must pay these prices without question. An estimated 266,000 people with AIDS are Medicaid beneficiaries (Kaiser Family Foundation 2006). In 2006, Medicaid accounted for 51% ($6.3 billion) of federal spending on HIV/AIDS care (Kaiser Family Foundation 2006). Lack of insurance and underinsurance represent formidable financial barriers to HIV/AIDS care.

The US government also invests substantial amounts of money in research and development through research supported at NIH and CDC. Government programs spend money in several areas for HIV (Figure 11–12).

Much of the cost of medical care for a person infected with HIV is concentrated in the relatively brief period after a diagnosis

Figure 11–12 Federal Spending for HIV, 2000.

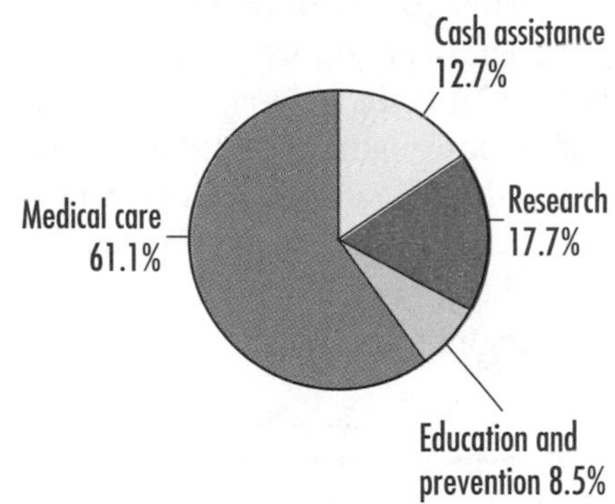

Source: Data from *Health, United States, 2002*, p. 306.

of full-blown AIDS. The best current estimate of medical care costs is $119,000 per person expended from diagnosis of HIV until death. Approximately $69,000 of the total direct costs are expended shortly after the diagnosis of AIDS. Most direct AIDS care costs (72 of 82%) are for inpatient hospital care (Aday 1993). Indirect costs include lost productivity, largely because of worker morbidity and mortality. However, other factors affect cost projections associated with the HIV epidemic, including the level of employment of HIV-positive people; regional differences in the cost of care, which is often associated with the lack of subacute care in many parts of the country; and the rate at which HIV spreads.

Containment of escalating medical costs (including the coordination of medical care) is the objective of two HIV-specific efforts: the Medicaid waiver program and the Ryan White Comprehensive AIDS Resources Emergency (CARE) Act. Through the ***Medicaid waiver program***, states may design packages of services to specific populations, such as the elderly, the disabled, and those who test HIV-positive. The waiver is an alternative to some form of institutional care. For the mentally retarded, the waiver is an alternative to the level of care in an intermediate care facility. For the HIV-positive, the level of care is the acute care hospital. State administrators who have evaluated these programs have said that certain needs remain unmet for highly marginalized populations. Clients of these services have spoken approvingly of case management, a core service in states' waivers, mainly because case managers have been advocates for client interests. At this time, it is unknown whether these programs are cost-efficient.

The passage of the Ryan White CARE Act in 1990 by the US Congress provided much-needed federal money to develop treatment and care options for persons with HIV and AIDS (Summer 1991). This legislation's main purpose was to provide emergency assistance to cities significantly affected by HIV/AIDS, allowing them to provide an array of testing, counseling, and other services, including case management, to people with HIV/AIDS. Title II of this legislation is administered by states and has been used to establish HIV clinics and related services in areas lacking the resources needed to offer this specialty care. Some public health systems have used Ryan White money to provide HIV and AIDS services in rural communities in which poor or medically underserved persons lack access to adequate care. Through the allocation of Ryan White funds, persons with HIV infection have been provided medical care, medicines, and care coordination within the public health system. The act focuses on the development of cost-efficient service schemes by funding innovative and existing services. Some services funded through the CARE Act are cost-efficient. For example, use of CARE Act funds to allow individuals to continue their private insurance plans deters them from becoming dependent on Medicaid and, essentially, forces the private sector to remain responsible for the cost of their care. Federal spending for Ryan White is estimated to total $2.1 billion in 2007 (Kaiser Family Foundation 2007).

AIDS and the US Health Care System

The course of AIDS is characterized by a gradual decline in a patient's physical, cognitive, and emotional function and well-being. Such a comprehensive decline requires a continuum of care, including emergency care, primary care, housing and supervised living, mental health and social support, nonmedical services, and hospice care. The continuum can encompass elements like outreach and case finding; primary, secondary, and tertiary prevention (see Chapter 2); primary, secondary, and tertiary health care; coordination of long-term care, primary care, therapy, nonmedical services, public benefits, and insurance; and legal services.

As HIV disease progresses, many persons become disabled or lose their jobs and rely on public entitlement or private disability programs for income and health care benefits. These programs include Social Security Disability Income and Supplemental Security Income, administered by the Social Security Administration. Medicare and Medicaid become primary payers for health care because of the onset of disability and depletion of personal funds.

Summary

This chapter examines the major characteristics of certain US population groups that face challenges and barriers in accessing health care services. These population groups are racial/ethnic minorities, children and women, those living in rural areas, the homeless, the mentally ill, and those with HIV/AIDS. The health needs of these population groups are summarized, and services available to them are described. The gaps that currently exist between these population groups and the rest of the population indicate that the nation must make significant efforts to address the unique health concerns of US subpopulations.

Test Your Understanding

Terminology

AIDS
chronic
dependency
developmental vulnerability
disability
HIV
homophobia
Medicaid waiver program
mental health system
new morbidities
opportunistic infections
psychiatrists
psychologists

Review Questions

1. What are the racial/ethnic minority categories in the United States?
2. Compared with White Americans, what are the health challenges faced by minorities?
3. Who are the AAPIs?
4. What is the Indian Health Service?
5. What are the health concerns of children?
6. Which childhood characteristics have important implications for health system design?
7. Which health services are currently available for children?
8. What are the health concerns of women?
9. What are the roles of the Office on Women's Health?
10. What are the challenges faced in rural health?
11. What measures are taken to improve access to care in rural areas?
12. What are the characteristics and health concerns of the homeless population?
13. How is mental health provided in the United States?
14. Who are the major mental health professionals?
15. How does AIDS affect different population groups in the United States?
16. Which services and policies currently combat AIDS in America?

REFERENCES

Aday, L.A. 1993. *At risk in America: The health and health care needs of vulnerable populations in the United States*. San Francisco: Jossey-Bass Publishers.

Aday, L.A. 1994. Health status of vulnerable populations. *Annual Review Public Health* 15: 487–509.

American Public Health Association. 1998. Survey: Americans don't see poverty, health care as children's most pressing problems. *The Nation's Health*, January, 6.

Barker, P.R. et al. 1989. *Serious mental illness and disability in the adult household population: United States, 1989*. Hyattsville, MD: National Center for Health Statistics.

Bennefield, R. 1995. Current population reports: Health Insurance Coverage 1995. Bureau of the Census. [Online]. Available: *http://www.census.gov/prod/99pubs/p60–208.pdf [October 10, 1999]*.

Benson, V., and M.A. Marano. 1998. Current estimate from the National Health Interview Survey, 1995. National Center for Health Statistics. *Vital Health Statistics* 10, no. 199: 5.

Branson, B.M., et al. 2006. Revised recommendations for HIV testing of adults, adolescents, and pregnant women in health care settings. *MMWR* 55 (RR14): 1–17.

Burks, L.J. 1992. Community health representatives: The vital link in Native American health care. *The IHS Primary Care Provider* 16, no. 12: 186–190.

Castor, M.L., et al. 2006. A nationwide population-based study identifying health disparities between American Indians/Alaska Natives and the general populations living in select urban counties. *Am J Public Health* 96, no.8:1478–84.

Centers for Disease Control and Prevention (CDC). 1995a. *Facts about women and HIV/AIDS*. Atlanta, GA.

Centers for Disease Control and Prevention (CDC). 1995b. *HIV/AIDS Surveillance Report*, February.

Centers for Disease Control and Prevention (CDC). 1998. Update: HIV counseling and testing using rapid tests—United States, 1995. *MMWR* 47, no. 11: 211–215.

Centers for Disease Control and Prevention (CDC). 1999a. Guidelines for national human immunodeficiency virus case surveillance, including monitoring for human immunodeficiency virus infection and acquired immunodeficiency syndrome. *MMWR* 48, no. RR-13: 2–7.

Centers for Disease Control and Prevention (CDC). 1999b. *Rapid HIV tests: questions/answers*. *http://www.cdc.gov/nchstp/hiv_aids/pubs/rt/rapidqas.htm* [December].

Centers for Disease Control and Prevention (CDC). 1999c. Anonymous or confidential HIV counseling and voluntary testing in federally funded testing sites—United States, 1995–1997. *MMWR* 48, no. 24: 509–513.

Centers for Disease Control and Prevention (CDC). 1999d. *CDC fact sheet: HIV/AIDS among US women: Minority and young women at continuing risk. http://www.cdc.gov/nchstp/hiv_aids/pubs/facts.htm* [December].

Centers for Disease Control and Prevention (CDC). 1999e. *CDC fact sheet: Recent HIV/AIDS treatment advances and the implications for prevention. http://www.cdc.gov/nchstp/hiv_aids/pubs/facts.htm* [December].

Centers for Disease Control and Prevention (CDC). 1999f. *CDC fact sheet: Status of perinatal HIV prevention: US declines continue. http://www.cdc.gov/nchstp/hiv_aids/pubs/facts.htm* [December].

Centers for Disease Control and Prevention (CDC). 1999g. *CDC fact sheet: The deadly intersection between TB and HIV. http://www.cdc.gov/nchstp/hiv_aids/pubs/facts.htm* [December].

Centers for Disease Control and Prevention (CDC). 2001. National Center for HIV, STD, and TB Prevention. Commentary. *http://www.cdc.gov/hiv/stats/hasrsupp62/commentary.htm.*

Centers for Disease Control and Prevention (CDC). 2002. HIV/AIDS Update: A glance at the HIV epidemic. *http://www.cdc.gov/nchstp/od/news/At-a-Glance.pdf*. Accessed April 20, 2003.

Centers for Disease Control and Prevention (CDC). 2002. CDC fact sheet: HIV/AIDS among African-Americans, key facts. *http://www.cdc.gov/hiv/pubs/facts/afam.pdf*. Accessed April 20, 2003.

Centers for Disease Control and Prevention (CDC). 2002. CDC fact sheet: HIV/AIDS among US women: Minority and young women at continuing risk. *http://www.cdc.gov/hiv/pubs/facts/women.htm*. Accessed April 20, 2003.

Centers for Disease Control and Prevention (CDC). 2002. CDC fact sheet: Chronic disease overview. *http://www.cdc.gov/nccdphp/overview.htm*. Accessed April 20, 2003.

Centers for Disease Control and Prevention (CDC). 2002. CDC fact sheet: Burdens posed by chronic disease. *http://www.cdc.gov/washington/overview/chrondis.htm*. Accessed April 20, 2003.

Centers for Disease Control and Prevention (CDC). 2002. CDC fact sheet: Young people at risk: HIV/AIDS among America's youth. *http://www.cdc.gov/hiv/pubs/facts/youth.htm*. Accessed April 20, 2003.

Centers for Disease Control and Prevention (CDC). 2005. HIV/AIDS Surveillance Report, 2004. Vol. 16. Atlanta: US Department of Health and Human Services.

Centers for Disease Control and Prevention (CDC). 2006. HIV/AIDS Surveillance Report, 2005. Vol. 17. Atlanta: US Department of Health and Human Services.

Cohen, S.E. et al. 1994. The geography of AIDS: Patterns of urban and rural migration. *Southern Medical Journal* 85, no. 6: 599.

Department of Health and Human Services, Office of Minority Health. 2003. *HIV impact, AIDS in Rural America*. Washington, DC: Government Printing Office, p.10–11.

Donelan, K. et al. 1996. Whatever happened to the health insurance crisis in the United States? *Journal of the American Medical Association* 276, no. 16: 1346 1350.

Fitzwilliams, J. 1977. Critical health manpower shortage areas: Their impact on rural health planning. *Agricultural Economic Report* No. 361. Washington, DC: Economic Research Service, Department of Agriculture, March.

Freeman, H.E., and C.R. Corey. 1993. Insurance status and access to health services among poor persons. *Health Services Research* 28: 531–541.

Gray, S. 1996. *Health of native people of North America*. Lanhan, MD and London: The Scarecrow Press.

Greenberg, P.E., et al. 2003. The economic burden of depression in the United States: How did it change between 1990 and 2000? *J Clin Psychiatry* 64, no.12, 1465–76.

Greenwald, J.L., et al. A rapid review of rapid HIV antibody tests. *Current Infectious Disease Reports* 8: 125–31.

Gross, E.J., and M.H. Larkin. 1996. The child with HIV in day care and school. *Nursing Clinics of North America* 31, no. 1: 231–241.

Health Resources and Services Administration (HRSA), Bureau of Health Professions. 2003. National Health Service Corps. *http://nhsc.bhpr.hrsa.gov/about/*.

Health Resources and Services Administration (HRSA), Bureau of Health Professions. 2007a. About NHSC. *http://nhsc.bhpr.hrsa.gov/about/history.asp*.

Health Resources and Services Administration (HRSA), Bureau of Health Professions. 2007b. Shortage designation. *http://bhpr.hrsa.gov/shortage/*.

Health Resources and Services Administration (HRSA), Bureau of Health Professions. 2007c. Health Professional Shortage Area Primary Medical Care Designation Criteria. *http://bhpr.hrsa.gov/shortage/hpsacritpcm.htm*.

Health Resources and Services Administration (HRSA), Bureau of Primary Health Care. 2007a. Migrant Health Centers. *http://bphc.hrsa.gov/migrant/*.

Health Resources and Services Administration (HRSA), Bureau of Primary Health Care. 2007b. America's Health Centers. *http://bphc.hrsa.gov/chc/charts/healthcenters.htm*.

Health Resources and Services Administration (HRSA), Office of Rural Health Policy. 2007. Strategic Plan 2005–2010. *http://ruralhealth.hrsa.gov/policy/StrategicPlan.asp*.

HHS Rural Task Force, July 2002. *Report to the Secretary: One department serving rural America. http://ruralhealth.hrsa.gov/PublicReport.htm#2001.*

Herzog, D.B., and P.N. Copeland. 1985. Medical progress: Eating disorders. *New England Journal of Medicine* 313, no. 5: 295–303.

Iglehart, J.K. 1996. Health policy report—Managed care and mental health. *New England Journal of Medicine* 334, no. 2: 131–135.

Indian Health Service (IHS). 1987. *A comprehensive care program for American Indians and Alaska Natives*. Washington, DC: Public Health Service.

Indian Health Service (IHS). 1999a. A quick look. Washington, DC: *Public Health Service*, September: 1.

Indian Health Service (IHS). 1999b. *Fact sheet: Comprehensive health care program for American Indians and Alaskan Natives*. Washington, DC: Public Health Service, October: 1.

Indian Health Service (IHS). 2001. *Indian Health Service, An Agency Profile*. Washington, DC: Public Health Service. February.

Indian Health Service (IHS). 2003. *Year 2003 Profile*. Washington, DC: Public Health Service, January.

Indian Health Service (IHS). 2006a. Facts on Indian Health Disparities. *http://info.ihs.gov/Files/DisparitiesFacts-Jan2006.pdf.*

Indian Health Service (IHS). 2006b. Indian Health Service Fact Sheet. *http://info.ihs.gov/Files/IHSFacts-June2006.pdf.*

Indian Health Service (IHS). 2006c. Indian Health Service Year 2006 Profile. *http://info.ihs.gov/Files/ProfileSheet-June2006.pdf.*

Johnson, J.P., and P.E. Vink. 1992. Diagnosis and classification of HIV infection in children. In *Management of HIV infection in infants and children*, eds. R. Yogev and E. Connor, 117–128. St. Louis: Mosby–Year Book.

Kaiser Commission on Medicaid and the Uninsured. 2006. *The uninsured: A primer. http://www.kff.org/uninsured/upload/7451-021.pdf.*

Kaiser Family Foundation. 2007. Fact sheet: The Ryan White Program. *http://www.kff.org/hivaids/upload/7582_03.pdf.*

Kaiser Family Foundation. 2006. Fact sheet: Medicaid and HIV/AIDS. *http://www.kff.org/hivaids/upload/7172-03.pdf.*

Kaiser Family Foundation. 2005. Women and health care: A national profile. *http://www.kff.org/womenshealth/7336.cfm.*

Kaiser Family Foundation. 2004. Health care and the 2004 elections: Women's health policy. *http://www.kff.org/womenshealth/7184.cfm#repro.*

Kaiser Family Foundation 2002. Memorandum. *Latest findings on employer-based coverage of contraception. http://www.kff.org/womenshealth/loader.cfm?url=/commonspot/security/getfile.cfm&PageID=14079.*

King, M.P. 1997. *Year of the child in health care: A new state program will give states $24 billion to help poor, uninsured children get health care.* State Legislatures National Conference of State Legislatures: 20–22.

Klerman, G.L., and M.M. Weisman. 1989. Increasing rate of depression. *Journal of the American Medical Association* 261, no. 24: 2229–2235.

Kozoll, R. 1986. Indian health care. In *New dimensions in rural policy: Building upon our heritage*, 447–480. Washington, DC: Government Printing Office.

Kraus, L.E., et al. 1996. *Chartbook on disability in the United States, 1996*. An InfoUse Report. Washington, DC: US National Institute on Disability and Rehabilitation Research.

Kronick, R., and T. Gilmer. 1999. Explaining the decline in health insurance coverage, 1979–1995. *Health Affairs* 18, no. 2: 30–47.

Kuo, J., and K. Porter. 1998. Health status of Asian Americans: United States, 1992–94. Advance data from vital and health statistics. Hyattsville, MD: *National Center for Health Statistics*, no. 298: 1–3.

Lam, N., and K. Liu. 1994. Spread of AIDS in rural America, 1982–1990. *Journal of Acquired Immune Deficiency Syndrome* 7, no. 5: 485–490.

Lurie, N. 1997. Studying access to care in managed care environment. *Health Services Research* 32: 691–701.

Mail, P.D. 1988. Hippocrates was a medicine man: The health care of Native Americans in the twentieth century. *Annals of the Academy of Political and Social Science* 436, no. 1: 40–49.

Merson, M.H. 1996. Returning home: Reflections on the USA's response to the HIV/AIDS epidemic. *Lancet* 347, no. 9016: 1673–1676.

Misra, D. ed. 2001. *Women's health data book: A profile of women's health in the United States*, 3rd ed. Washington, DC: Jacobs Institute of Women's Health and the Henry J. Kaiser Family Foundation.

Morrison, C. 1993. Delivery systems for the care of persons with HIV infection and AIDS. *Nursing Clinics of North America* 28, no. 2: 317–333.

Myers, J.K. et al. 1984. Six-month prevalence of psychiatric disorders in three communities. *Archives of General Psychiatry* 41, no. 10: 959–967.

National Association of Community Health Centers (NACHC). 2006. A Sketch of Community Health Centers: Chartbook 2006. Washington, DC: NACHC.

National Association of Rural Health Clinics (NARHC). 2007. *http://www.narhc.org/about_us/about_us.php*.

National Center for Health Statistics (NCHS). 1999. *Health, United States, 1999*. Hyattsville, MD: Department of Health and Human Services.

National Center for Chronic Disease Prevention and Health Promotion. 2005. Chronic Disease: Overview. *http://www.cdc.gov/nccdphp/overview.htm*.

National Center for Health Statistics. 2006. *Health, United States, 2006*. Hyattsville, MD: Department of Health and Human Services.

National Coalition for the Homeless. 2006a. *NCH fact sheet #2: How many people experience homelessness? http://www.nationalhomeless.org/publications/facts/How_Many.pdf*.

National Coalition for the Homeless. 2006b. *NCH fact sheet #3: Who is homeless? http://www.nationalhomeless.org/publications/facts/Whois.pdf*.

National Institute of Allergy and Infectious Diseases. 2006. Fact sheet: HIV infection in women. *http://www.niaid.nih.gov/factsheets/womenhiv.htm*.

National Institute of Allergy and Infectious Diseases. 2002. Fact sheet: HIV infection in women. *http://www.niaid.nih.gov/factsheets/womenhiv.htm*. Accessed April 21, 2003.

National Institute of Health (NIH). July 9, 2002. News Release: NHLBI Stops Trial of Estrogen Plus Progestin Due to Increased Breast Cancer Risk, Lack of Overall Benefit. *http://www.nhlbi.nih.gov/new/press/02-07-09.htm*.

National Institute of Mental Health (NIMH). 2007. Statistics. *http://www.nimh.nih.gov/healthinformation/statisticsmenu.cfm*.

National Institute of Mental Health (NIMH). 2006. The numbers count. *http://www.nimh.nih.gov/publicat/numbers.cfm#Schizophrenia*.

Newacheck, P.W., and N. Halfon. 1998. Prevalence and impact of disabling chronic conditions in childhood. *American Journal of Public Health* 88, no. 4: 610–617.

Nolan, L.J. et al. 1996. Local research: Needed guidance for the Indian Health Services urban mission. *Public Health Reports* 111, no. 4: 320.

Office on Women's Health (OWH). 2007. Campaigns and events. *http://www.4woman.gov/owh/campaigns/*.

O'Hara, M.J., and D. D'Orlando. 1996. Ambulatory care of the HIV-infected child. *Nursing Clinics of America* 31, no. 1: 179–205.

Ostir, G.V., et al. 1999. Disability in older adults 1: Prevalence, causes, and consequences. *Behavioral Medicine* 24: 147–154.

Patton, L., and D. Puskin. 1990. *Ensuring access to health care services in rural areas: A half century of federal policy*. Essential Health Care Services Conference Center at Georgetown University Conference Center. Washington, DC.

Pell, J. et al. 1996. Management of HIV infected health care workers: Lessons from three cases. *British Medical Journal* 312, no. 7039: 1150–1152, discussion 1152–1153.

Pevar, S.L. 1992. *The rights of Indians and tribes: The basic ACLU guide to Indian and tribal rights*. 2nd ed. Carbondale and Edwardsville, IL: Southern Illinois University Press.

Pleasant, R. 2003. Minority health. In *The Department of Health and Human Services: 50 Years of Service*. DHHS, pp.92–95.

Priscilla, D.A. et al. 1996. Women living with HIV infection. *Nursing Clinics of North America* 31, no. 1: 97–104.

Regier, D.A. et al. 1988. One month prevalence of mental disorders in the United States: Based on five epidemiologic catchment area sites. *Archives of General Psychiatry* 45, no. 11: 977–986.

Rhodes, E.R. 1987. The organization of health services for Indian people. *Public Health Reports* 102, no. 4: 361–365.

Robertson, L.S. et al. 1974. *Changing the medical care system: A controlled experiment in comprehensive care*. New York: Praeger Publishers.

Romanoski, A.J. et al. 1992. The epidemiology of psychiatrist-ascertained depression and DSM-III depressive disorders. Results from the Eastern Baltimore Mental Health Survey Clinical Reappraisal. *Psychological Medicine* 22, no. 3: 629–655.

Rosenbaum, S., and J. Darnell. 1997. *An analysis of the Medicaid and health-related provisions of the Personal Responsibility and Work Opportunity Reconciliation Act of 1996* (P.L. 104–193). Washington, DC: The Kaiser Commission on the Future of Medicaid.

Rumby, R.L. et al. 1991. AIDS in rural Eastern North Carolina. Patient migration: A rural AIDS burden. *AIDS* 5, no. 11: 1373–1378.

Salazar, W.H. 1996. Management of depression in the outpatient office. *Medical Clinics of North America* 80, no. 2: 431–455.

Satcher, D. 1999. Mental Health: A Report of the Surgeon General. [Online]. Available: *http://www.surgeongeneral.gov/library/mentalhealth/home.html* [January 4, 2000].

Schroeder, S.A. et al. 1997. The medically uninsured—Will they always be with us? *The New England Journal of Medicine* 334, 17: 1130–1133.

Schutt, R.K., and S.M. Goldfinger. 1996. Housing preferences and perceptions of health and functioning among homeless mentally ill persons. *Psychiatric Services* 47, no. 4: 381–386.

Sechzer, J.A. et al. 1996. *Women and mental health*. New York: New York Academy of Sciences.

Selike, R.M. et al. 1993. HIV infection as leading cause of death among young adults in US cities and states. *Journal of the American Medical Association* 269, no. 23: 2991–2994.

Shi, L., et al. 2007. Health center financial performance: National trends and state variation, 1998–2004. *J Public Health Management Practice* 13, no.2: 133–50.

Shortell, S.M., et al. 1996. *Remaking health care in America*. San Francisco: Jossey-Bass Publishers.

Solis, J.M. et al. 1990. Acculturation, access to care, and use of preventive services by Hispanics: Findings from HHANES 1982–84. *American Journal of Public Health* 80 (Supplement): 11–19.

Stratton, T. et al. 1993. *A demographic analysis of nurse shortage counties: Implications for rural nursing policy*. Grand Forks, ND: University of North Dakota Rural Health Research Center.

Summer, L. 1991. *Limited access: Health care for the rural poor*. Washington, DC: Center on Budget and Policy Priorities.

The Robert Wood Johnson Foundation. 1996 (November). Chronic care in America: A 21st century challenge. *http://www.rwjf.org/files/publications/other/ChronicCareinAmerica.pdf?gsa=1*.[O1]

Ungvarski, P.J. 1996. Challenges for the urban home health care provider. *Nursing Clinics of North America* 31, no. 1: 81–95.

United Nations. 2007. The State of the World's Children 2007. *http://www.unicef.org/sowc07/docs/sowc07.pdf[O2]*.

US Census Bureau. 2000. *Racial and ethnic classifications used in Census 2000 and beyond*. Washington, DC: Government Printing Office.

US Census Bureau. 2007. Statistical Abstract of the United States, 2007: The National Data Book. Washington, DC: Government Printing Office.

US Department of Veteran Affairs. 2006. Fact sheet: VA programs for homeless veterans. *http://www1.va.gov/opa/fact/hmlssfs.asp*.

Weissman, M.M., and G.L. Klerman. 1977. Sex differences and the epidemiology of depression. *Archives of General Psychiatry* 34, no. 1: 98–111.

Weissman, M.M., and J.K. Klerman. 1992. Depression: Current understanding and changing trends. *Annual Review of Public Health* 13: 319–339.

Wenzel, M. 1996. A school-based clinic for elementary school in Phoenix, Arizona. *Journal of School Health* 66, no. 4: 125–127.

Williams, S.J. 1995. *Essentials of health services*. Albany, NY: Delmar Publishers.

World Health Organization (WHO). 2006. UNAIDS/WHO Epidemic Update: December 2006. *http://www.unaids.org/en/HIV_data/epi2006/default.asp*.

World Health Organization (WHO). 2004. Women and AIDS: Have you heard us today? *http://www.who.int/features/2004/aids/en/*.

Yoon, E., and F. Chien. 1996. Asian American and Pacific Islander health: A paradigm for minority health. *Journal of the American Medical Association* 275, no. 9: 736–737.

Yu, S.M., et al. 2004. Health status and health services utilization among US Chinese, Asian Indian, Filipino, and other Asian/Pacific Islander children. *Pediatrics* 113, no. 1 part 1: 101–7.

PART IV

System Outcomes

Chapter 12

Cost, Access, and Quality

Learning Objectives

- To understand the meaning of health care costs and review recent trends
- To examine the factors that have led to cost escalations in the past
- To become familiar with both regulatory and market-oriented approaches to contain costs
- To understand why some regulatory cost-containment approaches were unsuccessful
- To appreciate the framework and various dimensions of access to care
- To learn about access indicators and measurement
- To understand the nature, scope, and dimensions of quality
- To understand the difference between quality assurance and quality assessment

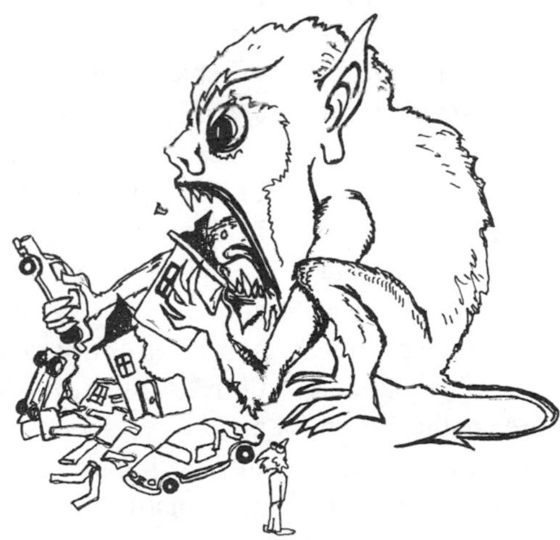

The health care sector of the economy is like a monster with a voracious appetite that needs to be controlled.

Introduction

Cost, access, and quality are three major cornerstones of health care delivery (Al-Assaf 1993a). For many years, employers and third-party payers in the United States have been preoccupied with controlling the growth of health care expenditures. One reason past attempts to bring universal access into the United States have failed is the concern that such a move would be extremely costly in terms of national health care expenditures. This fear is founded on the premise that cost and access go hand in hand. Although cost and access have remained the primary concerns within the US health care delivery system, quality of health care is increasingly taking center stage. At the same time, rising systemwide costs will remain the focus of attention for a long time to come.

The cost of health care, people's ability to obtain health care when needed, and the quality of services are interactively related. From a macro perspective, costs of health care are commonly viewed in terms of national expenditures for health care. A widely used measure of national health care expenditures is the proportion of the gross domestic product (GDP) a country spends on the delivery of health care services. In simple terms, it refers to the proportion of its national income a country spends on health care. From a micro perspective, health care expenditures refer to costs incurred by employers to purchase health insurance and out of pocket costs incurred by individuals when they receive health care services. Improving access to health care and equal access to quality health care are contingent on expenditures at both the macro and micro levels. High-quality care is also the most cost-effective care. Hence, cost is an important factor in the evaluation of quality. On the other hand, quality is achieved when accessible services are provided in an efficient, cost-effective, and acceptable manner (Al-Assaf 1993a).

This chapter discusses some major reasons for the dramatic rise in health care expenditures. Costs are compared with those in other countries, and the impact of cost-containment measures is examined. A considerable proportion of the US population is not assured basic access, and that is a serious problem. The government has played a significant role in cost containment and quality improvement, but extension of universal access to all Americans has remained an elusive dream.

Cost of Health Care

The term "cost" can carry different meanings in the delivery of health care. The meaning of health care costs depends on one's perspective. It has three different meanings: (1) When consumers and financiers speak of the "cost" of health care, they usually mean the "price" of health care. This could refer to the physician's bill, the price of a prescription, or the premiums employers pay to purchase health insurance for their employees. (2) From a national perspective, health care costs refer to how much a nation spends on health care services. In this context, health care costs are also commonly referred to as health care expenditures or health care spending. They primarily reflect the consumption of economic resources in the delivery of health care. The economic resources include health insurance, the skills of health care professionals, organizations and institutions of health care delivery, pharmaceuticals, medical equipment and supplies, public health functions, and new medical discoveries. Since expenditures (E) equals price (P) times quantity (Q), growth in health care spending can be accounted for by growth in prices charged by the providers of health services and by increases in the utilization of services (see Figure 6–1). (3) A third perspective is that of the providers. For these suppliers of health care, the notion of cost refers to the cost of producing health care services. Staff salaries, capital costs for buildings and equipment, rental of space, purchase of supplies, etc. constitute the costs of production.

Trends in National Health Expenditures

Chapter 6 discussed national and personal health expenditures, their composition, and the proportional share between the private and public sectors. Health care spending spiraled upward at double digit rates during the 1970s. This was right after the Medicare and Medicaid programs created a massive growth in access in 1965. By 1970, government expenditures for health care services and supplies had grown by 140%, from $7.9 to $18.9 billion (DHHS 1996). During much of the 1980s, average annual growth in national health spending continued in the double digits, but the rate of increase slowed down considerably (Figure 12–1). In the 1990s, medical inflation was finally brought under control, down to a single digit rate of growth, mainly due to control over medical care costs and utilization through managed care. Recently, the rate of growth has started to accelerate, but at a relatively slow pace (Table 12–1).

Trends in national health expenditures are commonly evaluated in two different ways. One is to compare medical inflation to general inflation in the economy, which is measured by annual changes in the consumer price index (CPI). Except for a brief period

Figure 12–1 Average Annual Percentage Growth in National Health Care Spending During Five-Year Periods, 1960–2002.

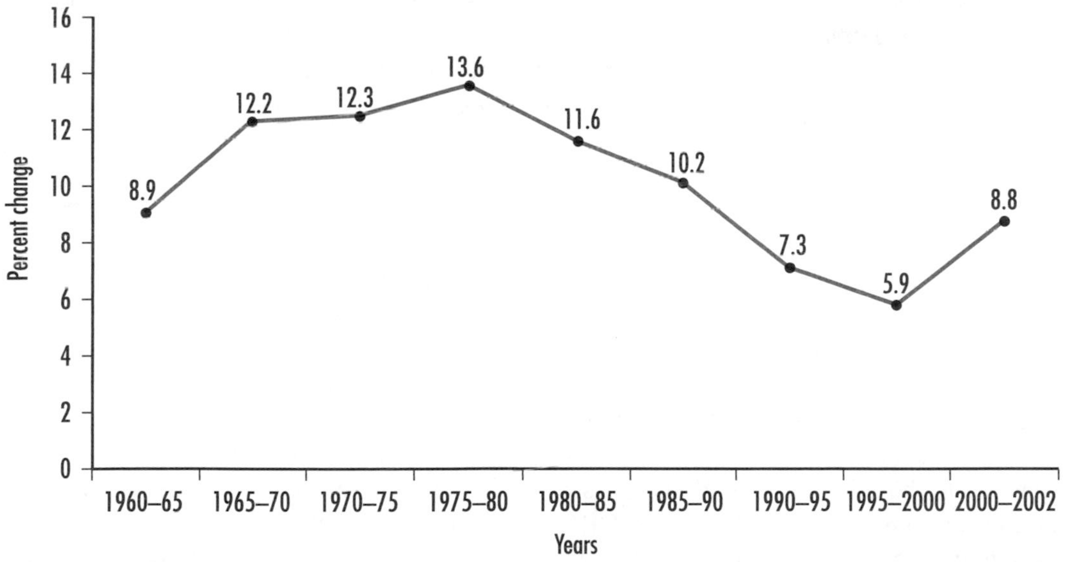

Sources: Data from *Health, United States, 1995*, p. 244; *Health, United States, 2002*, p. 291; *Health, United States, 2006*, p. 377, Department of Health and Human Services.

Table 12–1 Average Annual Percentage Increase in National Health Care Spending, 1975–2004

Periods	% Increase	Periods	% Increase
1975–1980	13.6	1990–1995	7.2
1975–1976	14.7	1990–1991	9.2
1976–1977	13.7	1991–1992	9.5
1977–1978	11.9	1992–1993	6.9
1978–1979	12.9	1993–1994	5.1
1979–1980	14.8	1994–1995	4.9
1980–1985	11.6	1995–2000	5.5
1980–1981	16.1	1995–1996	4.6
1981–1982	12.5	1996–1997	4.7
1982–1983	10.0	1997–1998	5.4
1983–1984	9.7	1998–1999	5.7
1984–1985	9.9	1999–2000	6.9
1985–1990	10.2	2000–2004	8.3
1985–1986	7.6	2000–2001	8.7
1986–1987	8.5	2002–2003	8.2
1987–1988	11.9	2003–2004	7.9
1988–1989	11.2		
1989–1990	12.1		

Sources: Data from *Health, United States, 1996–97,* p. 249, 1997; *Health, United States, 1995,* p. 243; National Center for Health Statistics, 1996–97, *Health, United States, 1999,* p. 284; *Health, United States, 2000,* p. 322; *Health, United States, 2002,* p. 288; *Health, United States, 2006,* p. 374; and K. Levit et al., Trends in US health care spending, 2003. *Health Affairs,* Vol. 22, no. 1: 154–164.

between 1978 and 1981 when the US economy was experiencing hyperinflation, the rates of change in medical inflation have remained consistently above the rates of change in the CPI (Figure 12–2). The second method compares changes in national health spending to those in the GDP. With only isolated exceptions (in 1983 to 1984, after DRG implementation for payment to hospitals; and in 1995 to 1998, after significant managed care penetration), health care spending growth rates have consistently surpassed growth rates in the general economy (Figure 12–3). When spending on health care grows at a faster rate than GDP, it means that health care consumes a larger share of the total economic output. Put another way, a growing share of total economic resources is devoted to the delivery of health care.

Compared to other nations, the United States uses a larger share of its economic resources for health care (Table 12–2). In

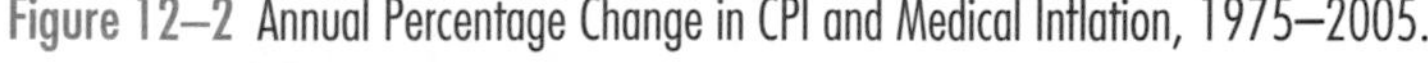

Figure 12–2 Annual Percentage Change in CPI and Medical Inflation, 1975–2005.

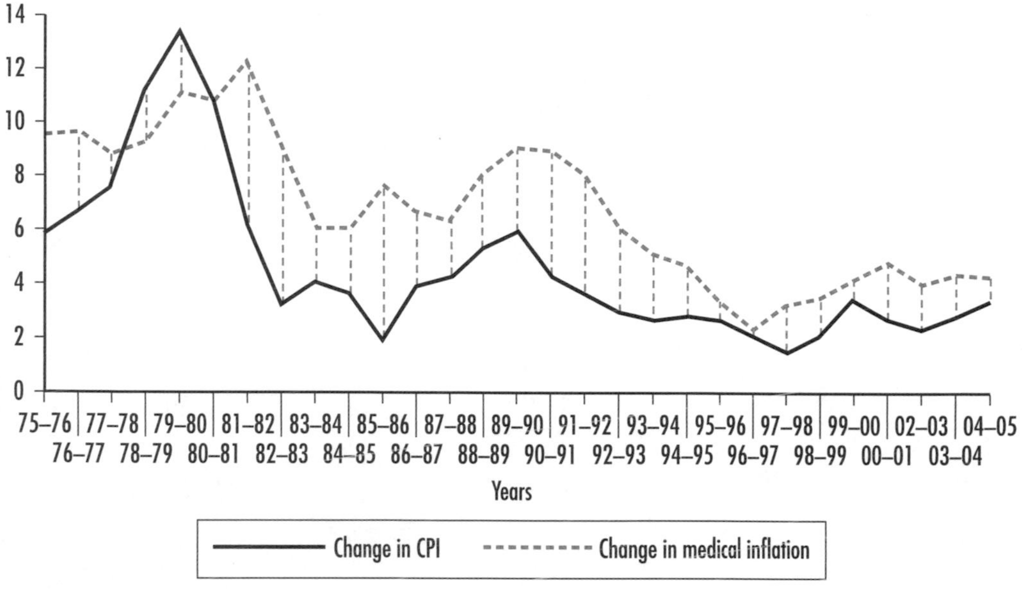

Sources: Data from *Health, United States, 1995,* p. 241; *Health, United States, 1996–97,* p. 251; *Health, United States, 2002,* p. 289; and *Health, United States, 2006,* p. 375.

Figure 12–3 Annual Percentage Change in US National Health Care Expenditures and GDP, 1980–2004.

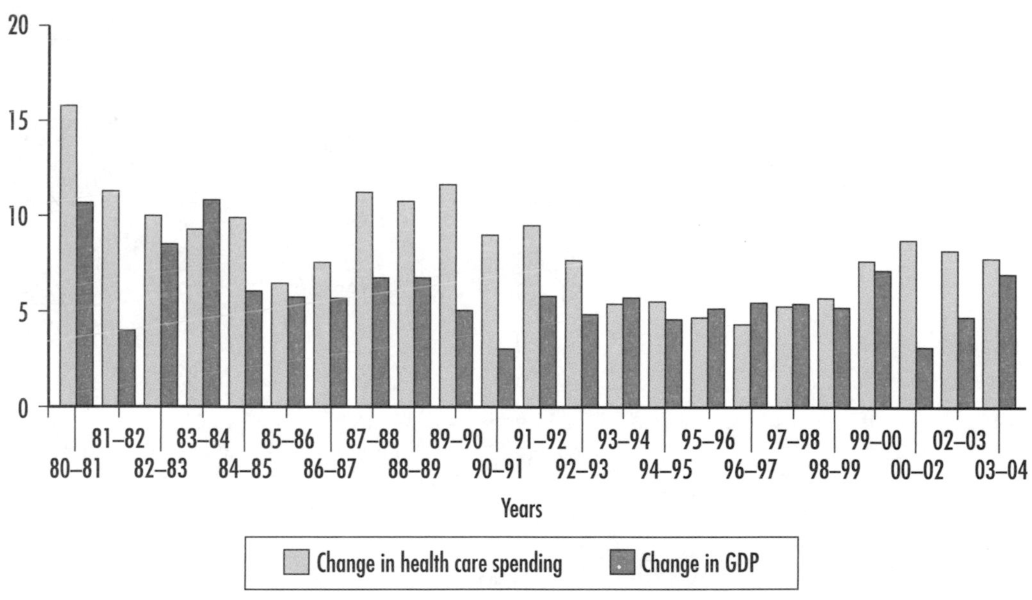

Sources: Data from *Health, United States, 1996–97,* p. 249; *Health, United States, 2002,* p. 288; *Health, United States, 2006,* p. 374; and National Center for Health Statistics, 2002.

Table 12–2 Total Health Care Expenditures as a Proportion of GDP and Per Capita Health Care Expenditures (Selected Years, Selected OECD Countries; Per Capita Expenditures in US Dollars)

	1990	1995	2000	2002
Australia	7.8	8.2	9.0	9.3
	$1,307	$1,745	$2,220	$2,521
Austria	7.0	8.0	7.6	7.6
	$1,338	$1,870	$2,184	$2,280
Belgium	7.4	8.4	8.7	9.1
	$1,345	$1,820	$2,279	$2,607
Canada	9.0	9.2	8.9	9.6
	$1,737	$2,051	$2,503	$2,845
Denmark	8.5	8.2	8.4	8.8
	$1,567	$1,848	$2,382	$2,655
Finland	7.8	7.5	6.7	7.2
	$1,422	$1,433	$1,718	$2,013
France	8.6	9.5	9.3	9.7
	$1,568	$2,033	$2,456	$2,762
Germany	8.5	10.6	10.6	10.7
	$1,748	$2,276	$2,761	$2,916
Italy	7.9	7.3	8.1	8.4
	$1,391	$1,535	$2,049	$2,248
Japan	5.9	6.8	7.6	7.9
	$1,115	$1,538	$1,971	$2,139
Netherlands	8.0	8.4	8.3	9.3
	$1,438	$1,826	$2,259	$2,775
Sweden	8.4	8.1	8.4	9.2
	$1,579	$1,738	$2,273	$2,594
United Kingdom	6.0	7.0	7.3	7.7
	$986	$1,374	$1,833	$2,231
United States	11.9	13.3	13.1	13.8
	$2,738	$3,654	$4,539	$5,287

[1]Proportion of GDP.

[2]Per capita expenditures adjusted to US dollars using GDP purchasing power parities.

Sources: Data from *Health, United States, 2006,* p. 373.

addition, the United States has outpaced the growth in health care spending in other countries (Figure 12–4). Numerous reasons have been given for the growth of health care expenditures, and several different measures have been undertaken over the years to prevent these costs from mushrooming to previously projected levels. These topics are discussed a little later in the chapter.

The rate of growth in health spending came down to its lowest levels in four decades (5.7% average annual growth) between 1993 and 2000 as managed care proliferated (Levit et al. 2003). However, the good news ended as the year 2001 recorded the fastest annual growth (8.7%) since 1991 (see Table 12–1). In 2004, the average annual percentage increase in national health care spending declined slightly to 7.9%. The main culprits for this recent rise in expenditures are hospital services, prescription drugs, and physician services (Levit et al. 2003). Once again, the US health care delivery system has come to a crossroads, which will require some difficult decisions in the near future. The rise in private health insurance premiums, coupled with growing Medicare and Medicaid expenditures, will force private employers and the government to take some drastic steps to prevent any uncontrolled rise in health care costs. As discussed in Chapter 9, current trends may force a restructuring of managed care plans toward more tightly managed models.

In 2005, the United States spent $2 trillion on health care. This amounted to a per capita spending of $6,697 and consumed 16% of the GDP (Catlin et al. 2007). According to current projections, national health care expenditures will grow to 20% of GDP by 2015 (Borger 2006). These forecasts portend that the health care sector will remain one of the fastest growing components of the US economy. Increased demand for services will expand job opportunities, including those for health services administrators. On

Figure 12–4 Health Care Spending as a Percentage of GDP for Selected OECD Countries, 1985 and 2000.

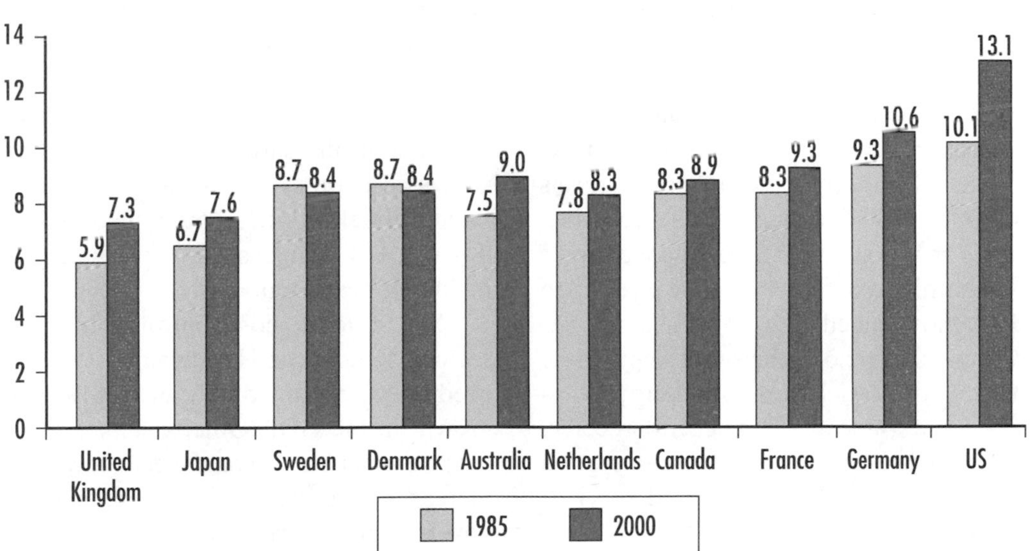

Source: Data from *Health, United States, 2002,* p. 287; *Health, United States, 2006,* p. 373; and National Center for Health Statistics.

the other hand, we can expect to see policy debates and new initiatives to keep costs from getting out of control.

Do Health Care Costs Need to Be Contained?

Americans view growth in expenditures in other sectors of the economy, such as manufacturing, much more favorably than expenditures on medical care. Increased medical expenditures create new health care jobs, do not pollute the air, save rather than destroy lives, and alleviate pain and suffering. Why shouldn't society be pleased that more resources are flowing into a sector that cares for the aged and the sick? It would seem to be a more appropriate use of a society's resources than spending those same funds on faster cars, fancy clothes, or other consumable items. Yet, increased expenditures on these other industries do not cause the concern that arises when medical expenditures increase (Feldstein 1994, 12).

Even though rising health care expenditures may seem innocuous to some, they need to be controlled for several reasons. First, rising health care costs consume greater portions of the total economic output. Because economic resources are limited, rising health care costs mean that Americans have to forgo other goods and services when more is spent on health care. Second, limited economic resources should be directed to their highest valued uses, but consumers decide how much should be spent to purchase a product or service based on their perception of the value they expect to receive, knowing that an expenditure on one good means forgoing other goods and services (Feldstein 1994, 13). As discussed in Chapter 1, health care delivery does not follow the principles of free markets. In the United States, individual patients want maximum expenditures incurred while receiving health care because out-of-pocket payments amount to only a small fraction of the costs of services. They want to get the maximum returns out of prepaid expenditures or health insurance benefits. In countries with national health insurance, patients want to get the maximum in return for the taxes they have paid toward their health coverage. Hence, in either system, unless deliberate attempts are made to control costs, the total health care expenditures will far exceed what they would be under free market conditions.

In the United States, employer-financed health benefits represent a substantial cost of doing business (operating cost). These costs are believed to be the third highest expense category in US corporations after salaries and raw materials (Loubeau and Maher 1996). In 2004, the costs of employer-sponsored coverage was about $575.5 billion. Of this, the employer paid about 77% ($443.2 billion) and employees and retirees paid about 23% ($132.3 billion) (Sheils and Haught 2004). For a business to stay profitable, these costs must be incorporated into the pricing structure and passed on to consumers in higher prices. Some observers think that health care costs are placing businesses at a competitive disadvantage in the international market. To compete internationally, US businesses must reduce costs, including health care costs.

In addition to cost control in the private sector, Medicare and Medicaid expenditures need to be restrained at a level close to the growth in the GDP. Otherwise, health care puts a greater burden on the economy, which increases pressure on the federal and state governments to raise taxes. From time to time, serious concerns have been expressed regarding the long-term solvency of the

Medicare Hospital Insurance Trust Fund that finances Part A benefits. The Balanced Budget Act of 1997 was intended to slow down the rapid rise in Medicare spending. According to the latest estimates based on the most probable economic and demographic assumptions, Medicare trustees project that the trust fund will be depleted by 2018 (Van de Water 2006). In past years, these projections have shifted significantly. The conclusion, however, is that at some point the Medicare trust fund will not have adequate funds to pay for the growing health care needs of an aging population, unless steps are taken now to address this issue. According to Representative David Obey, a member of the House Budget Committee, Medicare will absolutely have to be cut in a few years. "When the time comes, there is no way out of it." That time will come as baby boomers move into the system (Tucker 1997). The same is true for countries that have national health care programs. Governments cannot continue to raise taxes indefinitely. Various mechanisms must therefore be employed to contain ever-rising health care costs. One proposal already floated in the US Congress is to raise the eligibility age for Medicare from 65 years to 67 or higher. The downside is that it would leave many elderly uninsured.

Reasons for Cost Escalation

Numerous factors have been attributed to rising health care expenditures. They interact in complex ways. Hence, one cannot just point to one or two main causes. General inflation in the economy is a more visible cause of health care spending because it affects the cost of producing health care services through higher wages, cost of supplies, etc. But, apart from the effects of general inflation, medical cost inflation is influenced by the following factors:

- third-party payment
- imperfect market
- growth of technology
- increase in elderly population
- medical model of health care delivery
- multipayer system and administrative costs
- defensive medicine
- waste and abuse
- practice variations

Third-Party Payment

The notion of moral hazard was introduced in earlier chapters. Health care is among the few services for which a third party, not the consumer, pays for most services used. Whether payment is made by the government or by a private insurance company, individual patients pay a price far lower than the actual cost of the service (Altman and Wallack 1996). Since they have to bear only a fraction of the financial burden out of pocket, the patients are not too concerned about the cost of care. The patient has no incentive to be cost conscious when someone else is paying the bill. Introduction of prospective payment methods and capitation have, to a large extent, minimized provider-induced demand. However, the backlash against managed care (see Chapter 9) from consumers and providers alike has, in a sense, kept the door open to overuse of high-cost technologies and other services. Also, fee-for-service reimbursement and its discounted fee variation are still widely used. Hence, provider-induced demand has not been expunged from the system.

The number of persons with health insurance jumped dramatically after World War II, and so did the spending for health care services. The passage of Medicare and Medicaid in 1965 added third-party protection for an additional 50 million elderly and poor Americans (Altman and Wallack 1996). The Rand Health Insurance Experiment empirically demonstrated the theoretical connection between health insurance and costs. The most comprehensive study of its type, the experiment ran from 1974 through 1981. It enrolled more than 7,000 people into one of 14 different health plans. They included a free plan carrying no deductible or co-payments. The other plans involved varying degrees of cost sharing. It was found that cost sharing resulted in lower costs compared to the free plan. Coinsurance rates of 25% resulted in a 19% decline in expenditures because out of pocket costs reduced health care utilization. Increased coinsurance rates resulted in further declines in utilization and expenditures. Another important finding of the Rand Experiment was that lower utilization due to cost sharing did not affect most measures of health status. People enrolled in the free plan did better in three areas: vision, blood pressure, and dental health, but the average appraised mortality risk for people on the free plan was close to the risk for those with cost sharing (Feldstein 1993, 93–95).

Imperfect Market

Prices charged by providers for health care services are likely to be much closer to the cost of producing the services in a highly regulated or highly competitive market (Altman and Wallack 1996). The US health care market is neither. Because the US health care delivery system does not consist of a national health care program, it is not highly regulated as are the single-payer systems in other countries. Health care delivery in the United States also does not represent a highly competitive market because of various market imperfections discussed in Chapter 1. In an imperfect market, utilization of health care is driven by need rather than economic demand, the quantity of health care services produced and delivered is likely to be much higher than in a competitive market, and the prices charged for health care services will be permanently higher than the true economic costs of production (Altman and Wallack 1996). Because E 5 Q 3 P (see Figure 6–1), it is not difficult to see why an unregulated quasi-market would result in increased health care expenditures because both Q and P remain unchecked. One reason for an imperfect market is the existence of third-party payments. Third-party payments insulate patients from higher prices and higher utilization. This and other market imperfections also insulate providers against the possibility of facing lower demand from higher prices. In other words, because of the imperfect nature of the health care market, demand is not sensitive to changes in prices, as it would be under free-market conditions* (see Figure 1–3).

Growth of Technology

The United States has been characterized as following an early-start-fast-growth pattern

*Chiropractic care and outpatient mental health services are more sensitive to prices than overall medical and dental care. Access to free chiropractic care among health maintenance organization (HMO) enrollees increased chiropractic use ninefold compared with a contemporaneous sample of HMO enrollees who faced 95% cost sharing. When patients have to share 25% or more of the cost, they decrease their chiropractic expenses by one half. (P.G. Shekelle, W.H. Rogers, and J.P. Newhouse. 1996. The effect of cost sharing on the use of chiropractic services. *Medical Care* 34, 9: 863–872.)

in the adoption and diffusion of intensive procedures (TECH Research Network 2001). Growth and intensive use of technology have a direct impact on the escalation of health care costs (see Chapter 5). New technology is expensive to develop, and costs incurred in research and development (R&D) are included in the total health care expenditures. One reason Canada and European nations, compared to the United States, have incurred lower costs is because they have proportionally invested far less in R&D. They have been able to buy or duplicate American breakthroughs (Easterbrook 1987).

Once technology is developed, it drives up demand for its use. Compared to other nations, the overall diffusion and utilization of technology is greater in the United States, although countries like Japan, Austria, and Switzerland have more magnetic resonance imagers (MRIs) and computed tomography (CT) scanners (Reinhardt et al. 2002). Development of new technology raises the expectations of consumers about what medical science can do to diagnose and treat diseases and prolong life.

As discussed in Chapter 4, technology has been at least partly responsible for the surplus of specialists in the United States. Specialty services are more technology intensive and, consequently, more expensive than primary care services. Since disease prevalence is too low to support all the specialists, many high-tech procedures are overused.

Technology has substantially increased diagnosis and treatment and improved quality of life, but it is also used simply to keep people alive with little or no chance of recovery. Third-party insurance has generally paid for almost all diagnostic tests and procedures with few questions asked. Attempts to limit diffusion of certain expensive technologies in the United States have been largely unsuccessful. Hence, many more cost-increasing technologies have been developed than cost-reducing technologies (Weisbrod 1991).

Increase in Elderly Population

Since the early part of the 20th century, life expectancy in the United States has consistently risen (see Figure 12–5). Life expectancy at birth increased by over 30 years from 47.3 years in 1900 to 77.5 years in 2003 (National Center for Health Statistics 2006). Consequently, the United States and other industrialized nations are also experiencing an aging boom. Growth in the US elderly population has outpaced growth in the nonelderly population since 1900. Figure 12–6 shows changes in the makeup of the US population from 1970 to 2004. Most remarkable is the growth in the age group 85 years and older while the youngest age group is shrinking. Growth of the elderly population is projected to continue through the middle of the 21st century. Between 2000 and 2030, the proportion of the US population that is 65 years of age and older is expected to rise from 12.4% to 20%, or one in five. The number in the 85-and-older category is projected to more than double. The swelling of the elderly population will result from the aging of the baby-boom generation of roughly 77 million Americans born between 1946 and 1964. The youngest of the baby boomers will be 66 years old in 2030.

Elderly people consume more health care than younger people. In 2003, the average medical expenses for people 65 years of age and older was $8,209 per person compared to $2,837 per person for those under the age of 65 (National Center for Health Statistics 2006). In other words, health care

Figure 12–5 Life Expectancy of Americans at Birth, Age 65, and Age 75, Selected Years 1900–2003.

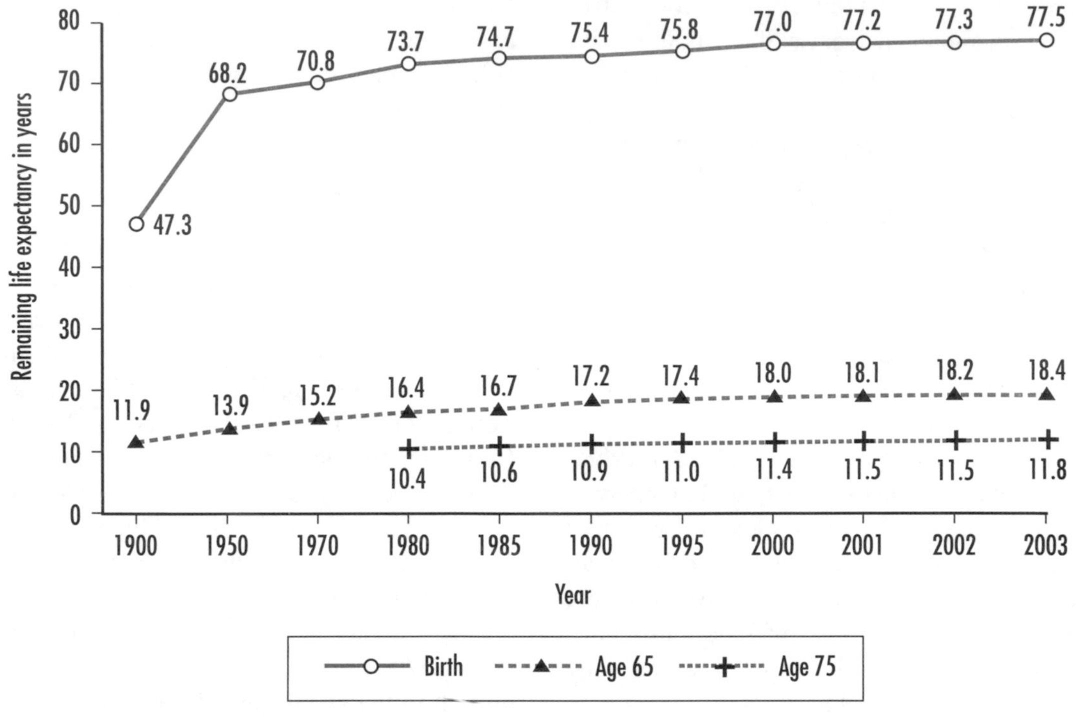

Sources: Data from *Health, United States, 2002,* p. 116 and *Health, United States, 2006,* p. 176.

costs for the elderly are nearly three times more than those for the nonelderly. Total Medicare expenditures are projected to increase from 2.7% of GDP in 2005 to 9% of GDP in 2050 (Van de Water 2006). A growing elderly population and expansion of Medicare by adding prescription drug coverage will seriously affect future health care expenditures.

Medical Model of Health Care Delivery

As discussed in Chapter 2, the medical model emphasizes medical interventions after a person has become sick and plays down prevention and lifestyle behavior changes to promote health. Although health promotion and disease prevention are not the answer to every health problem, these principles have not been accorded their rightful place in the US health care delivery system. Consequently, more costly health care resources must be deployed to treat health problems that could have been prevented. For example, smoking-related illnesses are estimated to cost the United States $75.5 billion annually for direct medical care and an additional $167 billion in lost productivity (CDC 2005). However, evidence suggests the costs of smoking cessation programs pose a minimal burden to insurers and employers with potential for significant cost savings in subsequent years (Levy 2006). Although the prevalence of cigarette smoking has been slowly declining, in 2004, 23% of American adult males and 18.7% of women were smokers (National Center for Health Statistics 2006).

Figure 12–6 Change in US Population Mix between 1970 and 2000, and Projections for 2030.

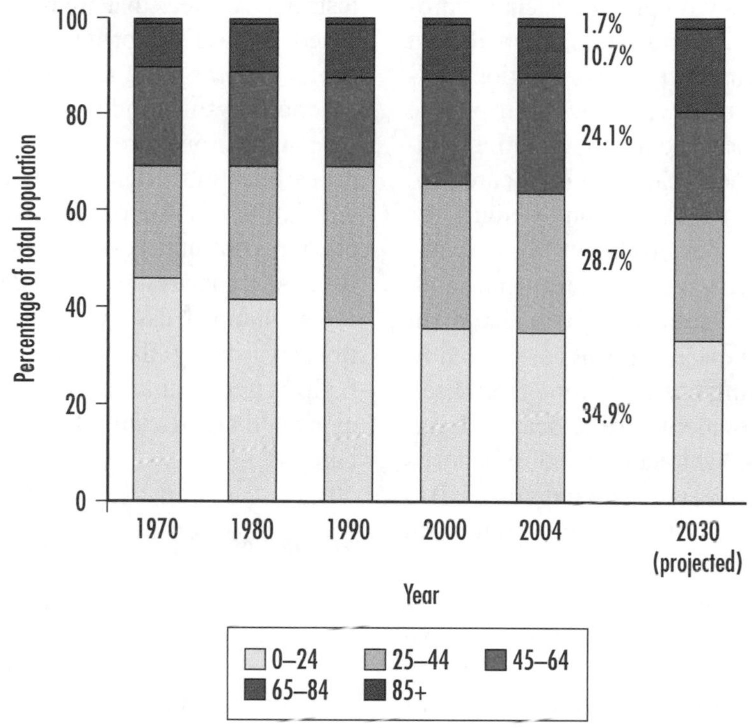

Sources: Data from *Health, United States, 2006*, p. 127, National Center for Health Statistics; *Census 2000*, US Census Bureau; *Projections of the Total Resident Population by 5-Year Age Groups, and Sex with Special Age Categories: Middle Series, 2025 to 2045*, US Census Bureau.

Overweight conditions and obesity have reached alarming rates in the United States and in many other developed nations. In 2004, 66% of Americans age 20 and over were overweight with 31.4% obese (National Center for Health Statistics 2006). Overweight and obesity substantially elevates the risk of heart disease, diabetes, some types of cancers, musculoskeletal disorders, and gallbladder problems.

Consequently, overweight and obesity are contributing to the nation's health care spending at a growing rate. Recent estimates suggest that of the total medical spending in the United States, 9.1% could be attributed to overweight and obesity, rivaling that attributable to smoking. Total health care expenditures attributable to overweight and obesity may be as high as $92.6 billion in 2002 dollars. Both Medicare and Medicaid spend a disproportionate share to treat overweight- and obesity-related health problems (Finkelstein et al. 2003). Even though considerable preventive efforts have been targeted at smoking cessation, to date very little has been done to combat overweight and obesity among both children and adults.

Multipayer System and Administrative Costs

Administrative costs are associated with the management of the financing, insurance, delivery, and payment functions. They include management of the enrollment process, setting up contracts with providers, claims processing, utilization monitoring, denials and appeals, and marketing and promotional expenses. The enrollment process in private employer-financed health plans and in publicly financed Medicaid and Medicare programs includes determination of eligibility, enrollment, and disenrollment. Each activity has associated costs. Insurers and managed care organizations (MCOs) also incur enrollment and disenrollment costs, in addition to marketing costs to promote and sell their plans. Providers have to deal with numerous plans in which the extent of benefits and reimbursement are not standardized. It is difficult and costly to remain current with the numerous and frequently changing rules and regulations. Denials of payment result in appeals and follow-up. Utilization monitoring has become commonplace in the delivery of health care services. Review and authorization of care incur additional costs for payers. They also incur additional costs for providers, who must provide the required information to payers. Denial of hospitalization and specialist referrals may result in appeals, which again create additional costs.

Due to the complexity of a multi-payer system, costs are often duplicated. It is estimated that administrative costs associated with the delivery of health care in the United States may be as high as 24% to 25% of total health care expenditures. A single-payer health care system might cut health care administrative costs by one-half (Hellander et al. 1994).

Defensive Medicine

The US health care delivery system is characterized by legal risks for providers, which promote defensive medicine (see Chapter 1). The practice of ***defensive medicine*** leads to tests and services that are not medically justified but are performed by physicians to protect themselves against potential malpractice lawsuits. Induction of labor and cesarean sections are commonly overused procedures in the United States. Fear of legal liability is one of the main reasons for carrying out unnecessary cesarean sections because it makes it easier to defend a potential birth injury case. Unrestrained malpractice awards by the courts and increased malpractice insurance premiums for physicians add significantly to the cost of health care.

Waste and Abuse

The previous discussions pinpoint some of the inefficiencies in the US health care delivery system. These inefficiencies are wasteful. Another type of waste is fraud and abuse within the system. In general terms, ***fraud*** involves a knowing disregard of the truth. Fraudulent activities are both illegal and immoral. Fraud generally occurs when billing claims or cost reports are intentionally falsified. A mere oversight or an inadvertent error will not rise to the level of fraud; however, a pattern of oversights or errors may be tantamount to fraud (Lovitky 1997). Health care fraud has been identified as a major problem in the Medicare and Medicaid programs.

Fraud may also occur when more services are provided than are medically necessary or when unprovided services are billed. The latter practice may include billing for a higher priced service when a lower priced service is actually delivered. In the managed care sector, some providers may not deliver necessary services even though they are included in the capitated fees. Another type of fraud involves misallocation of costs to increase Medicaid and/or Medicare reimbursement. As some services still continue to be reimbursed on a cost-plus basis, disguising a nonallowable cost as an allowable cost to increase reimbursement is fraudulent.

It is illegal to provide any remuneration to any individual or entity in exchange for a referral for services to be paid by the Medicare or Medicaid program. Knowingly providing such financial inducements amounts to a federal crime punishable by imprisonment. Under the Anti-Kickback Act, several physicians have been prosecuted for accepting payments from hospitals to which the doctors referred Medicare patients. Similar types of prosecutions have occurred with respect to illegal payments to nursing homes and home health agencies made by durable medical equipment suppliers. The Stark Law prohibits physician self-referral for laboratory or other designated health services. This law prevents physicians from referring a patient to laboratories in which they or members of their immediate families have a financial interest (Lovitky 1997).

Practice Variations

The work of John Wennberg and others brought to the fore a disturbing aspect of physician behavior accounting for wide variations in treatment patterns for similar patients. Numerous studies, in the United States and abroad, have documented notable differences in utilization rates for hospital admissions and surgical procedures among different communities as well as for the same specialties (Feldstein 1993, 204). These practice variations are referred to as ***small area variations*** (SAV) because the differences in practice patterns have only been associated with geographic areas of the country. For example, in earlier studies, variations in the rate of tonsillectomies in New England counties could not be explained by differences in the demographics or other characteristics of the populations studied (Wennberg and Gittelsohn 1973); the overall inpatient hospital utilization by an aged population in East Boston was higher than that by an equivalent population in New Haven, after controlling for several variables (Wennberg et al. 1987). More recent investigations on regional differences in Medicare spending demonstrated that higher rates of inpatient-based care and specialist services were associated with higher costs but not with improved quality of care, health outcomes, access to services, or satisfaction with care (Fisher et al. 2003a; Fisher et al. 2003b). This variation, which can be as great as twofold, cannot be explained by age, gender, race, pricing variations, or health status (Baucus and Fowler 2002). Geographic variations, as discussed here, signal gross inefficiencies in the US health care delivery system because they increase costs without yielding appreciably better outcomes. This variation is also unfair because workers and Medicare beneficiaries in low-cost, more efficient regions subsidize the care of those in high-cost regions (Wennberg 2002). SAVs cannot be explained by demand inducement. For example, no incentives are provided for physicians to induce demand in Canada or Britain, yet variations similar to those in the United States also exist in those countries. SAVs indicate that patients in some parts of the country are receiving too much treatment, whereas others may be receiving too little. Medical opinions often differ on the appropriateness of clinical interventions because physicians use different criteria for hospital admissions and surgical interventions (Gittelsohn and Powe 1995).

Cost Containment—Regulatory Approaches

Many attempts to control health care spending have been undertaken in the United States; however, most of these attempts have met with only limited success mainly because the United States has never been able to implement a systemwide cost-control initiative. An ***all-payer system***, in which centralized controls would allow cost-containment efforts to sweep through the entire health care delivery system, has never been tried in the United States, because that would require a major overhaul of the system. Cost-containment measures have been piecemeal, affecting only certain targeted sectors of the health care delivery system at a time. So, for instance, when prices have been regulated, utilization has been left untouched; when capital expenditures have required preapprovals, operating costs of production have been exempted; when reimbursement rates have been set for inpatient services, the outpatient sector has remained free of cost-cutting regulation. In a fragmented system, it is impossible to implement cost-control measures in a systematic and global manner.

Other industrialized nations have created national regulatory mechanisms to keep their health care spending in line with their national income. Many of these countries follow what is referred to as ***top-down control*** over total expenditures. They establish budgets for entire sectors of the health care delivery system. Funds are distributed to providers in accordance with these global budgets. Thus, total spending remains within established budget limits. The downside to this approach is that, under fixed budgets, providers are not as responsive to patient needs, and the system provides little incentive to be efficient in the delivery of services. Once budgets are expended, providers are forced to cut back services, particularly for illnesses that are not life threatening or do not represent an emergency. This top-down approach is in sharp contrast to the "bottom-up" approach used in the United States, where each provider and MCO establishes its own fees or premiums (Altman and Wallack 1996). Competition, created by employers shopping for the best premium rates and by MCOs contracting with providers who agree to favorable fee arrangements, determines what the total expenditures will be. To some extent, the United States also uses regulatory cost control, although it is not as comprehensive as it is in countries with national health care programs.

Cost-control efforts in the United States are characterized by a combination of government regulation and market-based competition. As a result of this fragmented approach, only short-lived successes have been achieved to date. The main reason for this lack of success is cost shifting between programs and/or sectors when cost-control measures are not comprehensive. ***Cost shifting*** refers to the ability of providers to make up for lost revenues in one area by increasing utilization or charging higher prices in areas free of controls. For example, when regulatory controls are employed to squeeze costs out of the inpatient sector, providers experience reduced revenues from inpatient services. To make up for the lost revenues, they increase utilization of outpatient services if that sector is free of controls. In another scenario, when the government implements cost-control measures, providers may start charging higher prices to private payers. This practice is very common in the nursing home industry, in which reimbursement is restricted under Medicaid rate setting criteria. In this case, nursing home administrators make a conscious attempt to make up for the lost revenues by admitting more private-pay residents and by establishing higher private-pay charges.

Regulatory approaches to cost containment typically control the capacity of the supply-side, prices, and utilization (Exhibit 12–1). Supply-side constraints are accomplished through "health planning." Planning enables policymakers to limit the number of hospital beds and diffusion of costly technology, but regulatory limits on the health care system's capacity inevitably create monopolies on the supply-side. To make sure that these artificially created monopolies do not exploit their economic power, health planning is always coupled with stiff price and budgetary controls (Reinhardt 1994). Countries with national health care programs

Exhibit 12–1 Regulation-Based and Competition-Based Cost-Containment Strategies

Regulation-Based Cost-Containment Strategies	
Supply-side controls	Restrictions on capital expenditures (new construction, renovations, and technology diffusion) Example: Certificate of need Restrictions on supply of physicians Example: Entry barriers for foreign medical graduates
Price controls	Artificially determined prices Examples: Reimbursement formulas Prospective payment systems Diagnosis-related groups Resource utilization groups Global budgets
Utilization controls	Peer review organizations
Competition-Based Cost-Containment Strategies	
Demand-side incentives	Cost sharing Sharing of premium costs Deductibles and co-payments
Supply-side regulation	Antitrust regulation
Payer-driven competition	Competition among insurers Competition among providers
Utilization controls	Managed care

tightly control supply. Demand-side constraints are used in the form of utilization control. These countries also use global budgets to restrict payments to hospitals and physicians, and place limitations on total expenditures. This simultaneous and comprehensive approach cannot work in the United States due to the system's fragmentation because of multiple payers (see Chapter 1). Instead, the United States can only implement piecemeal programs.

Health Planning

Health planning refers to a government undertaking to align and distribute health care resources so that in the eyes of the government, it will achieve desired health outcomes for all people. The planning function becomes critical in a centrally controlled national health care program so that the basic health care needs of the population are met and expenditures are maintained at predetermined levels. Health planning employs supply-side constraints to control health care expenditures. The central planning function does not fit so well in a system that is largely private because of the absence of a central administrative agency to monitor the system (see Chapter 1). Instead, the system is governed by market forces, and the types of health care services, their geographic distribution, access to these services, and the prices charged by providers develop independently of any preformulated plans. Levels of expenditures cannot be predetermined, and such a system is not conducive to achieving broad social objectives. Nevertheless, the United States has tried some forms of health planning on voluntary or mandated bases, but these efforts have met with limited success.

Some of the early efforts to control health care costs in the United States took the form of voluntary health planning. The goal was to minimize duplication of services. Early forms of health planning—in the 1930s and 1940s—were primarily the result of communitywide voluntary organizations, called hospital councils, which were established by hospitals in some of the largest cities. Hospitals agreed to share or consolidate services, or they traded the closing of a service in one hospital for the expansion of another service (Williams 1995, 154). Voluntary planning worked only on a limited basis and only in instances where participating hospitals could gain an advantage through cooperative planning. Consequently, voluntary planning contributed little to overall efficiency (Gottlieb 1974).

The federal government got involved in health planning after the passage of Medicare and Medicaid in the 1960s. These programs were designed to achieve broad social objectives by extending health care access to the underprivileged, but the passage of these programs generated an explosion in health care spending. Recognizing the increasing dollars that the federal government was putting into health care, Congress believed that it had the right to control escalating costs (Williams 1995, 154). The comprehensive health planning legislation of the mid-1960s mandated the establishment of local and state health planning agencies. These agencies assessed local health care needs and advocated better coordination and distribution of resources. However, the agencies had little or no actual regulatory power and were largely ineffective (Williams 1995, 154). When these agencies were evaluated, planned and unplanned areas had the same amount of duplication of facilities and services, and the rate of increase in hospital costs was the same (May 1974). The Health Planning and Resource Development Act of 1974 was enacted to provide incentives and penalties that would encourage states to adopt ***certificate-of-need*** (CON) legislation (Feldstein 1993, 273) in an attempt to implement an enhanced regulatory approach.

As discussed in Chapter 5, CON statutes were state-enacted legislation whose primary purpose was to control capital expenditures by health facilities. The CON process required prior approval from a state government agency for construction of new facilities, such as hospitals and nursing homes. Similar approvals were required for the expansion of existing facilities or the acquisition of expensive equipment. Approvals were based on the demonstration of a community need for additional services. Although the reasons given for the CON legislation were better planning of resources and control of increasing expenditures, in reality, the adoption of CON was easier in states having greater competition among hospitals (Wendling and Werner 1980), indicating that hospitals supported CON legislation when it was to their own benefit. These hospitals did not want additional capital spending on new construction and equipment by their competitors. On the other hand, CON laws did not seem to lower hospital expenditures on a per patient day basis. CON also represented a conservative approach to containing the rise in hospital costs because it did not address reimbursement and provided no incentives to change utilization behavior in patients or physicians (Feldstein 1993, 273). In the case of nursing homes, however, CON regulations have been used to contain Medicaid costs. In the face of a growing demand for nursing home beds, the CON regulations have restricted the supply of nursing home beds that otherwise would have been utilized. Because Medicaid plays a significant role in financing nursing home care, the added utilization would have increased overall Medicaid costs. The downside is that for years CON regulations have restricted genuine competition in the nursing home industry.

In the early 1980s, the US government moved away from its commitment to health care planning. The Health Planning and Resource Development Act was repealed in 1986. Between 1983 and 1988, 11 states followed the federal government and dropped their CON programs (Altman and Wallack 1996). By 2007, 19 states no longer had CON regulation (Ross 2007). However, several states have retained their programs, and others have reactivated them as a boom in outpatient care and ambulatory surgery centers has led to fears of oversaturation.

Price Controls

In 1971, President Nixon imposed the Economic Stabilization Program (ESP) as an economywide measure to contain general inflation through wage and price controls. The ESP limited the amount by which hospitals could raise their prices from year to year (Williams and Torrens 1993). Although controls on most of the economy were dropped by the end of 1971, the special problems of health care inflation led the administration to keep tight controls on the health care sector through 1974 (Altman and Wallack 1996). The ESP controls did generate a moderating influence on price increases for most medical services; however, the program had placed no limits on the quantity of services (Altman and Eichenholz 1976). For example, the quantity of services delivered to Medicare patients increased by about 10% during the first year of the ESP and between 8% and 15%, depending on physician specialty, during the second year (Gabel and Rice 1985). Also, the costs of production remained relatively unchanged. Therefore, once controls were lifted, inflation returned to its precontrol levels (Altman and Eichenholz 1976). ESP demonstrated that, although price increases can be limited for a short period, effective controls on total spending require much more extensive limits on the costs of production as well as on the quantity of services utilized (Altman and Wallack 1996).

During 1984 and 1986, Medicare froze physician fees; however, during each year fees were frozen, per-enrollee physician expenditures increased by at least 10% (Mitchell et al. 1988) because physicians could induce demand and thus increase the quantity of services provided. Similar results from price controls have been demonstrated in other countries. Perhaps the most important effort to control prices of inpatient hospital care was the conversion of hospital Medicare reimbursement from cost-plus to a prospective system based on diagnosis-related groups (DRGs) authorized under the Social Security Amendments of 1983 (see Chapter 6). The DRG-based reimbursement significantly reduced growth in inpatient hospital spending, but had little impact on total per capita Medicare cost inflation because costs were shifted from the inpatient to the outpatient sector (Figure 12–7). Use of per capita spending data in Figure 12–7 controls for the growth in Medicare population; hence, the increased rate of spending in the outpatient sector and the corresponding decline in the inpatient sector are mainly attributable to the types of services.

Most states have also employed price-control measures to control their Medicaid expenditures. Both retrospective and prospective methods have been used to define pay-

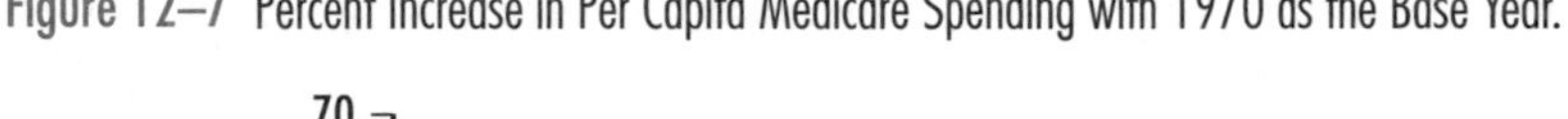
Figure 12–7 Percent Increase in Per Capita Medicare Spending with 1970 as the Base Year.

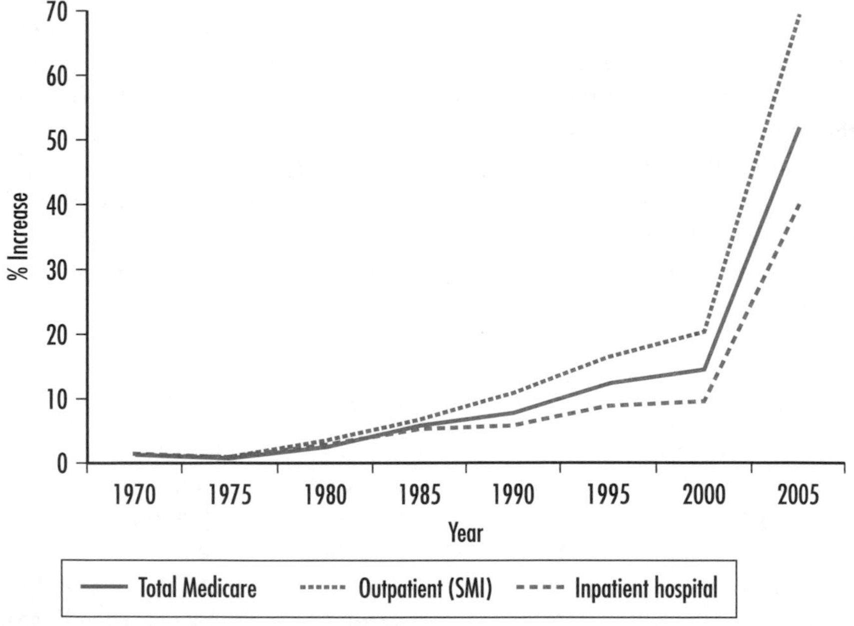

Sources: Data from *Health, United States, 1995,* p. 263; *Health, United States, 2002,* p. 322; *Health, United States, 2006,* p. 404, National Center for Health Statistics.

ment rates for hospitals and nursing homes. Often, complex formulas are used which, in essence, produce arbitrary reimbursement rates and rate ceilings. For example, two neighboring states can have sizable differences in Medicaid reimbursement for practically the same level of services.

Another rate-setting mechanism instituted the most significant change in the way Medicare pays physicians. It was the Omnibus Budget Reconciliation Act (OBRA) of 1989, which was implemented in 1992. The law authorized Medicare's Physician Payment Reform Program (MPPRP) to establish a national Medicare Fee Schedule (MFS). The MFS is based on a resource-based relative value scale (RBRVS) (see Chapter 6). In other words, physicians are paid according to relative value units established for more than 7,000 covered services. A volume performance standard (VPS) was implemented to contain the annual rate of growth in Medicare physician payments. The program seems to have had some success. Between 1992 and 1997, the average annual growth in total Part B expenditures was 9.2%, compared to 6.1% for physician services. Between 1999 and 2005, total Part B expenditures increased from $82.3 to $152.4 billion (National Center for Health Statistics 2006).

The most sweeping price-control initiatives were authorized by the Balanced Budget Act (BBA) of 1997 for Medicare postacute services, namely, home health and skilled nursing facility services, which had been left untouched by the earlier prospective payment system for inpatient hospital care (see Chapter 6 for details).

Another recent development in Medicare reimbursement is the move toward pay-for-performance. Pay-for-performance, which is receiving attention in both the private and public sectors, aims to align provider payments with the quality of care provided. In 2003, as part of the Medicare Prescription Drug, Improvement, and Modernization Act, the US Congress asked the Institute of Medicine (IOM) to assess the potential for implementing pay-for-performance in the Medicare program (IOM, 2004). Specifically, the IOM studied the performance measure set that could be used, the payment policy that could be used, and the key implementation issues involved, such as data and information technology requirements. The IOM found mixed evidence regarding the effectiveness of pay-for-performance demonstration programs, and it noted that unintended adverse consequences of pay-for-perfomance could include decreased access to care, increased disparities in care, and impediments to innovation. However, the IOM concluded that careful monitoring of pay-for-performance could minimize these adverse consequences. Further, the IOM argued that if Medicare payment structures were left unchanged, they would pose a barrier to improved quality of care. The IOM recommended a phased approach to implementing pay-for-performance in Medicare, consisting of small-scale implementation initially, allowing for adjustments as needed before launching large-scale changes.

The Medicare program is not alone in considering pay-for-performance strategies. At least 12 states have instituted pay-for-performance in their Medicaid programs (CMS, 2007). While these programs are in the early stages of development, the Centers for Medicare and Medicaid Services is offering technical assistance to states who are implementing and evaluating pay-for-performance.

Peer Review

The term ***peer review*** refers to the general process of medical review of utilization and quality when it is carried out directly or under the supervision of physicians (Wilson and Neuhauser 1985, 270). Based on this concept, the Social Security Amendments of 1972 required the establishment of professional standards review organizations (PSROs). These associations of physicians reviewed professional and institutional services provided under Medicare and Medicaid. The stated purpose was monitoring and control of cost and quality. When Congress evaluated the performance of PSROs for their cost-control effectiveness, the program had not produced any net savings. Because of their questionable effectiveness, the PSROs were replaced in 1984 by a new system of peer review organizations (PROs). ***PROs*** are statewide private organizations composed of practicing physicians and other health care professionals who are paid by the federal government to review the care provided to Medicare beneficiaries. Each state has a PRO. To control utilization, PROs determine whether care is reasonable, necessary, and provided in the most appropriate setting. PROs also decide whether care meets standards of quality generally accepted by the medical profession. PROs can deny payments if care is not medically necessary or not delivered in the most appropriate setting (Health Care Financing Administration [HCFA] 1996). PROs are now referred to as Quality Improvement Organizations (***QIOs***).

Cost Containment—Competitive Approaches

Competition refers to rivalry among sellers for customers (Dranove 1993). In health care delivery, it means that providers of health care services will try to attract patients who can choose among several different providers. Although competition more commonly refers to price competition, it may also be based on technical quality, amenities, access, or other factors (Dranove 1993). Because competition is an essential element for the operation of free markets, competitive approaches are also referred to as market-oriented approaches.

During the Reagan presidency in the 1980s, competitive reforms were given preference because of growing interest in market-oriented approaches in many sectors of the economy. These reforms were accompanied by waning interest in comprehensive health care reform at the national level. Market-oriented reforms were accompanied by mounting cost-containment efforts in the private sector and the growth of managed care. Competitive reforms have been diverse and have often entailed simultaneous reforms in the regulation of health care markets (Arnould et al. 1993). Competitive strategies fall into four broad categories: demand-side incentives, supply-side regulation, payer-driven price competition, and utilization controls (Exhibit 12–1).

Demand-Side Incentives

The underlying notion of cost sharing (discussed in Chapter 6) is that if consumers pay more of the insurance cost, they will be more cost-conscious in selecting the insurance plan that best serves their needs. They will not automatically opt for the most comprehensive plan. Also, when consumers pay a larger share of the cost of health care services they use, they will consume services more judiciously. In essence, cost sharing encourages consumers to ration their own health care. By foregoing unnecessary services, health care consumers can save money. Their cost-conscious behavior then leads to lower costs within the health delivery system as unnecessary utilization is minimized and the system becomes more cost-efficient.

Findings of the Rand Health Insurance Experiment, discussed earlier, have been confirmed by more recent evidence. In addition, Wong and colleagues (2001) demonstrated that, as a result of cost sharing, people are more likely to forego professional services for minor ailments than for more serious problems. Only very high levels of cost sharing deterred the use of medical care considered appropriate and necessary.

Supply-Side Regulation

As pointed out in Chapter 9, US antitrust laws prohibit business practices that stifle competition among providers. These practices include price fixing, price discrimination, exclusive contracting arrangements, and mergers the Department of Justice deems anticompetitive. The purpose of antitrust policy is to ensure the competitiveness, and thus the efficiency, of economic markets. In a competitive environment, MCOs, hospitals, and other health care organizations have to be cost-efficient to survive.

Payer-Driven Price Competition

Generally speaking, consumers drive competition. However, because health care markets are imperfect, patients are not typical consumers in the marketplace because insured patients lack the incentive to be good shoppers and because patients face information barriers that prevent them from being efficient shoppers. Despite the information boom, it is extremely difficult for individual patients or their surrogates to obtain needed information on cost and quality. Payer-driven competition in the form of managed care has overcome the drawbacks of patient-driven competition (Dranove 1993). Payer-driven competition occurs at two different points. First, employers shop for the best value in terms of the cost of premiums and the benefits package (competition among insurers). Second, MCOs shop for the best value from providers of health services (competition among providers).

Utilization Controls

Managed care also helps overcome some of the other inefficiencies of an imperfect health care market. The utilization controls in managed care (discussed in Chapter 9) have cut through some of the unnecessary or inappropriate services provided to consumers. Managed care is designed to intervene in the decisions made by care providers to ensure that they give only appropriate and necessary services, and that they provide the services efficiently. MCOs base this intervention on information that is not generally available to consumers. MCOs thus act on the consumer's behalf (Dranove 1993).

Access to Care

In broad terms, ***access*** to care is the ability to obtain needed, affordable, convenient, acceptable, and effective personal health services in a timely manner. Access has several key implications for health and health care delivery.

- Access to medical care is one of the key determinants of health, along with environment, lifestyle, and heredity factors (see Chapter 2).

- Access is a significant benchmark in assessing the effectiveness of the medical care delivery system. For example, access can be used to evaluate national trends against specific goals, such as those proposed in Healthy People 2010 (see Chapter 2), or to evaluate the performance and accountability of health care plans and providers.
- Measures of access reflect whether or not the delivery of health care is equitable.
- Recently, with the growth of managed care and the ensuing integration of health care delivery functions (financing, insurance, delivery, and payment), access is increasingly linked to quality of care and the efficient use of needed services.

Although "access" is a familiar term often employed by popular and academic media, it can indicate several different concepts. It may refer to whether an individual has a usual source of care (such as a primary care physician), the actual use of health services (based on availability, convenience, referral, etc.), or it may reflect the acceptability of particular services (according to an individual's preferences and values). In the 1970s, it was commonly perceived that more use was better, and the policy objective was to overcome barriers to access and to increase utilization. In the 1980s, under resource constraints, this belief was seriously challenged. The beginning of DRGs and prospective reimbursement mechanisms marked the end of unlimited use.

Framework of Access

The conceptualization of access to care (see Figure 12–8) can be traced to Andersen (1968) and was later refined by Aday and Andersen (1975) and Aday and colleagues (1980). Andersen (1968) believed that in addition to need, predisposing and enabling conditions also prompt some people to use more medical services than others. Predisposing conditions include an individual's sociodemographic characteristics, such as age, sex, education, marital status, family size, race and ethnicity, and religious preference. These factors indicate a person's propensity to use medical care. For example, holding everything else constant, elderly people are more likely to use medical care than young people are. The enabling conditions are income, socioeconomic status, price of medical services, financing of medical services, and occupation. They focus on the individual's means enabling that person to use medical care. For example, holding everything else constant, those with high incomes are more likely to use medical care than those with low incomes, particularly in countries where no national health insurance is provided.

The distinction between predisposing and enabling conditions can be applied to assess the equity of a health care system (Aday et al. 1993). To the extent that significant differences in medical care utilization can be explained by need and certain predisposing characteristics (e.g., age, gender), the delivery of medical care is considered equitable. When enabling characteristics create significant differences in medical care utilization, the delivery of medical care is considered inequitable.

This access to care model has been expanded to include characteristics of health policy and the health care delivery system (Aday et al. 1980). Examples of health policy include major health care financing initiatives (Medicare, Medicaid, State Children's Health Initiative) and organization of health services delivery (Medicaid managed care, community health centers). Character-

Figure 12–8 The Expanded Behavioral Model.

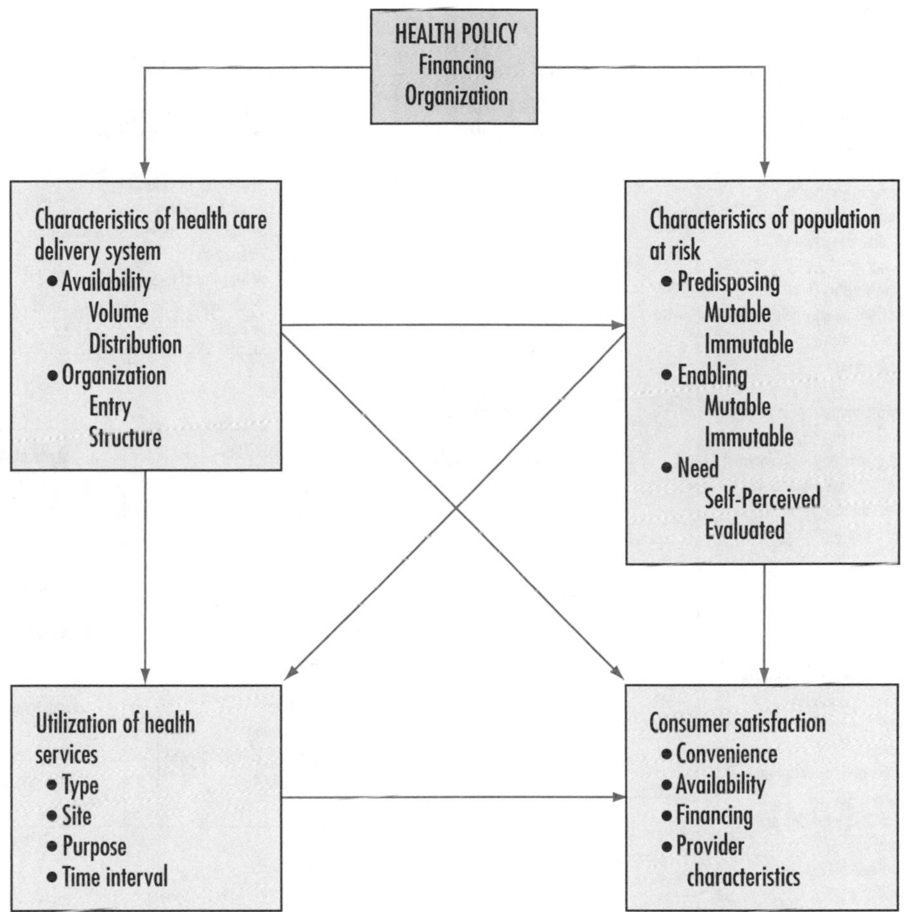

Source: L.A. Aday, R. Anderson, and D.V. Flaming, *Health Care in the US: Equitable for Whom?* p. 49, Copyright © 1980 by Sage Publications, Inc. Reprinted by permission of Sage Publications, Inc.

istics of the health care delivery system include availability (volume and distribution of services) and organization (mechanisms of entry into, and movement within, the system). Both health policy and the health care delivery system are aggregate components in contrast to the individual components of predisposing, enabling, and need characteristics. The expanded model recognizes the importance of systemic and structural barriers to access and is useful in comparing access to care among countries with different health policies and health care delivery systems.

Managed care's growth and the ensuing integration of the health care delivery functions represent a fundamental change in health care delivery. Accordingly, the access framework must be updated to reflect the new paradigm under managed care. Gold contributed a revised framework for access in the context of managed care (Docteur et al. 1996) (see Figure 12–9). According to this framework, access to care is a two-stage process in a managed care environment. In the first stage, individuals select among the health plans available to them, constrained

Figure 12–9 Framework for Access in the Managed Care Context.

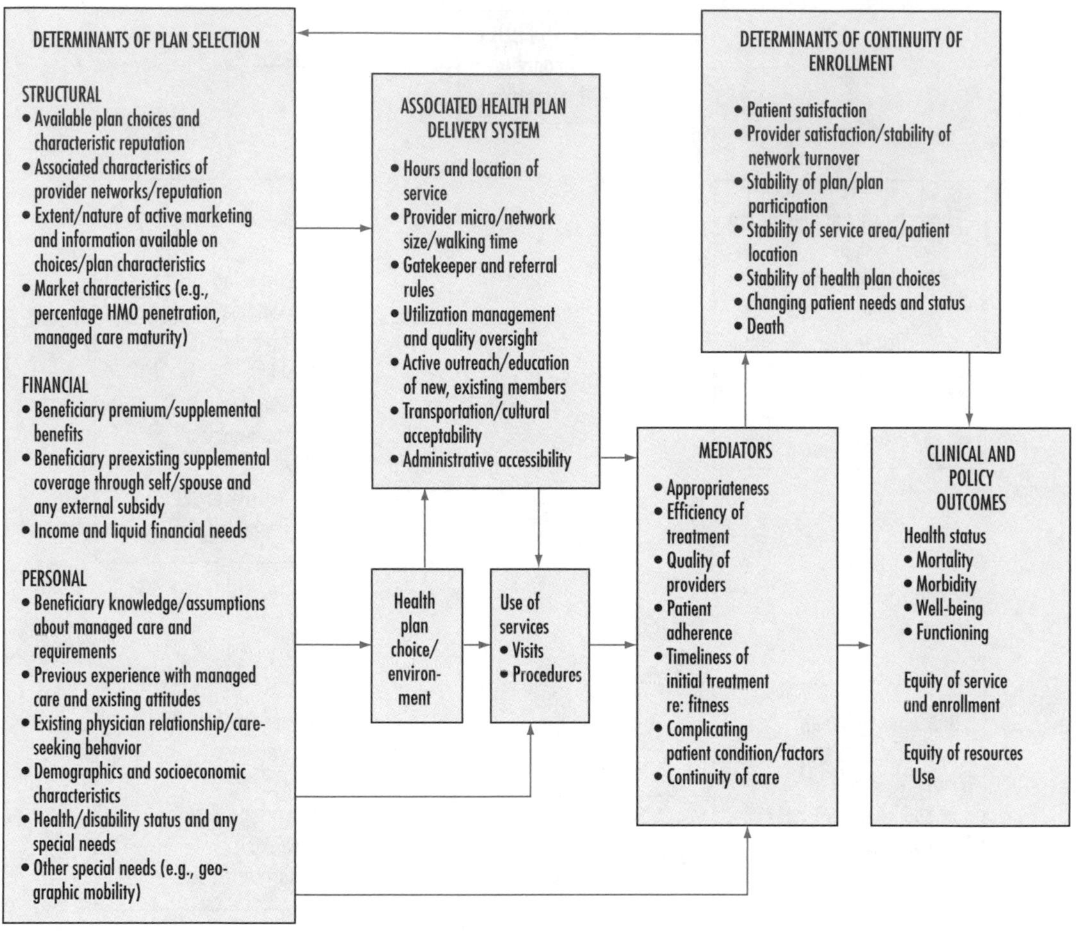

Source: Reprinted from E. Docteur and M. Gold, "Shifting the Paradigm," *Health Care Financing Review* 17, no. 4 (1996): p. 12.

by structural, financial, and personal characteristics. In the second stage, individuals seek medical care, constrained by both plan-specific and nonplan factors. The framework accounts for people enrolling and staying with the plan or disenrolling. It also links actual utilization with clinical and policy outcomes. Although comprehensive models are useful in conceptualizing access to care, they are difficult to test because of the range of variables and the differing levels of analysis they require. Empirical research is more likely to focus on specific dimensions of access.

Dimensions of Access

Penchansky and Thomas (1981) described access to care as consisting of five dimensions: availability, accessibility, accommodation, affordability, and acceptability.

Availability refers to the fit between service capacity and individuals' requirements. Availability-related issues include whether primary and preventive services are available to patients; whether enabling services, such as transportation, language, and social services, are made available by the provider;

whether the health plan has sufficient specialists to care for patients' needs; and whether access to primary care services is provided 24 hours a day, 7 days a week.

Accessibility refers to the fit between the locations of providers and patients. It is likely that individuals with different enabling conditions (e.g., transportation) may have different perceptions of accessibility. Accessibility-related issues include convenience (Can the provider be reached by public or private transportation?), design (Is the provider site designed for convenient use by disabled or elderly patients?), and payment options (Will the provider accept patients regardless of payment source, e.g., Medicare, Medicaid?).

Affordability refers to individuals' ability to pay. Even individuals with insurance often have to consider deductibles and copayments prior to utilization. Affordability-related questions include: Are insurance premiums too high? Are deductibles and copayments reasonable for the services covered under the plan? Are prescription prices affordable?

Accommodation refers to the fit between how resources are organized to provide services and the individual's ability to use the arrangement. Accommodation-related questions include: Can a patient schedule an appointment? Are scheduled office hours compatible with most patients' work and way of life? Can most of the urgent cases be seen within one hour? Can most patients with acute, but nonurgent, problems be seen within one day? Can most appropriate requests for routine appointments, such as preventive exams, be met within one week? Does the plan permit walk-in services?

Acceptability is based on the attitudes of patients and providers and refers to the compatibility between patients' attitudes about providers' personal and practice characteristics, and providers' attitudes toward their clients' personal characteristics and values. Acceptability issues include waiting time for scheduled appointments; whether patients are encouraged to ask questions and review their records; and whether patients and providers are accepted regardless of race, religion, or ethnic origin.

Types of Access

Andersen (1997) described four main types of access: potential access, realized access, equitable or inequitable access, and effective and efficient access.

Potential access refers to both health care system characteristics and enabling characteristics. Examples of health care system characteristics include capacity (e.g., physician–population ratio), organization (e.g., managed care penetration), and financing mechanisms (e.g., health insurance coverage). Enabling characteristics include personal (e.g., income) and community resources (e.g., residence).

Realized access refers to the type, site, and purpose of health services (Aday 1993). The type of utilization refers to the category of services rendered: physician, dentist, or other practitioners; hospital or long-term care admission; prescriptions; medical equipment; and so on. The site of utilization refers to the place where services are received (e.g., inpatient setting, such as short-stay hospital, mental institution, or nursing home; or ambulatory setting, such as hospital outpatient department, emergency department, physician's office, staff HMO, public health clinic, community health center, freestanding emergency center, or patient's home). The purpose of utilization refers to the reason medical care was sought: for health maintenance in the absence of symptoms (primary prevention), for the diagnosis or treatment of illness to return to well-being (secondary prevention or illness related), or for rehabilitation or maintenance in the case of a chronic health problem (tertiary prevention or custodial care).

Equitable access refers to the distribution of health care services according to the patient's self-perceived need (e.g., symptoms, pain, physical and functional status) or evaluated need as determined by a health professional (e.g., medical history, test results). Inequitable access refers to services distributed according to enabling characteristics (e.g., income, insured status).

Effective and efficient care links realized access to health outcomes (Institute of Medicine 1993). For example, does adequate prenatal care lead to successful birth outcomes, as measured by birth weight? Is immunization related to reduction of vaccine-preventable childhood diseases, such as diphtheria, measles, mumps, pertussis, polio, rubella, and tetanus? Are preventive services related to the early detection and diagnosis of treatable diseases? The concepts of effectiveness and efficiency link access to quality of care.

Measurement of Access

Using the conceptual models, access can be measured at three different levels: individual, health plan, and the delivery system. Access indicators at the individual level include (1) measures of medical services utilization relative to enabling and predisposing factors while controlling for need for care (Aday and Andersen, 1975) and (2) the patient's assessment of the interaction with the provider. Examples include differences in physician visits by race/ethnicity, gender, age, income, and insurance. Patients' perceived level of access is closely related to patient satisfaction with care and is part of the access framework (Aday et al. 1984).

At the health plan level, indicators include (1) plan characteristics that affect enrollment, such as cost of premium, deductibles, co-payments, coverage for preventive care, authorization of new and expensive procedures, physician referral incentives, and out-of-plan use; (2) plan practices that affect access, such as travel time to a usual source of care and waiting time to see a physician (accessibility), whether an appointment is necessary, hours of operation, language and other enabling services (accommodation), the content of encounters, including tests ordered and done, and referral to specialists (contact); and (3) plan quality as measured by the Health Plan Employer Data and Information Set (HEDIS) (discussed later) and patient satisfaction surveys.

Indicators of access at the level of the health care delivery system comprise ecological measures that affect populations rather than individuals. System indicators help study access in an environmental context; that is, how context affects the access of persons and groups. Examples of system access indicators include health policies or programs related to access, physician–population ratio, hospital beds per 1,000 population, percentage of population with insurance coverage, median household income, state per capita spending on welfare and preventive care, and percentage of population without access to primary care physicians.

Population-based surveys supported by federal statistical agencies are the major sources of data for conducting access-to-care analyses. Large national surveys, such as the National Health Interview Survey, the Medical Expenditure Panel Survey (MEPS), and the Community Tracking Survey are the leading data sources used to monitor access trends and other issues of interest. MEPS is a series of surveys that contain data on health care use and expenditures (e.g., inpatient, outpatient, and office-based care; dental care; and prescription medications), health insurance coverage, access to care, sources of payment, health status and disability, medical conditions, health care quality, and socioeconomic and demographic measures.

Other well-known national surveys include the Current Population Survey and Survey of Income and Program Participation (Bureau of the Census), which collects information on population characteristics. The Area Resource File (Bureau of Health Professions) pools information on characteristics of population and the health care delivery system. The National Health and Nutrition Examination Survey (National Center for Health Statistics [NCHS]) collects information on demographics, prevalence of selected diseases, nutrition, and behavioral risk factors. The National Hospital Discharge Survey (NCHS) provides data on short-stay hospital discharges and utilization. The Ambulatory Medical Care Survey (NCHS) provides data on ambulatory medical encounters. The National Hospital Ambulatory Medical Care Survey (NCHS) provides data on ambulatory hospital encounters. The National Nursing Home Survey (NCHS) provides data on nursing homes and utilization, nursing home residents, and nursing home staff. The Behavioral Risk Factor Survey (Centers for Disease Control and Prevention) provides data on health practices and behavioral risks of illness.

In addition, the federal government also collects data on special topics. Human immunodeficiency virus (HIV) and acquired immune deficiency syndrome (AIDS) were studied in the AIDS Cost and Services Utilization Survey 1991 to 1992 and the HIV Cost and Services Utilization Study 1994 to 1998. Managed care was studied in the Consumer Assessment of Health Plans Study 1996, and mental health is being examined in the Mental Health Care Services Study. Health care utilization by veterans, military staff, and dependents has been researched in the National Survey of Veterans 1994; the Patient Satisfaction Survey, Patient Treatment File; and AQCESS CHAMPUS. The Medicare Current Beneficiary Survey, the Medicare Statistical System, the Medicaid Data System, and the Medicaid Demonstration Projects (1983–1984, 1992–1996) have collected data relevant to Medicare and Medicaid. Other studies report on community health centers (Bureau of Common Reporting Requirement and Uniform Data System), immunization (National Immunization Survey), ambulatory surgery (National Survey of Ambulatory Surgery), home and hospice care (National Home and Hospice Care Survey), inpatient facilities (National Health Provider Inventory), aging (Longitudinal Survey on Aging), nursing homes (National Nursing Home Survey Follow-Up), insurance (National Employer Health Insurance Survey), and vital statistics (Vital Statistics of the US). The Bureau of Primary Care, Health Resources and Services Administration, collects information on vulnerable populations served by community health centers. In addition to the Uniform Data System, which collects center-specific financial, patient, and provider information, the Bureau regularly launches large-scale data collection on individual users. The Community Health Center Visit Survey, modeled after the National Ambulatory Medical Care Survey, collects information on patient visits to community health centers. The Community Health Center User Survey, modeled after the National Health Interview Survey, collects information from users of community health centers on a wide range of topics associated with health care and health practices.

In addition to the federal government, states, associations, and research institutions also regularly collect data on topics of interest to them. Examples of state-based initiatives include state health services utilization data (all-payer hospital discharge data systems), state managed care data (managed care encounter data), and state Medicaid enrollee satisfaction data (Medicaid enrollee satisfaction surveys). Examples of association-based initiatives include data on physicians (American Medical Association's Physician Masterfile and the Periodic Survey of Physicians 1969 to present) and hospitals (American Hospital Association's Annual Survey of Hospitals 1946 to present). Examples of research institution-based initiatives include collecting data on the health care delivery system (Center for Evaluative Clinical Sciences: Dartmouth Atlas of Health Care in the US), women's health (Kaiser Family Foundation: Women's Health Survey 2004), minority health (Commonwealth Fund: Minority Health Survey 1997), family health (Urban Institute National Survey of America's Families 1997, 1999, 2002), health insurance (Commonwealth Fund Bienniel Health Insurance Survey 2005), and access to care (Robert Wood Johnson Foundation National Access Surveys).

With the growth of managed care, encounter databases have become increasingly critical in recording and evaluating access. Good encounter databases combine electronic medical records (which contain diagnostic information based on ICD-9 and CPT codes) with administrative data (which contain plan, individual, payment, and cost information). In addition to the federal government, private nonprofit research centers also collect information on managed care. Examples are the National Health Maintenance Organization Census (1977 to the present, sponsored by Interstudy) and the HEDIS (sponsored by the National Committee for Quality Assurance [NCQA]).

Access to care data for vulnerable populations is systematically collected by the Sentinel Centers Network (SCN) initiative. The SCN is a partnership among the Bureau of Primary Health Care (BPHC), HRSA, the Johns Hopkins Bloomberg School of Public Health, and Morehouse School of Medicine. They are all participants in the SCN and BPHC health center grantees. The SCN is currently composed of 37 participants located in the majority of states in the United States. Approximately 650 health care practitioners provide services to 1 million registered users within the SCN. The SCN data system is the first primary care administrative database that focuses exclusively on care delivery and outcomes for medically underserved populations.

Current Indicators of Access

In the United States, significant barriers to access still exist at both the individual and the system level. People without health insurance, minorities, low-income individuals, those with little formal education, or those with special needs defined by disability and chronic illness continue to face greater barriers to access than the rest of the population. Access is best predicted by race, income, and occupation. These three factors are interrelated. People belonging to minority groups tend to be poor, not well educated, and more likely to work in jobs that pose greater health risks.

Geographic disparities in access are also present, and individuals from rural areas face greater access barriers than those residing in urban areas. Rural Americans have higher

Table 12–3 Visits to Office-Based Physicians, 2004

Characteristic	Number of Visits (million)	Percentage Distribution	Visits per 100 Persons/Year
All visits	910.9	100.0	315.9
Age			
Under 15 years old	147.9	16.2	243.4
15–44 years old	264.9	29.1	410.3
45–64 years old	264.1	29.0	376.2
65–74 years old	113.4	12.4	622.6
75 years old and over	120.6	13.2	733.6

Source: Data from US Bureau of the Census. *Statistical Abstracts of the United States, 2007,* Washington, DC, p. 112.

mortalities and morbidities and shorter life expectancies than their urban counterparts (Cordes 1989; DeFriese and Ricketts 1989; Rowland and Lyons 1989; Sherman 1991). Rural Americans are more likely to be poor, to suffer from chronic impairment, to be uninsured if under 65 years of age and to be elderly than their urban counterparts (Norton and McManus 1989). The health care system available to address these problems, however, faces severe limitations, including maldistribution of physicians, lack of sufficient primary care services, and lack of access to care for geographic, financial, or discrimination/cultural reasons (Freeman et al. 1982; Sardell 1988). Tables 12–3 and 12–4 summarize physician contacts by categories of age, sex, race, income, and geographic location. Table 12–5 summarizes dental visits. These results are not adjusted for health need, however, and therefore are not true indicators of access. Rather, they provide utilization measures as a proxy for access.

It is society's duty to ensure that all have equitable access to an adequate level of health care. According to one view, economic scarcity is a relative measure. Scarcity in the US medical delivery system is largely the result of distributive practices that limit access for

Table 12–4 Physician Contracts, According to Selected Patient Characteristics, 1996

Characteristic	Physician Contacts per Person
Total	5.8
Sex	
Male	5.0
Female	6.5
Race and age	
White	5.8
Black	5.7
Family income	
Less than $16,000	7.5
$16,000–$24,999	5.5
$25,000–$34,999	5.6
$35,000–$44,999	5.9
$50,000 or more	5.3
Geographic region	
Northeast	5.7
Midwest	5.7
South	6.1
West	5.3
Location of residence	
Within MSA	5.8
Outside MSA	5.7

Source: Data from *Health, United States, 1999,* p. 229, National Center for Health Statistics, Division of Health Interview Statistics, 1999.

Table 12–5 Dental Visits in the Past Year among Persons 18–64 Years of Age, 2004

Characteristic	Percentage of Persons
All persons	64.0
Poverty status	
Poor	44.5
Near poor	47.6
Nonpoor	71.3
Race and Hispanic origin	
White, non-Hispanic	65.2
Black, non-Hispanic	56.9
Hispanic	49.6
Sex	
Male	60.5
Female	67.4

Source: Data from *Health, United States, 2006,* p. 329, National Center for Health Statistics.

those who are poor and those who live in rural areas. In the overall system, a surplus exists, for instance, of hospital beds and physicians practicing in urban areas. The problem is that these surpluses are not generally shifted to respond to need (Brown 1992).

Earlier chapters discussed the lack of access for the uninsured. Access, however, is also limited because of underinsurance and, for a few people, because of lifetime caps on health insurance. For years, these lifetime caps have been arbitrarily set at about $1 to $2 million. A number of otherwise insured Americans are affected by lifetime caps because of a costly catastrophic injury or illness. For example, the average lifetime cost of care for a person with a spinal cord injury who is ventilator-dependent can be more than $5 million. When the cap is reached, insurance companies stop coverage, although the need for medical care continues.

Quality of Care

One reason why the pursuit of quality in health care has trailed behind the emphasis on cost and access is the difficulty of defining and measuring quality. On the other hand, growth of managed care and the emphasis on cost containment have produced a heightened interest in quality because of the intuitive concern that control of costs may negatively impact quality. Indeed, changes occurring within the US health care delivery system in recent years have created fears of diminished quality because these changes have brought about disruptions in the way health care professionals are allowed to provide care and the way in which patients may seek care. Since the 1990s, quality has taken center stage in the delivery of health care. However, a great deal of ambiguity still exists about the definition of quality. There is still a long road ahead to specify what constitutes good quality in medical care, how to ensure it for patients, and how to reward providers and health plans whose outcomes indicate successes in quality improvement. One challenge in achieving such a goal is that patients, providers, and payers each define quality differently, which translates into different expectations of the health care delivery system and thus differing evaluations of its quality (McGlynn 1997).

The Institute of Medicine (IOM) has defined ***quality*** as "the degree to which health services for individuals and populations increase the likelihood of desired health outcomes and are consistent with current professional knowledge" (McGlynn 1997). The definition has several implications: (1) Quality performance occurs on a continuum, theoretically ranging from unacceptable to excellent. (2) The focus is on services provided by the health care delivery system (as opposed to individual behaviors). (3) Quality may be evaluated from the perspective of individuals and populations or communities. (4) The emphasis is on desired health outcomes. Research evidence must identify the services that improve health outcomes. (5) In the absence of scientific evidence regarding appropriateness of care, professional consensus can be used to develop criteria for the definition and measurement of quality (McGlynn 1997).

Although complete in many respects, the IOM definition leaves out the role of cost in the evaluation of quality. Even though the United States spends more of its national income on health care than other nations, Americans are not the healthiest people in the world. For example, based on comparative data on 37 countries, 27 nations had better outcomes than the United States on infant mortality rates in 2003, and 25 countries had better outcomes on life expectancy at birth for both males and females in 2002 (National Center for Health Statistics 2006). Clearly, more health care expenditures or a greater intensity of medical services does not produce better health. In other words, more is not better, and more does not represent better quality.

Another element missing from the IOM definition is the relationship between access and quality. Perhaps a key reason why the United States, despite its tremendous advances in medical technology, trails behind other industrialized nations in broad population measures of health is lack of access to basic health care for many Americans. Hence, unless access to primary care and preventive services is improved, population-based indicators of health are unlikely to improve. In other words, amelioration of the overall quality of the US health care delivery system would require universal access to basic health care.

Dimensions of Quality

Quality needs to be viewed from both micro and macro perspectives. The microview focuses on services at the point of delivery and their subsequent effects. It is associated with the performance of individual caregivers and health care organizations. The macroview looks at quality from the standpoint of populations. It reflects the performance of the entire health care delivery system.

The Microview

The micro dimension of health care quality encompasses the clinical aspects of care delivery, the interpersonal aspects of care delivery, and quality of life.

Clinical Aspects

Clinical aspects of care deal with technical quality, which evaluates the appropriateness of care according to several criteria. Some of the key criteria evaluated to determine clinical appropriateness of care are the facilities where care is delivered, the qualifications and skills of caregivers, the processes and interventions used, cost-efficiency of care, and the results or effects on patients' health.

Small area variations, discussed earlier in this chapter, compromise clinical quality. Geographic variations also indicate widespread inefficiencies. Hence, addressing the problem of clinical variations would result in improved cost as well as quality. The variability in the delivery of care cannot be blamed on physicians alone. The variations do not reflect negatively on the sincerity, honesty, or diligence of most physicians. One of the main causes of variability is that physicians often have to make decisions about phenomenally complex problems under difficult circumstances. Often, they are in the impossible position of not knowing the outcomes of different actions, but having to act anyway (Eddy 1994).

Incidents of medical errors in hospitals have been widely reported. For example, the IOM reported that 44,000 to 98,000 patients die in American hospitals each year because of medical errors, making "adverse events" the eighth leading cause of death in the United States (IOM 2000). Even though medical errors and adverse events in outpatient settings have not received as much emphasis, concerns do exist. One reason the outpatient sector has not come under the spotlight is that only a handful of states have implemented reporting systems for it (Lapetina and Armstrong 2002). Yet, evidence is slowly gathering for adverse occurrences in outpatient settings. For example, death and brain damage due to adverse anesthesia administration for children have been found to be more than twice as high in outpatient settings as in hospitals (Coté 2000). The mortality rate for lipoplasty, a cosmetic procedure for remodeling fat tissue under skin, is higher than it is for motor vehicle deaths and homicides; most of the deaths occur in outpatient settings (Minino and Smith 2001). As an increasing number of surgical procedures are now being performed in ambulatory clinics, surgi-centers, and physicians' offices, medical errors in the outpatient sector are likely to come under increased scrutiny.

Interpersonal Aspects

When quality is viewed from the patient's perspective, clinical quality remains important, but interpersonal aspects of care take on added significance. Patients generally lack technical expertise and often judge the quality of technical care indirectly by their perceptions of the practitioner's interest, concern, and demeanor during clinical encounters (Donabedian 1985). Interpersonal relations and satisfaction become even more important when placed within the holistic context of health care delivery. Positive interactions between patients and practitioners are major contributors to treatment success through greater patient compliance and return for care (Svarstad 1986). Expressions of love, hope, and compassion can enhance the healing effects of medical treatments. Without these elements, the quality of health care remains incomplete.

Interpersonal aspects of quality are also important from the standpoint of organizational management. Consumers—that is, patients and their surrogates—gain lasting impressions of organizational quality from the way they are treated by an organization's employees. Such employee–customer interactions include not just the direct caregivers but a variety of other employees associated with the health care organization, such as receptionists, workers in the cafeteria, housekeeping employees, and billing clerks.

To measure interpersonal aspects of quality, patient satisfaction surveys have been widely used by various types of health care organizations. Ratings by consumers provide the most appropriate method for evaluating interpersonal quality (McGlynn and Brook 1996). Satisfaction surveys have been used to give physicians feedback on important dimensions of interpersonal communication and service quality. Evidence suggests that such feedback has achieved widespread acceptance by physicians, with more than three-fourths of the physicians affected by such surveys reacting positively to their use (Reed et al. 2003).

Quality of Life

The concept of quality of life has received a great deal of attention in recent years because patients with chronic and/or debilitating diseases are living longer but in a declining state of health. Chronic problems often impose serious limitations on patients' functional status (including physical, social, and mental functioning), access to community resources and opportunities, and sense of well-being (Lehman 1995). In a composite sense, during or subsequent to disease, a person's own perception of health, ability to function, role limitations stemming from physical or emotional problems, and personal happiness are referred to as health-related quality of life (***HRQL***).

An even narrower definition of quality of life has been proposed. Although a few basic measurements might be applicable to everyone in every situation (general HRQL), many more are relevant only to a particular patient or to patients suffering from a specific disease (disease-specific HRQL). General HRQL refers to the essential or common components of overall well-being. Disease-specific HRQL is associated with the potential quality of life impacts of a specific disorder and its treatment. Disease-specific HRQL focuses entirely on impairments that are caused by a specific disorder and the effects and side effects of treatments for that disorder. For example, arthritis quality of life is concerned with joint pain and mobility and the side effects of antiinflammatory agents; depression quality of life deals with the symptoms of depression (such as suicidal thoughts) and such medication side effects as blurred vision, dry mouth, constipation, and impotence (Bergner 1989); and cancer-specific HRQL may include anxiety about cancer recurrence (Ganz and Litwin 1996) and pain management.

Institution-related quality of life is also an important attribute of quality in addition to the clinical and interpersonal aspects. It refers to a patient's quality of life while confined in an institution as an inpatient. Factors contributing to institutional quality of life can be classified into three main groups: environmental comfort, self-governance, and caregiver attitudes. Cleanliness, safety, noise levels, odors, air circulation, environmental temperature, and furnishings are some of the key comfort factors that are particularly relevant to the physical aspects of institutional living. Factors associated with self-governance and staff attitudes, in particular, influence the emotional well-being of institutionalized patients. Self-governance means autonomy to make decisions, freedom to air grievances without fear of reprisal, and reasonable accommodation of personal likes and dislikes. Factors associated with caregiver attitudes are privacy and confidentiality, treatment from staff in a manner that maintains respect and dignity, and freedom from physical and/or emotional abuse.

The Macroview

The macroview encompasses systemwide efficiencies and outcomes, which include cost, access, and population health. Some of the other indicators of macro level quality are life expectancy, mortality rates, cause-specific mortality, low birth weight deliveries, and incidence and prevalence of specific diseases or chronic conditions. Access to health care has considerable influence on population health. The prospects of universal access in the United States are contingent on drastic reductions in health care expenditures. Without significant improvements in access, the US health care delivery system will continue to be rated behind most others in the developed world. From a systems standpoint, this predicament requires national policy initiatives, but it does not diminish the need to pursue quality improvements at the micro level over which practitioners, ancillary workers, and health care managers have more control.

Quality Assurance

The terms "quality assessment" and "quality assurance" are often encountered in literature on health care quality. Yet, these terms are not always well defined or differentiated. ***Quality assessment*** refers to the measurement of quality against an established standard. It includes the process of defining how quality is to be determined, identification of specific variables or indicators to be measured, collection of appropriate data to make the measurement possible, statistical analysis, and interpretation of the results of the assessment (Williams and Brook 1978). ***Quality assurance*** is synonymous with quality improvement. It is the process of institutionalizing quality through ongoing assessment and using the results of assessment for continuous quality improvement (CQI) (Williams and Torrens 1993). Quality assurance, then, is a step beyond quality assessment. It is a systemwide or organizationwide commitment to engage in the improvement of quality on an ongoing basis. Although the two activities—quality assessment and quality assurance—are related, quality assurance cannot occur without quality assessment. Quality assessment becomes an integral part of the process of quality assurance. On the other hand, it is possible to conduct quality assessment without engaging in quality assurance.

In the past, quality assurance focused on observing deviations from established standards by means of inspection techniques and was used in conjunction with punitive actions for noncompliance. The nursing home industry presents a typical case. Standards of patient care in nursing homes and the system for evaluating performance were developed mainly in conjunction with the certification of facilities for Medicare and/or Medicaid. Federal regulations developed by HCFA (now Centers for Medicare and Medicaid Services) are viewed as minimum standards or baseline criteria for defining quality of resident care in certified facilities. Compliance with the standards is monitored through annual inspections of the facilities (Singh 1997, 33–34), and serious noncompliance is punishable by monetary fines and threats of expulsion from Medicare and Medicaid. Although such external monitoring of quality is necessary (Lohr 1997), it is not quality assurance in the true sense. Rather, it is a rudimentary form of quality assessment that would be more appropriately referred to as "periodic monitoring of quality."

Quality assurance is based on the principles of total quality management (TQM), also referred to as CQI. The philosophy of TQM was developed and used in other industries before it was adapted for health care delivery. ***TQM*** is an integrative management concept of continuously improving the quality of delivered goods and services through the participation of all levels and functions of the organization (Evans 1993) to meet the needs and expectations of the customer. TQM encompasses five main elements: (1) Quality is an integrative concept. It must permeate everything that a health care organization does. In other words, it is not simply confined to the delivery of health services to patients, but applies equally to activities that support clinical care. Examples of supportive services include business office, housekeeping, and building and equipment maintenance functions. TQM must also have the support and commitment of the top management and managers at all levels. (2) The organization is committed to ongoing improvement. This means that the standards against which quality is assessed do not remain static. As soon as the current standards of performance are achieved, higher standards are set. The ultimate goal is to achieve a zero error rate or a 100% success rate. Even though such a state of perfection may never be attained, goals must nevertheless be set toward its achievement. (3) Everyone working in the organization plays a part in the production of quality goods and services. (4) TQM emphasizes the value of striving to exceed prevailing standards. This suggests an imperative to study the processes throughout the organization by which health care is produced and provided (Laffel and Blumenthal 1993). (5) TQM needs to be customer driven. The efforts of TQM are directed toward customer satisfaction. In a general sense, customers are the recipients (not necessarily the purchasers) of a service or product. From the organizational perspective, there are both internal and external customers. The organization's internal customers are the users of products or services that ultimately influence the quality of patient care. For example, nursing units are customers of the pharmacy, which must furnish the right medications as ordered by the physicians. The pharmacy is the customer of the physicians, who must prescribe legibly and correctly. Patients and communities are the external customers who ultimately benefit from the results of TQM. The adoption of TQM by many hospitals and health systems has streamlined administration, reduced lengths of stay, improved clinical outcomes, and produced higher levels of patient satisfaction (HCIA Inc. and Deloitte & Touche 1997).

Quality Assessment

Quality assessment is particularly difficult because it requires the measurement of phenomena that are often subjective or qualitative. They must be quantified to be measured and compared. Measurement scales are developed to assess quality defined by qualitative concepts. Before these scales are used, their validity and reliability must be established. The ***validity*** of a scale is the extent to which it actually assesses what it purports to measure. If a measure is supposed to reflect the quality of care, one would expect improvements in quality to affect the measure positively. In other words, the measurement scale would show a higher score for improved quality and vice versa. ***Reliability*** reflects the extent to which the same results occur from repeated applications of a measure. The following sections survey some of the main criteria and mechanisms used to evaluate quality.

The Donabedian Model

In his well-known model to help define and measure quality in health care organizations, Donabedian proposed three domains in which health care quality should be examined: structure, process, and outcomes. Donabedian noted that all three domains are equally important. He also emphasized that these three approaches are complementary and should be used collectively to monitor care quality (Al-Assaf 1993b).

Structure, process, and outcomes are closely linked (Figure 12–10). The three

Figure 12–10 The Donabedian Model.

Final Results

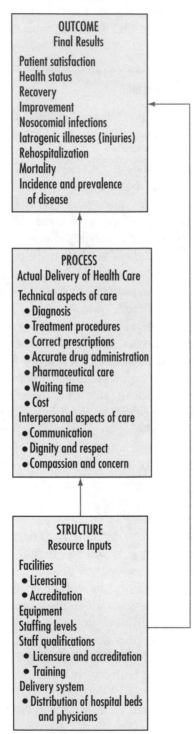

domains are also hierarchical. Structure is the foundation of the quality of health care. Good processes require a good structure. In other words, deficiencies in structure generally have a negative effect on the processes of health care delivery. Structure and processes together influence quality outcomes. Structure primarily influences process and has only a secondary direct influence on outcome. The model views quality strictly from the delivery system's perspective. It does not account for social and individual lifestyle and behavior factors that also have a significant influence on health status.

• Compassion and concern
Structure

Structure has been defined as "the relatively stable characteristics of the providers of care, of the tools and resources they have at their disposal, and of the physical and organizational settings in which they work" (Donabedian 1980, 81). Structural criteria refer to the resource inputs, such as facilities, equipment, staffing levels, staff qualifications, programs, and the administrative organization (Guralnik et al. 1991; McElroy and Herbelin 1989). Structural measures indicate the extent to which health care organizations have the capability to provide adequate levels of care (Williams and Torrens 1993). Hence, structure provides an indirect measure of quality, under the assumption that a good structure enables health delivery professionals to employ good processes that would lead to good outcomes.

In the past, it was common to rely mostly on the evaluation of structural measures for quality assessment. As such, they were designed to ensure that certain minimum standards were met. Examples are licensing of facilities, accreditation of facilities by the Joint Commission on Accreditation of Healthcare Organizations (Joint Commission), and licensing and certification of health care professionals to ensure that they meet certain minimum qualifications. Training of personnel is designed to improve the structural elements of quality. From a system-wide macroperspective, structural elements include the number of physicians and hospital beds available per 1,000 population; the geographic distribution of physicians, hospitals, and nursing home beds; and the mix between primary care and specialist physicians.

Process

Process refers to the specific way in which care is provided. Examples of process are correct diagnostic tests, correct prescriptions, accurate drug administration, pharmaceutical care (see Chapter 4), waiting time to see a physician, and interpersonal aspects of care delivery. Peer review, discussed earlier in this chapter, was designed to serve a dual purpose: control costs and ensure that quality does not suffer. The activities of PROs rely mainly on process indicators in evaluating the quality of care provided to Medicare patients (Al-Assaf 1993a).

Like structure, process relates to patient care outcomes. In other words, structures and processes should be employed to achieve better outcomes. Some significant initiatives toward process improvement have been undertaken. Some main developments are clinical practice guidelines, cost-efficiency, critical pathways, and risk management.

Clinical Practice Guidelines

As discussed earlier, small area variations bring into question the appropriateness of care. In response, various professional groups, MCOs, and the government have embarked on the development of standardized practice guidelines. ***Clinical practice guidelines*** (also called medical practice guidelines) are explicit descriptions representing preferred clinical processes for specified conditions. A clinical practice guideline constitutes a plan to manage a clinical problem based on evidence whenever possible, and on consensus in the absence of evidence (Larsen 1996). Hence, clinical practice guidelines are designed to provide scientifically-based protocols to guide physicians' clinical decisions. Proponents believe that these guidelines simultaneously promote lower costs and better outcomes. Critics view guidelines as an administrative mechanism to reduce utilization. By the mid-1990s, 75 national organizations had developed approximately 1,800 sets of guidelines, and individual hospitals, MCOs, private researchers, and pharmaceutical manufacturers developed thousands of others (Firshein 1996).

The US Congress established the Agency for Health Care Policy and Research in 1989. This agency was reauthorized under the Healthcare Research and Quality Act of 1999, and was renamed Agency for Healthcare Research and Quality (AHRQ). Although the agency has a broad research agenda, one of its primary mandates is to build the scientific base of which health care practices work and which do not. In this role, the agency develops the information, tools, and strategies that decision-makers can use to make good clinical choices necessary to provide high-quality health care based on evidence. These activities have been mandated in the belief that they will eliminate inappropriate medical interventions and reduce health care costs (IOM 1990). AHRQ has established a National Guideline Clearinghouse (NGC) in partnership with the American Medical Association and the American

Association of Health Plans. The NGC is a comprehensive database of evidence-based clinical practice guidelines and related documents. It facilitates access to information produced by different organizations by making it all available at one site.

After some initial reluctance by physicians, current evidence suggests that clinical practice guidelines are being viewed positively. According to one report, among physicians affected by this care management tool, 66% expressed a positive view (only 8% were negative) on its overall effect on quality and efficiency of medical practice (Reed et al. 2003).

Cost-Efficiency

Also referred to as cost-effectiveness, ***cost-efficiency*** (discussed in Chapter 5 in conjunction with technology assessment) is an important concept in quality assessment. A service is cost-efficient when the benefit received is greater than the cost incurred to provide the service. Cost-efficiency uses the health production function to evaluate the relationship between increasing medical expenditures (or health risks) and improvements in health levels. As medical interventions and expenditures are increased, there is a curvilinear, rather than a constant, effect on improved health (Feldstein 1994, 26). At the start of medical treatment, each unit is likely to deliver benefits exceeding its costs, or benefits exceeding the potential risks. The marginal (i.e., additional) health benefits become smaller and risks become bigger, as more care is delivered and greater costs are incurred (see Figure 5–2). An optimum point is reached when additional health benefits approximately equal the additional costs (or risks). Beyond this point, additional interventions result in fewer benefits in relation to the additional costs, or the risks are greater than the benefits. In economic terms, additional services beyond the optimum point produce diminishing marginal returns. This point also represents optimal quality, which serves as a point of demarcation between underutilization and overutilization.

Underutilization (underuse) occurs when the benefits of an intervention outweigh its risks or costs, and yet it is not used (Chassin 1991). Potential adverse health outcomes related to underutilization include hospitalizations that could be avoided by providing better medical access and timely care, low birth weight due to lack of prenatal care, infant mortality due to lack of early pediatric care, and low cancer survival rates due to lack of early detection and treatment. On the other hand, ***overutilization*** (overuse) occurs when the costs or risks of treatment outweigh its benefits, and yet additional care is delivered. When health care is overused, precious resources are wasted. Hence, inefficiency can be regarded as unethical because it deprives someone else of the potential benefits of health care. The principles of cost-efficiency indicate that health care costs can be reduced without lowering quality of care. Conversely, quality can be improved without increasing costs. A trade-off does not have to occur between cost and quality. Introduction of the prospective payment system (PPS) by Medicare is an example. The resulting discharge of patients "quicker and sicker" triggered by PPS initially raised some alarm concerning decreased quality, but it was found that processes of care in hospitals actually improved and mortality rates were unchanged or lower (Rogers et al. 1990). Other potential negative health outcomes that can be avoided by curtailing overuse include life-threatening drug interactions, nosocomial infections, and iatrogenic illnesses.

Critical Pathways

Critical pathways are outcome-based and patient-centered case management tools that are interdisciplinary, facilitating coordination of care among multiple clinical departments and caregivers. In the last few years, critical pathways have been used across multiple delivery settings. A critical pathway is a timeline that identifies planned medical interventions along with expected patient outcomes for a specific diagnosis or class of cases, often defined by a DRG. The outcomes and interventions included in the critical pathway are broadly defined. In addition to technical outcomes, pathways may measure such factors as patient satisfaction, self-reported health status, mental health, and activities of daily living (ADL). Interventions include treatments, medications, diagnostic tests, diet, activity regimens, consultations, discharge planning, and patient education. The critical pathway serves as a plan of action for all disciplines caring for the patient and incorporates a system for documenting and evaluating variances from the critical path plan. Critical pathways are unique to the institutions that develop them because they are based on the particular practices of that facility and its caregivers. A pathway also is customized to the patient population being served and the available patient care resources. Finally, critical pathways are meant to promote interdisciplinary collaboration within the environment of the hospital and its market. The latter occurs by making patients and families active participants in the process. For these reasons, critical pathways are difficult to replicate from one organization to another. Use of critical pathways reduces costs and improves quality by reducing errors, improving coordination among interdisciplinary players, streamlining case management functions, providing systematic data to assess care, and reducing variation in practice patterns (Giffin and Giffin 1994).

Risk Management

Risk management consists of proactive efforts to prevent adverse events related to clinical care and facilities operations and is especially focused on avoiding medical malpractice (Orlikoff 1988). Malpractice lawsuits are a deterrent to poor technical quality of care and provide redress for patients experiencing such care (Williams and Torrens 1993). In response to the threat of lawsuits, initiatives undertaken by a health care organization to review clinical processes and establish protocols for the specific purpose of reducing malpractice litigation can actually enhance quality. Because malpractice concerns also result in defensive medicine, risk management approaches should employ the principles of cost-efficiency along with standardized practice guidelines and critical pathways.

Threat of malpractice litigation also has a downside. Fear of litigation actually leads to a reluctance by hospitals and physicians to disclose preventable harm and actual medical errors. In this respect, it is believed that fear of litigation may actually conceal problems that may compromise patient safety (Lamb et al. 2003).

Outcomes

Outcomes refer to the effects or results obtained from utilizing the structure and processes of health care delivery. Outcomes are viewed by many as the bottom-line measure of the effectiveness of the health care delivery system (McGlynn and Brook 1996).

Positive outcomes suggest recovery from disease and improvement in health. They also suggest an overall improvement in health status through health promotion and disease prevention and adequate access to health care services. Outcomes are often gauged through a comparative assessment—between two time intervals—of the measures of morbidity, mortality, and health status presented in Chapter 2. Other outcome measures include postoperative infection rates, nosocomial infections, iatrogenic illnesses, and rates of rehospitalization. Malpractice litigation is sometimes used as an outcome indicator because litigation seeks damages for negative outcomes. Another indicator of positive outcome is patient satisfaction (discussed earlier), which is assessed through questionnaires completed by patients and/or surrogates.

Quality outcomes are also evaluated using interview techniques and self-administered questionnaires to report on functional status, neuropsychiatric function, social function, and emotional and spiritual health. Determination of HRQL is an example. Typically, HRQL data are collected with self-report questionnaires, called "instruments," using survey research techniques. These instruments contain questions or items organized into scales. Each scale measures a different aspect or domain of HRQL. Some scales comprise dozens of items, whereas others may include only one or two items (Ganz and Litwin 1996). HRQL domains can be general, disease-specific, or institution-related.

None of the outcome measures provides a perfect assessment. Each measure focuses on a particular aspect of quality. Hence, using a combination of measures is likely to produce more objective results, but there is a cost and benefit trade-off. The greater the number of measures used for evaluating quality, the more costly the assessment process.

Quality Report Cards

The growing predominance of managed care raised concerns that efforts to control costs may jeopardize quality. The move to develop quality report cards for health plans responded to these concerns. The report cards can be used by employers and their employees to make health plan choices. Health Plan Employer Data and Information Set ***(HEDIS)*** has become the standard for reporting quality information on managed care health plans. This quality tool is a product of a partnership established in 1989 among health plans, employers, and the National Committee for Quality Assurance (NCQA), which now manages the HEDIS program. The latest edition is HEDIS 2007. Originally designed for private employers' needs as purchasers of health insurance, HEDIS has been adapted for use by the public, public insurers, and regulators. HEDIS 2007 contains over 70 measures across eight domains of care: effectiveness of care, access and availability of care, satisfaction with care, health plan stability, use of services, cost of care, informed health care choices, and health plan descriptive information (NCQA 2007). The HEDIS program has been criticized because disclosure is voluntary. In the absence of a national requirement, the voluntary aspect of reporting affords health plans the ability to restrict public disclosure and allows poorly performing health plans to escape public scrutiny (Thompson et al. 2003). Such selective nondisclosure undermines both informed consumer decision-making and public accountability (McCormick et al. 2002). However, MCOs seeking accreditation from NCQA (see Chapter 9) are required to provide HEDIS results, which are audited by an NCQA certified auditor (NCQA 2003).

Summary

Increasing costs, lack of access, and concerns about quality pose the greatest challenges to health care delivery in the United States. To some extent, the three issues are interrelated. Increasing costs limit the system's ability to expand access, and without universal coverage for all Americans, they may never match the health status of populations in other developed countries. Despite spending the most resources on health care, the United States continues to rank in the bottom quartile among developed countries on outcome indicators, such as life expectancy and infant mortality. In fact, its relative ranking has been declining since 1960 (Anderson 1997).

Nations that have national health insurance can control systemwide costs through top-down controls, mainly in the form of global budgets. This approach is not possible in the United States because it has a multi-payer system. In the United States, regulatory approaches have been used to try to constrain the supply-side, but the major emphasis has been on constricting reimbursement to providers. Several competitive approaches have been used, mainly through the expansion of managed care. A move toward prospective payments and the growth of managed care can be largely credited with the brakes put on rising health care spending during the 1990s. However, the best current forecasts are for accelerated spending growth in the future, which means that a growing share of economic resources will be devoted to the delivery of health care.

Access to medical care is one of the key determinants of health status, along with environment, lifestyle, and heredity factors. Access is also regarded as a significant benchmark in assessing the effectiveness of the medical care delivery system. Access is explained in terms of enabling and predisposing factors, as well as factors related to health policy and health care delivery. Access has five dimensions: availability, accessibility, accommodation, affordability, and acceptability. Measures of access can relate to individuals, health care plans, and the health care delivery system.

Quality in health care has been difficult to define and measure, although it is receiving increasing emphasis. At the micro level, health care quality encompasses the clinical aspects of care delivery, the interpersonal aspects of care delivery, and quality of life. Indicators of quality at the macro level are commonly associated with life expectancy, mortality, and morbidity. Quality assessment is the measurement of quality against an established standard. Quality assurance emphasizes improvement of quality using the principles of CQI. Donabedian proposed that quality should be assessed along three dimensions: structure, process, and outcomes. These three approaches are complementary and should be used collectively to monitor quality of care. Reliability and validity are important concepts in the measurement of quality.

Test Your Understanding

Terminology

access
administrative costs
all-payer system
certificate-of-need
clinical practice guidelines
competition
cost-efficiency
cost shifting
critical pathways
defensive medicine
fraud
health planning
HEDIS
HRQL
institution-related quality of life
outcomes
overutilization
peer review
PRO
QIO
quality
quality assessment
quality assurance
reliability
risk management
small area variations
top-down control
TQM
underutilization
validity

Review Questions

1. What is meant by the term "health care costs"? Describe the three different meanings of the term "cost."
2. Why should the United States control the rising costs of health care?
3. How do findings of the Rand Health Insurance Experiment reinforce the relationship between growth in third-party reimbursement and increase in health care costs? Explain.
4. Explain how, under imperfect market conditions, both prices and quantity of health care are higher than they would be in a highly competitive market.
5. What are some of the reasons for increased health care costs that are attributed to the providers of medical care?
6. What are some of the main differences between broad cost-containment approaches used in the United States and those used in countries with national health insurance?
7. Discuss the effectiveness of CON regulation in controlling health care expenditures.
8. Discuss price controls and their effectiveness in controlling health care expenditures.
9. Discuss the role of PROs (QIOs) in cost containment.
10. What are the four competition-based cost-containment strategies?
11. What are the implications of access for health and health care delivery?
12. What is the role of enabling and predisposing factors in access to care?
13. Briefly describe the five dimensions of access.
14. What are the four main types of access described by Anderson?

15. Describe the measurement of access at the individual, health plan, and delivery system levels.
16. What are some of the implications of the definition of quality proposed by the Institute of Medicine? In what way is the definition incomplete?
17. Discuss the dimensions of quality from the micro and macro perspectives.
18. Discuss the two types of health-related quality of life.
19. Distinguish between quality assessment and quality assurance.
20. What are the basic principles of TQM (or CQI)?
21. Give a brief description of the Donabedian model of quality.
22. Discuss the main developments in process improvement that have occurred in recent years.

REFERENCES

Aday, L.A. 1993. Indicators and predictors of health services utilization. In *Introduction to health services*. 4th ed., eds. S.J. Williams and P.R. Torrens, 46–70. Albany, NY: Delmar Publishers.

Aday, L.A., and R. Andersen. 1975. *Development of indices of access to medical care*. Ann Arbor, MI: Health Administration Press.

Aday, L.A. et al. 1980. *Health care in the US: Equitable for whom?* Newbury Park, CA: Sage.

Aday, L.A. et al. 1984. *Access to medical care in the US: Who has it, who doesn't?* Research Series No. 32. Chicago, IL: Center for Health Administration Studies, University of Chicago, Pluribus Press Inc.

Aday, L.A. et al. 1993. *Evaluating the medical care system: Effectiveness, efficiency, and equity*. Ann Arbor, MI: Health Administration Press.

Al-Assaf, A.F. 1993a. Introduction and historical background. In *The textbook of total quality management*, eds. A.F. Al-Assaf and J.A. Schmele, 3–12. Delray Beach, FL: St. Lucie Press.

Al-Assaf, A.F. 1993b. Outcome management and TQ. In *The textbook of total quality management*, eds. A.F. Al-Assaf and J.A. Schmele, 221–37. Delray Beach, FL: St. Lucie Press.

Altman, S.H., and J. Eichenholz. 1976. Inflation in the health industry: Causes and cures. In *Health: A victim or cause of inflation?* ed. M. Zubkoff, 1–32. New York: Milbank Memorial Fund.

Altman, S.H., and S.S. Wallack. 1996. Health care spending: Can the United States control it? In *Strategic choices for a changing health care system*, eds. S.H. Altman and U.E. Reinhardt. Chicago: Health Administration Press.

Andersen, R. 1968. *A behavioral model of families' use of health services*. Research Series No. 25. Chicago, IL: Center for Health Administration Studies, University of Chicago.

Andersen, R. 1997. Too big, too small, too flat, too tall: Search for "just right" measures of access in the age of managed care. Paper presented at the Association for Health Services Research Annual Meeting. Chicago, IL.

Anderson, G.F. 1997. In search of value: An international comparison of cost, access, and outcomes. *Health Affairs* 16, no. 6: 163–71.

Arnould, R.J. et al. 1993. Competitive reforms: Context and scope. In *Competitive approaches to health care reform*, eds. R.J. Arnould, R.F. Rich, and W.D. White, 3–18. Washington, DC: The Urban Institute Press.

Baucus, M., and E.J. Fowler. 2002. Geographic variation in Medicare spending and the real focus of Medicare reform. *Health Affairs Web Exclusives* 2002: W115–W117.

Bergner, M. 1989. Quality of life, health status, and clinical research. *Medical Care* 27, no. 3 (Supplement): S148–S156.

Borger, C., et al. 2006. Health spending projections through 2015: Changes on the horizon. *Health Affairs* 25, no.2: w61–w73.

Brown, K. 1992. Death and access: Ethics in cross-cultural health care. In *Choices and conflict: Explorations in health care ethics*, ed. E. Friedman. Chicago: American Hospital Publishing.

Catlin, A., et al. National health spending in 2005: The slowdown continues. *Health Affairs* (Millwood) 26, no.1:142–53.

Centers for Disease Control and Prevention (CDC). 2005. Annual Smoking-Attributable Mortality, Years of Potential Life Lost, and Productivity Losses—United States, 1997–2001. *MMWR* 54, no.25:625–8. Available at: *http://www.cdc.gov/mmwr/preview/mmwrhtml/mm5425a1.htm*.

Centers for Medicare & Medicaid Services. 2007. Pay for performance. *http://www.cms.hhs.gov/MedicaidSCHIPQualPrac/04_P4P.asp*.

Chassin, M.R. 1991. Quality of care—Time to act. *Journal of the American Medical Association* 266, no. 24: 3472–3.

Cordes, S.M. 1989. The changing rural environment and the relationship between health services and rural development. *Health Services Research* 23, no. 6: 757–84.

Coté, C.J. 2000. Adverse sedation events in pediatrics: A critical incident analysis of contributing factors. *Pediatrics* 105, no. 4: 805–14.

DeFriese, G.H., and T.C. Ricketts. 1989. Primary health care in rural areas: An agenda for research. *Health Services Research* 23, no. 6: 931–74.

Department of Health and Human Services (DHHS). 1996. *Health, United States, 1995*. Hyattsville, Maryland: National Center for Health Statistics.

Department of Health and Human Services (DHHS). 2002. *Health, United States, 2002*. Hyattsville, Maryland: National Center for Health Statistics.

Docteur, E.R. et al. 1996. Shifting the paradigm: Monitoring access in Medicare managed care. *Health Care Financing Review* 17, no. 4: 5–21.

Donabedian, A. 1980. *Explorations in quality assessment and monitoring: The definition of quality and approaches to its assessment*. Vol. 1. Ann Arbor, MI: Health Administration Press.

Donabedian, A. 1985. *Explorations in quality assessment and monitoring: The methods and findings of quality assessment and monitoring*. Vol. 3. Ann Arbor, MI: Health Administration Press.

Dranove, D. 1993. The case for competitive reform in health care. In *Competitive approaches to health care reform*, eds. R.J. Arnould, R.F. Rich, and W.D. White, 67–82. Washington, DC: The Urban Institute Press.

Easterbrook, G. 1987. The revolution. *Newsweek*, 26 January, 40–74.

Eddy, D.M. 1994. Clinical decision making: From theory to practice. In *The nation's health*. 4th ed., eds. P.R. Lee and C.L. Estes, 315–21. Boston: Jones & Bartlett Publishers.

Evans, J.R. 1993. *Applied production and operations management*. 4th ed. Minneapolis/St. Paul, MN: West Publishing Co.

Feldstein, P.J. 1993. *Health care economics*. 4th ed. Albany, NY: Delmar Publishers.

Feldstein, P. 1994. *Health policy issues: An economic perspective on health reform*. Ann Arbor, MI: AUPHA Press/Health Administration Press.

Finkelstein, E.A. et al. 2003. National medical spending attributable to overweight and obesity: How much, and who's paying? Health Affairs Web Exclusive, May 14. *http://www.healthaffairs.org/WebExclusives/Finkelstein_Web_Excl_051403.htm*.

Firshein, J. 1996. Measuring progress toward practice guidelines. *Business and Health* 14, no. 5: 38–42.

Fisher, E.S. et al. 2003a. The implications of regional variations in Medicare spending. Part 1: The content, quality, and accessibility of care. *Annals of Internal Medicine* 138, no. 4: 273–87.

Fisher, E.S. et al. 2003b. The implications of regional variations in Medicare spending. Part 2: Health outcomes and satisfaction with care. *Annals of Internal Medicine* 138, no. 4: 288–98.

Freeman, H.E. et al. 1982. Community health centers: An initiative of enduring utility. *Milbank Memorial Fund Quarterly/Health and Society* 60, no. 2: 245–67.

Gabel, J., and T. Rice. 1985. Reducing public expenditures for physician services: The price of paying less. *Journal of Health Politics, Policy and Law* 9, no. 4: 595–609.

Ganz, P.A., and M.S. Litwin. 1996. Measuring outcomes and health-related quality of life. In *Changing the US health care system: Key issues in health services, policy, and management*, eds. R.M. Anderson et al. San Francisco: Jossey-Bass Publishers.

Giffin, M., and R.B. Giffin. 1994. Market memo: Critical pathways produce tangible results. *Health Care Strategic Management* 12, no. 7: 1–6.

Gittelsohn, A., and N.R. Powe. 1995. Small area variation in health care delivery in Maryland. *Health Services Research* 30, no. 2: 295–317.

Gottlieb, S.R. 1974. A brief history of health planning in the United States. In *Regulating health facilities construction*, ed. C.C. Havighurst. Washington, DC: American Enterprise Institute for Public Policy Research.

Guralnik, J.M. et al. 1991. Morbidity and disability in older persons in the years prior to death. *American Journal of Public Health* 81, no. 4: 443–7.

HCIA Inc. and Deloitte & Touche. 1997. *The comparative performance of US hospitals: The sourcebook*. Baltimore, MD: HCIA Inc.

Health Care Financing Administration (HCFA). 1996. Overview of the Medicare program. *Health Care Financing Review: Medicare and Medicaid Statistical Supplement* 5.

Heffler, S. et al. 2002. Health spending projections for 2001–2011: The latest outlook. *Health Affairs* 21, no. 2: 207–18.

Hellander, I. et al. 1994. Health care paper chase, 1993: The cost to the nation, the states, and the District of Columbia. *International Journal of Health Services* 24, no. 1: 1–9.

Institute of Medicine (IOM). 1990. *Clinical practice guidelines: Directions for a new program*. Washington, DC: National Academy Press.

Institute of Medicine (IOM). 1993. *Access to health care in America*, ed. M. Millman. Washington, DC: National Academy Press.

Institute of Medicine (IOM). 2000. *To err is human: Building a safer health system*, eds. L.T. Kohn, J.M. Corrigan, and M.S. Donaldson. Washington, DC: National Academy Press.

Institute of Medicine (IOM). 2004. *Rewarding provider performance: Aligning incentives in Medicare*. Washington, DC: National Academy Press.

Laffel, G., and D. Blumenthal. 1993. The case for using industrial quality management science in health care organizations. In *The textbook of total quality management*, ed. A.F. Al-Assaf and J.A. Schmele, 40–50. Delray Beach, FL: St. Lucie Press.

Lapetina, E.M., and E.M. Armstrong. 2002. Preventing errors in the outpatient setting: A tale of three states. *Health Affairs* 21, no. 4: 26–39.

Lamb, R.M. et al. 2003. Hospital disclosure practices: Results of a national survey. *Health Affairs* 22, no. 2: 73–83.

Larsen, R.R. 1996. Narrowing the gray zone: How clinical practice guidelines can improve the decision-making process. *Postgraduate Medicine* 100, no. 2: 17–24.

Lehman, A.F. 1995. Measuring quality of life in a reformed health system. *Health Affairs* 14, no. 3: 90–101.

Levit, K. et al. 2003. Trends in US health care spending, 2001. *Health Affairs* 22, no. 1: 154–64.

Levy, D.E. 2006. Employer-sponsored insurance coverage of smoking cessation treatments. *American Journal of Managed Care* 12, no.9: 553–62.

Lohr, K.N. 1997. How do we measure quality? *Health Affairs* 16, no. 3: 22–5.

Loubeau, P.R., and V.F. Maher. 1996. Any-willing-provider laws: Point and counter point. *Medical Law* 15, no. 2: 219–26.

Lovitky, J.A. 1997. Health care fraud: A growing problem. *Nursing Management* 28, no. 11: 42, 44–5.

May, J. 1974. The planning and licensing agencies. In *Regulating health facilities constructions*, ed. C.C. Havighurst. Washington, DC: American Enterprise Institute for Public Policy Research.

McCormick, D. et al. 2002. Relationship between low quality-of-care scores and HMOs' subsequent public disclosure of quality-of-care scores. *Journal of the American Medical Association* 288, no. 12: 1484–90.

McElroy, D., and K. Herbelin. 1989. Assuring quality of care in long-term care facilities. *Journal of Gerontological Nursing* 15, no. 7: 8–10.

McGlynn, E.A. 1997. Six challenges in measuring the quality of health care. *Health Affairs* 16, no. 3: 7–21.

McGlynn, E.A., and R.H. Brook. 1996. Ensuring quality of care. In *Changing the US health care system: Key issues in health services, policy, and management*, eds. R.M. Andersen, T.H. Rice, and G.F. Kominski, San Francisco: Jossey-Bass Publishers.

Minino, A.M., and B.L. Smith. 2001. Deaths: Preliminary data for 2000. *National Vital Statistics Reports* 49, no. 12. National Center for Health Statistics.

Mitchell, J. et al. 1988. *Impact of the Medicare fee freeze on physician expenditures and volume: Final report*. Baltimore, MD: Health Care Financing Administration.

National Center for Health Statistics. 2002. *National Vital Statistics Reports* 49, no. 12. Centers for Disease Control and Prevention.

National Center for Health Statistics. 2006. Health, United States, 2006. Hyattsville, MD: US Department of Health and Human Services.

National Committee for Quality Assurance (NCQA). 2007. HEDIS 2007 Summary Table of Measures and Product Lines. *http://www.ncqa.org/programs/hedis/2007/MeasuresList.pdf.*

National Committee for Quality Assurance (NCQA). 2003. Managed care organization accreditation. *http://web.ncqa.org/tabid/67/Default.aspx.*

Norton, C.H., and M.A. McManus. 1989. Background tables on demographic characteristics. *Health Services Research* 23, no. 6: 807–48.

Orlikoff, J.E. 1988. *Malpractice prevention and liability control for hospitals*. 2nd ed. Chicago: American Hospital Publishing.

Penchansky, R., and J.W. Thomas. 1981. The concept of access: Definition and relationship to consumer satisfaction. *Medical Care* 19: 127–40.

Public Health Service. 1997. *Smoking cessation: A systems approach*. Rockville, MD: Department of Health and Human Services (AHCPR Publication No. 97–0698), April.

Reed, M. et al. 2003. Physicians and care management: more acceptance than you think. *Issue brief* [Center for the Study of Health System Change], January (60): 1–4.

Reinhardt, U.E. 1994. Providing access to health care and controlling costs: The universal dilemma. In *The nation's health*. 4th ed., eds. P.R. Lee and C.L. Estes, 263–78. Boston: Jones & Bartlett Publishers.

Reinhardt, U.E. et al. 2002. Cross-national comparisons of health systems using OECD data, 1999. *Health Affairs* 21, no. 3: 169–81.

Rogers, W.H. et al. 1990. Quality of care before and after implementation of the DRG-based prospective payment system: A summary of effects. *Journal of the American Medical Association* 264, no. 15: 1989–94.

Ross, J.S., et al. 2007. Certificate of need regulation and cardiac catheterization appropriateness after acute myocardial infarction. *Circulation* 115, no. 8:1012–19.

Rowland, D., and B. Lyons. 1989. Triple jeopardy: Rural, poor, and uninsured. *Health Services Research* 23, no. 6: 975–1004.

Sardell, A. 1988. *The US experiment in social medicine, the Community Health Center Program, 1965–1986*. Pittsburgh, PA: University of Pittsburgh Press.

Sheils, J., and Haught, R. 2004. The cost of tax-exempt benefits in 2004. *Health Affairs* (Millwood) W4: 106–12.

Shekelle, P.G., and D.L. Schriger. 1996. Evaluating the use of the appropriateness method in the Agency for Health Care Policy and Research clinical practice guideline development process. *Health Services Research* 31, no. 4: 453–68.

Sherman, A. 1991. *Falling by the wayside: Children in rural America*. Washington, DC: Children's Defense Fund.

Singh, D.A. 1997. *Nursing home administrators: Their influence on quality of care*. New York: Garland Publishing.

Svarstad, B.L. 1986. Patient-practitioner relationships and compliance with prescribed medical regimens. In *Applications of social sciences to clinical medicine and health policy*, eds. L.H. Aiken and D. Mechanic. New Brunswick, NJ: Rutgers University Press.

TECH Research Network. 2001. Technology change around the world: Evidence from heart attack care. *Health Affairs* 20, no. 3: 25–42.

Thompson, J.W. et al. 2003. Health plan quality-of-care information is undermined by voluntary reporting. *American Journal of Preventive Medicine* 24, no. 1: 62–70.

Tucker, J. 1997. Obey says future Medicare cuts inevitable. *PT Bulletin*, 27 June, 10.

Van de Water, P.N., Lavery, J. 2006. Medicare finances: Findings of the 2006 trustees report. *Medicare Brief* 13: 1–8.

Weisbrod, B. 1991. The health care quadrilemma: An essay on technological change, insurance, quality of care, and cost containment. *Journal of Economic Literature* 29 (June): 523–52.

Wendling, W., and J. Werner. 1980. Nonprofit firms and the economic theory of regulation. *Quarterly Review of Economics and Business* 20, no. 3: 6–18.

Wennberg, J.E. 2002.Unwarranted variations in healthcare delivery: Implications for academic medical centres. *British Medical Journal* 325, no. 7370: 961–4.

Wennberg, J.E. et al. 1987. Are hospital services rationed in New Haven or over-utilized in Boston? *Lancet* 1, no. 8543: 1185–9.

Wennberg, J.E., and A. Gittelsohn. 1973. Small area variations in health care delivery. *Science* 183: 1102–8.

Williams, S.J. 1995. *Essentials of health services*. Albany, NY: Delmar Publishers.

Williams, K.N., and R.H. Brook. 1978. Quality measurement and assurance. *Health Medical Care Services Review* 1: 3–15.

Williams, S.J., and P.R. Torrens. 1993. Influencing, regulating, and monitoring the health care system. In *Introduction to health services*. 4th ed., eds. S.J. Williams and P.R. Torrens, 377–396. Albany, NY: Delmar Publishers.

Wilson, F.A., and D. Neuhauser. 1985. *Health services in the United States*. 2nd ed. Cambridge, MA: Ballinger Publishing Co.

Wong, M.D. et al. 2001. Effects of cost sharing on care seeking and health status: Results from the medical outcomes study. *American Journal of Public Health* 91, no. 11: 1889–94.

Chapter 13

Health Policy

Learning Objectives

- To understand the definition, scope, and role of health policy in the United States
- To recognize the principal features of US health policy
- To comprehend the process of legislative health policy
- To become familiar with some of the critical health policy issues in the United States

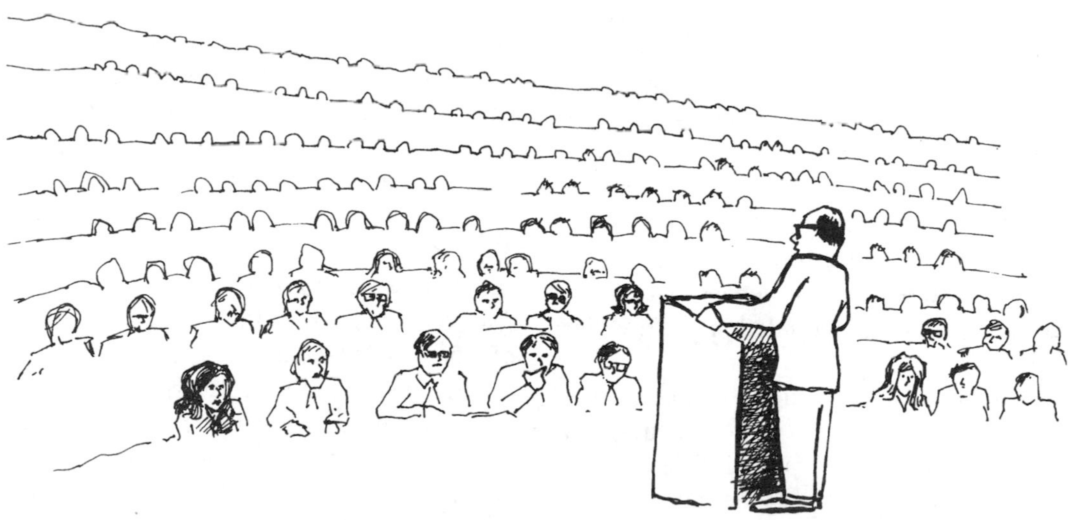

"Ladies and Gentlemen, to come up with a uniform health policy, we will now break up into 31 different groups."

Introduction

Even though the United States does not have a centrally controlled system of health care delivery, it does have a history of federal, state, and local government involvement in health care and health policy. Americans possess an incredible desire to be healthy. They contend that their individual health contributes to the overall health of the nation and, consequently, to the economy. It is, therefore, not surprising that the government is so keenly interested in health policy. This chapter first defines what health policy is and explores the principal features of health policy in the United States. Next, it describes the development of legislative policy and gives examples of critical health policy issues. Finally, it provides an outlook for the future of health policy in the United States.

What Is Health Policy?

Public policies are authoritative decisions made in the legislative, executive, or judicial branches of government intended to direct or influence the actions, behaviors, or decisions of others (Longest 1994). When public policies pertain to or influence the pursuit of health, they become health policies. Therefore, ***health policy*** can be defined as "the aggregate of principles, stated or unstated, that . . . characterize the distribution of resources, services, and political influences that impact on the health of the population . . ." (Miller 1987, 15).

Public policies are supposed to serve the interests of the public; however, the term "public" has been interpreted differently in the political landscape. At the most general level, the term "public" refers to all Americans. "Public" also can refer to voters or likely voters; that is, the subset of Americans who directly determine the outcomes of political elections. Finally, the term can refer to only those who are politically active. The latter group consists of those Americans who communicate directly with their representatives by either writing or calling, contribute money to politicians or political groups, attend protests or other forums on behalf of a particular interest or candidate, or in other ways make their voices and policy preferences heard. Legislators and policymakers are most responsive to the views or wishes of these active Americans, particularly when they are constituents from within their legislative districts. People who are older, have more years of education, and have strong party identification are more likely to be politically active.

Different Forms of Health Policies

Health policies often come as a by-product of public social policies enacted by the government. For example, important changes in the US health care system came about after World War II due to policies that excluded fringe benefits from income or Social Security taxes and a Supreme Court ruling that employee benefits, including health insurance, could be legitimately included in the collective bargaining process (see Chapter 3). As a result, employer-provided health insurance benefits grew rapidly in the mid-20th century (Health Insurance Association of America 1992). In 1965, adoption of the Medicare and Medicaid legislation expanded the health sector by providing publicly subsidized health insurance to the elderly and the indigent. In 1997, Congress approved the State Children's Health Insurance

Program (SCHIP), which extends health coverage to children whose families have incomes above the eligibility level for Medicaid, but who cannot afford private coverage. All of these developments in public policy have shaped the way health services are delivered in this country.

The American health care system has been developed under extraordinarily favorable public policies. For example, the nation has a long history of support for the development of medical technology through policies that directly support biomedical research and encourage private investments in such research. The National Institutes of Health (NIH) had a budget of about $10 million when the agency was established in the early 1930s. Today, following exponential growth, the proposed FY 2008 NIH budget is nearly $29 billion (NIH 2007). Encouraged by policies that permit firms to recoup their investments in research and development, private industry also spends a significant amount on biomedical research and development.

Health policies pertain to health care at all levels, including policies affecting the production, provision, and financing of health care services. Health policies affect groups or classes of individuals, such as physicians, the poor, the elderly, or children. They can also affect types of organizations, such as medical schools, health maintenance organizations (HMOs), nursing homes, medical technology producers, or employers. In the United States, each branch and level of government can influence health policy. For example, both the executive and legislative branches at the federal, state, and local levels can establish health policies, and the judicial branch can uphold, strike down, or modify existing laws affecting health and health care at federal, state, or local levels.

Health policies can be made through the private sector or the public policymaking process. An example of private-sector health policies is the decisions made by insurance companies regarding their product lines, pricing, and marketing. Their focus is to restrict the public policymaking process and the public-sector health policies that result from this process. Examples of public health policies include (1) major reforms in medical education, as suggested in the 1910 Flexner report, which encouraged a university/hospital-based model for education (see Chapter 3); (2) the 1965 legislation that established the Medicare and Medicaid programs; (3) an executive order regarding operation of federally funded family planning clinics; (4) a court's decision that the merger of two hospitals violates federal antitrust laws; (5) a state government's decision about its procedures for licensing physicians; (6) a county health department's decision about its procedures for monitoring sanitation standards in restaurants; (7) and a city government's enactment of an ordinance banning smoking in public places within the city. Thus, health policies can take several different forms.

Statutes or laws, such as the statutory language contained in the 1983 Amendments to the Social Security Act that authorized the prospective payment system (PPS) for reimbursing hospitals for Medicare beneficiaries, are also considered policies. Another example is the certificate-of-need (CON) programs through which many states seek to regulate capital expansion in their health care systems (see Chapters 5 and 12).

The scope of health policy is limited by the political and economic system of a country. In the United States, where pro-individual and pro-market sentiments dominate, public policies are likely to be fragmented, incremental, and noncomprehensive. National policies and programs are typically based on the notion that local communities are in the best position to identify strategies that will address their unique needs. However, the type of change that can be enacted at the community level is clearly limited.

Regulatory Tools

Health policies may be used as ***regulatory tools*** (Longest 1994). They call on government to prescribe and control the behavior of a particular target group by monitoring the group and imposing sanctions if it fails to comply. Examples of regulatory policies are abundant in the health care system. Federally funded peer review organizations (PROs), for instance, develop and enforce standards concerning appropriate care under the Medicare program (see Chapter 12). State insurance departments across the country regulate health insurance companies in an effort to protect customers from default on coverage in case of financial failure of an insurance company, excessive premiums, and mendacious practices.

Some health policies are "self-regulatory." For example, physicians set standards of medical practice, hospitals accredit one another as meeting the standards that the Joint Commission on Accreditation of Healthcare Organizations has set, and schools of public health decide which courses should be part of their graduate programs in public health (Weissert and Weissert 1996).

Allocative Tools

Health policies may also be used as ***allocative tools*** (Longest 1994). They involve the direct provision of income, services, or goods to certain groups of individuals or institutions. Allocative tools in the health care arena are distributive or redistributive. ***Distributive policies*** spread benefits throughout society. Typical distributive policies include funding of medical research through the NIH, the development of medical personnel (e.g., medical education through the National Health Service Corps), the construction of facilities (e.g., hospitals under the Hill-Burton program during the 1950s and 1960s), and the initiation of new institutions (e.g., HMOs). ***Redistributive policies***, on the other hand, take money or power from one group and give it to another. This system often creates visible beneficiaries and payers. For this reason, health policy is often most visible and politically charged when it performs redistributive functions. Redistributive policies include Medicaid, which takes tax revenue from the more affluent and spends it on the poor in the form of free health insurance. Other redistributive policies include the State Children's Health Insurance Program (SCHIP), welfare, and public housing programs. Redistributive policies, in particular, are believed to be essential for addressing the fundamental causes of health disparities.

The Principal Features of US Health Policy

Several features characterize US health policy, including government as subsidiary to the private sector; fragmented, incremental, and piecemeal reform; pluralistic (interest group) politics; the decentralized role of the states; and the impact of presidential leadership. These features often act or interact to influence the development and evolution of health policies.

Government as Subsidiary to the Private Sector

In much of the developed world, national health care programs are built on a consensus that health care is a right of citizenship and that government should play a leading role in the provision of health care. In the United States, however, health care is not seen as a right of citizenship or as a primary responsibility of government. Instead, the private sector plays a dominant role. Similar to many other public policy issues, Americans generally prefer market solutions as opposed to government intervention in health care financing and delivery. For this reason, a strong preference prevails to minimize the government's role in the delivery of health care.

Americans have typically harbored a general mistrust of government. The Declaration of Independence defined the new nation in a great protest over government intrusion on personal liberty. The United States is a capitalist nation where the presumption is that private markets best determine the production and consumption of goods and services, including health care services. One result is that Americans have developed social insurance programs far more reluctantly than most industrialized democracies. In addition, American public opinion often presumes these programs are overly generous.

Generally speaking, the government's role in US health care has grown incrementally, mainly to address perceived problems and negative consequences. Some of the most-cited problems associated with government involvement include escalating costs, bureaucratic inflexibility, excessive regulation, red tape, irrational paperwork, arbitrary and sometimes conflicting public directives, inconsistent enforcement of rules and regulations, and fraud and abuse. Other problems include inadequate reimbursement schedules, arbitrary denial of claims, insensitivity to local needs, consumer and provider dissatisfaction, and charges that government programs tend to promote welfare dependence rather than a desire to seek employment (Longest 1994).

The most credible argument for policy intervention in the nation's domestic activities begins with the identification of situations in which markets fail or do not function efficiently. Health care in the United States is a big industry, but certain specific characteristics and conditions of the health care market distinguish it from other businesses. The market for health care services in the United States violates the conditions of a competitive market in several ways. The complexity of health care services almost eliminates the consumer's ability to make informed decisions without guidance from the sellers (providers). Sellers' entry into the health care market is heavily regulated. Widespread insurance coverage also affects the decisions of buyers and sellers regarding cost and utilization. These and other factors determine that the markets for health care services do not operate competitively, thus inviting policy intervention (see Chapter 1 for a detailed discussion of violations of market principles in health care).

Government spending for health care has been largely confined to filling the gaps in the private sector. This intervention includes environmental protection, preventive services, communicable disease control, care of special groups, institutional care of the mentally and chronically ill, provision of medical care to the indigent, and support for research and training. With health coverage considered a privilege or even a luxury for those who are offered insurance through their employer, the government is left in a gap-filling role for the most vulnerable of the uninsured population.

Another important example of the subsidiary role of government was the enactment of the Hospital Survey and Construction Act in 1946 (also known as the Hill-Burton Act). This legislation expanded the availability of health services and improved hospital facilities after the unregulated markets had failed to provide adequate access to inpatient hospital care. The program, intended to provide funds for hospital construction, marked the beginning of extensive federal developmental subsidies to increase the availability of health services.

Fragmented, Incremental, and Piecemeal Reform

Public power in the United States is enormously fragmented. This system follows the design of the founding fathers, who developed a structure of "checks and balances" to limit government's power. Federal, state, and local governments pursue their own policies with little coordination of purpose or programs. The subsidiary role of the government and the attendant mixture of private and public approaches to the provision of health care also resulted in a complex and fragmented pattern of health care financing, in which: (1) The employed are predominantly covered by voluntary insurance provided through contributions that they and their employers make. (2) The aged are insured through a combination of coverage financed out of Social Security tax revenues (Medicare Part A) and government-subsidized voluntary insurance for physician, supplementary, and prescription drug coverage (Medicare Part B and Part D). (3) The poor are covered through Medicaid via federal, state, and local revenues. (4) Special population groups—for example, veterans, American Indians, members of the armed forces, Congress, and the executive branch—have coverage that the federal government provides directly.

US health policies have been incremental and piecemeal, resulting from compromises involving the resolution of a variety of competing interests. An example is the broadening of the Medicaid program since its start in 1965. Congress has enacted policies to expand Medicaid eligibility to enroll more children into the program. In 1984, the first steps were taken to mandate coverage of pregnant women and children in two-parent families who met income requirements and to mandate coverage for all children five years old or younger who met financial requirements. When the federal government mandates Medicaid eligibility or benefits, it is telling the states that they must expand their programs accordingly to continue receiving federal matching dollars.

In 1986, states were given the option of covering pregnant women and children up to five years of age in families with incomes below 100% of federal poverty income guidelines, regardless of their participation in the Aid to Families with Dependent Children (AFDC) program. In 1988, that option was increased to cover families at 185% of federal poverty income. In 1988, Congress required that Medicaid coverage for families leaving the AFDC program be continued for six months, and they gave states the option of adding another six months. In addition, as part of the Medicaid Catastrophic Act, which remains in effect today, Congress mandated coverage for pregnant women and infants in families with incomes below 100% of federal poverty guidelines. In 1989, it was expanded to 133% of the poverty income, and the age of covered children was raised to six. In the early 1990s, states began experimenting with waivers allowing for expansion of Medicaid managed care programs. In 1996, the Personal Responsibility and Work Opportunity Act (PRWORA) ended the formal link between AFDC benefits and Medicaid benefits. In 1997, the Balanced Budget Act created SCHIP, which allows states to use Medicaid expansion to extend insurance coverage to uninsured children who otherwise are not qualified for existing Medicaid programs. This illustrates how a program is reformed and/or expanded through successive legislative action. In typical American fashion, the Medicaid program has been reformed through incremental change, but without ensuring access to medical care for all of the nation's uninsured. Among the uninsured are millions of Americans who are not categorically eligible for services. These uninsured consist mostly of adults younger than 65 years of age with no dependent children. Congress has demonstrated the desire and political will to address the needs of a small number of the uninsured perceived to be the most vulnerable (e.g., pregnant women and children) but has not developed a consensus on more dramatic steps to move beyond incremental adjustments to existing programs.

Institutional fragmentation is vividly clear in the process of legislative development of health policy. Thirty-one congressional committees and subcommittees try to claim some fragment of jurisdiction over health legislation. The conglomeration of reform proposals that emerges from these committees faces a daunting political challenge—separate consideration and passage in each chamber, negotiations in a joint conference committee to reconcile the bills passed by the two houses, and then return to each chamber for approval. In the Senate, 41 of the 100 members can thwart the whole process at any point.

Once a bill has passed in Congress, however, it is not a fait accompli. Multiple levels of federal and state bureaucracy must interpret and implement the legislation. Rules and regulations must be written. During this process, politicians, interest groups, or project beneficiaries may influence the program's ultimate design. Sometimes, the result can differ significantly from its sponsors' intent. This complex and seemingly anarchic process of policy formulation and implementation makes fundamental, comprehensive policy reform extremely difficult. Ideology and government organization reinforce the tendency toward a standstill. It usually takes a great political event—a landmark election, a popular upheaval, a war, or a domestic crisis—to overcome the tilt toward inaction.

Pluralistic and Interest Group Politics

Perhaps the most common explanation for US health policy outcomes takes into full account the demands of interest groups and the incremental policies resulting from compromises struck to satisfy those demands. Traditionally, the policy community has included (1) the legislative committees with jurisdiction in a policy domain, (2) the executive branch agencies implementing policies, and (3) private interest groups. The first two supply the policies demanded by the third.

Established groups resist innovative, nonincremental policies because these measures undermine the bargaining practices that reduce threats to existing interests. The system's stability is ensured because most groups are satisfied with the benefits they receive; however, the result for any single group is less than optimal. Interest groups' pluralism affects health policy just as it does any other policy debate in American politics. Powerful interest groups involved in health care politics adamantly resist any major change (Alford 1975). Each group fights hard to protect its own best interests.

Well-organized interest groups are the most effective "demanders" of policies. By combining and concentrating their members' resources, organized interest groups can dramatically change the ratio between the costs and benefits of participation in the political markets for policy change. These interest groups represent a variety of individuals and entities, such as physicians in the American Medical Association; senior citizens allied with AARP (formerly called the American Association of Retired Persons); institutional providers such as hospitals belonging to the American Hospital Association; nursing homes belonging to the American Health Care Association; and the companies making up the Pharmaceutical Research and Manufacturers of America.

Physicians have often found it hard to lobby for their interests with a single voice because they include so many specialty groups. For example, the American Academy of Pediatrics is involved in advocacy for children's health issues. Other groups include Physicians for a National Health Program, the American Society of Anesthesiologists, and the Society of Thoracic Surgeons. Though driven by their specific interests, they can come together on issues that threaten the entire group, such as the 1992 decision by the Office of Management and Budget to reduce total Medicare payments when implementing a reimbursement system based on resource-based relative values.

Not only do the traditional members of the health policy community find themselves split over questions of optimal health policy, but the community has also grown considerably as new interest groups have formed and joined. Business is the major new member, although it too is split, mainly along the lines of large and small employers. Other, newer members of the health policy community represent consumer interests, but consumer interests are not uniform, nor are the policy preferences of their interest groups. Consumers often lack financial means to organize and advocate for their interests.

To overcome pluralistic interests and maximize policy outcomes, diverse interest groups form alliances among themselves and with legislators to protect and enhance the interests of those receiving benefits from government programs. Each alliance member receives benefits from current programs. Legislators can show their constituencies the economic benefits of government spending in their districts, agencies can expand their programs, and interest groups benefit directly from government programs.

The policy agendas of interest groups typically reflect their interests. For example, the AARP advocates programs to expand financing for long-term care for the elderly and was a major advocate for prescription drug coverage for Medicare beneficiaries, which went into effect on January 1, 2006. Organized labor has been among the staunchest supporters of national health insurance. The primary concerns of educational and research institutions and accrediting bodies are embedded in policies that would generate higher funding to support their educational and research activities. Other policy concerns of these groups include licensure and practice guidelines, and anything that may influence future demand for their graduates and affiliates. The Food and Drug Administration's job is to ensure that new pharmaceuticals meet safety and efficacy standards. Quality Improvement Organizations (QIOs) ensure that Medicare beneficiaries receive only needed and appropriate procedures.

Pharmaceutical and medical technology organizations are concerned with detecting changes in health policy and influencing the formulation of policies concerning approval and monitoring of drugs and devices. Three main factors drive health policy concerns about medical technology: (1) medical technology is an important contributor to rising health costs, (2) medical technology often provides health benefits, and (3) the utilization of medical technology also provides economic benefits. These factors are likely to remain important determinants of US policies on medical technology. Another factor driving US technology policy is the policymakers' desire to develop cost-saving technology and to expand access to it. The government is spending more and more money on outcome studies to identify the value of alternative technologies that promise to provide better care at lower cost.

American employers' health policy concerns are shaped mostly by the degree to which they provide health insurance benefits to their employees and their dependents, and to their retirees. Many small business owners adamantly oppose health policies requiring them to cover employees because they believe they cannot afford it. Employees also pay attention to health policies that affect worker health or the labor-management relations experienced by employers. For example, employers have to comply with federal and state regulations on employee health and well-being, and on the prevention of job-related illnesses and injuries. Employers are often inspected by regulatory agencies to ensure that they adhere to workplace health and safety policies.

The health policy concerns of consumers and the groups that represent them reflect the rich diversity of the American people. African Americans and, more recently, the rapidly growing numbers of Hispanic Americans face special health problems. Both groups are underserved by many health care services and underrepresented in all of the health professions in the United States. Their health policy interests include getting their unique health problems (e.g., higher infant mortality, higher exposure to violence among adolescents, higher levels of substance abuse among adults, and earlier deaths from cardiovascular disease and various other causes) adequately addressed. Exhibit 13–1 summarizes the major concerns of dominant interest groups.

Decentralized Role of the States

In the United States, individual states play a significant role in the development and implementation of health policies. The role of individual states has taken several forms: financial support for the care and treatment of the poor and chronically disabled, which includes the primary responsibility for the administration of the federal/state Medicaid and SCHIP programs; quality assurance and oversight of health care practitioners and facilities (e.g., state licensure and regulation); regulation of health care costs and insurance carriers; health personnel training (states pay most of the costs to train health care professionals); and authorization of local government health services.

Most of the incremental policy actions of recent years originated in state governments. One action, taken by 24 states, was to create a special program called an "insurance risk pool." These programs help people acquire private insurance otherwise unavailable

Exhibit 13–1 Interest Group Preferences

Federal and state governments
- Cost containment
- Access to care
- Quality of care

Employers
- Cost containment
- Workplace health and safety
- Minimum regulation

Consumers
- Access to care
- Quality of care
- Lower out-of-pocket costs

Insurers
- Administrative simplication
- Elimination of cost shifting

Practitioners
- Income maintenance
- Professional autonomy
- Malpractice reform

Provider organizations
- Profitability
- Administrative simplification
- Bad debt reduction

Technology producers
- Tax treatment
- Regulatory environment
- Research funding

to them because of the medical risks they pose to insurance companies. Most of these programs are financed by a combination of individual premiums and taxes on insurance carriers.

Other state-initiated programs have addressed additional vulnerable populations. New Jersey developed a program to ensure access to care for all pregnant women. Florida began a program, called Healthy Kids Corporation, which linked health insurance to schools. Washington developed a special program for the working poor that uses HMOs and preferred provider organizations to provide care within the state's counties. Maine established a program, MaineCare, to offer HMO-based coverage at moderate prices to small businesses with 15 or fewer employees. The state subsidized premiums on a sliding-fee scale based on the employer's ability to contribute (Lemov 1990). Minnesota created a program, Children's Health Plan, designed to provide benefits to children up to age nine who lived in families with incomes below 185% of the poverty level, but who do not qualify for Medicaid. Colorado and New York have also enacted similar legislation. Several states, including Massachusetts, Hawaii, and Oregon, have experimented with more comprehensive programs designed to provide universal access to care within their jurisdictions. Most notably, Massachusetts recently passed legislation requiring about 515,000 people (most of the state's uninsured) to obtain health insurance by July 1, 2007, or face penalties including the potential loss of a personal income tax deduction. To bring the plan to fruition, Massachusetts expanded Medicaid eligibility, reconfigured its $1 billion free care pool, and established rules to help insurance companies create more affordable health plans (Belluck 2007). Exhibit 13–2 lists the arguments often cited in favor of decentralizing health programs at the state level.

Arguments have also been made against too much state control over health policy de-

Exhibit 13–2 Arguments for Enhancing States' Role

- Americans distrust centralized government in general and lack faith in the federal government as an administrator in particular.
- The federal government has grown too large, intrusive, and paternalistic.
- The federal government is too impersonal, distant, and unresponsive.
- State and local governments are closer to the people and more familiar with local needs; therefore, they are more accessible and accountable to the public and better able to develop responsive programs than federal agencies.
- National standards reduce flexibility and seriously constrain the ability of states to experiment and innovate.
- States are equipped to take on such functions (i.e., more full-time legislators, more professional staffs and bureaucrats).
- States are more likely to implement and enforce programs of their own making.
- States have served as important laboratories for testing different structures, approaches, and programs and for providing insight into the political and technical barriers encountered in enactment and implementation.
- States respond to crises faster.
- It is easier to change a state law than a federal one.
- States are more willing to take risks.

cisions. The greater control states have, the more difficult it becomes to develop a coordinated national strategy. For example, it is difficult to plan a national disease-control program if all states do not participate, or if they do not collect and report data in the same way. Moreover, some argue that disparities among states may lead to inequalities in access to health services. This might, in turn, lead to migration from states with poor health benefits to those with more generous programs. Finally, states may interpret federal incentives in ways that jeopardize the policy's original intent. For example, many states took advantage of federal matching grants for Medicaid programs by including a number of formerly state-funded services under an "expanded" Medicaid program. This allowed states to gain increased federal funding while providing exactly the same level of services they had provided before. This phenomenon, called Medicaid maximization, although pursued by only a few states, had an impact outside of those states and may have contributed nationally to rising health care costs in the early 1990s (Coughlin et al. 1999).

Impact of Presidential Leadership

Americans often look to strong presidential leadership in the search for possible sources of major change in health policies. President Lyndon Johnson's role in the passage of Medicare and Medicaid is often cited as a prime example. Presidents have important opportunities to influence congressional outcomes through their efforts to develop compromises that get bills passed with at least some of their preferred agendas.

Some important health policies have been passed since President Harry Truman's administration. The major piece of health legislation passed under Truman was the Hill-Burton Hospital Construction Act. In 1965, Johnson achieved the passage of Medicare and Medicaid because of an unusually favorable level of political opportunity and his leadership skills. Two major pieces of health legislation were passed during Nixon's presidency: (1) the actions leading to federal support of HMOs in 1973 and (2) the enactment of the National Health Planning and Resources Development Act of 1974 (CON legislation). This act represented an additional effort to restrain rapidly rising health care costs and included a fairly elaborate system of required approvals for new equipment and new hospital construction. Under Reagan, new Medicare cost-control approaches for hospitals and physicians were created, and additional Medicare coverage for the elderly was established. Even though Clinton's comprehensive reform efforts failed, his incremental initiatives have succeeded. Examples include the Health Insurance Portability and Accountability Act of 1996 and SCHIP.

Many political lessons can be learned from the failure of Clinton's health care reform initiative (Litman and Robins 1997). Presidents can achieve landmark changes in health policies only when political opportunity, political skill, and commitment converge. Opportunities were uniquely abundant for Johnson in 1965, and he effectively handled his legislative role. Presidents Truman, Kennedy, and Carter might have promoted their proposals with greater skill but were fundamentally thwarted by the lack of a true window of opportunity. Clinton enjoyed a uniquely high level of public interest in health care reform but failed in part because of other weaknesses in his level of opportunity, especially his failure to act within the "window of opportunity" (the first 100 days after his election). The complexity of the ever-changing details of his proposal was another major flaw and ultimately proved too hard for the public to grasp and too easy for adversaries to distort.

As described in Chapter 2, the health policy agenda of President George W. Bush has focused less on broad, sweeping reform, and more on market-based, individualistic, incremental policies, such as health savings accounts and implementation of health information technology.

The Development of Legislative Health Policy

The making of US health policy is a complex process that involves private and public sectors (including multiple levels of government) and reflects (1) the relationship of the government to the private sector, (2) the distribution of authority and responsibility within a federal system of government, (3) the relationship between policy formulation and implementation, (4) a pluralistic ideology as the basis of politics, and (5) incrementalism as the strategy for reform.

The Policy Cycle

The formation and implementation of health policy occurs in a policy cycle comprising five components: (1) issue raising, (2) policy design, (3) public support building, (4) legislative decision-making and policy support building, and (5) legislative decision-making and policy implementation. These activities are likely to be shared with Congress and interest groups in varying degrees.

Issue raising is clearly essential in the policy formation cycle. The enactment of a new policy is generally preceded by a variety of actions that first create a widespread sense that a problem exists and needs to be addressed. The president may form policy concepts from a variety of sources, including campaign information; recommendations from advisers, cabinet members, and agency chiefs; personal interests; expert opinions; and public opinion polls.

The second component of policymaking is the design of specific policy proposals. Presidents have substantial resources to develop new policy proposals. They may call on segments of the executive branch of government, such as the Centers for Medicare and Medicaid Services and policy staffs within the Department of Health and Human Services (DHHS). The alternative preferred by both Kennedy and Johnson was the use of outside task forces.

In building public support, presidents can choose from a variety of strategies, including major addresses to the nation and efforts to mobilize their administration to make public appeals and organized attempts to increase support among interest groups.

To facilitate legislative decision-making and policy support building, presidents, key staff, and department officials interact closely with Congress. Presidents generally meet with legislative leaders several mornings each month to shape the coming legislative agenda and to identify possible problems as bills move through various committees.

Suppliers of Policy

All three branches of government—legislative, executive, and judicial—are suppliers of policy. Of these, the legislative branch is the most active in policymaking, which is particularly evident from policies that take the form of statutes or laws. Legislators play central roles in providing policies demanded by their various constituencies.

Members of the executive branch also act as suppliers of policies. Presidents, governors, and other high-level public officials propose policies in the form of proposed legislation and push legislators to enact their preferred policies. Top executives, as well as executives and managers in charge of departments and agencies of government, make policies in the form of rules and regulations used to implement statutes and programs. In this manner, they interpret congressional interest and thereby become intermediary suppliers of policies.

The judicial branch of government also is a policy supplier. Whenever a court interprets an ambiguous statute, establishes judicial precedent, or interprets the US Constitution, it makes policy. These activities are not conceptually different from legislators enacting statutes or members of the executive branch establishing rules and regulations for the implementation of the statutes. All three activities concur with the definition of policy in that they are authoritative decisions made within government to influence or direct the actions, behaviors, and decisions of others.

Legislative Committees and Subcommittees

The legislative branch creates health policies and allocates the resources necessary to implement them. Congress has three important powers that make it extremely influential in the health policy process. First, the Constitution grants Congress the power to "make all laws which shall be necessary and proper for carrying into execution." The doctrine of implied powers states that Congress may use any reasonable means not directly prohibited by the Constitution to carry out the will of the people. This mandate gives it great power to enact laws influencing all manner of health policy. Second, Congress possesses the power to tax, which allows it to influence and regulate the health behavior of individuals, organizations, and states. Taxes on cigarettes, for example, are intended to reduce individual cigarette consumption, whereas tax relief for employer benefits is designed to promote increased insurance coverage for working people. Third, Congress possesses the power to spend. This ability allows for direct expenditures on the public's health through federal programs, such as Medicare and the NIH, but the power to allocate resources also gives Congress the ability to induce state conformance with federal policy objectives. Congress may prescribe the terms with which it dispenses funds to the states, such as mandating the basic required elements of the federal/state-funded Medicaid program.

At least 14 committees and subcommittees in the House of Representatives, 24 in the Senate, and more than 60 other such legislative panels directly influence legislation (Falcone and Hartwig 1991). Of these, five committees—three in the House and two in the Senate—control most of the legislative activity in Congress (Longest 1994) and are discussed below.

House Committees

The US Constitution provides that all bills involving taxation must originate in the US House of Representatives. The organization of the House gives this authority to the Ways and Means Committee. Hence, the Ways and Means Committee is the most influential by distinction of its power to tax. This committee was the launching pad for much of the health financing legislation passed in the 1960s and early 1970s under the chairmanship of Representative Wilbur Mills (D-AR). Ways and Means has sole jurisdiction over Medicare Part A, Social Security, unemployment compensation, public welfare, and health care reform. It also shares jurisdiction over Medicare Part B with the House Commerce Committee. This committee, formerly Energy and Commerce, has jurisdiction over Medicaid, Medicare Part B, matters of public health, mental health, health personnel, HMOs, foods and drugs, air pollution, consumer products safety, health planning, biomedical research, and health protection.

The Committee on Appropriations is responsible for funding substantive legislative provisions. Its subcommittee on Labor, Health and Human Services, Education, and Related Agencies is responsible for health appropriations. Essentially, this committee holds the power of the purse. The committee and the subcommittee are responsible for allocating and distributing federal funds for individual health programs (except for Medicare and Social Security, which are funded through the Social Security Trust Fund).

Senate Committees

The Committee on Labor and Human Resources has jurisdiction over most health bills, including the Public Health Service Act, the Federal Drug and Cosmetic Act, HMOs, health personnel, and mental health legislation (e.g., Community Mental Health Centers Act). This committee formerly included a subcommittee on Health and Scientific Research, which was used by its then chairman Senator Edward Kennedy (D-MA) as a forum for debate on whether the United States should have a national health care program. When the full committee came under Republican control in the 1980s, the subcommittee was abolished.

The Committee on Finance and its Subcommittee on Health, similar to the Ways and Means Committee in the House, has jurisdiction over taxes and revenues, including matters related to Social Security, Medicare,

Medicaid, and Maternal and Child Health (Title V of the Social Security Act). It is responsible for many of the Medicare and Medicaid amendments, such as professional standards review organizations, PPS, and amendments controlling hospital and nursing home costs.

The Legislative Process

When a bill is introduced in the House of Representatives, the Speaker assigns it to an appropriate committee. The committee chair forwards the bill to the appropriate subcommittee. The subcommittee forwards proposed legislation to agencies that will be affected by the legislation, holds hearings ("markup") and testimonies, and may add amendments. The subcommittee and committee may recommend, not recommend, or recommend tabling the bill. Diverse interest groups, individuals, experts in the field, and business, labor, and professional associations often exert influence on the bill through campaign contributions and intense lobbying. The full House then hears the bill and may add amendments. The bill can be approved with or without amendments. The approved bill is sent to the Senate.

In the Senate, the bill is sent to an appropriate committee and next forwarded to an appropriate subcommittee. The subcommittee may send the bill to agencies that will be affected. It also holds hearings and testimonies from all interested parties (e.g., private citizens, business, labor, agencies, experts). The subcommittee votes on and forwards the proposed legislation with appropriate recommendations. Amendments may or may not be added. The full Senate hears the bill and may add amendments. If the bill and House amendments are accepted, the bill goes to the president. If the Senate adds amendments that have not been voted on by the House, the bill must go back to the House floor for a vote.

If the amendments are minor and noncontroversial, the House may vote to pass the bill. If the amendments are significant and controversial, the House may call for a Conference Committee to review the amendments. The Conference Committee consists of members from equivalent committees of the House and Senate. If the recommendations of the Conference Committee are not accepted, another Conference Committee is called.

After the bill has passed both the House and Senate in identical form, it is forwarded to the president for signature. If the president signs the legislation, it becomes law. If the president does not sign the legislation, at the end of 21 days it becomes law unless the president vetoes the legislation. If less than 21 days are left in the congressional session, presidential inaction results in a veto. This is called a "pocket veto." The veto can be overturned by a two-thirds majority of the Congress; otherwise the bill is dead.

Once legislation has been signed into law, it is forwarded to the appropriate agency for implementation. The agency publishes proposed regulations in the Federal Register and holds hearings on how the law is to be implemented. A bureaucracy only loosely controlled by either the president or Congress writes (publishes, gathers comments about, and rewrites) regulations. Then the program goes on to the 50 states for enabling legislation, if appropriate. There, organized interests hire local lawyers and lobbyists and a completely new political cycle begins. Finally, all parties may adjourn to the courts, where long rounds of litigation shape the final outcome.

Critical Policy Issues

Government health policies have been enacted to resolve or prevent perceived deficiencies in health care delivery. Over the last four decades, most health policy initiatives have focused on access to care, cost of care, and quality of care (Falcone and Hartwig 1991). Some Americans contend that they have the right (access) to the best care (quality) at the least expense (cost), despite their level of income or social class. Legislative efforts have been specific to issues in access (expanding insurance coverage, outreach programs in rural areas), cost containment (PPS, relative-value scales), and quality (creating the Agency for Health Care Policy and Research [now Agency for Health Care Research and Quality] and calling for clinical practice guidelines, see Chapter 12).

With the publication of Healthy People 2010, elimination of health disparities across sociodemographic subpopulations has emerged as a bold policy objective. Since health disparities are caused primarily by nonmedical factors (see Chapter 2), the advancement of this goal signals a new policy direction that integrates health policy with broader public policy. Although it is highly unlikely this goal will be fulfilled within the first decade of the 21st century, the promotion of this policy objective reflects a significant government commitment. In the remainder of this section, critical policy issues related to access to care, cost of care, and quality of care, the three areas of greatest health policy concerns, are highlighted.

Access to Care

Underlying support for government policies enhancing access to care is the social justice principle that access to health care is a right that should be guaranteed to all American citizens (see Chapter 2). There are two variations on this argument: (1) All citizens have a right to the same level of care, and (2) all citizens have a right to some minimum level of care. The latter is more prevalent in the United States. However, significant debate exists over which health care services ought to be included in a basic tier. However, the conclusion that all citizens are entitled to a minimum level of services remains intact. Policies on access are aimed primarily at providers and financing mechanisms to expand care to the most needy and underserved populations, including the elderly, children, minorities, rural residents, those of low-income, and persons with acquired immune deficiency syndrome (AIDS) (see Chapter 11).

Providers

Several groups of providers deliver health care. Policy issues include ensuring a sufficient number and desirable geographic distribution of each. The debate over the supply of physicians is an important public policy issue because policy decisions influence the number of persons entering the medical profession, and that number, in turn, has implications for other policies. The number of new entrants into the profession is influenced by programs of government assistance for individual students and by government grants made directly to educational institutions. An increased supply of physicians, particularly specialists, may result in increased health care expenditures because of increased demand for care induced by the physicians. An increased supply of physicians, particularly primary care physicians, may help alleviate shortages in certain regions of the country. Programs enacted to expand delivery of care, particularly to the underserved, have included the National Health Service Corps, legislation supporting rural health clinics to expand geographic access, student assistance programs to expand the pool of health care workers, legislation to expand a system of emergency medical services, and the establishment of community health centers in inner cities and rural areas.

Public Financing

Although a national health care program is seen by many people as the best way to ensure access, the United States focuses instead on the needs of particular groups. As early as the Truman administration, and certainly by 1958, congressional attention turned to the health care needs of the elderly (Marmor 1973). In 1960, Congress enacted the Kerr-Mills program (P.L. 86–778), which provided federal grants to state government programs assisting the elderly. Medicare, and its companion program Medicaid (care for the poor was added to Medicare in part to compromise with a physician-drafted proposal), established the precedent that government should facilitate access to health care among those unable to secure it for themselves. Over the years, policies have been enacted to provide access to health care for specific groups otherwise unable to pay for and receive care. These groups include the elderly (Medicare), poor children (Medicaid and SCHIP), poor adults (Medicaid and local or state general assistance), the disabled (Medicaid and Medicare), veterans (Department of Veterans Affairs), Native Americans (Indian Health Service), and patients with end-stage renal disease (Social Security benefits for kidney dialysis and transplants).

Access continues to be a problem in many communities, partly because health policies enacted since 1983 have focused on narrowly defined elements of the delivery system. The United States has not had a unified strategy of reforming the system based on a policy of integrated services. Since the diminution of health planning in the early 1980s, the United States has approached the access problem on a piecemeal basis—one group, one type of geographic location, and one type of service at a time. The fact that many Americans remain uninsured is reason to expect ongoing debate toward a public policy on this issue.

Access and the Elderly

Two main concerns dominate the debate about Medicare policy. First, spending should be restrained to keep the program viable. Current emphasis is on using market-based mechanisms to deliver services more efficiently. Second, the program needs to be made truly comprehensive by adding services not currently covered (e.g., comprehensive nursing home coverage). Both concerns originate from the assumption that the elderly need public assistance to finance their health care.

Access and Minorities

Minorities are more likely than Whites to face access problems and to warrant special attention. Hispanics, African Americans, Asian Americans, and Native Americans, to name the most prevalent minorities, all face barriers accessing the health care delivery system. In some instances, the combination of low-income and minority status creates difficulties; in others, the interaction of special cultural habits and minority status causes problems. With the exception of Native Americans, no other minority population has programs specifically designed to serve its needs. Resolving the problems confronting minority groups would require policies designed to target the special needs of minorities, to encourage professional education programs sensitive to their special needs, and to develop programs to expand the delivery of services to areas populated by minorities. Many of these areas are known to be short of health care professionals.

Access in Rural Areas

Delivery of health care services in rural communities has always raised the question of how to bring advanced medical care to residents of sparsely settled areas. Financing high-tech equipment for a few people is not cost efficient, and finding physicians who want to live in rural areas is difficult. The medical model of health services delivery evident in large teaching institutions makes specialists and expensive diagnostic equipment readily available. This is not the case in rural medical practices, making those practices less desirable to many medical school graduates. Reimbursement systems based on average costs make it difficult for rural hospitals with few patients to survive financially.

In the Omnibus Budget Reconciliation Act (OBRA) of 1986, Congress began to address the particular problems of rural hospitals with three important provisions. The act separated the urban and rural pools of funds used to pay for outliers, those cases in which excessive expenditures above the PPS allotment are incurred. This ended the practice of using revenues otherwise intended for rural hospitals to reimburse expensive cases in urban hospitals. It provided early payments to hospitals with fewer than 100 beds. It also changed the criteria for rural referral centers to allow more hospitals to qualify for funds.

The OBRA of 1987 included provisions that (1) provided a greater increase in reimbursement to rural hospitals than to urban hospitals, (2) allowed rural hospitals located adjacent to metropolitan statistical areas to be defined as urban hospitals, (3) authorized a rural health care transition program to provide assistance to hospitals and others wishing to adopt new service delivery strategies, (4) required a report on the appropriateness of separate urban and rural rates, (5) and authorized small rural hospitals to serve as residency training sites for physicians (Patton 1988).

Shortages of personnel translate into access problems for rural residents. The federal government designates certain areas as health professions shortage areas, based on having a population-to-primary care physician ratio of at least 3,500:1 and being an area adjacent to others in which primary medical care personnel are overused.

Providing funding for the National Health Service Corps is another major step toward redressing the problem of personnel shortages in rural areas. The Corps affects only the percentage of graduating physicians practicing in shortage areas, and then only for a limited period for each student. Additional programs increase the total supply of physicians and create incentives for permanent practice in rural areas as needed.

Access and Low Income

Low-income mothers and their children have problems accessing the health care system, because they lack insurance and because they generally live in medically underserved areas. Limited access among children creates problems of untreated chronic health conditions that lead to increased medical expenditures and loss of productivity to society.

Low-income mothers face the same problems as their children in accessing medical services. Pregnant women in low-income families are far less likely to receive prenatal care than are women in higher income categories. The SCHIP program, signed into law August 5, 1997, gave states some flexibility in how to spend federal funds allocated for children's health coverage over five years (States Face a Welcome Dilemma 1997). After a period of enthusiastic outreach efforts and program expansion, a severe economic downturn, beginning in 2002, forced states to implement enrollment barriers for SCHIP (and Medicaid). As of January 2007, approximately 9 million children remain uninsured, despite the fact that a majority of them are eligible for Medicaid or SCHIP (Kaiser Family Foundation 2007a). As SCHIP undergoes federal reauthorization in 2007, funding decisions will critically affect whether this number of uninsured children can be reduced.

Access and Persons with AIDS

Persons with AIDS, who have progressed from infection by human immunodeficiency virus to actually having the disease and therefore needing more expensive treatment, also have problems obtaining health care. People with AIDS have difficulty obtaining insurance coverage, and their illness leads to catastrophic health care expenditures. Financial access can be a barrier, particularly for persons without adequate health insurance benefits. The AIDS epidemic presents a special challenge to policymakers committed to universal access to health care services. The services required are expensive, and the population in need is relatively small. Further, the care is directed toward patients who are terminally ill. In 2003, President Bush pledged $15 billion over five years to combat HIV/AIDS in the developing countries, with a particular focus on Africa. As of September 2006, the President's Emergency Plan for AIDS Relief (PEPFAR) supported prevention of mother-to-child transmission of HIV in over 6 million pregnancies and antiretroviral treatment for 822,000 people (US President's Emergency Plan for AIDS Relief 2007). On the other hand, funding to help AIDS victims at home remains inadequate by many accounts. According to The Foundation for AIDS Research (amfAR), Congress has provided significant increases for HIV/AIDS research, care, treatment, and prevention in the United States; however, domestic agencies still lack adequate resources to effectively combat the HIV/AIDS epidemic (Foundation for AIDS Research 2007).

Cost of Care

The strengths of the US health care delivery system also contribute substantially to its weaknesses. The United States has the latest developments in medical technology and well-trained specialists, but these advances amount to the most expensive means possible to provide care to patients, making the US health care system the most costly in the world. No other aspect of health care policy has received more attention during the past 20-plus years than efforts to contain increases in health care costs. Cost containment has become a major policy priority because of the government's increasing role in financing of health care services. Government programs, especially Medicare, Medicaid, Veterans Affairs, armed services, and federal employee benefit programs, are under constant pressure from Congress to keep costs down.

The National Health Planning and Resources Development Act of 1974 (P.L. 93–641) became law in 1975. This act marked the transition from improvement of access to cost containment as the principal theme in federal health policy. Advocates for both objectives supported health planning; however, the purpose rapidly became defined solely in terms of containing health care expenditures by the 1970s and health service researchers showed that the increased supply of health care facilities also increased expenditures. When Congress was considering expanding programs such as the Hill-Burton construction grants for health facilities through comprehensive health planning, policy analysts concluded that unneeded health care facilities were causing increases in health expenditures. In health care, unneeded supply generates demand. Therefore, it seemed logical to enact a policy that would allow construction of only those facilities that were actually needed. Need for facilities could be determined through a planning process, and final decisions would include some input from the citizens of the community.

Health planning, through CON review, was used as a policy tool to contain hospital costs; however, hospital charges continued to increase throughout the 1970s. The 1980 election signaled formal changes in the policy environment. One major change in the health policy environment was a new system of paying hospitals for Medicare clients, the PPS, enacted in 1983 (Mueller 1988). By 1982, members of Congress and the administration were convinced that voluntary efforts to contain hospital expenditures were failing. Congress used the Tax Equity and Fiscal Responsibility Act of 1982 as the legislative vehicle to reduce reimbursement for hospitals by $5 billion over three years. Congress commissioned the DHHS to develop a new system for reimbursement that would pay hospitals on a prospective basis rather than a retrospective basis. In lieu of tight regulation of charges established by individual hospitals, the PPS serves as a general fee schedule and establishes a prospective payment for general categories of treatment (based on diagnosis-related groups) that applies to all short-stay hospitals. PPS has proved to be the most successful tool for controlling hospital expenditures. As cost containment continued to be the dominant theme in the 1980s, health planning was no longer viewed as a national policy priority.

The election of Ronald Reagan in 1980 marked a general shift in policy that was geared to a reduction of federal government activity in domestic policy issues and toward an acceleration of deregulation throughout the domestic economy. The CON program, the cornerstone of cost containment through health planning, was retained by 38 states after Congress repealed the national law requiring such a program. The targets of CON laws may not always be hospitals, which were the subject of debates and legislation in the 1970s. Instead, the concerns of the 1990s became nursing homes, psychiatric facilities, and long-term hospitals. The owners of these facilities are less powerful than hospitals in influencing fiscal policy.

States use health planning in ways other than the review of petitions to add capital expenditures. More than 35 states have established state offices of rural health. Many of these programs use methods of health planning (i.e., needs assessment and consideration of alternative strategies for delivering services) to assist medical care providers and rural communities. A few states have used a direct regulatory approach to determine how much hospitals and nursing homes would be reimbursed. A variety of methods have been used, including limiting payments to a fixed percentage of the institution's charges, reimbursing only what the state determines is a reasonable amount for a given service, and determining in advance the total expenditures to be paid to hospitals and nursing homes for the coming year.

The policy focus on cost containment is also influenced by the private sector. Major corporations have awakened from the habit of passively paying medical bills. They are now aggressively pursuing ways to restrain the escalation of medical costs. These large purchasers are buying medical services in volume, at wholesale prices, and even dictating the terms of service. This method is a radical change from the long-held custom of individuals or their insurers paying for health care retail on a case-by-case basis. Institutional buyers want to know what they are getting for their money. The answers require detailed data, close scrutiny, and, ultimately, outside judgment of whether the services are worth their cost.

Expenditures are a function of the price of services times the quantity of services delivered (see Chapter 6). Most policies enacted to date have focused on the price of services. Policymakers are reluctant to consider restricting the quantity of services, fearful of interpretations that they are sacrificing quality of care for cost containment. These concerns are warranted as the media fuel the frenzy over denial of services by managed care organizations.

Increased debate over the right to die and the value of life-extending services provides an opportunity to discuss limiting reimbursable services. So far, the federal government has been reluctant to adopt an explicit rationing strategy to contain expenditures, but state governments can be expected to experiment with various means of cost containment. Interest in Oregon's rationing policies of the 1990s indicates that the issue may be addressed by state legislatures seeking to contain rising medical expenditures.

The fragmented multi-payer system in the United States does not lend itself to a centralized policy of cost containment. This is one main reason why health care expenditures in the United States will remain above per capita expenditures in other countries.

Quality of Care

Along with access and cost, quality of care is the third main concern of health care policy. Funding to evaluate new treatment methods and diagnostic tools is increasing dramatically. Funding for research to measure the outcome of medical interventions has also increased. This research is focused on the question of appropriateness of medical procedures.

The federal government began its actions to relieve the malpractice crisis and devoted greater attention to policing the quality of medical care with the Health Care Quality Act of 1986. This legislation mandated the creation of a national database within the DHHS to provide data on legal actions against health care providers. This information helps people recruiting physicians in one state to know of actions against those physicians in other states. Additional national legislation has been suggested to reform legal proceedings to lower the cost of malpractice claims and, therefore, reduce the premiums charged to providers.

In 1989, the federal government embarked on a major effort to sponsor research to establish guidelines for medical practice. In the OBRA of 1989, Congress created a new agency, the AHCPR, formerly called the

National Center for Health Services Research, and more recently called the Agency for Healthcare Research and Quality (AHRQ), and mandated it to conduct and support research with respect to the outcomes, effectiveness, and appropriateness of health care services and procedures (House of Representatives 1989). In the late 1980s, AHCPR (now AHRQ) established funding for patient outcomes research teams (PORTs) that focus on particular medical conditions. The PORTs are part of a broader effort, the medical treatment effectiveness program, which "consists of four elements: medical treatment effectiveness research, development of databases for such research, development of clinical guidelines, and the dissemination of research findings and clinical guidelines" (Salive et al. 1990). Today, the PORTs continue to produce valuable and applicable research findings on quality of care for various diseases and conditions, such as schizophrenia, diabetes, and stroke prevention. In March 2001, the Institute of Medicine (IOM) issued a comprehensive report, Crossing the Quality Chasm. Building on the extensive evidence collected by the IOM committee, the report identified six areas for quality improvement: (1) Safety. Patients ought to be as safe in health care facilities as they are in their homes. (2) Effectiveness. The health care system should avoid overuse of ineffective care and underuse of effective care. (3) Patient-centeredness. Respect for the patient's choices, culture, social context, and special needs must be incorporated into the delivery of services. (4) Timeliness. Waiting times and delays should be continually reduced for both patients and caregivers. (5) Efficiency. Health care should engage in a never-ending pursuit to reduce total costs by curtailing waste, such as waste of supplies, equipment, space, capital, and the innovative human spirit. (6) Equity. The system should seek to close racial and ethnic gaps in health status (Berwick 2002).

Policies designed to increase activities that promote good health are targeting individual behavior. Smoking cessation programs are designed to eliminate a specific behavior known to be related to the onset of several critical illnesses, including cancer, heart problems, and chronic obstructive lung disease. Data on the nation's health behavior indicators are published regularly by the US Office of Disease Prevention and Health Promotion. The US Environmental Protection Agency continues to monitor the quality of the air and water, and reports on cities and states not complying with federal standards.

Research and Policy Development

The research community can influence health policymaking through documentation, analysis, and prescription (Longest 1994). The first role of research in policymaking is documentation; that is, the gathering, cataloging, and correlating of facts that depict the state of the world that policymakers face. This process may help define a given public policy problem or raise its political profile. A second way in which research informs, and thus influences, policymaking is through analysis of what does and does not work. Examples include program evaluation and outcomes research. Often taking the form of demonstration projects intended to provide a basis for determining the feasibility, efficacy, or practicality of a possible policy intervention, analysis can help define solutions to health policy problems. The third way in which research influences policymaking is through prescription. Research that demonstrates that a course of action being contemplated by policymakers may (or may not) lead to undesirable or unexpected consequences can contribute significantly to policymaking.

The Future of Health Policy

Many of the problems confronted in US health care policy exist because policymakers have not adopted a comprehensive approach. Instead, single issues have been approached individually, and not all dimensions of any one issue have been considered when developing specific policies. Given the political system, the future of health policy is likely to continue in a piecemeal, fragmented, disjointed, and largely state-based manner aimed at enhancing access, containing cost, and improving quality. The recent policy goal of elimination of health disparities could not be realized without concerted efforts and coordinated strategies across health and non-health sectors.

Health Insurance Reform

The US health care system is criticized for many reasons. One common criticism is that the United States is the only industrialized nation that fails to assure universal access to basic health care. Over 44 million people—mostly adults and children in wage-earning families—lack health insurance. Nor does holding onto a job guarantee coverage. Seven out of every 10 Americans depend on their employers for their insurance, but in today's tight economy employers are chipping away at benefits, compelling employees to pay more of the cost and even eliminating coverage entirely. Being without health insurance often means being without medical care, especially for many of the adult poor and minorities (Freeman et al. 1990). One critical future policy concern is to ensure that most, if not all, Americans have adequate health insurance. If and when the time comes for a comprehensive reform of the current health care system, policy debate is likely to include several different proposals. These proposals are addressed in Chapter 14.

States as Leaders

From the 1930s through the 1950s, states' involvement in health care was limited to basic public health functions, such as control of communicable diseases, direct delivery of certain services, such as care for the chronically mentally ill, and administration of federal grants-in-aid. With the start of the health insurance industry in the 1940s and 1950s, states also began to regulate both Blue Cross and Blue Shield plans and commercial policies.

The states' role in health care diminished considerably in the 1970s as Medicare and Medicaid grew well beyond most of their creators' predictions and as other federal programs, such as support for community health centers, expanded in scope.

During the 1980s, President Reagan ushered in a new era characterized by an effort to return greater control and discretion over the financing, delivery, and regulation of health care to the states. ***Block grants***, which consolidate funds from many different categorical programs into one lump sum that is distributed to the states on a formula basis, became a key vehicle to achieve all three goals.

By the mid-1990s, states faced the prospect of gaining even greater control and flexibility for the administration and financing of health and human service programs. In 1995, Congress seriously considered a proposal to turn the entire Medicaid program over to state governments by giving them a block grant with few federal strings attached.

States are vested with broad legal authority to regulate almost every facet of the health care system. They license and regulate health care facilities and health professionals; restrict the content, marketing, and price of health insurance (including professional liability or malpractice insurance); set and enforce environmental quality standards; and enact a variety of controls on health care costs.

All states bear a large responsibility for financing health services for the poor, primarily through the Medicaid program, for which financing is shared with the federal government. States also pay the costs of providing health coverage to state employees and retirees, and sometimes for other publicly employed workers, such as teachers and police. In addition, most states also help subsidize some costs of delivering health services to those without any coverage at all. An example is Oregon, which, in 1989, embarked on a controversial experiment that expands Medicaid coverage to more than 100,000 additional people by reducing the Medicaid benefit package (Bodenheimer 1997).

By far, however, the states' most significant effort to contain costs was to increase enrollment of Medicaid beneficiaries into HMOs and other managed care arrangements, starting in the 1990s. By 2001, over half of Medicaid beneficiaries received services via managed care (Kaiser Family Foundation 2001). A review of studies on the effects of Medicaid managed care programs confirmed cost savings of 10% to 15% below those of the regular fee-for-service system; however, this cost savings may now be in jeopardy because many states, as part of their Medicaid maximization strategies, have crafted their programs to include safety net providers and mental health benefits. As the federal government closes the loopholes that allow for Medicaid maximization, this strategy may lead to higher costs for states, which could ultimately undermine the purpose of moving Medicaid beneficiaries to managed care: to increase access and quality of care (Coughlin et al. 1999).

Medicaid's inability to cover all the poor is one reason that approximately 44.6 million Americans lack health coverage (Kaiser Family Foundation 2007b). Often, it falls on the state governments, along with city and county governments, to help subsidize the costs of caring for those who lack health insurance coverage. Although many of these individuals are served by public health agencies or public hospitals that provide direct care to those without health insurance, many states also administer programs to provide coverage to these people.

One of the oldest and most fundamental state roles has been protecting the public's health. Originally, this meant controlling the spread of communicable diseases. The roles have expanded exponentially over the past several decades to include protecting the environment, workplace, housing, food, and water; preventing injuries and promoting health behaviors; responding to disasters and assisting communities in recovery efforts; ensuring the quality, accessibility, and accountability of medical care and providing basic health services when otherwise unavailable; monitoring population health status and changes in the health care system; and developing policies and plans that support individual and community health improvement. The Institute of Medicine (1988), in its study of the future of public health, condensed these various activities into three basic functions: assessment of health status and systems; policy development; and assurance of personal, educational, and environmental health services.

The biggest challenge facing state public health agencies today is strengthening their capacity to protect and promote the public's health while ensuring that basic health services are still available to those who cannot pay. Personal health services funded or provided by states, often in cooperation with local governments, range from public health nursing and communicable disease control to family planning and prenatal care, to nutritional counseling and home health services.

The challenge before state public health agencies is to seek partnerships with the private sector or with local governments. The goal is not merely to decrease their role in direct care but rather to engage private-sector and local government partners in efforts that will improve overall health status. One of the benefits of a managed care approach in the private health care market is managed care's emphasis on population-based services.

As discussed previously in this chapter, states are already undertaking their own comprehensive reforms. They have made important strides in expanding coverage to low-income uninsured groups through SCHIP, subsidy programs, Medicaid expansions, and insurance reforms. Many states have implemented effective cost-containment programs, such as hospital rate setting and setting limits on insurance premium increases.

Growth Initiative for Health Centers

One of the few goals that Republicans and Democrats seem to agree upon is preserving Community Health Centers as a safety-net health care provider for the uninsured. Acting on the recommendation of President Bush, Congress passed a significant increase in health center funding in the Omnibus Appropriations Act of 2003. The federal Health Centers program received $1.5 billion, $161 million more than the previous year. The President, who has pledged to double the size of the health center program, has continued to support increased funding for the health center program each year since then. In 2006, federal health center program allocations totaled $1.78 billion (NACHC 2006).

In addition to the President's request for 1,200 new and expanded sites, the increased health center funding will stabilize present health centers financially; they had been deteriorating in the light of state and local funding reductions, the rising number of uninsured, and the full impact of mandated Medicaid managed care in a more competitive health care marketplace. Significant progress toward the President's goals has been accomplished: as of 2004, the President's initiative had resulted in more than 600 new or expanded health center sites (Shi 2007).

Medical Malpractice

President Bush has asked Congress to set a $250,000 cap on noneconomic or so-called pain-and-suffering damages. Doctors in some parts of the country are facing double-digit increases in their malpractice insurance premiums and blaming the problem on runaway jury verdicts in malpractice suits. According to DHHS, the malpractice litigation "crisis" threatens access to health care. Many states have already limited damage awards in malpractice cases. But trial lawyers and consumer groups say malpractice suits are not out of control. They claim that insurance companies are raising premiums because of poor underwriting decisions and low investment returns. They also warn that limiting lawsuits hurts victims of egregious medical mistakes and reduces incentives to protect patient safety. Doctors contend that high liability expenses drive up health care costs, thus reducing access to treatment.

Mental Health Benefits

More than 30 million Americans suffer from schizophrenia, severe depression, and other mental disorders. Historically, employers' insurance has paid much lower treatment benefits for mental problems than for medical illness. The 1996 Mental Health Parity Act (MHPA) requires that annual or lifetime dollar limits on mental health benefits be no lower than any such dollar limits for medical and surgical benefits offered by a group health plan or health insurance issuer offering coverage in connection with a group health plan (US Dept of Labor 2007). Congress has considered broadening the MHPA, but conservative lawmakers and business lobbies claim the cost of parity is too high.

Steps to a Healthy United States

To advance President Bush's goal of helping Americans live longer, better, and healthier lives, the DHHS has launched the Steps to a Healthy US initiative. The initiative unites all relevant programs of the Health and Human Services agencies, including the Centers for Disease Control and Prevention, the Centers for Medicare and Medicaid Services, the Food and Drug Administration, and the National Institutes of Health. The initiative will also highlight health promotion programs to motivate and support responsible health choices, community initiatives to promote and enable healthy choices, health care and insurance systems that put prevention first by reducing risk factors and complications of chronic disease, state and federal policies that invest in the prevention for all Americans, and cooperation among policymakers, local health agencies, and the public to invest in disease prevention. Although the initiative's goals are lofty and worthy, concrete, workable strategies are yet to be developed and implemented.

Summary

Health policies are developed to serve the public's interests; however, public interests are diverse. The public often holds conflicting views. A 2007 New York Times/CBS News poll found a majority of Americans support access to health insurance for all. Sixty percent of respondents said they would be willing to pay more in taxes to support such a policy (NY Times 2007). However, while the public supports the goal of national health insurance, it also rejects the idea of the federal government running the health care delivery system. Similarly, while the public wants the government to control health care costs, it also believes that the federal government already controls too much of Americans' daily lives.

In the future, policymakers' challenge will be to find a balance between governmental provisions and control and the private health care market to improve coverage and affordability of care. Successful health policies are more likely to be couched in terms of cost containment (a market justice, economic, business, and middle-class concern) than improved or expanded access, and reducing or eliminating health disparities (a social justice, liberal, labor, low-income issue). However, cost-related policies are unlikely to significantly affect the quality of care or reduce health disparities.

Test Your Understanding

Terminology

allocative tools
block grants
distributive policies
health policy
public policies
redistributive policies
regulatory tools

Review Questions

1. What is health policy? How can health policies be used as regulatory or allocative tools?
2. What are the principal features of US health policy? Why do these features characterize US health policy?
3. Identify health care interest groups and their concerns.
4. What is the process of legislative health policy in the United States? How is this process related to the principal features of US health policy?
5. Describe the critical policy issues related to access to care, cost of care, and quality of care.
6. What do you think the future of health policy will look like in the United States?

REFERENCES

Alford, R.R. 1975. *Health care politics: Ideology and interest group barriers to reform*. Chicago: University of Chicago Press.

Belluck P. Jan. 9, 2007. Massachusetts could serve as a guide in California's health insurance bid. New York: *The New York Times*.

Berwick, D.M. 2002. A user's manual for the IOM's "Quality Chasm" report. *Health Affairs* 21, no. 3: 80–90.

Bodenheimer, T. 1997. The Oregon health plan—Lessons for the nation. *New England Journal of Medicine* 337, no. 9: 651–655.

Coughlin, T. et al. 1999. A conflict of strategies: Medicaid managed care and Medicaid maximization. *Health Services Research* 34, no. 1: 281–293.

Falcone, D., and L.C. Hartwig. 1991. Congressional process and health policy: Reform and retrenchment. In *Health policies and policy.* 2nd ed., eds. T. Litman and L. Robins, 126–144. New York: John Wiley & Sons.

Foundation for AIDS Research (amFAR). 2007. Public Policy. *http://www.amfar.org/cgi-bin/iowa/programs/publicp/record.html?record=9.*

Freeman, H.E. et al. 1990. Uninsured working-age adults: Characteristics and consequences. *Health Services Research* 24 (February): 811–823.

Health Insurance Association of America. 1992. *Source book of health insurance data.* Washington, DC.

House of Representatives. 1989. Omnibus Budget Reconciliation Act of 1989: Conference report to accompany H.R. 3299. Washington, DC: Government Printing Office, 21 November.

Institute of Medicine, Committee for the Study of the Future of Public Health. 1988. *The future of public health*. Washington, DC: National Academy Press.

Kaiser Family Foundation, Commission on Medicaid and the Uninsured. 2007a. State Children's Health Insurance Program at a Glance. *http://www.kff.org/medicaid/upload/7610.pdf.*

Kaiser Family Foundation, Commission on Medicaid and the Uninsured. 2007b. Characteristics of the uninsured. *http://www.kff.org/uninsured/upload/7613.pdf.*

Kaiser Family Foundation, Commission on Medicaid and the Uninsured. 2001. Medicaid and managed care fact sheet. *http://kff.org/medicaid/loader.cfm?url=/commonspot/security/getfile.cfm&PageID=13724.*

Lemov, P. 1990. Health insurance for all: A possible dream? *Governing* (November): 56–62.

Litman, T., and L. Robins. 1997. The relationship of government and politics to health and health care—A sociopolitical overview. In *Health politics and policy*. 3rd ed., eds. T. Litman and L. Robins, 3–45. New York: John Wiley & Sons.

Longest, B.B. 1994. *Health policymaking in the United States*. Ann Arbor, MI: Health Administration Press.

Marmor, T. 1973. *The politics of Medicare.* Chicago: Aldine Publishing Co.

Miller, C.A. 1987. Child health. In *Epidemiology and Health Policy*, eds. S. Levine and A. Lillienfeld. New York: Tavistock Publications.

Mueller, K.J. 1988. Federal programs do expire: The case of health planning. *Public Administration Review* 48 (May/June): 719–735.

National Association of Community Health Centers (NACHC). 2006. A sketch of community health centers: Chart book 2006. *http://www.nachc.com/research/Files/Chart%20Book%202006.pdf.*

National Institutes of Health. 1991. *NIH data book*. Washington, DC.

National Institutes of Health. 2007. Summary of the FY 2008 President's Budget. *http://officeofbudget.od.nih.gov/PDF/Press%20info-2008.pdf.*

Patton, L.T. 1988. *The rural health care challenge*. Staff Report to the Special Committee on Aging, US Senate. Washington, DC: Government Printing Office, October.

Salive, M.E. et al. 1990. Patient outcomes research teams and the Agency for Health Care Policy and Research. *Health Services Research* 25 (December): 697–708.

Shi, L., P.B. Collins, and K.F. Aaron. 2007. Health center financial performance: National trends and state variation, 1998–2004. *J Public Health Management and Practice* 13(2):133–50.

States face a welcome dilemma: How to best spend $24 billion to cover nation's uninsured children. 1997. *State Health Watch* 4, no. 8: 1, 4.

US Department of Labor. 2007. Mental Health Parity Fact Sheet. *http://www.dol.gov/ebsa/newsroom/fsmhparity.html.*

US President's Emergency Plan for AIDS Relief. 2007. *http://www.pepfar.gov/.*

Weissert, C., and W. Weissert. 1996. *Governing health: The politics of health policy*. Baltimore: Johns Hopkins University Press.

PART V

System Outlook

Chapter 14

The Future of Health Services Delivery

Learning Objectives

- To assess the trends in private and public health insurance
- To evaluate the challenges faced by managed care
- To discuss future financing and insurance options in the current system
- To discuss various options for a universal health insurance system
- To understand future challenges in wellness and prevention, chronic care, and long-term care
- To identify trends in the spread of infectious diseases attributed to globalization
- To foresee the evolving role of public health under new threats
- To explore the future outlook of US hospitals
- To address issues pertaining to the future needs for a well-prepared health care workforce.
- To understand the value of collaborative teamwork and cross-training in the delivery of health care
- To appreciate the emphasis on customer service and potential barriers
- To get an overview of new frontiers in clinical technology
- To survey the unfolding era of evidence-based health care

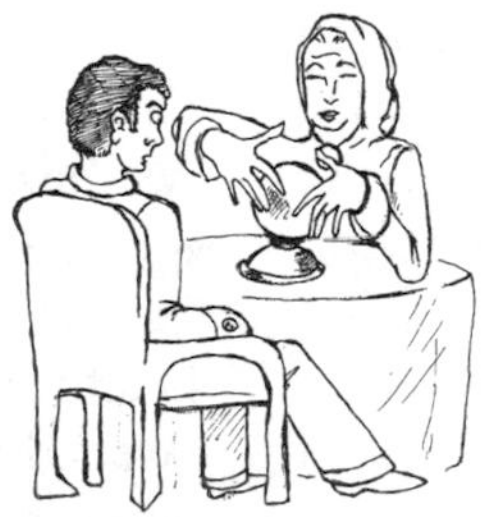

"Will the U.S. have universal health insurance?"

Introduction

Predicting the future direction of health care delivery in the United States is predicated upon major current developments and the course they might take in the foreseeable future. Future change also relies on historical precedents and a society's fundamental values (see Chapters 2 and 3). These elements come into play particularly when any kind of a sweeping transformation is proposed. For instance, in 1993, President Clinton proposed his national health care initiative in an economic, social, and political environment in which health care expenditures were getting out of hand and a significant number of Americans were without health insurance. However, the majority of Americans did not think that nationalized health insurance was the right way to address these issues. Most Americans were opposed to uninvited government intervention. The insured Americans were particularly fearful of losing their existing coverage with which they were reasonably satisfied. Middle-class Americans have also held a widespread belief that they pay more than their reasonable share of taxes to support Medicare and Medicaid programs to help the underprivileged. Besides the American middle class, the Clinton Plan was also opposed by most providers, particularly by physicians in private practice.

Rejection of the Clinton plan based on ingrained American values provided the impetus for a widespread shift toward managed care, which at that time had already started to emerge as a growing force. Managed care became the natural choice for injecting competition into the financing, insurance, delivery, and payment functions of health care.

At this point, the foundational values of American society remain intact. Hence, no sweeping changes are expected. However, medical cost escalation and cost of health insurance premiums continue to outpace both general inflation and general economic growth. For example, premiums for family coverage have risen by 87% since 2000 (Claxton et al. 2006). Faced with such a cost burden, fewer employers are offering health insurance coverage to their workers. The percentage of firms offering health insurance has fallen from 69% in 2000 to 61% in 2006 (Claxton et al. 2006). Also, since the mid-1990s, there has been steady erosion in retiree health benefits. Buchmueller and colleagues (2006) estimated that in 2003 only about 25% of private-sector employees worked at establishments that offered retiree health benefits, down from 32% in 1997. At the same time, Americans' appetite for new medical breakthroughs remains unabated. Amid these transitions, any major health care reform on a national scale has remained a nonissue. But, in April 2006, Massachusetts restructured its own health insurance markets, imposed assessments on employers who did not provide health insurance to their workers, and pooled private and public resources to cover many of the uninsured. If successful, this model may open the way for other states to initiate health insurance reforms.

At the time of this writing, the United States has also undergone a major political change with the Democrats gaining majority in both houses of Congress and control of the powerful Ways and Means Committee in Fall 2006. The presidential election of 2008 will be of significant interest because of major uncertainties on several fronts.

Any attempts to project the future of health care provoke more questions than answers. Even though precise forecasts cannot be made, certain fundamental features of health care delivery in the United States are assured at least for the foreseeable future. The stable features of US health care essentially recapitulate some of the points made in earlier chapters. In addition, this chapter provides some insights into current directions that might impact the future financing and delivery of health care. Other discussions revolve around what might be achievable, given the right configuration of broader socioeconomic, cultural, and technological forces, particularly in view of some of the major issues that must be addressed.

Trends in Private and Public Health Insurance

Trends in Employment-Based Insurance

During the era marked by the rapid growth of managed care, the proportion of nonelderly who had employment-based health insurance increased from 64.4% in 1994 to 66.8% in 2000. This was also a period of economic expansion and shortage of skilled workers that created stiff competition for labor. Since then, employment-based coverage has been eroding. It went down to 62.4% in 2004, which is below the level in 1994 (Gold 2006). Between 2000 and 2004, declines in employment-based coverage were the steepest for younger and low-income people (Holahan and Cook 2005). In addition, as the US workforce continues to age, the composition of enrollees in employment-based insurance will shift toward older adults, which portends an acceleration in the rate of premium growth. Well before we see the effects of baby boomers' enrollment in Medicare, rising premiums in private health plans could place more pressure on an already strained employment-based health insurance system (Keenan et al. 2006).

Public sector employers, particularly state and local governments, also face challenges similar to those in the private sector. As are major private employers, the public sector is experimenting with numerous cost-containment strategies, including disease and case management, aggressive management of pharmacy benefits, and contracting with managed care (McKethan et al. 2006).

Given the existing conditions, at least some commentators regard employers as ineffective and unenthusiastic managers of the health benefits they sponsor (Galvin et al. 2005). It is suggested that, if possible, employers would like to get out of the business of offering health benefits altogether, but it is unlikely to happen (Galvin and Delbanco 2006). Research suggests that employers, both large and small, hold a positive view of the value of health benefits in attracting and retaining workers, improving morale, and increasing workers' productivity. The same employers also believe that all employers should share in the cost of health insurance (Whitmore et al. 2006). It appears that employers are sensitive to having to carry the cost burden of those employed elsewhere, such as spouses of employees.

High-Deductible Health Plans

Faced with escalating health insurance premiums, employers appear to be embracing increased responsibility and higher cost sharing by the employees as strategies for reducing their health care costs (Claxton et al. 2005a). One emerging health plan type, the high-deductible health plan (HDHP), seems to be gaining some initial momentum. For example, in 2006, among firms that offered employment-based health insurance, 7% offered a HDHP. It was estimated that out of 155 million Americans covered under employment-based health insurance, as many as 2.7 million may be covered under a HDHP (Claxton et al. 2006). However, these plans may become more popular in the future because they carry the lowest premium compared to HMO, PPO, and POS plans, they offer tax advantages to workers and give the insured control over how the money is spent. Hence, these plans are also loosely referred to as consumer-directed health plans.

There are two basic types of HDHPs. The first type, called health reimbursement arrangements (HRAs), grew out of federal regulations made by the Internal Revenue Service in 2002. The second type, health savings accounts (HSAs), were authorized in the Medicare Prescription Drug, Improvement, and Modernization Act (MMA) of 2003.

An ***HRA*** is a medical care reimbursement plan sponsored by an employer. HRAs are typically offered in conjunction with a health plan that carries a high deductible. Generally, health plans that carry at least $1,000 deductible for a single plan and $2,000 for a family plan are considered ***high-deductible health plans***. In this arrangement, employers typically commit a predetermined amount of funds that the employee (and eligible dependents) can use to pay for medical expenses and for premium costs for the HDHP. Once the allocated funds are exhausted, the HDHP health insurance kicks in, in which the employee must first meet the deductible requirements out of pocket. Once the deductible is met, the plan becomes similar to a traditional health plan (Claxton et al. 2005b).

An ***HSA*** is a savings account created by an individual to pay for health care. To be eligible to create an HSA, a person must be covered by a "qualified health plan," which is a HDHP but also meets other legal requirements. Employers can offer qualified health plans, and both employers and employees can contribute to an HSA, but employer contributions are optional. An HSA offers certain tax advantages to the employee. Any contributions made by the employer are nontaxable. Employee contributions are on a pre-income tax basis. Funds in the HSA are invested and the earnings from investments are tax free. Withdrawals from the account to pay for health care are nontaxable; only withdrawals for nonmedical purposes are taxable. The savings account can build up over time, it belongs to the employee, and is portable (Claxton et al. 2005b). HSAs are an improvement over medical savings accounts (MSAs) that were authorized under the Health Insurance Portability and Accountability Act of 1996, but were available only to small businesses, the self-employed, and the uninsured.

The major problem with HDHPs as a reform effort is that they do not achieve universal coverage, and no one knows their impact on the control of health care cost growth. Poor families and individuals with limited tax liability are unlikely to benefit from HSAs' tax incentives. Also, people may skimp on care and delay seeking medical treatment for fear of depleting their accounts, thus jeopardizing their health.

Insurance Restructuring in Massachusetts

In April 2006, Massachusetts became the first state to break the gridlock between Democrats and Republicans, and passed a bipartisan plan that would achieve nearly universal coverage in the state. The plan was implemented in July 2007. The "individual mandate" part of the legislation requires all state residents to have health insurance or face legal penalties. The "employer mandate" part of the legislation requires all employers with more than 10 workers to offer at a minimum a Section 125 cafeteria plan that permits workers to purchase health insurance with pre-tax dollars (The Henry J. Kaiser Family Foundation 2006a). Large government subsidies would enable low-income individuals to buy insurance. People whose incomes are less than the federal poverty level will have their premiums paid by the state. Those earning up to 300% of the federal poverty level will pay a subsidized premium.

At the core of the plan is the reorganization of a large part of the state's private insurance system into a "single market" structure with uniform rules and a central clearinghouse or "Connector" to facilitate the purchase and administration of private health insurance coverage. The Connector relieves employers of the burden of obtaining and administering health insurance coverage. Only plans approved by the state's insurance department may be sold through the Connector (Haislmaier and Owcharenko 2006).

The plan is expected to cost $1.2 billion over three years. This funding will be derived from redistribution of existing funding that includes federal Medicaid payments that were previously paid to safety net providers under a federal waiver. Actually, the potential loss of this federal funding is what prompted the state to reform its health care system. Also noteworthy is the fact that Massachusetts had enacted a play-or-pay (see explanation of this option later in this chapter) mandate in 1988, but it was never implemented.

Unknown at this point are some key questions regarding the availability of private plans that the state would consider "affordable," whether employers would continue to offer current health insurance or switch to the Section 125 plan, which would be cheaper, and whether the plan can be financed over the long term.

The key features of what the program offers are quite appealing. If successful, the plan is likely to be emulated by other states. The plan has three main desirable features, as described by Haislmaier and Owcharenko 2006: (1) Insurance through the Connector is available to all residents of the state. (2) Coverage can become portable among employers within the state, and the coverage can be retained during periods of unemployment, part-time employment, or self-employment. (3) The program will provide a choice of plans. Once a year, participants will be allowed to switch coverage on a guaranteed-issue basis at standard prices. However, the plan faces many challenges and unknowns, and its full effects will not become known for several months.

Trends in Medicare and Medicaid

The Medicare Part D prescription drug benefit requires beneficiaries to receive drug coverage through private plans. The MMA of 2003 also provides new incentives, including sizable payment increases, to expand the role of private managed care plans to provide all Medicare covered services under the Medicare Advantage option (Biles et al. 2004). The policy is intended to attract more beneficiaries into managed care from the traditional fee-for-service option. Although only 14% of Medicare beneficiaries have chosen to enroll in Medicare Advantage, the Centers for Medicare and Medicaid Services estimates that by 2013 the proportion of beneficiaries in Medicare Advantage will rise to 30%. This estimate is perhaps based on the current levels of increased payments to private plans, but there is no certainty that Congress will maintain the payment increases when faced with future budget constraints. The program will very likely face budget constraints as, by 2015, annual Medicare expenditures are projected to reach $792 billion, which is more than double the amount of spending in 2005, and represents an average annual increase of 9%. In comparison, national health expenditures are expected to grow at an average rate of 7.2% between 2005 and 2015 (Borger et al. 2006).

The MMA has also attached a means-test feature to Medicare for both Part B and Part D premiums. In Part B, for example, single beneficiaries earning less than $80,000 per year ($160,000 per couple) will pay the standard premium, whereas those earning more will pay a higher income-based premium. As originally crafted, Medicare was not to be a means-tested program. Means-tested premiums may have opened the way for future reforms in which the wealthy would be asked to share a greater cost burden for financing the program.

Total enrollment in Medicaid has increased from 33.5 million in 2000 to 44.5 million in 2005 (Sanofi-Aventis US 2006), and expenditures have jumped from $118 billion to $179 billion (Catlin et al. 2007), or from $3,522 to $4,022 on a per capita basis, during the same period. Between 2005 and 2015, Medicaid spending is projected to grow at an average annual rate of 7.8%. Spending is projected to reach $384.4 billion in 2015 (Borger et al. 2006), which is more than double the amount spent in 2005. In 2005, 10 states had at least 90% of their Medicaid recipients enrolled in managed care. Nationwide, 62.2% of Medicaid recipients were in managed care, up from 58.4% in 2003 (Sanofi-Aventis US 2006). There is some evidence that Medicaid recipients enrolled in HMOs incur less overall expenditures (Kirby et al. 2003). Hence, it is expected that more states will mandate HMO enrollment in the future.

Future Options in Financing and Insurance

National health expenditures are projected to reach $4 trillion by 2015, approximately double the total spending in 2005, despite the fact that health care expenditures are expected to grow at a moderate rate of 7.2% annually. The amount of spending is projected to consume 20% of the gross domestic product (GDP) in 2015 (Borger et al. 2006), up from 16% in 2005. Although 88% of insured Americans rate their own health insurance coverage as excellent or good, approximately 20% are dissatisfied with the costs. Also, among the insured, 60% are at least somewhat worried about being able to afford the cost of their health insurance over the next few years, mainly if they lost their jobs. People's inability to pay for care when needed is on the rise; one in four Americans indicated they had a problem paying for care sometime during the previous year (The Henry J. Kaiser Foundation 2006b).

Some innovative approaches in health care financing and insurance have already started to emerge. This section also includes proposals that might reduce the number of uninsured through innovative financing policies. Given that one out of every five dollars would be consumed by health care, Americans will have to forego some other goods and services. This will likely lower, at least to some degree, the overall standard of living that Americans have become accustomed to. Erosion in the standard of living is perhaps best reflected in the growing number of poor in the United States. This is simply another social ill effect that unrestrained growth in health care will bring.

Defined Contribution Plans

Currently, the majority of employers offer what is referred to as a ***defined benefit plan***. The employer selects a health insurance plan and commits to providing the health benefits package, generally on a cost sharing basis. Large employers generally offer a choice of plans that vary in cost. Employees can choose from more expensive and less expensive plans. In the defined benefit health insurance arrangement, consumers have no financial incentives to be prudent purchasers, and patients are almost totally removed from the cost of care. But, the consumer of health insurance and health care is likely to bear more responsibility in the future. The defined contribution approach holds this promise. Defined contribution health insurance products that make use of Internet technologies are also getting some attention. Under a ***defined contribution plan***, employers commit to a fixed dollar amount for health benefits rather than to a predetermined package of health benefits.

The model for a defined contribution approach has, for some time, been used for retirement benefits. A shift occurred in the 1980s on the retirement benefits front when employers began moving away from defined benefit (or pension) plans toward defined contribution (or savings) plans (White 2001). Many employers see adoption of the defined contribution approach for health care benefits as compatible with the need to give employees a greater role in purchasing health insurance as well as health care services (Christianson et al. 2002). Actually, both HRAs and HSAs, discussed earlier, use certain features of defined contribution arrangements. In the future, other variations of defined contribution arrangements are likely to emerge.

A defined contribution plan could take one of two basic forms. On the more conservative side, employees would simply use the defined contribution to choose among several health plans selected by their employer. On the more radical side, employees could take their defined contribution dollars and purchase their own health insurance. In either case, the employer's share of premium costs is capped at a predetermined fixed dollar amount. One way to ensure that the money is actually applied to health care is to directly deposit the employer's contribution into employees' HSAs, which the employees are responsible for managing (White 2001).

In the future, the Internet is likely to play a major role in the purchase of health insurance and in the management of HSAs. Internet-based ***e-health plans*** will enable consumers to tailor plans according to individual needs, obtain instant quotes, and make online purchases. Managed care organizations are likely to play a major role by adapting their existing structures to meet the new demand. On the other hand, many of the emerging e-health plans have secured partners, such as Merrill Lynch, Chase Capital Partners, Hewitt Associates, Pricewaterhouse Coopers, and even the Mayo Clinic. These developments may indicate the emergence of the next wave of health care financing (White 2001). In any event, "consumer choice," "affordability," "cost effectiveness," and "better value" are going to be tomorrow's buzzwords.

Defined contribution plans also have implications for the health insurance market.

With consumers in the driver's seat, aided by the ability to shop on the Web, insurers will have to come up with differentiated plans that would serve a variety of needs and fit different budgets.

Public Entitlement Programs

Care for the future elderly, particularly as the first wave of baby boomers turns 65 in 2011, has serious implications for the Medicare program. Today's elderly account for 13% of the US population, yet they get more than 60% of all federal social spending (Lamm and Blank 2005). By 2020, the elderly will constitute 16% of the population, which will put unprecedented financial strains on the younger generations.

The RAND Corporation, in collaboration with Stanford University and the VA system of Greater Los Angeles, explored how changes in medical technology, disease, and disability would affect health care spending for the elderly population. Their key finding: Medical innovations will result in better health and longer life, but they will likely increase, not decrease, Medicare spending. Even though the health of the population over age 65 has been improving since the early 1980s, cumulative Medicare spending is relatively unaffected by the health status of new beneficiaries because healthier people live longer and have more years in which to accumulate costs. As in the past, new technologies will increase health care expenditures even though such technologies may improve health. The reason is that the reduction in spending resulting from better health will be outweighed by the costs of technologies themselves and by health expenditures during the additional years of life that the technologies may make possible. In short, there are no silver bullets for Medicare's fiscal crisis on the foreseeable horizon (RAND 2005). Given the grim prospects, Medicare will require a major reform effort and political will to carry out the needed reforms. Means testing has already been addressed earlier. Other reforms will most likely be coordinated along with reforms for the Social Security system which will also face severe financial shortfalls. Since there is no single magic bullet to cure these programs, the main options will likely include a combination of raising eligibility age, increasing premiums and other mechanisms to shift costs from the program to the beneficiaries, reducing reimbursement to providers, and curtailing benefits. Given the expansion of benefits in recent years, the latter option will be the most controversial, but will likely become necessary.

Given the cost projections presented earlier, the Medicaid program will also have to choose various options to curtail spending, similar to the ones just discussed, but for a couple of exceptions. Age limitation does not apply because eligibility is means tested, and there is perhaps little room, if any, to raise income-based eligibility thresholds. Secondly, shifting costs to the beneficiaries will be impractical because the program serves the indigent. Experiences of some states during the 2001–2003 recession might provide some lessons for the future. A study by Coughlin and Zuckerman (2005) concluded that states relied on a range of short-term solutions instead of reassessing their basic tax structures and policies. By resorting to short-term approaches, some states have created structural deficits that will profoundly influence state policymaking for many years to come (Coughlin and Zuckerman 2005). The implication here is that Medicaid reform will require tax hikes at both the federal and state levels.

Tax Credits and Vouchers

McClellan and Baicker (2002) argued that President Bush's proposal to introduce tax credits for the purchase of health insurance would enable millions of Americans to purchase private health insurance. It would also improve the functioning of private markets, empower patients to make informed decisions, and increase the use of high-value health care while reducing inappropriate use. To this effect, Congress passed the Trade Adjustment Assistance Act of 2002, which includes health insurance tax credits for displaced workers and retirees who have lost their employer coverage. The work of Patel (2002) suggests that affordable individual health insurance is available for most Americans, but one main barrier is the lack of consumer awareness. A variation of this approach is to issue the tax credits in advance in the form of vouchers that enable people, particularly the poor, to purchase insurance.

High-Risk Pools

Tax credits would still leave some people uninsured, particularly those who are considered high risk due to severe illnesses or chronic conditions. ***High-risk pools*** target groups that cannot purchase health insurance on their own because of poor health. Over 30 states currently have set up high-risk pools that enable hard-to-insure people to purchase subsidized coverage. In almost all cases, premium rates are capped at 125% to 150% of the average market rate. Deductibles are generally $1,000 or less, and an 80–20 coinsurance is common. Proposals that the federal government should help states establish these pools are based on the premise that the federal government already is the insurer of last resort in case of major natural catastrophes, and in the housing mortgage market through loan guarantees (Swartz 2002). Under the Trade Adjustment Assistance Reform Act of 2002, the Centers for Medicare and Medicaid Services (CMS) awarded the entire $80 million dollars that the bill had appropriated. The Deficit Reduction Act of 2005 reauthorized federal funds through fiscal year 2010. Federal grants provide seed money to create new high-risk pools and to cover operational losses.

Future Challenges for Managed Care

The role of managed care, as we know it, is assured in American health care at least for the foreseeable future. For now, status quo has been maintained in employer-sponsored health insurance as employers have been able to pass increased insurance costs to the employees through higher cost sharing in insurance premiums and higher deductibles and co-payments. However, pressures to control health care costs are beginning to mount. Once again, managed care will have to adapt and change to remain competitive.

Management of Risk

The greatest challenge in insurance is maintaining a balance between healthy and sick enrollees. However, 30% of persons 21 to 24 years of age are uninsured compared to 13.7% of people 55 to 64 years of age (Serota 2002). With the shifting demographics of the health insurance pool, managed care in the future will have to focus on managing the risk of an increasing number of people with potentially debilitating chronic illnesses, and also the sickest people in society. As discussed earlier, a growing number of Medicaid and Medicare beneficiaries, most of whom are high risk, are receiving care through managed care plans. Reforms in Medicaid, Medicare, and managed care will be necessary for MCOs to do a better job of managing health risk and for keeping costs under control. Future trends point to managed care as a risk-driven health care payment system. Instead of diagnosis and treatment as its principal business, the health care system will have to predict health risk and try to manage that risk before it turns into illness and cost (Institute of Medicine 1996, 54). Managing risk will involve population-based efforts to improve overall health status and an increased emphasis on prevention.

Accountability

MCOs in the future will have to be more accountable to both employers and enrollees. Although the choice of health plans by employers is driven primarily by the cost of premiums, accountability measures will be useful for enrollees in making informed decisions about which plan to choose. Such measures would be necessary if e-health programs catch on with the implementation of defined contribution benefits. Clinical practice guidelines to assess and improve the quality of care in MCOs will also become more common.

Comprehensive Reform: If and When It Occurs

At some point, debate over comprehensive reforms leading to universal coverage is likely to arise again. In a system driven by incremental reforms, experimentation with additional ad hoc arrangements is eventually likely to run out of viable options. Comprehensive reform may come up for debate, particularly if employer-based health coverage continues to erode, or if powerful politicians believe Americans are ready for comprehensive reform. The last situation occurred in 1992 when Clinton became president. Past proposals likely to be considered again have included a single-payer system, managed competition, and employer-based play-or-pay (see Exhibit 14–1 for summaries of major approaches to finance health care).

Exhibit 14–1 General Approaches for Health Care Financing Reorganization

Option 1: A laissez-faire, free-market approach ("piecemeal")

Pros:
- Builds on the current system rather than replacing it.
- Promotes managed care concepts (HMOs, PPOs) that incorporate mechanisms to control costs.
- Gives people an incentive to price-shop for insurance and medical care, improving individual choice and reducing personal costs.
- Maintains private market-based approach.
- Significantly restricts government involvement and regulation compared with the other approaches.

Cons:
- Does not mandate coverage for everyone.
- Requires consumers to have a sophisticated knowledge of insurance plans.

Exhibit 14–1 continued

- Relies primarily on questionable cost-control strategies already in place.
- Does not address administrative waste.
- Continues a two-tier medical system in which those who can afford it have greater coverage, while low income people receive minimum coverage.
- Lacks coverage for long-term care services.

Option 2: Government-financed public health care system ("single-payer" or "national health insurance")

Pros:
- Guarantees access to care for all individuals.
- Ensures coverage regardless of health status, economic status, job loss, or job change.
- Reduces or eliminates many out of pocket costs.
- Controls costs by setting payment rates and global limits on total health care spending.
- Removes employers' responsibility to provide health insurance, though they continue to pay for coverage through taxes.
- Greatly reduces multiple payers, thus lowering administrative costs.
- Spreads risk and cost across entire population.

Cons:
- Requires a substantial increase in taxes.
- Puts government in charge of whole system, which could lead to budgetary constraints affecting choice, quality, and use of new technologies.
- May result in waiting lists and shortages due to supply-side rationing.
- Significantly curbs need for private insurance coverage, resulting in thousands of lost jobs throughout the insurance industry.
- Could allow political and ideological biases to influence scientific decisions.

Option 3: Employer-based regulatory approach ("play-or-pay")

Pros:
- Provides coverage for everyone.
- Builds on the current system rather than replacing it.
- Eliminates exclusions for preexisting conditions.
- Reduces out of pocket costs substantially for many groups of people.
- Maintains competition among private-market insurance companies.
- Spreads risk and cost across entire population.

Cons:
- May offer no real incentive for some employers to "play" because tax route may be cheaper, which could shift millions of employed people into government pool.
- Mandates small businesses to pay, through either health insurance ("play") or higher taxes ("pay").
- Enables many insurance companies to continue to operate, which means some of the administrative costs (e.g., advertising) also continue.
- Increases taxes, although less than for government-based approaches.

Assuming that a major reform of the US health care system does occur in the future, the single-payer proposal is the least likely to be adopted because this will be the most drastic of the three approaches. Employer mandates enacted in Hawaii in 1974 are also discussed in this section, but are unlikely to be an option today because they will be highly resisted by employers.

Although a universal health insurance program will cover all citizens, access will be restricted to essential care. People wanting access to services beyond what is determined to be essential will have to pay for them (Ginzberg 1999). Besides, those who currently have good coverage will have to settle for a system that imposes supply-side rationing, and the delivery system will quickly become overburdened with an unanticipated surge in demand for services. Cost-effectiveness criteria will become thc gold standard for rationing medicine. There are three major problems with proposals for universal health insurance. (1) To financially sustain such a system Americans will have to "give up a cherished dream: the dream of total, universal care for any ailment freely available on demand" (Lamm and Blank 2005). (2) Proposed options (discussed below) only deal with insurance financing. They do not address the potential problem with access—how an overburdened system will meet increased demand for services. (3) Americans will have to be willing to pay increased taxes to sustain such a system.

Single-Payer

A ***single-payer health plan*** would place the responsibility for financing health care with a central agency (most likely the federal government). One major advantage of this system is that all Americans and lawful residents would be entitled to benefits regardless of individual or family income. Private insurance plans and government entitlement programs (Medicaid, Medicare, TriCare, and the Federal Employee Health Benefits Program) would no longer be necessary under a single-payer system, although the market for some private insurance will remain for those desiring coverage beyond what a basic government plan might offer.

According to one proposal, financing would come from an employer excise tax (8.7%) on annual revenues and a payroll tax levied on employees' salaries (2.2%), similar to federal or state income tax (LAPSR 1996). Additionally, the unemployed, disabled, and elderly would be subsidized through federal and state funds based on their ability to pay (LAPSR 1996, 1). Health care providers would be reimbursed on a fee-for-service scale. Hospitals, nursing homes, and other institutional facilities would be given an annual prospective budget to provide all required care.

A single-payer system could accomplish two major goals of health care reform: (1) provide universal coverage and (2) contain costs. By eliminating private health insurance, the single-payer system can lower administrative costs. But, the bulk of savings will come from supply-side rationing, which is the hallmark of all national health insurance programs.

A single-payer system has other drawbacks. Financing this type of plan primarily with an employer tax would place a financial burden on small businesses. Very likely, an increase in general taxes will also become necessary to support a burgeoning system. In addition, a single-payer system will likely create bureaucratic problems associated with the centralized administrative process. These problems include lack of flexibility and enhanced power and control over providers and businesses. Open rationing of health services will be highly resisted by the American public.

Managed Competition

President Clinton's proposed Health Security Act of 1993 was based largely on the principles of ***managed competition***. The plan proposed to guarantee every citizen the right to receive a comprehensive package of health care benefits. Under the proposal, regional alliances would be established to ensure that every citizen was enrolled in a plan. The alliances would function very much like the Connector in the Massachusetts health plan discussed earlier, that is, act as the fiscal intermediary between the plans and enrollees. Financing for the proposed program was based on cost sharing between employers (80%) and employees (20%).

The advantage of adopting a managed competition arrangement is that the medical infrastructure is already in place, and the private insurance industry, the would-be administrator of care, is well established in the United States. This could facilitate a smooth transition, whereas the single-payer system would require redesigning the entire health care delivery system. Also, compared to a single-payer system, managed competition calls for a smaller government bureaucracy.

Unfortunately, managed competition cannot guarantee that everyone would have equal access to care. Inner cities and rural areas in particular would have difficulty attracting enough health plans. A fundamental problem with managed competition is that unless several plans are competing against each other in a given geographic area, the system cannot drive down the cost of health care.

Play-or-Pay

Employer-based ***play-or-pay*** was introduced as a Senate bill in 1989 to achieve universal coverage. Under this system, employers must either provide their employees health insurance (play) or pay into a public health insurance program. The plan requires private or public insurance entities to provide identical benefits to working Americans and their dependents. Medicaid and Medicare would remain to provide care to the elderly, disabled, and poor.

If the employer chooses to pay, financing is through a payroll tax paid by the employer and the employee. The employee is still responsible for co-payments, premiums, and deductibles. Employees could also purchase supplemental health care benefits privately or through their employers.

Because an employer-based system is already in place, this type of plan is less disruptive than a single-payer system. Since many Americans who are uninsured are actually employed, this program could considerably reduce the number of uninsured.

Much like a single-payer system, play-or-pay would place an undue economic burden on small businesses because of mandatory employer financing. However, given the choice of "not to play, but pay" many employers, including those who currently provide health insurance to their workers, will choose to pay because, as the recent experience in Massachusetts indicates, it will be cheaper to pay than to play. Consequently, a greater cost burden would fall on the public who will have to pay higher taxes. This was precisely the reason why Massachusetts did not implement its 1988 enactment of a play-or-pay mandate. California is another state that passed a play-or-pay mandate in 2003, but the law was repealed through a ballot referendum. Another drawback of a play-or-pay system is that it focuses only on the financing of care, and does not address other areas of concern, such as access to care, utilization of services, and quality of care.

Employer Mandates

Employer mandates require employers to help pay for their employees' coverage. Despite the seeming appeal of an employer mandate, only Hawaii has implemented this type of reform. States' ability to adopt employer mandates has been thwarted by the federal Employee Retirement Income Security Act (ERISA), which exempts self-insured businesses from state insurance regulations and taxes. Hawaii is the only state that received a Congressional exemption from ERISA for its employer mandate. In spite of employer mandates, almost 10% of the population in Hawaii is uninsured (DHHS 2006, 420).

Most employers not offering health insurance to their workers would actually like to offer it, but they find it too costly. Other employers do not offer health insurance because most of their employees already have coverage (often from a spouse's employer) or because health insurance is not regarded as necessary to attract or retain the types of employees needed (Friedland 1996). This is often the case in low-skill jobs.

National and Global Challenges

To restrain the mounting burden of health care spending, wellness and disease prevention will have to be incorporated into health care delivery. On the other hand, the demands of chronic care and new and resurgent infectious diseases must also be incorporated into medical practice. New health care roles are required to coordinate the needs of people with chronic illnesses. Health care institutions and private practitioners must coordinate their efforts with public health agencies to identify emergent diseases and contain the spread of infection.

Future of Wellness, Prevention, and Health Promotion

Because of the changing causes of death, disease patterns, and the economic burden of disease, future health care emphasis will shift from acute to preventive care. To keep health benefit costs under control, employers are likely to promote employee health. Coile (2002) proposed that employers might have to take a long-term view instead of depending on short-term solutions. Employers would have to proactively identify employees and dependents with health risk factors, and support health promotion strategies to reduce health risks through smoking cessation, weight reduction, and stress management programs (Coile 2002, 14). Hospitals and managed care plans must continue as the leaders in integrating wellness and health promotion into medical care delivery. The goals and objectives laid out in Healthy People 2010 (see Chapter 2) are also consistent with this kind of shift in emphasis. However, the epidemic of overweight and obesity threatens to undo much of the progress that has been made in controlling cardiovascular disease, diabetes, and cancer (Satcher 2006).

The former US Surgeon General, David Satcher, laid out a three-point plan to increase investment in prevention: (1) At the first level, labeled "downstream," the focus is on the individual and his or her lifestyle and behaviors. For example, regular physical activity, good nutrition, and scheduled immunizations are emphasized here, as well as the importance of avoiding toxins such as tobacco, alcohol, and harmful drugs. (2) At the second level, labeled "midstream," the focus is on the community. For example, investments are needed in public infrastructures that support walking, biking, and physical recreation. Schools should provide physical education. (3) At the third level, labeled "upstream," the focus is on health policy that supports prevention. An example is legislation that promotes physical activity and good nutrition programs in schools (Satcher 2006). Although putting such a plan into practice will be a challenge, it will require public-private partnership.

Challenges of Chronic Illness Care

In one century, the United States and most other nations have made significant gains in health status and life expectancy—mainly by conquering communicable diseases and developing more affluent lifestyles. However, with a higher life expectancy, such chronic disorders as heart disease and cancer have become the major causes of death. Future trends project an increase in affluence-related diseases, including cardiovascular, oncotic, and degenerative diseases. The more successful health care is at vanquishing disease symptoms and prolonging life, the more people will have to face the inevitable physical deterioration of the aging process.

Changing patterns of diseases are occurring in the shift to more chronic and multifaceted illnesses—a shift that will affect the demand for services and the type of services required. The future health care delivery system will have to be configured to meet these impending challenges. At a fundamental level, the shift will be from a reactive approach that responds to illness and its accompanying complications to a proactive approach that focuses on managing the underlying medical conditions. (See Chapter 10 for future projections of the number of people with chronic conditions in the United States.)

Approximately one-third of Americans with chronic illnesses report that they are in fair to poor health, and too many chronically ill patients are not equipped to deal with their medical problems. According to one report, only 30% of patients with chronic illnesses felt very confident about their ability to decide something as basic as when it is appropriate to see a physician, 20% were not very confident about taking their medications in an appropriate manner, almost 50% had low levels of confidence about eating right, and about 50% could count on a high level of social support. On the other hand, people who suffer from chronic illnesses continue to engage in risky behaviors at rates comparable to the general population, despite the higher risks to their health. The chronically ill also face barriers because of affordability and physical access even though the vast majority has private or public insurance. The frequently expressed need for home care and special transportation services remains unmet for the vast majority of patients (Foundation for Accountability 2001). On the other hand, expenditures for long-term care are projected to increase at 2.6% annually above inflation to $154 billion in 2010, $195 billion in 2020, and a staggering $270 billion in 2030 (Congressional Budget Office-CBO-1999). Clearly, the future's health care delivery system will need to improve drastically to meet the growing demand for effective chronic care. The system needs to shift decisively from the current acute care model to a chronic care model.

Some of the main initiatives to improve the quality of care and reduce costs of care for the chronically ill have occurred through Medicare policy. For example, Section 721 of the MMA establishes the Chronic Care Improvement Program (CCIP). The CCIP, a new service that is predicated on disease management (see Chapter 9), is being introduced on a pilot basis with the fee-for-service option in Medicare. Other demonstration programs called for by previous legislative action such as the Medicare, Medicaid, and State Children's Health Insurance Program Benefits Improvement and Protection Act of 2000 are in various stages of planning and implementation. However, past demonstration projects have had a less than optimal record of achieving their intended objectives. Hence, more comprehensive, multifaceted innovations that simultaneously address provider practice, patient education, and patient self-management are necessary. Also, given the well-established influence of reimbursement on physician behavior, payment strategies should be restructured to facilitate transition of chronic care principles to the health care delivery system (Wolff and Boult 2005). Reimbursement systems must change in a way that also includes compensation for the services of nonphysician providers, such as nurse practitioners and community health nurses. In addition, health care professionals, including physicians, need to receive appropriate training in the management and coordination of the special needs of people suffering from chronic illnesses.

Challenges in Long-Term Care

The financing and delivery of long-term care will remain a major challenge. The good news is that long-term care is typically needed later in life. Even though the first wave of baby boomers will start retiring in 2011, they are not likely to need professional long-term care services until 2025 or later. However, the system must be reformed before that time comes. In their report to the National Commission for Quality Long-Term Care, Miller and Mor (2006) identified six main areas of concern that must be addressed: financing, resources, infrastructure, workforce, regulation, and information technology.

Financing

Currently, most middle-class families are unprepared to meet long-term care expenses. Most people think that Medicare would pay for their long-term care needs. But, as pointed out in Chapters 6 and 10, Medicare covers only short-term post-acute care. It is estimated that less than 10% of the elderly have private long-term care insurance (Burke et al. 2005). Unless policy initiatives are established to promote long-term care health insurance plans, the public sector will see its expenditures grow rapidly. Purchasing long-term care insurance is both expensive and confusing. The Congressional Budget Office (CBO 2004) recommended improving the way private markets for LTC insurance currently function. For instance, private insurance could be made more attractive to consumers by standardizing insurance policies to allow competing policies to be more easily compared. Currently, state insurance regulations do not require insurance carriers to offer policies that conform to particular design standards. Standardized policies could also stimulate price competition among insurers and help keep premiums lower than they would otherwise be. However, reform is also needed in a public financing system, particularly Medicaid, that pays for the bulk of long-term care costs. The Deficit Reduction Act (DRA) of 2005 tightened Medicaid eligibility rules. The law also extended the time period for asset transfers (called the look-back period) to qualify for Medicaid (Crowley 2006). In 2004, Medicaid and Medicare financed roughly 60% of all long-term care costs (CBO 2004). Without reform, these programs will put enormous financial pressure on the future working population.

Resources

Currently, financing for long-term care in the United States is tilted quite heavily in favor of institutional services rather than community-based services. Costs can be reduced if people who otherwise would be placed in nursing homes can have their needs met using community-based care. However, the Home and Community Based Waiver (HCBW) (see Chapter 10) program has been too restrictive. Some provisions have been made in the DRA to extend community-based care to a larger number of people.

Infrastructure

The institutional long-term care sector has been going through a cultural change that has led to the creation of enriched living environments in nursing homes. New architectural designs, living arrangements, and worker and patient empowerment are improving the quality of life in nursing facilities that have adopted the innovative models such as Eden Alternative, Green House Project, and Wellspring. Over time, traditional living and care arrangements will be replaced by these and other innovative models. (For an overview of these models, the reader is referred to Singh 2005, Chapter 6.)

Workforce

The aging of America will shrink the overall pool of workers. Experts think that this will have a particularly drastic effect on the health care sector, and long-term care in particular because of low pay and hard work. It is estimated that between 2000 and 2010 alone, when the baby boomers are about to reach retirement age, an additional 1.9 million direct care workers will be needed in long-term care settings (Department of Health and Human Services 2003). Another issue that must be addressed is a lack of training in geriatrics among the current workforce (discussed later).

Regulation

Currently, many experts see fundamental contradictions between the existing regulatory mechanisms that address quality issues in nursing facilities through periodic inspections and sanctioning, and regulations that require the same nursing facilities to implement quality improvement programs. Also, one of the most disconcerting aspects of government regulation of long-term care is its inconsistent application both within and across regions over time (Miller and Mor 2006). These issues need to be resolved.

Information Technology

Interoperable IT systems (discussed in Chapter 5) will enable providers to track patients' care across hospitals, nursing homes, home health agencies, and physicians' offices. Such systems are particularly critical in long-term care because the elderly frequently make transitions between long-term care and non-long-term care settings. Currently, such transitions rarely occur smoothly because of high rates of missing or inaccurate information (Miller and Mor 2006).

Infectious Diseases and Challenges of Globalization

The much-needed shift to chronic disease and disability does not mean that infectious disease prevention and control efforts will become unnecessary. In fact, intensified efforts will be required to combat emergent and resurgent infectious diseases. For instance, the sudden appearance in the early 1980s of a previously unknown disease we now call AIDS challenged the widely held belief that infectious diseases were under control. Since then, other deadly bacterial infections, such as Lyme disease, have appeared. Even though some of the newer infections have not created the panic that AIDS did, the scientific community is baffled by some ordinary bacterial infections that have turned lethal. Another cause of concern is that certain strains of bacteria have become antibiotic-resistant from the inadvertent overuse of antibiotics, which presents fresh challenges from infectious diseases, new and old. New forms of influenza virus have periodically raised alarms in the United States. Hantavirus, which is believed to have originated in Korea, has caused some lethal infections in the United States. National public health alerts made headlines in 2002 when encephalitis cases in New York were attributed to the West Nile Virus, which then traveled 3,000 miles west to California. This infection had never before been identified in the Western Hemisphere (Novick 2001), and its emergence in the United States has been attributed to global flow of goods, services, and people. Increase in air travel resulted in the spread of Severe Acute Respiratory Syndrome (SARS) from China to Canada in 2003, and of polio virus from India to northern Minnesota in 2005 (Milstein et al. 2006).

The above examples demonstrate that infectious diseases and health care must be viewed from a global perspective. The HIV/AIDS epidemic, for instance, has so far affected Africa the most. The African epidemic received little attention from the United States until very recently when it was recognized that the epidemic posed growing risks to US interests due to increasing globalization. Immigration of people from other countries to the United States, international travel to and from the United States, and shipments coming to the United States from other countries have made it increasingly possible for deadly infections to cross international borders. Data show that the US death rate from infectious diseases has doubled since 1980, and treatment of these diseases uses 15% of total US health spending (Kassalow 2001). HIV/AIDS, Hepatitis C, and other infectious diseases, some currently known and some as yet unknown, will pose growing threats to US interests, particularly as the AIDS crisis is expected to spread rapidly through India, Russia, China, and Latin America, which make up almost 40% of the world's population (Gow 2002).

The global aspect of infectious diseases emphasizes the need to link together the nation's foreign policy and public health policy. Globalization presents social and economic opportunities from which nations can benefit, but it also holds the potential for a global catastrophe. International cooperation, sharing of information, and technical and financial assistance will be necessary to avert any major health mishaps that could affect millions of people around the world.

Bioterrorism and the Transformation of Public Health

Public health has always been about protecting the population's health. More recently, emphasis on homeland security has lifted public health to a new level of respect and recognition as an instrument to protect the public against new threats to their health and well-being. Actually, the interest in public health in America has been like a seesaw, going up during times of danger to people's health and safety, and coming down when no present dangers loom. The importance of public health and deficiencies in the existing public health system received national attention during terrorism-related attempts to bring about an anthrax epidemic in October 2001, soon after the terrorist attacks and destruction of the World Trade Center in New York City on September 11, 2001. Since then, a heightened awareness of potential threats posed by chemical and biological weapons, and low-grade nuclear materials has prompted public officials nationwide to review and revamp the system. Most experts believe that the threat of terrorism on American soil will remain with us for the foreseeable future. The nation's central public health agency, the Centers for Disease Control and Prevention (CDC), will continue to play a vital role in recognizing emerging threats and in developing measures to contain any unexpected outbreaks. Public health agencies at local, state, and federal levels have been identifying infrastructure weaknesses and reevaluating plans to protect the American public (Baker and Koplan 2002). Public health must prepare for threats other than those posed by "imported" infectious diseases (discussed earlier); possible use of chemical, biological, and nuclear agents; and natural disasters such as Hurricanes Katrina and Rita in the Gulf Coast. Safeguarding the nation's food and water supplies is equally important.

The future effectiveness of public health will involve cooperation among public health agencies at the federal, state, and local levels; other departments of the government, such as the Department of Justice, and the Food and Drug Administration; private and public organizations, such as hospitals, clinics, and nursing homes; private practitioners, such as physicians and nurses; volunteer agencies, such as the American Red Cross and numerous other voluntary organizations; civil defense agencies, such as police and fire departments; businesses; and individuals and groups within communities.

To protect the health and safety of American communities, public health agencies will need to strengthen the 10 core public health functions enumerated by the National Association of County Health Officials (1994) in its *Blueprint for a Healthy Community: A Guide for Local Health Departments*:

1. ***Conduct a community diagnosis.*** Collect, manage, and analyze health-related data for information-based decision-making.
2. ***Prevent and control epidemics.*** Investigate and contain diseases and injuries.
3. ***Provide a safe and healthy environment.*** Maintain clean and safe air, water, food, and facilities.
4. ***Measure performance, effectiveness, and outcomes of health services.*** Monitor health care providers and the health care system.

5. ***Promote healthy lifestyles.*** Provide health education to individuals and communities.
6. ***Provide laboratory testing.*** Identify disease agents.
7. ***Provide targeted outreach and form partnerships.*** Assure access to services for all vulnerable populations and the development of culturally appropriate care.
8. ***Provide personal health care services.*** Treat illness, injury, disabling conditions, and dysfunction (ranging from primary and preventive care to specialty and tertiary treatment).
9. ***Promote research and innovation.*** Discover and apply improved health care delivery mechanisms and clinical interventions.
10. ***Mobilize the community for action.*** Provide leadership and initiate collaboration.

Effective public health responses will also require revamping the infrastructure and improving skills. Some priorities include workforce development; technical leadership skills for top-level public health professionals; modern information and communication systems; state-of-the-art disease surveillance systems, including early-warning systems; resources to maintain front-line public health response teams in a state of readiness; and rapid deployment of antidotes and vaccines when needed. In addition, periodic readiness assessment, ongoing research, and the upgrading of laboratory capabilities will be needed to ensure readiness for new and yet unknown challenges.

Local and state public health agencies will remain safety-net providers by continuing to deliver certain health care services to those in need. Increasingly, however, these governmental agencies will form partnerships with organized health care providers to ensure that population-based prevention is available to everyone. To increase efficiencies, consolidation will be effected by regionalizing public health jurisdictions. This would diminish the number of local public health jurisdictions from approximately 3,000 to somewhere between 500 and 1,000 (Mays et al. 2000). In some jurisdictions, the privatization of public health services using contractual arrangements with private providers will continue in ways that improve efficiency (Baker and Koplan 2002).

The Future Outlook for US Hospitals

It appears that a nationwide hospital construction boom is under way to expand capacity, replace aged facilities, or build new full-service or specialty hospitals. Many hospitals are replacing existing semi-private patient rooms with all private rooms. In many instances, hospitals are also increasing capacity in operating rooms, diagnostic radiology, telemetry observation beds, critical care for newborns and children, and outpatient services. For increasing capacity, the most notable market factor is population growth, particularly in areas where such populations are well insured. At this point, there is little evidence, however, as to how the benefits of increased capacity will balance with the increased costs (Bazzoli et al. 2006). Recent research shows that contrary to popular opinion, the aging of the baby boomers and increased longevity in general will have less of an impact on the future of hospital demand than local population trends and changing practice patterns attributable to advancing medical technology (Strunk et al. 2006).

Cost increases in the health care system have also been primarily attributed to hospitals. For example, it is estimated that hospitals were responsible for about 28% of the $528 billion increase in health care spending between 1998 and 2003 (D'Cruz and Welter 2005). Hence, hospitals will come under increased scrutiny to contain costs and improve efficiencies.

Hospitals will also be expected to continue to respond to other pressures from their external environments. They will increasingly develop a continuum of medical care services, and will continue to engage in providing one-stop shopping for all health care needs. Hospitals will also continue to reinvest capital in the development of integrated delivery networks, including joint ventures with other hospitals, physician practices, and managed care organizations.

The hospital of the future will be a health center, not just a medical center. Keeping people healthy will continue to receive a great deal of emphasis, and hospitals will increasingly engage in offering valuable resources to the community on matters of health and well-being, and will be held increasingly accountable for the community's health status. Hospitals will work not only to improve community health services but also to develop better programs to measure outcomes.

Other freestanding institutions of health care delivery will continue to exert competitive pressures on hospitals. On the other hand, concerns about Medicare's solvency and pick up in cost escalation will impose fiscal pressures. With the growing number of uninsured patients, the workloads of emergency departments are likely to increase, but without any additional reimbursement. Especially public hospitals and those located in urban centers will face increasing utilization and financial pressures because these hospitals end up sharing a larger burden of uncompensated care.

Cost pressures are likely to require hospitals to focus on greater labor productivity and reductions in overall staffing. This will require emphasis on multiskilled workers and labor-saving technology.

Future of the Health Care Workforce

Health care delivery influences, and is influenced by, the characteristics of the health care workforce. Some of the factors influencing the workforce include changes in the utilization of hospital-based and other health care services, an increasing elderly population, training and availability of skilled and semi-skilled workers, and more women and minorities entering the health care workforce. The future health care workforce will also be impacted by individual career choices and enrollments in training programs, and immigration of trained foreign workers in areas of high labor demand. Shortage of nurses is one of the dominant issues today. However, whether this shortage will continue is debated. Currently, pharmacists, technicians, and therapists are also in short supply (Coile 2002).

Supply and Demand for Physicians

The Council on Graduate Medical Education (COGME) assessed the likely future supply, demand, and need for physicians in the United States through 2020 for both generalist and specialist physicians. The report concluded that between 2000 and 2020, the number of practicing physicians would rise from approximately 781 thousand full-time equivalent (FTE) to 1.02 million FTEs under the most probable aggregate assumptions that take into account physician lifestyle factors such as working fewer hours, and increased productivity as a result of new technologies. These figures translate to 283 FTEs per 100,000 population in 2000, and 313 FTEs per 100,000 population in 2020 (Department of Health and Human Services 2005). On the surface, these figures may indicate a surplus of physicians. However, there are two main factors that suggest that the demand for physicians is likely to grow more rapidly than the supply (Department of Health and Human Services 2005): (1) A greater proportion of elderly in the population, and (2) the changing age-specific per capita physician utilization rates, with those age 45 and above using more services. When these assumptions are factored in, the demand for physicians in 2020 will be between 1.02 million and 1.24 million. Hence, there could actually be a shortage of physicians by 2020. Also, the problems of specialty maldistribution and geographic maldistribution (discussed in Chapter 4) are likely to continue. By 2010, the number of specialists is expected to reach 152 per 100,000 population (from 140 in 2000), and the number of generalists is expected to remain stable at 67 per 100,000 population (Institute for the Future 2000). These projections represent a generalist to specialist ratio of 31:69. The COGME forecasted a similar mix for 2020. A shortage of generalists will have serious consequences in a health care system that needs to focus more on addressing multiple chronic conditions. Two major forces will negatively affect the supply of generalist physicians in rural America—the number of residency graduates in primary care and the increasing feminization of the physician workforce. During the 1990s, growth of managed care had sparked a renewed interest among medical graduates in pursuing residencies in primary care because a shortage of generalists was widely forecast. Consequently, family practice residencies increased 54% between 1993 and 2000, a trend that would have had a sizable impact on the rural physician workforce (Colwill and Cultice 2003). However, the new century has seen a remarkable drop in student interest in primary care. The second factor, feminization of the physician workforce, is also believed to negatively affect the supply of rural practitioners because women have been less likely to select rural practice. The proportion of women in family medicine is expected to double to 40% by 2020 (Colwill and Cultice 2003).

Supply and Demand for Nurses

The recent shortage of RN-trained nurses in the United States has received much attention. Nurse shortages in the past have been cyclical. The current shortage began in 1998, and in 2006 entered its ninth year, making it the longest shortage in the past 50 years (Auerbach et al. 2007). In response, hospitals have used a mix of short-term and long-term strategies to deal with shortages. Among the long-term solutions are investments in training by expanding existing training capacity, opening new schools, and adding fringe benefits focused on education; and improvement of work environments through lengthening or redesigning of orientation programs for new nurses, increasing staffing levels, and work redesign (May et al. 2006). Only time will tell if these strategies will produce a lasting effect in alleviating the problem. Other factors, however, seem to suggest that the shortage of nurses will persist in the future. Unlike previous age cohorts of nursing students in the 1970s and 1980s, large numbers of people are entering the profession in their late 20s and early 30s. Based on revised projections taking into account this recent pattern of entry into nursing schools, the total RN workforce size is expected to be 2.45 million in 2012 and 2.47 million in 2020. The authors of these projections, Auerbach and colleagues (2007), used the demand data produced by the Health Resources and Services Administration, and estimated a shortfall of 340,000 nurses in 2020. The authors also comment that future changes in the economy, immigration, educational incentives, retirement trends among nurses, wages, delivery of health care, and societal values in general could affect future cohorts' propensities to enter nursing.

Deficits in Geriatric Training

Based on current trends, a shortage of health care professionals schooled in geriatrics is a critical challenge. It is estimated that only about 9,000 practicing physicians in the United States (2.5 geriatricians per 10,000 elderly) have formal training in geriatrics. This number is expected to drop down to 6,000 in the near future. Among nurses, less than 0.05% have advanced certification in geriatrics (CDC and Merck Institute of Aging and Health–CDC/Merck 2004).

The elderly use the majority of home health care services and nursing home care, about half of hospital inpatient days, and approximately a quarter of all ambulatory care visits. Growth of the elderly population will impose increased challenges on the health care delivery system, which has thus far ignored the need for specialized geriatrics training. Many elderly patients suffer from chronic conditions. Their care is complicated by the presence of comorbidities, use of multiple drug prescriptions, and an increased prevalence of mental conditions and dementia. Evidence shows that care of older adults by health care professionals prepared in geriatrics yields better physical and mental outcomes without increasing costs (Cohen et al. 2002a). Current trends in the education and training of health care professionals shows the future demand will far outstrip the supply of physicians, nurses, therapists, social workers, and pharmacists with geriatrics training. This problem is compounded due to a shortage of faculty in colleges and universities who are trained in geriatrics. Only 600 medical school faculty out of 100,000 list geriatrics as their primary specialty. Due to this and perhaps other reasons, only 3% of medical students take any elective geriatric courses. In other disciplines, such as nursing, pharmacy, medicine, and dentistry, the majority of educational curricula do not require geriatric training. For example, 60% of nursing schools have no geriatric faculty (CDC/Merck 2004). A shortage of workforce members prepared in geriatrics affects all settings, but it especially affects nursing facilities that serve large numbers of frail elderly. Geriatrics training is also important in other types of health services, such as oncology, neurology, rehabilitation, and critical care (Kovner et al. 2002). Even though there are some encouraging signs that initiatives are being taken by educational institutions in recognition of a critical deficit in geriatric training, it is not clear how the nation will deal with the impending need.

Workforce Diversity

Women's continual entry into the workforce in large numbers is likely to affect health services delivery. Although further research and time will clarify this impact, health services managers should be prepared to improve the work environment to accommodate the needs of female workers. Examples include day care services and flexible work schedules. MCOs are likely to select women for their staff physicians, nurses, social workers, and case managers. Female physicians are expected to prefer managed care to private practice because MCOs are more likely to provide secure income and regular hours.

The increase in the proportion of non-Whites, particularly in the most populous cities and states, is another change. Already, the states of California, Texas, New York, New Jersey, and Florida have significant minority populations. And estimates say near the middle of this century, more than half of US citizens will be non-White (US Census Bureau 2001, 17). Consequently, the future health care workforce will be much more diverse ethnically and racially. Preparation of a culturally competent health care workforce is a growing challenge. The term ***cultural competence*** refers to knowledge, skills, attitudes, and behavior required of a practitioner to provide optimal health care services to persons from a wide range of cultural and ethnic backgrounds. Development of cultural competence is necessary because most future health care professionals will be called upon to deliver services to many patients with backgrounds far different from their own. To do so effectively, health care providers need to understand how and why different belief systems, cultural biases, ethnic origins, family structures, and many other culture-based factors influence the manner in which people experience illness, comply with medical advice, and respond to treatment. These variations have implications for outcomes of care (Cohen et al. 2002b).

Changes in the racial/ethnic and gender makeup of the workforce will continue to influence the management of health services organizations. Managers will have to consider cultural backgrounds and attitudes toward work as well as employees' potential language and educational disparities. Having more women in the workforce will require awareness of gender pay disparities and the need to address family issues, such as childcare and maternity leave.

Work Organization

In many health care settings, multidisciplinary team approach, collaboration, and cross-training will be used to improve quality and productivity. These approaches improve communication, enable practitioners to address complex clinical cases from different perspectives, and improve productivity by avoiding duplication.

Collaborative Team Approach

Consistent with the concept of total quality management is the use of multidisciplinary teams to provide patient services. The team approach concept is intended to provide comprehensive care and to eliminate duplication of services. For example, diabetes is not only a growing health concern in the United States, but it is also a complex chronic disease. Care for diabetes requires significant daily self-care that includes medication management, proper diet, and physical activity. Insulin dependency creates additional daily tasks such as monitoring of blood glucose levels, administrating proper dosages of insulin, and managing hypoglycemic episodes. Further, depression is a common comorbidity accompanying diabetes that can lower physical and mental functioning, which can lead to decreased ability to adhere to the self-care regimens. The result can likely be complications that can eventually lead to serious problems such as blindness, heart disease, and kidney failure. In diabetes management, a collaborative team approach provides numerous benefits to patients and practitioners. Also, a collaborative approach can provide medical students valuable cross-training (Robinson et al. 2004). A multidisciplinary team approach is also indispensable in ethical decision-making. Most medium- and large-sized hospitals have ethics committees that generally include multiple disciplines, such as physicians, nurses, social workers, administrators, ethicists, and clergy. Development of medical science and new technology create new challenges regarding clinical decisions that defy straightforward answers.

Health services providers and managers are more likely to involve key stakeholders, including patients and the population, in decision-making (Issel and Anderson 1996, 82). By involving the patient in decision-making, health care organizations hope to improve customer service and control costs. In a wellness-care system, it will become apparent that dictating a treatment regimen that customers do not like, and will not comply with, will not meet the goals of the organization or the customer (Issel and Anderson 1996, 82).

Cross-Training

Cross-training of health service workers can include teaching an employee to assume additional clinical or clerical roles or training an employee to work in several different areas (D'Aunno et al. 1996). The ultimate objectives are to improve staff flexibility, realize greater efficiency, and reduce costs. However, cross-training also benefits the employees by furnishing them with a larger set of skills than they would otherwise have. Although licensure issues can hamper worker cross-training in a number of areas, in other areas licensure conflicts do not arise. For example, one tertiary care setting used a cross-training program to evaluate the feasibility of floating a medical/surgical floor nurse to the medical intensive care unit, and both units have been jointly managed (Gilbert and Counsell 2000).

Training workers to become multiskilled health practitioners (MHPs) has several advantages. MHPs are an asset to small rural hospitals that may have difficulty obtaining or maintaining staff in certain specialties. Workers trained in multiple areas can respond to changing needs and demands in the health services industry. Continuity of care may also be enhanced by the use of MHPs because cross-trained nurses can attend to patients throughout their care rather than attending to them in a specific care level setting (D'Aunno et al. 1996).

Enhanced Focus on Customer Service

Market forces have increased competition among health care providers and networks of providers. Competition has brought with it more input from payers as well as consumers, increased scrutiny of services, and accountability for outcomes. In response, the health care industry is placing more emphasis on patient satisfaction. In a consumer-choice market, an institution's client satisfaction ratings may be the best predictor of future success (Coile 2002). Health care organizations will undoubtedly become more service oriented because those regulations and economic factors that made the industry substantially immune to competition are being dismantled (Eisenberg 1997).

Health services will not make the transition to service orientation without challenge. Eisenberg (1997) cited four barriers that must be overcome: (1) Health care environments are highly regulated on everything from waste disposal to records maintenance. To comply with the extensive regulations requires a great deal of time and resources, which can impede focusing on the consumer. (2) The health care industry has a traditional resistance to entrepreneurship. Incentives for efficiency and cost management are uncommon. This is partly because of the large number and various types of payers and the traditional view of health services as a noble and charitable enterprise (Eisenberg 1997, 22). (3) Health services are typically paternalistic. Because hospitalization generally occurs not by choice but because of necessity, consumers are often in a subordinate role without much decision-making power about what happens to them in the hospital. (4) The traditional medical model tends to depersonalize the patient. Patients are categorized by their condition. Training for health careers predominantly focuses on scientific and technical levels, ignoring customer relations.

To compete in a changing health care environment, health services will have to overcome these barriers and make a commitment to customer satisfaction and patient relations. This goal can be accomplished by adopting customer service principles as part of the overall mission and philosophy, empowering staff, improving both internal and external communications, creating feedback systems measuring patient satisfaction, and making service environments more user-friendly (Eisenberg 1997).

New Frontiers in Clinical Technology

Technological progress is behind much of the growth in the health services industry. The Institute for the Future (2000) predicted that eight types of medical technologies would especially affect future delivery of patient care—rational drug design, advances in imaging, minimally invasive surgery, genetic mapping and testing, gene therapy, vaccines, artificial blood, and xenotransplantation.

1. Rational drug design is a step beyond the painstaking and costly random search for new pharmaceuticals that is characterized by trial and error. Now, scientists can study the structure and composition of a receptor or enzyme, and actually design new chemicals or molecular entities that bind to the receptors or enzymes. Rational drug design will shorten the drug discovery process. The chief candidates for this process are drugs to treat neurological and mental disorders, and antiretroviral therapies for HIV/AIDS, encephalitis, measles, and influenza.
2. Imaging technologies present an enhanced visual display of tissues, organ systems, and their functions. Current research focuses on four areas: (a) Finding new energy sources and focusing an energy beam to avoid damage to adjacent tissue and to minimize residual damage. (b) Use of microelectronics in digital detectors and advances in the contrast media for a finer detection of abnormalities. (c) Faster and more accurate analysis of images using 3-D technology. (d) Improvements in display technology to produce higher resolution displays.
3. The latest advances in minimally invasive surgery include image-guided

brain surgery, minimal access cardiac procedures, and the endovascular placement of grafts for abdominal aneurysms. The overall impact of minimally invasive procedures on cost-efficiency and the patients' quality of life from early recovery assures the growth of this technology and the growth of ambulatory surgi-centers.

4. Genetic mapping has enabled the identification of a wide range of genes that can cause complex diseases, such as diabetes, cancer, heart disease, Huntington's disease, and Alzheimer's disease. The discovery of genetic susceptibility to certain diseases will improve preventive techniques. The term ***genometrics*** is used for the association of genes with specific disease traits.
5. Gene therapy is a therapeutic technique in which a functioning gene is inserted into targeted cells to correct an inborn defect or to provide the cell with a new function. The future challenge in this area is to develop methods that discriminately deliver enough genetic material to the right cells. Cancer treatment is receiving much attention as a prime candidate for gene therapy since current techniques (surgery, radiation, and chemotherapy) are effective in only half the cases.
6. Vaccines have traditionally been used prophylactically to prevent specific infectious diseases, such as diphtheria, smallpox, and whooping cough. However, the therapeutic use of vaccines in the treatment of noninfectious diseases, such as cancer, has opened new fronts in medicine. At the same time, development of new vaccines for emerging infectious diseases remains on the research agenda. Making today's vaccines safer for wide-scale preventive use against bioterrorism, in which such agents as smallpox and anthrax may be used, will also be an ongoing challenge.
7. Research will continue on the development of fluids that, in many instances, could be used as substitutes for real blood in transfusions, particularly in war and in natural disasters when supplies may fall short.
8. Transplantation of organs is one of the 20th century's great medical advances. It treats a life-threatening chronic disease by replacing the diseased organ. However, a critical shortage of transplantable tissues remains a major concern. ***Xenotransplantation***, in which animal tissues are used for transplants in humans, is a growing research area. New knowledge and methods in molecular genetics, transplantation biology, and genetic engineering look promising.

The Era of Evidence-Based Health Care

Wide variations in clinical practice (see Small Area Variations in Chapter 12) have finally caught the attention of mainstream media in the United States, raising public awareness of the quality and cost implications of clinical variations (Schaeffer and McMurtry 2004). There is little evidence that high-spending providers deliver better outcomes. The goal of evidence-based medicine (EBM) is to increase the value of medicine. Even though consumers, as well as practitioners, often fear that reducing costs translates into lower quality, this is not necessarily true. Quality of care can be improved while reducing costs—thus increasing the value of medical care—by reducing misuse and overuse (Slawson and Shaughnessy 2001). The tools for the practice of evidence-based medicine have been developed for several years, mainly in the form of clinical practice guidelines. Evidence-based practice guidelines are intended to represent "best practices" and "proven therapies."

Several countries have undertaken some significant initiatives in the research and application of EBM. For example, in the United States, the Agency for Healthcare Research and Quality (http://www.ahrq.gov) leads national efforts in the use of evidence to guide health care decisions. The establishment of the National Institute for Health and Clinical Excellence (http://www.nice.org.uk) in England, the Scottish Intercollegiate Guidelines Network (http://www.sign.ac.uk), and the National Institute for Clinical Studies (http://www.nicsl.com.au) in Australia have similar responsibilities for developing evidence-based guidelines and for providing information on the clinical and cost-effectiveness of interventions (Gerrish et al. 2007).

There is at least some evidence that practitioners may have begun to incorporate EBM into their clinical decision-making. For example, Halm and colleagues (2007) reported a remarkable reduction in the proportion of patients undergoing carotid endarterectomy (a surgical procedure that removes the inner lining of the carotid artery if it has become thickened or damaged by plaque) for inappropriate reasons subsequent to the publication of several large international randomized controlled trials that rationalized the use of the procedure.

On the other hand, the use of guidelines is not widespread in the medical community. Even though the research community has known about clinical variations since the 1970s, and evidence has mounted since then, relatively little has been done to translate this research into actual practice. Many physicians think that guidelines and protocols are either too simple or too complicated, promote "cookbook care," lack creditable authors or evidence, are biased, decrease flexibility, reduce autonomy, and are not applicable to the practice population (Oeyen 2007).

Future strategies are needed to improve guidelines and protocols, and their adherence. At least six recommendations can be made for the future:

1. The issue of practice variations will require the attention of practitioners, payers, and policymakers.
2. Computer-based models will have to be developed to incorporate EBM into medical decision-making. Models that are easily usable and understandable are essential.
3. Ongoing clinical trials will be the backbone of EBM. Adherence to clinical guidelines is higher when the recommendations are supported by evidence from randomized controlled trials (Leape et al. 2003).
4. Guidelines and protocols must be revised and kept current to incorporate subsequent scientific evidence.
5. Future practice guidelines must incorporate economic analysis. Mounting health care expenditures will pressure society to make rational choices about when certain types of services become unwarranted. Treatments with cost-effectiveness ratios

greater than a widely agreed upon standard may have to be eliminated from recommended practice. Also, future technological change will be driven by assessments that show clear-cut clinical and economic advantages.

6. Financial incentives, including provider payments and patient cost sharing, must be restructured. Reimbursement methods should focus on paying for best achievable outcomes and the most effective care over the course of treatment instead of paying for units of service (Gauthier et al. 2006).

In the future, EBM will also transcend what physicians do. For example, the practice of nursing, pharmacology, and other disciplines allied with the practice of medicine will be governed by EBM. Eventually, EBM will become the standard that will govern the multidisciplinary process of health care delivery.

Summary

At the dawn of the 21st century, the only certainty facing health care is change. Future directions will be determined mainly by social, cultural, technological, and economic changes. Lack of access for the uninsured and cost inflation will continue to haunt the system. In the short run, greater cost shifting will move more expense from employers to employees. A defined contribution from employers is likely to replace the existing defined benefit program. To what extent this shift will occur and to what extent employers may actually abdicate their responsibility to be directly involved in purchasing health insurance will depend largely on the state of the economy and labor markets. Managed care's vast infrastructure will not be easily dismantled. Instead, it is more reasonable to assume that in a changing environment, managed care itself will have to evolve, since employers once again will be in a position to exert enough influence to bring about certain desired changes. Better management of risk and more accountability for cost and quality will be demanded. Given the right set of circumstances, universal health care could once again appear on the national policy agenda. If a national health care system becomes a reality, universal access will be restricted to essential care. Those wanting access to services beyond the essentials will have to pay for them.

Under growing cost pressures, wellness and public health will be more strongly emphasized. In a reformed health care system, a major challenge will be to forge partnerships between communities and all levels of government. Coordinating functions and developing needed infrastructures have become even more critical due to increased threats of bioterrorism and outbreaks of new infectious diseases.

A rapidly growing elderly population that requires care for chronic ailments and long-term care will pose increased challenges. Physicians will need training to function more effectively in a chronic care environment.

Composition of the health care workforce will undergo changes because of a decline in inpatient hospital care, an increasing elderly population, and more women and minorities entering the health care workforce. Despite recent efforts to bring about some parity, the problems associated with specialty maldistribution and geographic maldistribution will continue. Even though currently there is a surplus of physicians in the United States, by 2020, a shortage could exist. A shortage of nurses has also been projected, but factors such as economic conditions, immigration, and educational incentives could change the outlook.

As minority populations continue to increase and the workplace becomes increasingly diverse, health care managers face the challenge of preparing a culturally competent health care workforce. The health care workforce also needs to be schooled to give geriatric care. Additional workforce issues include cross-training and the team approach to addressing complex problems.

Health care is often seen as developing into a consumer-choice market. Client satisfaction and customer services will increasingly determine the success of health care organizations in a competitive market. However, industry regulations, lack of incentives, paternalism, and predominance of the medical model pose critical barriers to service orientation.

New frontiers will be opened in the application of clinical, informational, and telematics technology. Technologies such as new drugs, safer procedures, gene therapy, and therapeutic use of vaccines will strongly affect treatments for cancer, HIV/AIDS, and neurological diseases. Sharing of information among providers, intermediaries, and consumers will be necessary to achieve better efficiency and disease management. However, adoption of costly information technology will be driven by cost-benefit considerations.

Evidence-based medicine will play a growing role in the delivery of medical care that is both effective and cost-effective. Higher quality at lower cost can be achieved by reducing misuse and overuse based on clinical evidence. Hence, use of clinical practice guidelines that represent "best practices" and have been "proven" through clinical trials will become the standard for clinical care delivery.

Test Your Understanding

Terminology

cross-training
cultural competence
defined benefit plan
defined contribution plan
e-health plans
genometrics
high-deductible health plans
high-risk pools
HRA (health reimbursement arrangement)
HSA (health savings account)
managed competition
play-or-pay
single-payer health plan
xenotransplantation

Review Questions

1. Discuss the future direction of employer-based health insurance in the United States.
2. What are managed care's future challenges? How might MCOs address them?

3. What are some of the incremental changes in financing and insurance that the existing health care system might see?
4. What proposals might work in a universal access program in the United States, if and when the time comes to debate such proposals?
5. What main challenges regarding the future delivery of long-term care have been identified?
6. Discuss how the role of public health has been changing.
7. What challenges will the United States likely face in the future regarding the supply and demand of physicians and nurses?
8. What are some of the main reasons behind the deficits in geriatric training?
9. Discuss some of the changes in the areas of work organization in health care delivery.
10. Give an overview of what new technology might achieve in the delivery of health care.
11. What can be done to achieve greater adoption of evidence-based medicine in the delivery of health care?

REFERENCES

American Hospital Association. 1996. *American Hospital Association booklet*. Chicago.

Auerbach, D.I. et al. 2007. Better late than never: Workforce supply implications of later entry into nursing. *Health Affairs* 26, no. 1: 178–185.

Baker, E.L., and J.P. Koplan. 2002. Strengthening the nation's public health infrastructure: historic challenge, unprecedented opportunity. *Health Affairs* 21, no. 6: 15–27.

Biles, B. et al. 2004. Medicare advantage: Deja vu all over again? *Health Affairs Web Exclusive* 23, supplement 2: W4-586–W4-597.

Borger, C. et al. 2006. Health spending projections through 2015: Changes on the horizon. *Health Affairs Web Exclusive*, January–June 2006: W61–W73.

Buchmueller, T. et al. 2006. Trends in retiree health insurance, 1997–2003. *Health Affairs* 25, no. 6: 1507–1516.

Burke, S.P. et al. 2005. *Developing a better long-term care policy: A vision and strategy for America's future*. Washington, DC: National Academy of Social Insurance.

Catlin, A. at al. 2007. National health spending in 2005: The slowdown continues. *Health Affairs* 21, no. 1: 142–153.

CDC/Merck. 2004. *The state of aging and health in America, 2004*. Centers for Disease Control and Prevention/Merck Institute of Aging & Health. *http://www.cdc.gov/aging/*.

Christianson, J.B. et al. 2002. Defined-contribution health insurance products: Development and prospects. *Health Affairs* 21, no. 1: 49–64.

Claxton, G. et al. 2005a. *Employer health benefits: 2005 annual survey*. Washington, DC: The Kaiser Family Foundation and Health Research and Educational Trust.

Claxton, G. et al. 2005b. What high-deductible plans look like: Findings from a national survey of employers, 2005. *Health Affairs Web Exclusive* 24, Supplement 3: W5-434–W5-441.

Claxton, G. et al. 2006. *Employer health benefits: 2006 annual survey*. Washington, DC: The Kaiser Family Foundation and Health Research and Educational Trust.

Cohen, H.J. et al. 2002a. A controlled trial of inpatient and outpatient geriatric evaluation and management. *New England Journal of Medicine* 346, no. 12: 906–912.

Cohen, J.J. et al. 2002b. The case for diversity in the health care workforce. *Health Affairs* 21, no. 5: 90–102.

Coile, R.C. 2002. *Futurescan 2002: A forecast of healthcare trends*. Chicago: Health Administration Press.

Colwill, J.M., and J.M. Cultice. 2003. The future supply of family physicians: Implications for rural America. *Health Affairs* 22, no. 1: 190–198.

Congressional Budget Office (CBO). 1999. *CBO Memorandum: Projections of expenditures for long-term care services for the elderly*. Washington, DC.

Congressional Budget Office (CBO). 2004. *Financing long term care for the elderly*. Washington, DC: CBO.

Coughlin, T.A., and S. Zuckerman. 2005. Three years of state fiscal struggles: How did Medicaid and SCHIP fare? *Health Affairs Web Exclusive* 24, Supplement 3: W5-385–W5-398.

Crowley, J.S. 2006. *Medicaid long-term care services reforms in the Deficit Reduction Act*. Washington, DC: The Henry J. Kaiser Family Foundation.

D'Aunno, T. et al. 1996. Business as usual? Changes in health care's workforce and organization of work. *Hospital and Health Services Administration* 41, no. 1: 3–18.

Department of Health and Human Services. 2003. *The future supply of long-term care workers in relation to the aging baby boom generation, Report to Congress*. Washington, DC: Department of Health and Human Services.

Department of Health and Human Services. 2005. *Physician workforce policy guidelines for the United States, 2000–2020*. Washington, DC: Department of Health and Human Services.

Department of Health and Human Services (DHHS). 2006. *Health, United States, 2006*. Hyattsville, MD.

Eisenberg, B. 1997. Customer service in healthcare: A new era. *Hospital and Health Services Administration* 42, no. 1: 17–31.

Foundation for Accountability. 2001. *Portrait of the chronically ill in America, 2001*. Portland, OR: The Foundation for Accountability, and Princeton, NJ: The Robert Wood Johnson Foundation.

Friedland, R. 1996. The role of managed care in the future. *Generations* 20, no. 1: 37–41.

Galvin, R.S. et al. 2005. Has the Leapfrog Group had an impact on the health care market? *Health Affairs* 24, no. 1: 228–233.

Galvin, R.S., and S. Delbanco. 2006. Between a rock and a hard place: Understanding the employer mind-set. *Health Affairs* 25, no. 6: 1548–1555.

Gauthier, A. et al. 2006. *Toward a high performance health system for the United States*. New York: The Commonwealth Fund.

Gerrish, K. et al. 2007. Factors influencing the development of evidence-based practice: A research tool. *Journal of Advanced Nursing* 57, no. 3: 328–338.

Gilbert, M., and C. Counsell. 2000. Intensive care unit cross training: Saving dollars while retaining staff. *Journal of Nursing Administration* 30, no. 6: 308, 324.

Ginzberg, E. 1999. US health care: A look ahead to 2025. *Annual Review of Public Health* 20: 55–66. *http://biomedical.annual_reviews.org/cgi/content/full.*

Gold, M. 2006. Commercial health insurance: Smart or simply lucky? *Health Affairs* 25, no. 6: 1490–1493.

Gow, J. 2002. The HIV/AIDS epidemic in Africa: Implications for US policy. *Health Affairs* 21, no. 3: 57–69.

Halm, E.A. et al. 2007. Has evidence changed practice? Appropriateness of carotid endarterectomy after the clinical trials. *Neurology* 68, no. 3: 187–194.

The Henry J. Kaiser Family Foundation. 2006a. *Massachusetts health care reform plan*. April 2006. *http://www.kff.org*.

The Henry J. Kaiser Foundation. 2006b. *Health care in America 2006 survey*. October 2006. *http://www.kff.org.*

Holahan, J., and A. Cook. 2005. Changes in economic conditions and health insurance coverage, 2000–2004. *Health Affairs Web Exclusives* 24: w498–w508.

Haislmaier, E.F., and N. Owcharenko. 2006. The Massachusetts approach: A new way to restructure state health insurance markets and public programs. *Health Affairs* 25, no. 6: 1580–1590.

Institute for the Future. 2000. *Health and Health Care 2010: The forecast, the challenge*. San Francisco: Jossey-Bass Publishers.

Institute of Medicine. 1996. *2020 vision: Health in the 21st century*. Washington, DC: National Academy Press.

Issel, M., and R. Anderson. 1996. Take charge: Managing six transformations in health care delivery. *Nursing Economics* 14, no. 2: 78–85.

Kassalow, J.S. 2001. *Why health is important to US foreign policy*. New York: Council on Foreign Relations and Milbank Memorial Fund.

Keenan, P.S. et al. 2006. The "graying" of group health insurance. *Health Affairs* 25, no. 6: 1497–1506.

Kirby, J.B. et al. 2003. Has the increase in HMO enrollment within the Medicaid population changed the pattern of health service use and expenditures? *Medical Care* 41, (7 Supplement): III24–III34.

Kovner, C.T. et al. 2002. Who cares for older adults? Workforce implications of an aging society. *Health Affairs* 21, no. 5: 78–89.

Lamm, R.D., and R. H. Blank. 2005. The challenge of an aging society. *The Futurist*, July–August 2005: 23–27.

LAPSR (Los Angeles Physicians for Social Responsibility). 1996. *Health care reform: Information and commentary*. *http://www.labridge.com/psr.healthreform.html.*

Leape, L.L. et al. 2003. Adherence to practice guidelines: The role of specialty society guidelines. *American Heart Journal* 145, no. 1: 19–26.

May, J.H. et al. 2006. Hospitals' responses to nurse staffing shortages. *Health Affairs Web Exclusives* (January–June 2006): W316–W323.

Mays, G.P. et al. 2000. *Local public health practice: Trends and models*. Washington, DC: American Public Health Association.

McClellan, M., and K. Baicker. 2002. Reducing uninsurance through the nongroup market: Health insurance credits and purchasing groups. *Health Affairs Web Exclusives 2002:* W363–W366.

McKethan, A. et al. 2006. New directions for public health care purchasers? Responses to looming challenges. *Health Affairs* 25, no. 6: 1518–1528.

Miller, E.A., and V. Mor. 2006. *Out of the shadows: Envisioning a brighter future for long-term care in America*. Providence, RI: Brown University.

Milstien, J.B. et al. 2006. The impact of globalization on vaccine development and availability. *Health Affairs* 25, no. 4: 1061–1069.

National Association of County Health Officials. 1994. *Blueprint for a healthy community: A guide for local health departments*. Washington, DC.

Novick, L.F. 2001. Defining public health: Historical and contemporary developments. In *Public health administration: Principles for population-based management*, eds. L.F. Novick and G.P. Mays, 3–33. Gaithersburg, Maryland: Aspen Publishers Inc.

Oeyen, S. 2007. About protocols and guidelines: It's time to work in harmony! *Critical Care Medicine* 35, no. 1: 292–293.

Patel, V. 2002. Raising awareness of consumers' options in the individual health insurance market. *Health Affairs Web Exclusives 2002:* W367–W371.

RAND. 2005. *Future health and medical care spending of the elderly: Implications for Medicare.* Santa Monica, CA: RAND Corporation.

Robinson, W.D. et al. 2004. An interdisciplinary student-run diabetic clinic: Reflections on the collaborative training process. *Families, Systems, and Health* 22, no. 4: 490–496.

Sanofi-Aventis US. 2006. *Managed care digest series: Government digest*. Bridgewater, NJ: Sanofi-Aventis US.

Satcher, D. 2006. The prevention challenge and opportunity. *Health Affairs* 25, no. 4: 1009–1011.

Schaeffer, L.D., and D.E. McMurtry. 2004. When excuses run dry: Transforming the US health care system. *Health Affairs Web Exclusives* 2004: VAR117–VAR120.

Serota, S. 2002. The individual market: A delicate balance. *Health Affairs Web Exclusives 2002:* W377–W379.

Singh, D.A. 2005. *Effective management of long-term care facilities*. Sudbury, MA: Jones and Bartlett Publishers.

Slawson, D.C., and A.F. Shaughnessy. 2001. Using "medical poetry" to remove the inequities in health care delivery. *Journal of Family Medicine* 50, no. 1: 51–65.

Swartz, K. 2002. Government as reinsurer for very-high-cost persons in nongroup health insurance markets. *Health Affairs Web Exclusives 2002:* W380–W382.

US Census Bureau. 2001. *Statistical abstract of the United States, 2001*. Washington, DC: US Census Bureau.

White, B. 2001. The future of health care financing. *Family Practice Management* 8, no. 1: 31–36.

Whitmore, H. et al. 2006. Employers' views on incremental measures to expand health coverage. *Health Affairs* 25, no. 6: 1668–1678.

Wolff, J.L., and C. Boult. 2005. Moving beyond round pegs and square holes: Restructuring Medicare to improve chronic care. *Annals of Internal Medicine* 143, no. 6: 439–445.

Appendix A

Glossary

Academic medical center: The term is commonly used when one or more hospitals are organized around a medical school. Apart from the training of physicians, research activities and clinical investigations become an important undertaking in these institutions.

Access: The ability of persons needing health services to obtain appropriate care in a timely manner. Can you get medical care when you need it? If yes, you have access to medical care. Access is not the same as health insurance coverage, although insurance coverage is a strong predictor of access for **primary care** services.

Activities of daily living (ADL): The most commonly used measure of disability. ADLs determine whether an individual needs assistance to perform basic activities, such as eating, bathing, dressing, toileting, and getting into or out of a bed or chair. See **functional status**, and **IADLs**.

Actuary: A person professionally trained in the technical aspects of insurance and related fields, particularly in the mathematics of insurance, such as the calculation of premiums, reserves, and other values.

Acupuncture: Use of long, thin needles passed through the skin to specific reflex points to treat chronic pain or to produce regional anesthesia.

Acute care: Short-term, intense medical care for an illness or injury usually requiring hospitalization. See **subacute care**.

Administrative costs: Costs that are incidental to the delivery of health services. These costs are not only associated with the billing and collection of claims for services delivered but also include numerous other costs, such as time and effort incurred by employers for the selection of insurance carriers, costs incurred by insurance and managed care organizations to market their products, and time and effort involved in the negotiation of rates.

Adult day care (ADC): A community-based long-term care service that provides a wide range of health, social, and recreational services to elderly adults who require supervision and care while members of the family or other informal caregivers are away at work.

Advanced practice nurse (APN): A general name for nurses who have education and clinical experience beyond that required of an RN. APNs include four areas of specialization in nursing: clinical nurse specialists (CNSs), certified registered nurse anesthetists (CRNAs), nurse practitioners (NPs), and certified nurse midwives (CNMs).

Adverse selection: A phenomenon in which individuals who know they are most at risk of utilizing insurance benefits disproportionately purchase insurance. As health insurance becomes more and more expensive to buy, healthier subscribers drop out or switch to cheaper plans, whereas those who are more likely to use benefits retain coverage in **plans** providing better benefits.

Affective disorders: A group of disorders characterized by severe mood changes and often accompanied by a manic or depressive syndrome.

Agency for Healthcare Research and Quality (AHRQ): A federal agency within the Department of Health and Human Services whose mission is to improve the quality, safety, efficiency, and effectiveness of health care through research activities.

AIDS: Acquired immune deficiency syndrome. The occurrence of immune deficiency caused by the **HIV** virus.

Allied health: Includes professionals in many health-related areas, among them technicians, assistants, therapists, and technologists. The allied health professional's main function is to complement the work of physicians and other health care providers.

Allopathy: A philosophy of medicine that views medical treatment as active intervention to counteract the effects of disease through medical and surgical procedures that produce effects opposite to those of the disease. See **homeopathy** and **osteopathy**.

Alternative medicine: Nontraditional remedies, e.g., **acupuncture**, **homeopathy**, **naturopathy**, **biofeedback**, **yoga exercises**, **chiropractic**, and herbal therapy.

Alzheimer's disease: A progressive degenerative disease of the brain producing loss of memory, confusion, irritability, severe loss of functioning, and ultimately death. Named after German neurologist, Alois Alzheimer (1864–1915).

Ambulatory: Refers to the ability to move about at will.

Ambulatory care: Also referred to as **outpatient services**. Ambulatory care includes (1) care rendered to patients who come to physicians' offices, outpatient departments of hospitals, and health centers to receive care; (2) outpatient services intended to serve the surrounding community (community medicine); and (3) certain services that are transported to the patient.

Ancillary services: Hospital or other **inpatient services** other than room and board and professional medical services, such as physician and nursing care. Examples include radiology, pharmacy, laboratory, bandages and other supplies, physical therapy, etc.

Anesthesiology: Administration of drugs for the prevention of, or relief of, pain during surgery.

Angioplasty: The reconstruction or restructuring of a blood vessel by operative means or by nonsurgical techniques, such as balloon dilation or laser.

Anorexia nervosa: A mental disturbance characterized by self-imposed starvation because the patient may claim to feel fat even when emaciated.

Antiretroviral: A drug that stops or suppresses the activity of a retrovirus, such as HIV.

Antitrust: Federal and state laws that make certain anticompetitive practices illegal. These practices include price fixing, price discrimination, exclusive contracting arrangements, and mergers among competitors.

Arthroscope: An **endoscope** for examining the interior of a joint.

Assignment: Practice under which a physician agrees to accept whatever the insurer (generally **Medicaid** and **Medicare**) will pay. A physician not on assignment will **balance bill** the patient for the amount remaining after the insurer has paid.

Atherosclerosis: A form of hardening of the arteries caused by accumulation of substances such as fatty deposits.

Audiology: Identification and evaluation of hearing disorders and correction of hearing loss through **rehabilitation** and **prostheses**.

Baby boom: A sudden, large increase in the birth rate, especially the one in the United States after World War II from 1946 through 1964. Baby boomers, as this generation is often referred to, comprises about 77 million adults.

Balance bill: Billing of the leftover sum by the **provider** to the patient after insurance has only partially paid the charge initially billed.

Benefit period: Under **Medicare** rules, benefits for an inpatient stay are based on a benefit period. A benefit period is determined by a spell of illness beginning with hospitalization and ending when the beneficiary has not been an inpatient in a hospital or a skilled nursing facility for 60 consecutive days.

Biofeedback: A training program that uses relaxation and visualization to develop the ability to control one's involuntary nervous system as an aid to reducing stress, lowering blood pressure, and alleviating headaches.

Blue Cross: An independent, nonprofit membership corporation providing protection on a service basis against the cost of hospital care in a limited geographic area.

Blue Shield: An independent, nonprofit membership corporation providing protection on a service basis against the cost of surgical and medical care in a limited geographical area.

Bulimia: A mental disturbance that leads to bouts of overeating followed by induced vomiting.

Capitation: A reimbursement mechanism under which the provider is paid a set monthly fee per **enrollee** (sometimes referred to as per member per month or **PMPM** rate), regardless of whether or not an enrollee sees the provider and regardless of how often an enrollee sees the provider.

Cardiology: Medical science pertaining to study of the heart and its diseases.

Carve out: The assignment through contractual arrangements of specialized services to an outside organization because these services are not included in the contracts MCOs have with their providers, or the **MCO** does not provide the services.

Case management: An organized approach to evaluating the health care needs of a patient, identifying appropriate services to meet those needs, choosing the most cost-effective setting and **providers**, coordinating the delivery of services by maintaining communication among providers, patients, and payers, and monitoring progress.

Case mix: An aggregate of the intensity of conditions requiring medical intervention. Case-mix categories are mutually exclusive and differentiate patients according to the extent of resource use.

Catastrophic care: Medical care needed when a patient suffers a major injury or life-threatening illness that requires expensive long-term treatment.

Categorical programs: Public health care programs that are designed to benefit only a certain category of people.

CDC: Centers for Disease Control and Prevention. The federal public health agency in the United States.

Centers for Medicare and Medicaid Services (CMS): Federal agency that administers the Medicare and Medicaid programs.

Certificate of need (CON): Control exercised by a government planning agency over expansion of medical facilities, e.g., determination of whether a new facility should be opened in a certain location, whether an existing facility should be expanded, or whether a hospital should be allowed to purchase major equipment.

Certified nurse midwives: RNs with additional training from a nurse-midwifery program in areas such as maternal and fetal procedures, maternity and child nursing, and patient assessment. CNMs deliver babies, provide family planning education, manage gynecological and obstetric care. They can substitute for obstetricians/gynecologists in prenatal and postnatal care. See **Nonphysician practitioners** (NPPs).

Charge: The amount a **provider** bills for rendering a service. *See* **cost**.

Chiropractic: A system of medicine based on manipulation of the spine, physiotherapy, and dietary counseling to treat neurological, muscular, and vascular problems. Chiropractic care is based on the belief that the body is a self-healing organism.

Chiropractors: A licensed practitioner who has completed the Doctor of Chiropractic (DC) degree. Chiropractors must be licensed to practice. Requirements for licensure include completion of an accredited program that awards a Doctor of Chiropractic (DC) and an examination by the state chiropractic board.

Chronic condition (chronic disease): A medical condition that persists over time. Chronic diseases may lead to a permanent medical condition that is nonreversible and/or leaves residual disability.

Churning: A phenomenon in which people gain and lose health insurance coverage multiple times.

Claim: A demand for payment of covered medical expenses sent to an insurance company.

Clinical practice guidelines (medical practice guidelines): Standardized guidelines in the form of scientifically established protocols representing preferred processes in medical practice.

Clinical trial: A research study, generally based on random assignments, designed to study the effectiveness of a new drug, device, or treatment.

Closed panel: Sometimes also called "closed network," "in network," or "closed access." A health plan that pays for services only when they are provided by physicians and hospitals on the plan's **panel**.

Community health center (CHC): Local, non-profit, community-owned health care providers serving low-income and medically underserved communities.

Community hospital: Nonfederal (i.e., VA and military hospitals are excluded), short-term, general or special hospital whose services are available to the public.

Community rating: Same insurance rate for everyone, as opposed to medical underwriting or **experience rating**.

Comorbidity: Presence of more than one health problem in an individual.

Competition: Rivalry among sellers for the purpose of attracting customers.

Continuous quality improvement (CQI): See **total quality management**.

Continuum: A range or spectrum (of health care services) from basic to complex.

Copayment (coinsurance): A portion of health care charges that the insured have to pay under the terms of their health insurance policies. Technically, copayment is stated in dollar terms whereas coinsurance is stated as a percent. See **deductible**.

Cost: What it costs the provider to produce a service. See **charge**.

Cost-efficiency (cost-effectiveness): A service is cost-efficient when the benefit received is greater than the cost incurred to provide the service. See **efficiency**.

Cost-plus: Reimbursement to a **provider** based on **cost** plus a factor to cover the value of capital.

Cost sharing: Sharing in the cost of health insurance premiums by those enrolled, and/or payment of certain medical costs out of pocket, such as copayments and deductibles.

Cost shifting (cross-subsidizing): In general, shifting of costs from one entity to another. A way of making up losses in one area by charging more in other areas. For example, when care is provided to the uninsured, the **provider** makes up for it by charging more to the insured.

Covered lives: People enrolled in a managed care plan. See **enrollees**.

CPR (cardiopulmonary resuscitation): Medical procedure used to restart a patient's heart and breathing when the patient has suffered a heart failure.

Critical Access Hospital (CAH): Medicare designation for small rural hospitals, with 25 beds or less, that provide emergency medical services besides short-term hospitalization for patients with noncomplex health care needs. They receive **cost-plus** reimbursement.

Critical pathways: Outcome-based and patient-centered case management tools that are interdisciplinary, facilitating coordination of care among multiple clinical departments and caregivers. A critical pathway identifies planned medical interventions in a given case along with expected outcomes.

Cross-training: Cross-training of health service workers may include teaching an employee to assume additional clinical or clerical roles or training an employee to work in several different areas. The objectives are to improve staff flexibility, realize greater efficiency, and reduce costs.

Custodial care: Non-medical care provided to support and generally maintain the patient's condition and the essentials of daily living. It generally requires no active medical or nursing treatments.

Deductible: The portion of health care costs that the insured must first pay (generally up to an annual limit) before insurance payments kick in. Insurance payments may be further subject to **copayment**.

Deemed status: A designation used when a hospital, by virtue of its accreditation by the Joint Commission or the American Osteopathic Association, does not require separate certification from the DHHS to participate in the Medicare and Medicaid programs.

Defensive medicine: Excessive medical tests and procedures performed as a protection against malpractice lawsuits, otherwise regarded as unnecessary.

Delirium: A state of mental confusion and excitement that is often accompanied by disorientation, illusions, or hallucinations.

Dementia: A brain disorder that is characterized by progressive mental deterioration with loss of memory. **Alzheimer's disease** is one disorder that leads to severe dementia.

Denial of claim: Refusal by a **payer** to reimburse a **provider** for services rendered.

Dental assistants: Usually work for dentists in the preparation, examination, and treatment of patients.

Dental hygienists: Work under the supervision of dentists and provide preventive dental care, including cleaning teeth and educating patients on proper dental care.

Dentists: The major providers of dental care who must be licensed to practice. The licensure requirements include graduation from an accredited dental school that awards a Doctor of Dental Surgery (DDS) or Doctor of Dental Medicine (DMD) degree and successful completion of both written and practical examinations. Some states require dentists to obtain a specialty license before practicing as a specialist in that state. Their major roles are to diagnose and treat dental problems related to the teeth, gums, and tissues of the mouth. Many dentists are also involved in the prevention of dental decay and gum disease.

Dependency: Refers to the special circumstances children face in that others often have to recognize and respond to their health needs. Children depend on their parents, school officials, caregivers, and sometimes neighbors to discover their need for health care, seek health care services on their behalf, authorize treatment, and comply with recommended treatment regimens.

Dermatology: Medical science pertaining to the study of the skin and its diseases.

Developmental disability: A physical incapacity that generally accompanies **mental retardation** and often arises at birth or in early childhood.

Developmental vulnerability: Refers to the rapid and cumulative physical and emotional changes that characterize childhood and the potential impact that illness, injury, or untoward family and social circumstances can have on a child's life-course trajectory.

DHHS: Department of Health and Human Services. The principal US federal agency responsible for protecting the health of all Americans and providing essential human services.

Diagnosis-related group (DRG): Under the **prospective payment system (PPS)**, a preset fee is paid to the **provider** (generally a hospital), based on the patient's diagnostic category. Medicare has developed around 500 DRGS.

Diminishing marginal returns: A term used in economics that, in the health care context, means that at a certain point, additional deployment of health care resources in a given situation will become less effective in achieving the desired outcome.

Disability: Physical or mental handicap—partial or total—resulting from sickness or injury.

Discharge planning: Part of the overall treatment plan designed to facilitate discharge from an inpatient setting. It includes, for example, an estimate of how long the patient will be in the hospital, what the expected outcome is likely to be, whether any special requirements will be needed at discharge, and what needs to be facilitated.

Disease management: Used primarily by health **plan**s, this is a population-oriented strategy involving patient education, training in self-management, ongoing monitoring of the disease process, and follow-up aimed at people with chronic conditions such as diabetes, asthma, depression, and coronary artery disease.

Disparities: differences in the quality of healthcare or the health outcomes of different groups of people (e.g., racial/ethnic, socioeconomic, gender) that are not due to access-related factors or clinical needs, preferences, and appropriateness of interventions.

Do-not-resuscitate (DNR) orders: Advance directives telling medical professionals not to perform **CPR**. Through DNR orders, patients can have their wishes known regarding aggressive efforts at resuscitation.

DRG: See **Diagnosis-related group**.

Durable medical equipment (DME): Supplies and equipment that are not immediately consumed, such as **ostomy** supplies, wheelchairs, and oxygen tanks.

Durable power of attorney: A written document that provides a legal means for a patient to delegate authority to someone else to act on the patient's behalf even after the patient has been incapacitated.

Dyspnea: Difficult or labored respiration; shortness of breath.

Effectiveness (efficacy): Health benefits of a medical intervention.

Efficiency: Provision of higher quality and more appropriate services at a lower cost. It is generally measured in terms of benefits relative to costs. See **cost-efficiency**.

E-health: Health care information and services offered over the Internet by professionals and nonprofessionals alike.

Electronic health records: Electronically-stored medical records that include a patient's demographic information, problems and diagnoses, plan of care, progress notes, medications, vital signs, past medical history, immunizations, laboratory data and radiology reports.

Eligibility: The process of determining whether a patient qualifies for benefits, based on such factors as age, income, veteran status, etc.

Emergency department: Hospital facilities for the provision of unscheduled **outpatient** services to patients whose conditions require immediate care. They must be staffed 24 hours a day.

Emergent condition: An acute condition that requires immediate medical attention.

Enabling services: Services that enable people to receive medical care that otherwise would not be received despite insurance coverage, e.g., transportation, translation services.

Encephalitis: Inflammation of the brain.

Encephalography: X-ray examination of the brain.

Endemic: A disease restricted to a local region. See **epidemic** and **pandemic**.

Endoscope: An instrument consisting of a tube and an optical system used for observing the inside of a hollow organ or cavity.

Enrollee: A person enrolled in a health plan, especially in a managed care plan.

Enteral: Within or by way of the intestine.

Entitlement: A health care program to which certain people are entitled. For example, almost everyone at 65 years of age is entitled to Medicare because of contributions made through taxes. **Medicaid**, on the other hand, is a **welfare program**.

Epidemic: An outbreak of an infectious disease that spreads rapidly and affects many individuals within a population. See **endemic** and **pandemic**.

Epidemiology: The study of the distribution and determinants of health, health-related behavior, disease, disorder, and death in a population group.

Etiology: Study of the causes of disease or dysfunction.

Exclusive provider plan: A health plan that is very similar to ones offered by preferred provider organizations, except that use is restricted to in-network providers.

Experience rating: Setting of insurance rates based on a group's actual health care expenses in a prior period. This allows healthier groups to pay less.

Evidence-based medicine: Use of current best evidence from published research in medical decision making.

Family medicine: A branch of medical practice based on a core of knowledge that prepares the family physician to function as the primary provider of health care and to perform the roles of patient management, problem solving, counseling, and coordination of care.

Fee-for-service: Payment of separate fees to physicians for each service performed, such as examination, administering a test, hospital visit. The physician sets the fees.

Fee schedule: A schedule of fees for various health care services.

First-dollar insurance: Health care coverage with no **cost sharing**.

Flat-of-the-curve medicine: Medical care that produces relatively little or no benefit for the patient because of **diminishing marginal returns**.

Formulary: A list of acceptable prescription drugs approved by a health plan.

Fraud: Intentional filing of false billing claims or cost reports, and provision of services that are not medically necessary.

Fringe benefits: A term loosely denoting life insurance, health insurance, or pension benefits provided in whole or in part by an employer to its employees.

Functional status: A person's ability to cope with the **activities of daily living**.

Gatekeeper: A primary care physician who functions as the provider of first contact to deliver primary care services and to make referrals for specialty care.

Gatekeeping: The use of primary care physicians to coordinate health care services needed by an enrollee in a managed care plan.

Gene therapy: A therapeutic technique in which a functioning gene is inserted into targeted cells to correct an inborn defect or to provide the cell with a new function.

Generalist: A physician in family practice, general internal medicine, or general pediatrics. See **specialist**.

Genometrics: The association of genes with specific disease traits.

Geriatrics: A branch of medicine that deals with the problems and diseases that accompany aging.

Gerontology: Study of the aging process and of the special problems associated with aging.

Global budget: Setting the total volume of expenditures in a health care system in advance.

Globalization: A term referring to various forms of cross-border economic activities. Globalization is driven by global exchange of information, production of goods and services more economically in developing countries, and increased interdependence of mature and emerging world economies.

Gross domestic product (GDP): A measure of all the goods and services produced by a nation in a given year.

Group policy: An insurance policy purchased by an organization or association as a benefit to its employees or members. Typical groups are employers, union or trade organizations, and professional associations.

HCFA: Health Care Financing Administration. Now renamed Centers for Medicare and Medicaid Services.

Head Start: A federal government-funded program that provides child development services to children in low-income families, including services in education, health care, nutrition, and mental health.

Health informatics: The science that addresses how best to use information to improve health care. Health informatics requires the use of information technology (IT), but goes beyond IT by emphasizing the improvement of health care delivery

Health maintenance organization (HMO): A type of managed care organization that provides comprehensive medical care for a predetermined annual fee per enrollee.

Health Professional Shortage Area (HPSA): A federal designation indicating an area has shortages of primary medical care, dental, or mental health providers. HPSAs may be urban or rural areas, population groups, or medical or other public facilities.

Health Resources and Services Administration (HRSA): A federal agency of the Department of Health and Human Services whose mission is to improve access to health care services for people who are uninsured, isolated, or medically vulnerable

Health savings accounts (HSAs): A key element of President George W. Bush's health policy strategy, HSAs were created as part of the Medicare Prescription Drug, Improvement, and Modernization Act of 2003. Any adult covered by a high-deductible health plan may contribute money to an HSA through several tax-advantaged means. Funds distributed from the HSA are not taxed if they are used to pay qualified medical expenses.

Health technology assessment: Any process of examining and reporting properties of a medical technology used in health care, such as safety, effectiveness, feasibility, and indications for use, cost, and cost-effectiveness, as well as social, economic, and ethical consequences, whether intended or unintended.

HEDIS (Health Plan Employer Data and Information Set): The standard for reporting quality information on managed care plans. This quality tool is a product of a partnership established in 1989 among health plans, employers, and the National Committee for Quality Assurance (**NCQA**), which now manages the HEDIS program.

Hemiplegia: Paralysis of one half of the body.

Hemodialysis: A mechanical procedure used to cleanse the blood by removing toxic chemicals in patients who have lost the function of one or both kidneys.

HIV (human immunodeficiency virus): A virus that can destroy the immune system and lead to **AIDS**.

Holistic medicine: A philosophy of health care that emphasizes the well-being of every aspect of a person. It includes the physical, mental, social, and spiritual aspects of health.

Home health services: Services such as nursing, therapy, and health-related **homemaker** or social services brought to patients in their own homes because such patients are generally unable to leave their homes safely to get the care they need.

Homemaker services: Nonmedical support services given to a homebound individual, e.g., bathing, food preparation, house repairs, shopping.

Homeopathy: A system of medicine based on the theory that "like cures like," meaning that large doses of substances that produce symptoms of a disease in healthy people can be administered in small and diluted doses to cure the same illness. The system was founded in the late 18th century by a German physician, Samuel Hahnemann (1755–1843). See **allopathy**.

Horizontal integration: Merging of firms conducting the same or similar type of business. See **vertical integration**.

Hospice: A cluster of special services for the dying. It blends medical, spiritual, legal, financial, and family-support services. The venue can vary from a specialized facility to a nursing home to the patient's own home.

Hospitalist: A physician who specializes in the care of hospitalized patients.

HRQL (health-related quality of life): In a composite sense, HRQL includes a person's own perception of health, ability to function, role limitations stemming from physical or emotional problems, and personal happiness during or subsequent to disease experience.

Huntington's Disease: A disease of the central nervous system that slowly diminishes an individual's ability to walk, think, talk, and reason. Eventually, the person becomes completely dependent on others for care.

Hypertension: High blood pressure.

IADLs (instrumental activities of daily living): A person's ability to perform household and social tasks, such as home maintenance, cooking, shopping, and managing money. See **activities of daily living (ADLs)**.

Iatrogenic illness (injury): Illness or injury caused by the process of medical care.

ICD-9-CM: International Classification of Diseases, 9th Version, Clinical Modification. It is the official system of assigning codes to diagnoses and procedures.

Incidence: The number of new cases of a disease in a defined population, within a specified period.

Indemnity plan: An insurance plan that provides reimbursement to the insured, without regard to the expenses actually incurred. For example, a predetermined cash amount is paid to the beneficiary per procedure or per day in the hospital. The insured is responsible for paying the provider.

Independent practice association (IPA): A legal entity that physicians in private practice can join so that the organization can represent them in the negotiation of managed care contracts.

Information technology: Information technology (IT) deals with the transformation of data into useful information. IT involves determining data needs, gathering appropriate data, storing and analyzing the data, and reporting the information generated in a user-friendly format.

Informed consent: A fundamental patient right to make an informed choice regarding medical treatment based on full disclosure of medical information by the providers.

Inpatient services: Services delivered on the basis of an overnight stay in a health care institution.

Insurance carrier: The insurer.

Insured: The individual who is covered for risk by insurance.

Integrated health network: A local health services conglomerate, usually built around a major hospital that offers a continuum of health care services. Typically, these networks link hospitals, outpatient clinics, HMOs, and other services with a large pool of physicians.

Interest group: An organized sector of society, such as a business association, citizen group, labor union, or professional association, whose main purpose is to protect its members' interests through active participation in the policymaking process.

Internal medicine: General diagnosis and treatment for problems involving one or more internal organs in adults.

Job lock: People's inability to change jobs because they will not be able to get health insurance coverage if they do.

Joint Commission: Joint Commission on Accreditation of Healthcare Organizations (JCAHO). A private, nonprofit organization that sets standards and accredits most of the nation's general hospitals and many of the long-term care facilities, psychiatric hospitals, substance abuse programs, outpatient surgery centers, urgent care clinics, group practices, community health centers, hospices, and home health agencies.

Laparoscopy: A minimally invasive surgical procedure in which one or more tiny incisions are made instead of one large incision. Surgery is performed by inserting long, slender instruments through the openings, along with tiny cameras attached to special tubes, called endoscopes, to view the surgery. Examples of its use are gallbladder removal, appendectomies, and hernia repairs.

Licensed independent practitioners (LIPs): An individual licensed professional who is authorized to provide health care services without direction and supervision. Provision of services is limited by the scope of the practitioner's license. Examples are physicians, physical and occupational therapists, registered dietitians, dentists, clinical psychologists, and chiropractors.

Licensed practical nurses (LPNs): Called licensed vocational nurses (LVNs) in some states. Must complete a state-approved program in practical nursing and a national written examination. They often work under the supervision of RNs to provide patient care (see **Registered nurses**).

Life expectancy: Actuarial determination of how long, on average, a person of a given age is likely to live.

Lifetime cap: The maximum amount of money a health insurance policy will pay over the lifetime of the insured.

Lithotripsy: A technique in which kidney and gallbladder stones are pulverized by shockwaves. This procedure eliminates the need for invasive surgery.

Living will: A legal document in which a patient puts into writing what his or her preferences are about treatment during terminal illness and the use of life-sustaining technology. It is a directive instructing a physician to withhold or discontinue medical treatment when the patient is terminally ill and unable to make decisions.

Long-term care: A variety of individualized, well-coordinated services that are designed to promote the maximum possible independence for people with functional limitations, and these services are provided over an extended period of time to meet the patients' physical, mental, social, and spiritual needs while maximizing their quality of life.

Long-term care hospital: A special type of long-stay hospital described in section 1886(d)(1)(B)(iv) of the Social Security Act. LTCHs must meet Medicare's conditions of participation for acute (short-stay) hospitals, and must have an average length of stay greater than 25 days. LTCHs serve patients who have complex medical needs and may suffer from multiple chronic problems requiring long-term hospitalization.

Low birth weight: A weight of less than 2,500 grams at birth.

Magnetic resonance imaging (MRI): The use of a uniform magnetic field and radio frequencies to study body tissue and structure.

Maldistribution: Refers to an imbalance (i.e., surplus in some but shortage in others) of the distribution of health professionals, such as physicians, needed to maintain the health status of a given population at an optimum level. Geographic maldistribution refers to the surplus in some regions (such as metropolitan areas) but shortage in other regions (such as rural and inner city areas) of needed health professionals. Specialty maldistribution refers to the surplus in some specialties (such as physician specialists) but shortage in others (such as primary care).

Mammography: The use of breast X-ray to detect unsuspected breast cancer in asymptomatic women.

Managed care: A system that combines the functions of health insurance and the actual delivery of care, where costs and utilization of services are controlled by such methods as **gatekeeping, case management**, and **utilization review**. A large variety of arrangements can fall under this rubric.

Managed competition: A health care reform proposal that would foster competition among integrated networks of insurance companies and health **providers**. Large businesses and health insurance purchasing cooperatives would represent combined purchasing power to keep costs under control. The government would set certain basic standards, such as universal coverage and minimum benefits.

Margin: (Total revenues – Total costs)/Total revenues. Generally shown as a percentage.

Market justice: A distributional principle according to which health care is most equitably distributed through the market forces of supply and demand rather than government interventions. See **social justice**.

MCO: Managed care organization.

MDS: See **Minimum data set**.

Means-tested program: A program in which **eligibility** depends on income.

Medicaid: A joint federal–state program of health insurance for the poor.

Medical loss ratio: The ratio of benefit payments to premiums, indicating the proportion of the premiums spent on medical expenses.

Medical model: Delivery of health care that places its primary emphasis on the treatment of disease and relief of symptoms, instead of prevention of disease and promotion of optimum health.

Medical practice guidelines: See **clinical practice guidelines**.

Medical underwriting: Setting health insurance rates by estimating likely future claims based on the actual health status of individuals or groups.

Medically Underserved Area (MUA): A federal designation indicating an area has a shortage of personal health services for its residents. A MUA may be a whole county or a group of contiguous counties, a group of county or civil divisions, or a group of urban census tracts.

Medically Underserved Population (MUP). A federal designation indicating a group of persons who face economic, cultural, or linguistic barriers to health care.

Medicare: A federal program of health insurance for the elderly and some disabled persons.

Medigap: Commercial health insurance policies purchased by individuals covered by Medicare to pay for expenses not covered by Medicare.

Mental retardation: Significantly sub-average general intellectual functioning existing concurrently with deficits in adaptive behavior, and manifested during the developmental period.

Metropolitan statistical area (MSA): The US Bureau of Census has defined an MSA as a geographic area that includes at least (1) one city with a population of 50,000 or more, or (2) an urbanized area of at least 50,000 inhabitants and a total MSA population of at least 100,000 (75,000 in the New England Census Region).

Minimum data set (MDS): The MDS consists of a core of screening elements that must be assessed for each patient admitted to a **skilled nursing facility**. MDS protocols contain over 100 elements in the areas of patient care; functional, health, and mental status; and treatment.

Monopoly: A market dominated by a single supplier for a unique product or service.

Monopsony: A market dominated by a single buyer.

Moral hazard: Consumer behavior that leads to a higher utilization of healthcare services because people are covered by insurance.

Morbidity: Sickness.

Mortality: Death.

Myocardial infarction: A heart attack.

National Health Service Corps (NHSC): Administered by HRSA, the NHSC recruits health professionals to work in medically underserved rural and urban communities. Education loan repayment is a major incentive for providers to join the NHSC.

Naturopathy: A system of medicine based on such natural remedies as nutrition, use of herbs, massage, and **yoga exercises**.

NCQA: National Committee on Quality Assurance. An organization established by **HMOs** for their self-regulation, through a program of voluntary accreditation.

Neonatal: Refers to the first 28 days after birth.

Neurology: Branch of medicine that specializes in the nervous system and its diseases.

New morbidities: Include drug and alcohol abuse, family and neighborhood violence, emotional disorders, and learning problems from which older generations do not suffer. These dysfunctions originate in complex family or socioeconomic conditions rather than biological causes exclusively.

Nonphysician practitioners (NPPs): Refers to clinical professionals who practice in many areas similar to those in which physicians practice, but who do not have an MD or a DO degree. NPPs are sometimes called midlevel practitioners because they receive less advanced training than physicians but more training than RNs.

Nosocomial infections: Infections acquired while receiving health care.

Nurse practitioners (NPs): Individuals who have completed a program of study leading to competence as RNs in an expanded role. NP specialties include pediatric, family, adult, psychiatric, and geriatric programs. The primary function of NPs is to promote wellness and good health through patient education. Their traditional nursing role has expanded to include taking patients' comprehensive health histories, assessing health status, performing physical examinations, and formulating and managing a care regimen for acutely and chronically ill patients. See **nonphysician practitioners (NPPs)**.

Nursing facility (NF): A nursing home (or part of a nursing home) certified to provide services to Medicaid beneficiaries. See **skilled nursing facility**.

Obesity: For adults, it is defined as a body mass index (BMI) of 30 or greater. See **overweight**. BMI is calculated by dividing a person's body weight in kilograms by the square of his or her height in meters.

Obstetrics/gynecology: Diagnosis and treatment relating to the sexual and reproductive system of women, using surgical and nonsurgical techniques.

Occupational therapy: Therapy to help temporarily or permanently disabled individuals cope with psychological or physiological dysfunction.

OECD: Organization for Economic Cooperation and Development. A forum of about 30 countries including all Western European nations, the United States, Canada, New Zealand, Australia, Japan, and others committed to a market economy. Representatives of member nations meet and discuss global economic and social policies.

Oncology: Medical specialty dealing with cancers and tumors.

Ophthalmology: The branch of medicine specializing in the eye and its diseases.

Opportunistic infection: An infection that occurs when the body's natural immune system breaks down.

Optometrists: Possess a Doctor of Optometry degree and pass a written and clinical state board examination. They provide vision care, such as examination, diagnosis, and correction of vision disorders.

Organized medicine: Concerted activities of physicians, mainly to protect their own interests, through such associations as the American Medical Association (AMA).

Orphan drugs: Certain new drug therapies for conditions that affect fewer than 200,000 people in the United States.

Orthopedics: Branch of medicine dealing with the skeletal system (bones, joints, muscles, ligaments, and cartilage).

Osteopathy: A medical philosophy based on the holistic approach to treatment. It uses the traditional methods of medical practice, which include pharmaceuticals, laboratory tests, X-ray diagnostics, and surgery, and supplements them by advocating treatment that involves correction of the position of the joints or tissues and emphasizes diet and environment as factors that might destroy natural resistance. See **allopathy**.

Osteoporosis: Loss of bone density.

Ostomy: Surgically formed artificial opening for bowel discharge.

Otitis media: Inflammation of the middle ear.

Outcome: The end result of health care delivery; often viewed as the bottom-line measure of the effectiveness of the health care delivery system.

Out-of-pocket costs: Costs of health care to be paid by the recipient of care. For an individual covered by health insurance, these costs would generally include **deductibles**, **copayment**, cost of excluded services, and costs in excess of what the insurer has determined to be "customary, prevailing, and reasonable."

Outpatient services: As opposed to **inpatient services**, outpatient services include any health care services that are not provided based on an overnight stay in which room and board costs are incurred. See **ambulatory care**.

Overutilization (overuse): Utilization of medical services, the cost of which exceeds the benefit to consumers, or the risks of which outweigh potential benefits.

Overweight: For adults, it is defined as a body mass index (BMI) of 25 or greater. See **obesity**. BMI is calculated by dividing a person's body weight in kilograms by the square of his or her height in meters.

PACE: Program of All-Inclusive Care for the Elderly. PACE is an example of the integrated care model of long-term care case management for clients who have been certified to be eligible for nursing home placement. It has had a high success rate of keeping clients in the community.

Package pricing: Bundling of fees for an entire package of related services.

Palliative: Serving to relieve or alleviate, such as pharmacologic pain management and nausea relief.

Pandemic: Relating to the spread of disease in a large segment of the population. See **endemic** and **epidemic**.

Panel: Providers who are selected to render services to the members of a managed care plan constitute its panel. The plan generally refers to them as "preferred providers."

Paramedic: Paramedic personnel are health care workers other than physicians. However, the term is commonly used for emergency medical technicians.

Parenteral nutrition: The full name is total parenteral nutrition (TPN). It infuses nutrients and water into the veins through a catheter, bypassing the gastrointestinal tract.

Parkinson's disease: A chronic disease of the nervous system characterized by tremor and muscular debility. Named after the British physician James Parkinson (1755–1824).

Pathology: Study of the nature and cause of disease that involves changes in structure and function.

Patient-centered care: Delivery of health care that promotes patients' involvement in their treatment, grounding treatment decisions in patients' preferences, creating a caregiving environment in which staff solicit patients' inputs and patients' need for information and education.

Patient Outcomes Research Teams (PORTs): A set of multidisciplinary groups under the auspices of AHRQ whose purpose is to assess alternative treatments for medical conditions using a variety of outcome measures and to guide insurance coverage decisions.

Pay-for-performance: A reimbursement plan that links payment to quality and efficiency, as an incentive to improve the quality of health care as well as reduce systemwide costs.

Payer: The party who actually makes payment for services under the insurance coverage policy. In most cases, the payer is the same as the insurer.

Pediatrics: General diagnosis and treatment for children.

Peer review organizations (PROs): See **Quality Improvement Organization**.

Per diem: A type of reimbursement mechanism for inpatient care in a health care institution. The reimbursement comprises a flat rate for each day of inpatient stay.

Perinatal: Referring to the time period from the 28th week of pregnancy through 28 days after birth.

Pharmaceutical care: A mode of pharmacy practice in which the pharmacist takes an active role on behalf of patients, which includes giving information on drugs and advice on their potential misuse, and assisting prescribers in appropriate drug choices. In so doing, the pharmacist assumes direct responsibility, collaboratively with other health care professionals and with patients, to achieve the desired therapeutic outcomes.

Pharmacists: Pharmacists must have a state license to practice. The licensure requirements include graduation from an accredited pharmacy program that awards a Bachelor of Pharmacy or Doctor of Pharmacy degree, successful completion of a state board examination, and practical experience or completion of a supervised internship. Their major role is to dispense medicines prescribed by physicians, dentists, and podiatrists, and to provide consultation on the proper selection and use of medicines.

Pharmacology: Body of science dealing with drugs, their nature, properties, and effects.

Phlebotomy: Drawing of blood by using a syringe and needle.

Physical therapy: The evaluation and treatment of people with physical problems resulting from injury or disease, including assessment of joint motion, muscle strength and endurance, function of heart and lungs, and performance of activities required in daily living; and treatment, such as therapeutic exercise, cardiovascular endurance training, and training in **activities of daily living**.

Physician assistants (PAs): They work in a dependent relationship with a supervising physician to provide comprehensive medical care to patients. The major services provided by PAs include evaluation, monitoring, diagnostics, therapeutics, counseling, and referral. See **nonphysician practitioners (NPPs)**.

Physician extenders: They are also called **nonphysician practitioners** (NPPs).

Physician-hospital organization (PHO): A legal entity formed between a hospital and a physician group to achieve shared market objectives and other mutual interests.

Plan: A health insurance plan.

Plastic surgery: Surgery for the restoration, repair, or reconstruction of body structures.

Play-or-pay: A health care reform proposal under which employers must choose to provide health insurance (usually no less than a standard benefit plan) for their employees ("play") or to contribute, generally a certain percentage of payroll costs, to a government-administered fund ("pay") to provide health insurance for all who are not covered by their employers.

PMPM: Per member per month. Refers to a capitated rate. See **Capitation**.

Podiatrists: They treat patients with foot diseases or deformities, including performing surgical operations, prescribing medications and corrective devices, and administering physiotherapy.

Point-of-service (POS): A managed care plan that allows its members to decide at the time they need medical care (at the point of service) whether to go to a **provider** on the panel or to pay more and get services out of network.

Policy: The document that sets out the insurance contract.

Portability: The subscriber's ability to switch employers or **insurance carriers** without a gap in coverage. It prevents **job lock**.

Postneonatal: The period between 28 days and one year after birth. See **neonatal**.

Postpartum: Occurring after childbirth.

Practice profiling: Use of provider-specific practice patterns and comparing individual practice patterns to some norm.

Preadmission screening: The assessment of an individual's functional status by a trained health professional prior to institutional placement to determine whether alternative community services would be more appropriate.

Preexisting condition: Physical and/or mental condition that existed before the effective date of an insurance policy.

Preferred provider organization (PPO): A type of managed care organization that has a **panel** of preferred providers who are paid according to a discounted **fee schedule**. The enrollees do have the option to go to out-of-network providers at a higher level of **cost sharing**.

Premium: The insurer's charge for insurance coverage; the price for an insurance plan.

Prepaid plan: A contractual arrangement under which a provider must provide all needed services to a group of members (or enrollees) in exchange for a fixed monthly fee paid in advance to the provider on a per-member basis (called capitation)

Prevalence: The number of cases of a given disease in a given population at a certain point in time.

Primary care: Basic and routine health care that is provided in an office or clinic by a **provider** (physician, nurse, or other health care professional) who takes responsibility for coordinating all aspects of a patient's health care needs. An approach to health care delivery that is the patient's first contact with the health care delivery system and the first element of a continuing health care process.

Primary care case management (PCCM): A managed care arrangement in which a state contracts directly with primary care providers who agree to be responsible for the provision and/or coordination of medical services for Medicaid recipients under their care.

Primary prevention: In a strict epidemiological sense, it refers to prevention of disease, e.g., health education, immunization, and environmental control measures.

Prior approval: A form of **utilization review** in which an insurance company requires a **provider** to get permission from the insurance company before providing care (usually surgery).

Prospective payment system (PPS): Criteria for how much will be paid for a particular service is predetermined (as opposed to "retrospective payment," in which the amount of **reimbursement** is determined on the basis of costs actually incurred).

Prosthesis: An artificial device used to enhance lost functioning. Examples include artificial limbs, hearing aids, etc.

Provider: Any individual or organization that provides services generally covered under health insurance (including Medicaid and Medicare), e.g., physicians, hospitals, dentists, laboratories, pharmacies, and providers of durable medical equipment.

Provider-induced demand: Artificial creation of demand by providers that enables them to deliver unneeded services that boost their incomes.

Psychiatry: Branch of medicine that specializes in mental disorders.

Psychologists: Licensed or certified practitioners who deliver mental health care. Psychologists may specialize in such areas as clinical, counseling, developmental, educational, engineering, personnel, experimental, industrial, psychometric, rehabilitation, school, and social psychology.

Psychosomatic ailments: Disorders in which emotional distress is converted into physical symptoms.

Psychotropic medication: A category of medications that affect psychic function, behavior, or experience.

Public health: A wide variety of activities directed mainly at disease prevention and generally undertaken by state and local governments.

Quad-function model: The four key functions necessary for health care delivery: financing, insurance, delivery, and payment.

Quality-adjusted life year (QALY): The value of one year of high quality life, used as a measure of health benefit.

Quality assessment: Process of defining quality and deciding how it is to be measured, generally according to established standards.

Quality assurance: The process of ongoing quality measurement and using the results of assessment for ongoing quality improvement. See **total quality management**.

Quality Improvement Organization (QIO): Under the direction of CMS, the QIO Program consists of a national network of 53 QIOs, responsible for each US state, territory, and the District of Columbia. QIOs work with consumers, physicians, hospitals, and other caregivers to refine care delivery systems to make sure patients get the right care at the right time, particularly patients from underserved populations. The Program also safeguards the integrity of the Medicare Trust Fund by ensuring that payment is made only for medically necessary services, and investigates beneficiary complaints about quality of care. QIOs were formerly called PROs (Peer Review Organizations).

Quality of life: (1) Quality of life refers to factors considered important by patients, such as environmental comfort, security, interpersonal relations, personal preferences, and autonomy in making decisions when institutionalized. (2) It also includes overall satisfaction with life during and following a person's encounter with the health care delivery system.

R & D: Research and Development.

Radiology: The branch of medicine that involves the use of radioactive substances, such as X-rays, to diagnose, prevent, and treat disease.

Rationing: Process of limiting the utilization of all possible health care services. Rationing can be achieved by price, by waiting lists, or by deliberately limiting access to certain services.

RBRVS: Resource-based relative value scale. A system instituted by Medicare for determining physicians' fees. Each treatment or encounter by the physician is assigned a "relative value" based on the time, skill, and training required to treat the condition.

Registered nurses: Nurses who have completed an associate's degree (ADN), a diploma program, or a baccalaureate degree (BSN) and are licensed to practice. All states require nurses to be licensed to practice. Nurses can be licensed in more than one state through examination or endorsement of a license issued by another state. The licensure requirements include graduation from an approved nursing program and successful completion of a national examination. Nurses are the major caregivers of sick and injured patients, serving their physical, mental, and emotional needs.

Rehabilitation: Provision of therapies to restore lost functioning or maintain the current levels, preventing further deterioration.

Reimbursement: The amount insurers pay to a **provider**. The payment may only be a portion of the actual **charge**.

Reinsurance: Acceptance by an insurer, called the reinsurer, of all or part of the risk underwritten by another insurer.

Reliability: Reflects the extent to which repeated applications of a measure produce the same results.

Residency: Graduate medical education in a specialty that takes the form of paid on-the-job training, usually in a hospital.

Resident: (1) Patient in a nursing home or some other long-term care facility. (2) Physician in **residency**.

Resource utilization groups (RUGs): A classification system designed to differentiate nursing home patients by their levels of resource use. Among the variables differentiating resource utilization are such characteristics as principal diagnosis, limitations in the **activities of daily living**, and types of services received. Version 3 (RUG-III) is used to determine **per diem** rates for **skilled nursing facilities** under the **prospective payment system**.

Respiratory therapy: Treatment for various acute and chronic lung conditions using oxygen, inhaled drugs, and various types of mechanical ventilation.

Respite care: A service that provides temporary relief to informal caregivers, such as family members.

Retrospective reimbursement: Setting of reimbursement rates based on costs actually incurred.

Risk adjustment: Any adjustment made for people who are likely to be high users of health care services, for example, adjustment of payments based on the proportion of high-risk patients.

Risk contracting: In managed care, the concept of **capitation**, when applied to high-risk groups, such as the elderly, is sometimes referred to as risk contracting. All covered services are provided for a fixed monthly premium per enrollee.

Risk factor: An environmental element, personal habit, or living condition that increases the likelihood of developing a particular disease or negative health condition in the future.

Risk management: Limiting risks against lawsuits or unexpected events.

Risk pool: A pool of high-risk individuals who must be offered health insurance in some states.

Risk selection: Reducing costs of health insurance by enrolling healthier people and avoiding those who are likely to use more services.

RUGs: See **Resource utilization groups**.

Safety net: Programs (generally government-financed) that enable people to receive health care services when they lack private resources to pay for them. Without these programs, many people would have to forgo the services. For example, Medicaid becomes a safety net for **long-term care** services once a patient has exhausted private funds (see **spend-down**). Community health centers are safety net providers for many uninsured and vulnerable populations.

Secondary care: Routine hospitalization, routine surgery, and specialized outpatient care, such as consultation with specialists and **rehabilitation**. Compared to **primary care**, these services are usually brief and more complex, involving advanced diagnostic and therapeutic procedures.

Secondary prevention: Efforts to detect disease in early stages to provide a more effective treatment, e.g., screening.

Self-insure: A large company may act as its own insurer by collecting premiums and paying claims. Such businesses most often purchase **reinsurance** against unusually large claims.

Self-referral: Physicians order services from laboratories or other medical facilities in which they have a direct financial interest, usually without disclosing this conflict of interest to the patient.

Self-selection: Consumers choose among health insurance plans according to their particular health status. Low-risk consumers would rationally opt for low-cost plans; high-risk individuals would opt for plans offering comprehensive benefits.

Service plan: A service **plan** provides the **insured** with specified health care services. It pays the hospital or physicians directly, except for the **deductible** and **copayments**, which the insured pays.

S/HMO: Social health maintenance organization. S/HMO is an example of the integrated care model of long-term care case management that coordinates long-term care and acute care services for Medicare beneficiaries who voluntarily enroll in the program.

Single-payer system: A health care reform proposal to create a single organization, usually a government agency, to pay all medical claims. The United States currently has a multiple-payer system.

Skilled nursing care: Medically-oriented care provided mainly by a licensed nurse under the overall direction of a physician. Delivery of care includes assessment to determine the patient's care needs, monitoring of **acute** and unstable chronic conditions, and a variety of treatments that may include wound care, tube feedings, intravenous therapy, **oncology** care, HIV/AIDS care, etc.

Skilled nursing facility (SNF): A nursing home (or part of a nursing home) certified to provide services under Medicare.

Small area variations: Unexplained variations in the treatment patterns for similar patients and medical conditions.

Smart card: A credit card-like device with an embedded computer chip and memory to hold personal medical information that can be accessed and updated at a hospital or physician's office.

Social justice: A distribution principle, according to which health care is most equitably distributed by a government-run national health care program. See **market justice**.

Specialist: A physician who specializes in specific health care problems, for example, **anesthesiologists**, **cardiologists**, **oncologists**, etc. See **generalist**.

Speech therapy: Therapy focusing on individuals with communication problems, including using the voice correctly, speaking fluently, and feeding or swallowing.

Spend-down: A requirement under most Medicaid programs that individuals spend their assets down to a predetermined level to be eligible for benefits.

Spina bifida: A deformity of the spine.

SSI: Supplemental Security Income. A federal program of income support for the disabled (includes mental illness and some infectious diseases).

State Children's Health Insurance Program (SCHIP): A joint federal-state program, established as Title XXI of the Social Security Act under the 1997 Balanced Budget Act. SCHIP provides health insurance for children from low-income families who do not qualify for Medicaid.

Subacute care: Technically complex services that are beyond traditional **skilled nursing care**.

Supply-side rationing: Also called 'planned rationing' that is generally carried out by a government to limit the availability of health care services, particularly expensive technology.

Surgi-center: A freestanding ambulatory surgery center that performs various types of surgical procedures on an outpatient basis.

Swing bed: A hospital bed that can be used for acute care or skilled nursing care, depending on fluctuations in demand.

Teaching hospital: A hospital with an approved residency program for physicians.

Technology assessment: See health technology assessment.

Telehealth: Although in general the terms telemedicine and telehealth can be used interchangeably, in a stricter sense, telehealth encompasses educational, research, and administrative uses as well as clinical applications that involve nurses, psychologists, administrators, and other nonphysicians

Telematics: A term used to describe the combination of information and communications technology to meet user needs.

Telemedicine: Use of telecommunications technology that enables physicians to conduct two-way interactive video consultations or to transmit digital images, such as X-rays and MRIs, to other sites.

Telemetry: Remote monitoring (such as monitoring cardiac function) from a central station.

Tertiary care: The most complex level of care. Typically, tertiary care is institution-based, highly specialized, and highly technological. Examples are burn treatment, transplantation, and coronary artery bypass surgery.

Tertiary prevention: Efforts to prevent the progression of a disability to a state of dependency, e.g., rehabilitation.

Third-party administrator (TPA): An administrative organization other than the employee benefit **plan** or health care **provider** that collects premiums, pays **claims**, and/or provides administrative services.

Third-party payers: Under the current system, the **payers** for covered services, e.g., insurance companies, managed care organizations, and the government. They are called third parties because they are neither the **providers** nor the recipients of medical services.

Total parenteral nutrition (TPN): A liquid mixture pumped directly into the bloodstream, providing a balance of essential nutrients.

Total care: In the context of long-term care delivery, total care focuses on recognizing any health care need that may arise and ensuring that the need is evaluated and addressed by appropriate clinical professionals.

Total quality management (TQM): TQM creates an environment in which all aspects of health services within an organization are oriented to patient-related objectives and the production of desirable health outcomes. It holds the promise of not only improving quality but also increasing efficiency and productivity by identifying and implementing less costly ways to provide services. This system is viewed as an ongoing effort to improve quality. Hence, it is also referred to as **continuous quality improvement (CQI)**.

Trauma center: An emergency unit specializing in the treatment of severe injuries.

Triage: A system of prioritizing treatment when demand for medical care exceeds supply.

Two-tiered health care system: A system in which some people can afford to obtain medical services, conveniences, or amenities that others cannot. This kind of system exists in almost all countries.

Uncompensated care: Charity care provided to the uninsured who cannot pay.

Underinsurance: Medical insurance coverage inadequate to cover the costs of a major illness.

Underutilization: It occurs when medically needed health care services are withheld. This is especially true when the potential benefits are likely to exceed the cost or risks.

Underwriting: The process by which an insurance company determines medical risk and makes decisions about whom to cover and how much to charge.

Universal access: Health insurance coverage for all citizens, as in a national health care program. It is a misnomer because timely access to needed services may still be a problem because of supply-side rationing.

Urgent care center: A **walk-in clinic** that is generally open to see patients after normal business hours in the evenings and weekends, and without having to make an appointment.

Urology: The branch of medicine concerned with the urinary tract in both sexes and the sexual/reproductive system in males.

Utilization: Extent to which health care services are actually used. For example, the number of physician visits per person per year is a measure of utilization for primary care services.

Utilization review (UR): A process by which an insurer reviews decisions by physicians and other **providers** on how much care to provide.

VA: Department of Veterans Affairs.

Validity: The validity of a measure denotes the extent to which it actually assesses what it purports to measure. If a measure reflects the quality of care, improvements in quality should yield a higher score for improved quality, and vice versa.

Venous stasis: Stagnation of normal blood flow causing swelling and pain, generally in the legs.

Ventilator: A mechanical device for artificial breathing. The ventilator (or mechanical respirator) forces air into the lungs.

Vertical integration: Linking of services that are at different stages in the production process of health care. Examples include a hospital system that acquires a firm that produces medical supplies or a physician group practice or a hospital that launches hospice, long-term care, or ambulatory care services. See **horizontal integration**.

Voluntary hospital: A nonprofit hospital owned and operated by community associations or other nongovernment organizations to benefit the local community.

Voucher: The voucher approach to health insurance reform relies on individual decisions to purchase health insurance. Tax credits are issued in advance to individuals, typically the poor, as vouchers with which to offset the costs of purchasing health insurance.

Walk-in clinic: A freestanding **ambulatory** clinic. Patients are seen without appointments on a first come, first served basis.

Welfare program: A **means-tested program** for which only people below certain income levels qualify. Medicaid is a welfare program. See **entitlement**.

WIC: Supplemental Food Program for Women, Infants, and Children. The program was created on September 26, 1972, as an amendment to the Child Health Nutrition Act of 1966 with the express objective of providing sufficient nutrition for pregnant women, mothers, infants, and children. To reach that goal, target consumers must have access to food and infant formula.

Workers' compensation: Employer-paid benefit that compensates workers for medical expenses and wages lost due to work-related injuries or illnesses.

Xenotransplantation: Also called xenografting. Transplanting of animal tissue into humans.

Yoga exercises: Using physical postures and regulation of breathing to treat certain chronic conditions and to achieve overall health benefits.

Appendix B

Selected Web Sites

Agencies of the Federal Government

Department of Health and Human Services
http://www.dhhs.gov/

Administration for Children and Families
http://www.acf.dhhs.gov/

Administration on Aging
http://www.aoa.dhhs.gov/

Agency for Healthcare Research and Quality
http://www.ahrq.gov/

Centers for Disease Control and Prevention
http://www.cdc.gov/

National Center for Chronic Disease Prevention and Health Promotion
http://www.cdc.gov/nccdphp/

National Center for Environmental Health
http://www.cdc.gov/nceh/

Division of Birth Defects and Developmental Disabilities
http://www.cdc.gov/ncbddd/

Global Health Office
http://www.cdc.gov/nceh/globalhealth/default.htm

National Center for Health Statistics
http://www.cdc.gov/nchs/

Healthy People 2010 Web Site
http://www.healthypeople.gov/

National Center for Infectious Diseases
http://www.cdc.gov/ncidod/index.htm

Injury Center
http://www.cdc.gov/ncipc/default.htm

National Institute for Occupational Safety and Health
http://www.cdc.gov/niosh/

Centers for Medicare and Medicaid Services
http://www.cms.gov

Health Insurance Portability and Accountability Act
http://cms.hhs.gov/hipaa/

Medicaid
http://cms.hhs.gov/medicaid

Medicare
http://cms.hhs.gov/medicare

State Children's Health Insurance Program
http://cms.hhs.gov/schip

Food and Drug Administration
http://www.fda.gov/

Health Resources and Services Administration
http://www.hrsa.gov/

National Institutes of Health
http://www.nih.gov/

National Cancer Institute
http://www.nci.nih.gov/

National Institute of Environmental Health Sciences
http://www.cancer.gov/

National Institute of Mental Health
http://www.nimh.nih.gov/

National Institute on Aging
http://www.nia.nih.gov/

National Library of Medicine
http://www.nlm.nih.gov/

Other Government Agencies

Congressional Budget Office, US Congress
http://www.cbo.gov/

Department of Agriculture

Center for Nutrition and Policy Promotion
http://www.usda.gov/cnpp/

Office of Rural Health Policy
http://www.nal.usda.gov/

Food Safety and Inspection Service
http://www.fsis.usda.gov/

Department of Commerce, Census Bureau
http://www.census.gov/

Department of Energy
http://www.sc.doe.gov/

Office of Biological and Environmental Research
http://www.er.doe.gov/production/ober/ober_top.html

Office of Environment, Safety, and Health
http://www.doe.gov/environment/index.htm

Department of Justice, Health Care Antitrust Division
http://www.usdoj.gov/atr/public/health_care/health_care.htm

General Accounting Office
http://www.gao.gov/

Department of Labor
http://www.dol.gov/

Bureau of Labor Statistics
http://www.bls.gov/

Office of Workers' Compensation Programs
http://www.dol.gov/esa/owcp_org.htm

Department of Veterans Affairs
http://www.va.gov/

Veterans Health Administration
http://www1.va.gov/health/

National Center for Health Promotion and Disease Prevention
http://www.prevention.va.gov/

Private Agencies

AARP
http://www.aarp.org
Information on a wide variety of issues pertaining to people 50 years of age and older.

Abt Associates, Inc.
http://www.abtassoc.com
Health Watch newsletter and other information can be downloaded.

American College of Preventive Medicine
http://www.acpm.org
Provides links to other public health sites.

American Medical Association
http://www.ama-assn.org
Scientific journals and news. Links to other medical sites, national medical specialty societies, government sites, and search engines.

American Public Health Association
http://www.apha.org
Provides information on a broad set of issues affecting personal and environmental health.

Association of American Medical Colleges
http://www.aamc.org
Focuses on issues pertaining to medical education and academic medicine.

Center for Spirituality and Health
http://www.spiritualityandhealth.ufl.edu/websites/
Provides information on health and spirituality.

The Center for Studying Health System Change
http://www.hschange.org
A research organization dedicated to studying how the country's health care systems are changing and how those changes are affecting people at the community level.

The Commonwealth Fund
http://www.cmwf.org
Addresses many current issues in health care delivery.

Elderhope
http://www.elderhope.com/
Covers many topics dealing with health care of an aging population.

The Henry J. Kaiser Family Foundation
http://www.kff.org
Independent philanthropy focusing on major health care issues.

National Association of County and City Health Officials
http://www.naccho.org
Has a wide network, by health topics.

National Committee for Quality Assurance
http://www.ncqa.org
A diverse coalition of physicians, health plans, quality experts, consultants, and several of the nation's largest employers.

National Institute for Health Care Management
http://www.nihcm.org
The institute's research and educational foundation conducts research on health care issues, and disseminates research findings and analysis that promote and enhance access to health care and the efficiency and effectiveness of health care services and delivery.

PharmWeb
http://www.pharmweb.net
Information on pharmacology and alternative medicine.

The Rand Corporation
http://www.rand.org
Focuses on the nation's most pressing policy problems.

The Robert Wood Johnson Foundation
http://rwjf.org
The largest philanthropic organization devoted exclusively to health and health care in the United States. Publications can be viewed online.

The Urban Institute
http://www.urban.org/
A research organization working on a variety of health care issues.

Index